THE IMPACT OF
COMPUTERS ON NURSING

An International Review

IFIP-IMIA Workshop on
The Impact of Computers on Nursing
Church House, Westminster, London
8-9 September, 1982
and
Harrogate, England
10-15 September, 1982

sponsored by
IMIA - International Medical Informatics Association
National Staff Committee (Nurses and Midwives)
British Computer Society
Nursing Times of London
Department of Health and Social Security
Department of Industry
European Federation for Medical Informatics

NORTH-HOLLAND
AMSTERDAM ● NEW YORK ● OXFORD

THE IMPACT OF COMPUTERS ON NURSING

An International Review

Proceedings of the IFIP-IMIA Workshop on
The Impact of Computers on Nursing
held in Church House, Westminster, London
8-9 September, 1982
and in
Harrogate, England
10-15 September, 1982

edited by

Maureen SCHOLES
Director of Nursing Services
The London Hospital
Whitechapel, London
England

Yvonne BRYANT
Eastbourne, East Sussex
England

and

Barry BARBER
Chief Management Scientist
North Thames Regional Health Authority
London
England

1983

NORTH-HOLLAND
AMSTERDAM • NEW YORK • OXFORD

ISBN: 0 444 86682 5

Published by:
ELSEVIER SCIENCE PUBLISHERS B.V.
P.O. Box 1991
1000 BZ Amsterdam
The Netherlands

Sole distributors for the U.S.A. and Canada:
ELSEVIER SCIENCE PUBLISHING COMPANY, INC.
52 Vanderbilt Avenue
New York, N.Y. 10017
U.S.A.

Library of Congress Cataloging in Publication Data

IFIP-IMIA Workshop on the Impact of Computers on
    Nursing (1982 : London, England and Harrogate,
    North Yorkshire)
    The impact of computers on nursing.

    Includes index.
    1. Nursing--Data processing--Congresses. I. Scholes,
Maureen, 1929-   . II. Bryant, Yvonne, 1938-   .
III. Barber, Barry. IV. Information Federation for
Information Processing. V. International Medical
Informatics Association. VI. Title. [DNLM:
1. Computers--Congresses. 2. Nursing--Congresses.
WY 26.5 I34i 1982]
RT50.5.I34 1982   610.73'028'54   83-8239
ISBN 0-444-86682-5 (U.S.)

PRINTED IN THE NETHERLANDS

TABLE OF CONTENTS

Conference Portrait   xiii

Organizing Committee   xiv

Acknowledgements   xv

Preface   xvii

International Medical Informatics Association   xix

CHAPTER 1 : INTRODUCTION
            Maureen Scholes   1

CHAPTER 2 : PERSPECTIVES IN NURSING
            Keynote Address
            Dame Catherine Hall DBE   5

CHAPTER 3 : COMPUTER TECHNOLOGY IN HEALTH CARE   11

3.1. Getting Started
      Richard Turner   12

3.2. Microcomputers for Nursing: An Overview
      John Kwok   16

3.3. Computers Need Nursing
      Barry Barber   24

3.4. From the Computer Manager's Viewpoint
      John Rowson   34

3.5. The Importance of Nurses' Input for the Selection of Computerized
      Systems
      Constance M. Berg   42

3.6. An Overview of the Development of National Health Service
      Computing
      Doreen T. Redmond   59

3.7. Computer Technology in Health Care
      Discussion   70

CHAPTER 4 : CONFIDENTIALITY   73

4.1. Is Nursing Confidential?
      Josephine A. Plant   74

4.2. Confidentiality
      Discussion   82

CHAPTER 5 : NURSING RECORDS   83

5.1. Using Computers to Enhance Professional Practice
      (Nursing Times Lecture)
      Margo Cook   84

5.2. Computers in Support of Patient Care
      Shirley Hughes   91

5.3. Developing a Patient Care Program
      Anne N. Gebhardt   95

5.4. Caring for Patients within a Computer Environment
      Clare C. Ashton   105

5.5. Planning and Controlling Patient Care with the Exeter System
      Alison E. Head   115

5.6. The Computer as an Aid to Improving Patient Care
      Margaret Griffiths   120

5.7. Informatics and Clinical Nursing Records
John Anderson 126

5.8. Nursing Records
Discussion 133

CHAPTER 6 : MEASUREMENT OF CARE 135

6.1. Planning and Measuring Nursing Care — An Integrated Approach
Charles Tilquin, Diane Saulnier, Pierre Lambert, and Jocelyne Carle 136

6.2. Data Capture — From a Real Time Computerised Nursing System
Christine R. Henney and Lesley H. Stewart 147

6.3. Measurement of Care
Discussion 154

CHAPTER 7 : PATIENT MONITORING 155

7.1. Computers — Help or Hindrance to the Clinical Nurse?
Jill M. Martin 156

7.2. Nurses' Experience with a Computer in a Nephrology—Hypertension
Department
G.M. De Pooter, M.M. Elseviers, G.A. Verpooten, R.L. Lins,
J.P. Van Waeleghem, J. Van Pellicom, and M.E. De Broe 163

7.3. Patient Monitoring
Discussion 169

CHAPTER 8 : DRUG MANAGEMENT 171

8.1. Computerized Medication System
Margo Cook 172

8.2. A Computer System for Drug Prescribing and its Impact on Drug
Administration
Clare C. Ashton 175

8.3. Drug Management
Discussion   197

CHAPTER 9 : COMMUNITY BASED CARE   199

9.1. Community Nursing Information Systems
B.E.M. Warne OBE   200

9.2. A Comprehensive, Computer-Based System for Patient Information
in Primary Health Care
Pirjo Hynninen   207

9.3. Statistics, Computer Forms and Health Visitor Service Planning
Joyce Wiseman   215

9.4. PL Child Health Care Systems
Fumiko Ohata   222

9.5. Nurses in the Community — Preventive Medicine and the Computer
M.G. Sheldon   230

9.6. Community Based Care
Discussion   236

CHAPTER 10 : IMPLICATIONS FOR NURSE EDUCATION   239

10.1. Computers and Nursing Education: Change and Challenges
Mary Anne Sweeney   240

10.2. Educating Nursing Students about Computers
Judith S. Ronald   248

10.3. Nurse Education and Computers: Time for Change
Ron Hoy   257

10.4. Training Nurses in Computing in the United Kingdom
Brian Hambleton   265

10.5. Solution to a Dilemma: Computer Technology Facilitates Non-
Traditional, Post-Basic Nursing Education
Joan Cobin and Judith Lewis   269

10.6. Implication for Nursing Education
Discussion 277

CHAPTER 11 : COMPUTER ASSISTED LEARNING 279

11.1. Computer Assisted Learning in Nursing Education – A Macroscopic
Analysis
Kathryn J. Hannah 280

11.2. Learning Needs and Computers
Mary Anne Sweeney 288

11.3. Making the Most of the Microcomputer in Nursing Education
Susan Mirin 291

11.4. Nursing Education and the Computer Age in Retrospect and Prospect
Patricia Tymchyshyn 300

11.5. Protocols for Software Selection, Development and Evaluation for
Nursing Education
Susan J. Grobe 307

11.6. Computer Assisted Instruction in Nurse Education – An Approach
Susan E. Norman 327

11.7. The Second Coming – Resurrection or Reservation?
Ian Townsend 334

11.8. Computer Assisted Learning
Discussion 347

CHAPTER 12 : EDUCATION PROGRAMMES AND RECORDS 349

12.1. Computer Based Systems for Professional Education and Training
Sheila Collins OBE 350

12.2. A Step Towards Computerised Learner Nurse Allocation
Colin J. Fildes 356

12.3. Computerized Nurse Allocation and the Identification of Related
Service Tools
Jean Roberts 364

CHAPTER 13 : PLANNING THE NURSING SERVICE 369

13.1. The Use of Computers for Planning Nursing Services
Barbara Rivett 370

13.2. Computers in Health Service Management from a Nursing
Perspective
Patricia Hardcastle 374

13.3. The Nurse Manager and the Computer
Peter Squire 382

13.4. Nursing Demands on Distributed Computer Systems
Ulla Gerdin-Jelger 389

13.5. The Design and Implementation of Computer Programs for Order
Entry and Review
Dickey Johnson 394

13.6. Amending and Extending an Existing Patient Administration
System
Deirdre M. Gossington 406

CHAPTER 14 : RESOURCE MANAGEMENT 411

14.1. The Use of Computer Systems in Nursing Administration
Joy L. Brown 412

14.2. A Computerised Operating Theatre Management System
Elizabeth Butler 421

14.3. Computer-Assisted Training and Manpower Planning for Student
Nurses in Leiden Hospital
Elly Pluyter-Wenting 430

14.4. Computers and Nursing Administration
Sally Mizrahi 438

14.5. The Computer — A Tool for Nurse Managers to Improve
Standards of Care
Jean G. Jarvis 445

14.6. Present Practice and Potential of Computer Systems in Nursing
    — The State of the Art in One Health Board Area in Scotland
    Catherine V. Cunningham   457

14.7. Computers: A Resource in a Nursing Department Reorganization
    Fotine D. O'Connor   470

14.8. Budgetary Control System and the Development of Financial
    Management Systems
    Bernard Groves   476

CHAPTER 15 : MANAGEMENT SCIENCES IN THE NURSING SYSTEM   481

15.1. Why Nurse an Analyst?
    Barry Barber   482

15.2. Performance Criteria
    William Abbott   492

15.3. Understanding Data Capture in Nursing
    Kathryn Erat   496

15.4. Computer Based Quality Assurance for Nursing Management
    Lillian Eriksen   510

15.5. Combined Nursing Management
    Discussion   524

CHAPTER 16 : RESEARCH   529

16.1. Information Use in Nursing
    Margaret R. Grier   530

16.2. Some Thoughts on the Future Direction of Nursing
    Maureen Lahiff   544

CHAPTER 17 : CONCLUSIONS   551
    Barry Barber

CHAPTER 18 : GLOSSARY   553

CHAPTER 19 : BIBLIOGRAPHY
            Compiled by Yvonne M. Bryant   563

Author Index for Bibliography   579

Organizing Committee and Contributors   584

Author Index of Contributors   590

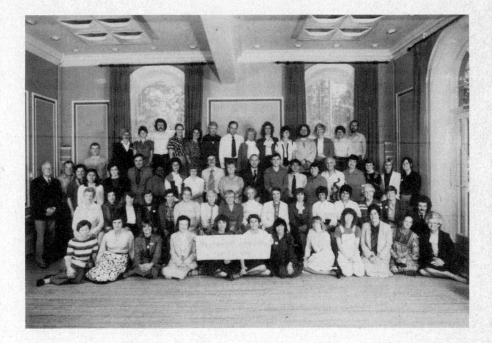

CONFERENCE PORTRAIT

From left to right;

Back row: Brian Hambleton, Pirjo Hynninen, Diane Saulnier, Brian Layzell, Maureen Lahiff, Susan Norman, Lillian Eriksen, Ron Hoy, Pat Tymchyshyn, Connie Berg, Ulla Gerdin-Jelger, Ian Townsend, Elly Pluyter-Wenting, Patricia Hardcastle, John Rowsen.

Third row: Jim Cartright, Bud Abbott, Mary Anne Sweeney, Fumiko Ohata, Margaret Griffiths, Peter Squire, Joy Brown, Valerie Wilkinson, Geraldine Ribbons, Bernard Groves, Joyce Wiseman, John Anderson, Colin Fildes, John Kwok, Kathryn Hannah, Barry Barber, Betty Anderson, Sally Mizrahi, Gerd de Pooter, Jean Roberts.

Second row: Beryl Warne, Fotine O'Connor, Kathryn Erat, Doreen Redmond, Dickey Johnson, Barbara Rivett, Elizabeth Butler, Maureen Scholes, Margaret Grier, Anne Gebhardt, Shirley Hughes, Deirdre Gossington, Joan Cobin, Sheila Collins, Margo Cook, Charles Tilquin.

Front row: E. M. Seager, Josephine Plant, Susan Mirin, Yvonne Bryant, Monica Baker, Dorothy Scott, Christine Henney, Clare Ashton, Penny Keeble, Susan Grobe, Catherine Cunningham, Judith Ronald.

ORGANIZING COMMITTEE

Miss Maureen Scholes	The London Hospital, Whitechapel, Chairman and Editor
Dr. Barry Barber	N.E. Thames Regional Health Authority, Secretary and Editor
Mr. William Abbott	N.E. Thames Regional Health Authority, Treasurer
Miss Clare Ashton	Queen Elizabeth Hospital, Birmingham, Joint Co-ordinator, Care Stream
Mrs. Yvonne Bryant	Eastbourne. Editor
Miss Elizabeth Butler	St. Thomas Hospital, London, Joint Co-ordinator, Management Stream
Mr. Jim Cartwright,	N.H.S. Training Centre, Harrogate, Yorks.
Mr. Brian Hambleton	D.H.S.S. London, Joint Co-ordinator, Management Stream
Mr. Ron Hoy	Middlesex Hospital, Joint Co-ordinator, Education Stream
Mr. Brian Layzell	D.H.S.S. London, Joint Co-ordinator, Management Stream
Miss Doreen Redmond,	D.H.S.S. London, Joint Co-ordinator, Care Stream.
Ms. Jean Roberts	Lancashire Royal Infirmary, Exhibition Organiser
Mrs. Jackie Streeter	London, Joint Co-ordinator, Management Stream,

ACKNOWLEDGEMENTS

The Committee wish to acknowledge the valuable assistance given by Data Recall Ltd to the working seminar. All the material in the book was prepared on Diamond word processors thus facilitating the editing and preparation for this book's production.

The Committee also wish to acknowledge the assistance received from "Word for Word" word processing bureau who specialise in the use of the Diamond systems, particularly for their preparation of the original texts.

The detailed administration of the Conference was handled by Dorothy Scott and the final processing and management of the text was carried out by Monica Baker and Penny Keeble. The Committee wishes to acknowledge their gratitude to them.

PREFACE

This book is the work of many nurses, and other health workers and computer professionals interested in Nursing. They came from a variety of countries to the United Kingdom to speak at an International Medical Informatics Association (I.M.I.A.) Working Conference on the Impact of Computers on Nursing. This event started with an 'Open Forum' held in London, 8th and 9th September, 1982 followed immmediately by a closed workshop held in Harrogate, Yorkshire. Here, intensive discussion sessions were held in order to describe the state of the art of the use of computers in Nursing and to try and predict future needs. The Forum, the Workshop and this publication were sponsored by I.M.I.A. and generously supported by The British Computer Society, The National Staff Committee (Nurses and Midwives), The Department of Industry, The Department of Health and Social Security, The European Federation for Medical Informatics and The Nursing Times of London. The bibliography undertaken by Yvonne Bryant was financed by The British Computer Society.

We are grateful to them all for making it possible for us to share ideas widely and hopefully to have furthered the development of Nursing Informatics. Computers are important tools for Nursing today and they will only be fully exploited for the benefit of patients if there is adequate discussion both nationally and internationally on all aspects of their usage in Nursing.

The Editors have attempted to weld together a great deal of material in a very short time. We hope that the authors of individual papers will accept our editing of their papers in the common enterprise and forgive any over simplifications we may have perpetrated in reducing the volume of material to manageable proportions and trying to render the text as readable as possible for an international readership.

Maureen Scholes
Barry Barber
Yvonne Bryant
12.12.82

INTERNATIONAL MEDICAL INFORMATICS ASSOCIATION

International Federation for Information Processing (IFIP) was formed in 1960 with its headquarters in Geneva. IFIP represents international cooperation in data processing. To accomplish this task it formed 10 technical committees, each with a specific interest.

Technical Committee Four (TC4) dealt with health data processing and biomedical research and soon became one of the largest and most active of these technical committees. After 10 years as a technical committee, TC4 reached maturity and looked for its own identity. It asked for and was accorded the status of a special interest group within the parent body of IFIP as of May, 1979.

This special interest group, known as International Medical Informatics Association (IMIA), has more autonomy than a technical committee, having as its membership the representatives of the various national Health (Medical) Informatics societies rather than the national computer societies. It also controls its own budget and is responsible for operating its own working conferences and affiliations.

The term "Medical Informatics" is a compromise between several descriptions and is considered synonymous with "Health Informatics". It covers the whole range of computing and operations analysis activities within the health care area.

IMIA is an international and world representative federation of national societies of Health Informatics and affiliated organisations. It does not have individual members although there may be several delegates from each country as observers, but each country has only one designated representative with one vote.

IMIA performs several functions on the international scene. Its prime function is the dissemination of knowledge regarding health information processing, In order to accomplish this IMIA organises:

1. Triennial MEDINFO series scientific congresses which were held in Stockholm (1974), Toronto (1977), Tokyo (1980) and will be held in Amsterdam (1983), and Washington (1986). These large general coverage congresses provide an excellent review of the state of the art of Medical Informatics.

2. Working groups on special topics such as education, EKG (ecg) processing, and confidentiality, security and privacy.

3. Working conferences, of which approximately 20 have been held in the last 10 years. Recent conferences have been held on such diverse subjects as hospital information systems, data security, doctors office systems, optimisation of EKG processing, ultrasonics and tomography, hospital statistics, and drug information.

IMIA also represents IFIP in the Health Information processing field to such organisations as World Health Organisation and World Medical Association and at world conferences such as the Alma Ata WHO/UNICEF conference on primary health care.

Finally, IMIA disseminates knowledge by means of the publication and distribution of MEDINFO and working conference proceedings.

Following the report of the working conference on the Impact of Computers on Nursing held in U.K., 8th - 15th September 1982, the IMIA General Assembly held in Melbourne, Australia agreed to the setting up of a working group on Nursing Informatics to assist in the world-wide development of this area of activity.

Further information, and the name and address of your national I.M.I.A. representative can be obtained from IMIA Headquarters, Enschedepad 41-43, NL - 1324 GB Almere, The Netherlands. Phone (0)3240 - 31341. Telex: 70424 ifsec.

The Impact of Computers on Nursing
M. Scholes, Y. Bryant and B. Barber (eds.)
Elsevier Science Publishers B.V. (North-Holland)
© IFIP-IMIA, 1983

CHAPTER 1

INTRODUCTION

Maureen Scholes

Living has never been easy and each century has had its share of dis-ease. The leader of a tribe or country has to be mindful of preserving the health of his people in order that the group will survive and flourish.

Every century has its methods of communication; the spoken word, the written word providing a source of knowledge to be drawn upon by those who follow. Paintings, photographs and television have all enhanced the words. Standing stones, beacons and satellites have marked the way. Bells, drums, and sirens have called our attention.

Every century has its methods of organisation, its laws and customs embodying individual rights. Religious orders and specialised groups have taken collective responsibility particularly for the weak and sick.

In the 20th century, communication is still by the spoken and written word, the radio, telephone or television, but more often it is now also by computer. Computers are to this century what steam was to the last. Computers can calculate and deal with large numbers. They can store enormous amounts of data - the contents of whole libraries, in a very small space. They can sort, and analyse these data and then allow one to retrieve just that element of data that is required immediately. They can also lead to new insight by the manipulation of the data.

In the 20th century, nurses are the specialised group caring for the sick and promoting health. There are greatly increased populations, diseases are better understood and there are known methods of prevention and treatment for many of them. Surgical techniques and drug therapy have advanced rapidly. In response, nursing has become more complex with specialised sub-groups. At one extreme the health visitor acting as counsellor and adviser about health, at the other extreme the intensive therapy nurse needing highly technical skills to care for critically ill people.

It is timely to explore the effect that computers have had on nursing and to consider the potential impact on nursing in the future. Nurses, like many of their fellow creatures, are now familiar with certain aspects of computers in daily living; - when, for example, using an automatic washing machine, visiting a bank or booking a flight. On the other hand, nurses have been slow to grasp the potential of computers for nursing.

In the last decade, a mere fragment in our history we have begun to recognise the possibilities and the problems. Leaders of the profession are confronted by recruits who know nothing about nursing but who are more knowledgeable about computers than they themselves. This has produced a sense of unease and an urgent desire for knowledge about computers, and the beginnings of some interesting research.

Nurses involved in direct care see the computer as a possible solution to some of their problems of nursing records. In order for a frequently changing team of nurses to give planned, systematic and consistently good care to an individual patient, whether in hospital or the community, there is a plethora of paperwork. The time taken up by this constantly makes inroads into the time needed to give the planned care. Will the computer tip the scales in the patients' favour?

Certainly one Japanese nurse, talking about the computer system she used, thought it did when she said "Nevertheless, the over-riding advantages were that it allowed the Intensive Care Nurse to consider the patient as a whole - to give calm loving care to a critically ill patient and in an environment which was quieter because data could be assessed by the doctors away from the bedside. The psychological advantage to the patient was an important factor in recovery".

Nurses involved in teaching see the computer as some solution to at least two of their problems - one of keeping the required training records and the other of ensuring that the student is actually learning what he or she needs to know to practice as a qualified nurse. The training records have to reflect the very strict statutory requirements for different programmes, each involving the student in specified amounts of theoretical instruction, and of clinical practice undertaken in defined specialties. The recording needs to be precise, often in hours, and computers lend themselves to this detailed cumulative process. The instruction of students and the assessment of their knowledge is varied and complex. The development of decision making skills is crucial to good nursing. Computer assisted instruction and computer managed learning are seen as important methods for the future.

Nurses involved in administration see the computer as a highly useful management tool. Too often they are required to provide a nursing service for a workload over which they have little control. Medical staff appointments are made without proper estimation of the nursing workload which will accrue to them. Alternatively the workload may have been predicted but the money needed for resources not agreed. Predictions based on a sound scientific basis are more acceptable to health authorities and management committees than those solely based on practical experience or intuition, mainly because they are susceptible to informed discussion and examination. Computer based nursing manpower systems have been developed and may incorporate and link student allocation programs, sickness, absence, sub-systems with pay-roll systems.

The central chapters of the book (5-15) develop many of these themes and they represent the three major streams of the workshop; patient care, nurse education and nursing management. They describe both the systems that have been implemented and also those that are planned but still have to be tried and tested. Each chapter begins with an introduction to the topic, followed by relevant individual papers. References are numbered and listed at the end of each paper. Those referred to by a letter and number in the text, for example (A2) are to be found in the bibliography, Chapter 19. The discussions which were held each day at the workshop are reported at the end of the appropriate chapter or section. Nurses are essentially practical people and are generally realistic. They, therefore, discuss the advantages and disadvantages, the hopes that have sometimes been dashed as well as the doubts that have sometimes proved unnecessary. The introductory chapters include a chapter in which Dame Catherine Hall sets the scene in her "Perspectives in Nursing". This is followed by a chapter giving some insight into computer technology both as the computer professional sees the requirements and also as the nurse begins to participate in the development of a computer system. The arguments for and against microcomputers and mainframes are touched upon here and referred to again in Chaper 15.

The introductory chapters are then concluded with a short but important one on confidentiality and data protection. It is essential that as a profession we ensure that moral and ethical values are not pushed aside by new technology.

The final chapters cover research aspects of the subject (Chapter 16), a brief conclusion together with a bibliography (Chapter 19) and glossary.

If we, as Nurses, can combine logic and precision with intuitiveness and generosity and if we have a sound knowledge base we can improve the quality of care.

The Impact of Computers on Nursing
M. Scholes, Y. Bryant and B. Barber (eds.)
Elsevier Science Publishers B.V. (North-Holland)
© IFIP-IMIA, 1983

CHAPTER 2

PERSPECTIVES IN NURSING

Keynote Address

Dame Catherine Hall D.B.E.

Introduction

It was with trepidation that I accepted the invitation to undertake this address. My experience of computers is limited to their use in maintaining organisational records and providing management information. The United Kingdom Central Council is currently engaged in developing a computer system to maintain a single professional register of nurses, midwives and health visitors. The system, which is being designed in collaboration with the National Boards in the four countries of the U.K., will have a capacity, inter alia, to record additional qualifications, to hold training records, information about continuing education and the payment of fees. Such a system will have a potential for providing valuable manpower information which is currently lacking. While as Chairman of the UKCC I am conversant with this work I remain a layman in the sphere of computer science and its application. I will, therefore, endeavour to set the scene, to put the topic into perspective, to identify some of the current issues in nursing, and to raise the question - can computer science assist in the development of nursing and so benefit indirectly the recipients of this major professional service?

The Historical Perspective

We live in an age which has seen science fiction become a reality. There has been an explosion of knowledge, particularly in the spheres of science and technology. Space travel has now ceased to be a seven days wonder and men have landed on the moon. The cost of these breath-taking achievements has been phenomenal, but the ingenuity of man which they represent is awe inspiring. The part played by computer science has been considerable and computers have now such universal application that their usage has its place in the curriculum of the school children of today.

However, developments of this magnitude give rise to major ethical issues - for instance the extent to which computers are now used to record information about individual citizens gives rise to concerns about the adequacy of controls to ensure confidentiality and proper usage. We are faced with a fundamental question namely, has man's ability to make moral judgements, effectively to control, and to use for right purposes, these tremendous scientific developments, progressed in parallel, or has it been outstripped and left us without a sound philosophy on which to base judgements.

The World Scene

The 'Declaration of Alma Ata', resulting from the International Conference on Primary Health Care, held under the aegis of the World Health Organisation in 1978, asserted:-

"A main social target of governments , international organisations and the world community in the coming decades should be the attainment by all peoples of the world by the year 2000 of a level of health that will permit them to lead a socially and economically productive life."

The Quadrennial Congress of the International Council of Nurses in 1981, took as its theme 'Health for all by the year 2000'. An informal meeting of nurses, convened by the World Health Organisation and held in November 1981, was addressed by Dr. Tejada-de-Rivero, Assistant Director General of W.H.O. He outlined the implications of primary health care for the health system and the need for a reorientation of that system. He went on to express the view that the place of nursing in bringing about essential change in that system was clear; in most countries nurses were the most important group of health workers in terms of numbers, closeness to prevailing health problems, and understanding of community needs.

This recognition of the key role of nursing by the Assistant Director General of W.H.O. is highly significant. W.H.O. has often been seen as a medically dominated body which has failed in its attitudes and structures to give adequate recognition to nursing and nurses.

The National Dimension

The national dimension is crucial in considering health care needs and health care resources. In this context I would concentrate on the position in the 'developed countries'. Irrespective of the health care system which pertains, health care has an insatiable appetite for funds. Governments, tax payers, the community at large, have to determine the money they are prepared to allocate to this vitally important social service. However, for the professionals engaged in health care the allocation is never likely to be regarded as sufficient.

The provision of health care is a labour intensive service; a service given by people to people. In the United Kingdom the National Health Service is the largest single employer. Health care now involves a range of professions, supported by ancillary workers.

It is the aim of each of the professions concerned to provide the highest possible standards of service, utilising to the full developments in knowledge and technology.

A higher level of general education and the increased emphasis on health education, have resulted in a more informed public and one more demanding of the totality of health care provision.

Advances in medical science and in pharmacology have resulted in the disappearance of many former 'killer' diseases; increased longevity and the 'nuclear family' have led to a change in the balance of need. The elderly frail and the psycho-geriatric make increased demands on health care resources while, at the same time, advances in technology enable 'miracle' surgery to be performed, but at a high cost.

Priorities have to be determined in the context of the finite resources of money and manpower. The ethical issues which arise demand careful study by all the health care professions, and debate by the community at large; it is not the prerogative of any one profession or any group of professions to 'play God'.

The most immediate issue for this international forum is that all health care professions have a responsibility constantly to address themselves to the ways and means by which the most effective use can be made of resources. This involves a willingness to take a new look, an analytical look, at traditional concepts and practices and to seek out new tools which may assist in the better utilisation of resources of both money and professional manpower.

Policy Making

It is essential that nurses are involved in policy making, at all the different levels, not only because they are the largest professional group in the health care delivery system but also because of their closeness to prevailing health needs.

In the United Kingdom the nursing profession is fortunate in that, in each of the four countries, there is a strong team of nurses within the relevant government departments, led by a Chief Nursing Officer; these teams have an input to the formation of government policies. And, within the National Health Service itself, the committee and management structures provide for nurse involvement at each level.

In order to be fully effective in their policy making role the nurses concerned must have available to them all relevant information, facts and figures. Opinions formed in the light of experience are not a sound base for policy formulation although, in the absence of adequate information systems, they have often had to serve in the past. The development of inter-linked computer systems can assist greatly in this sphere; they provide a valuable resource for nurses and others engaged in policy making.

The Delivery of Care

Moving from the policy level to the level of professional practice, it should be noted that it is of the nature of a profession that the professional provides a direct service to clients, and that there is a relationship of trust and confidentiality between the professional and the client.

Nursing has developed as an hierarchically structured profession. This is inevitable because nurses are employees within the health care system and the resources they require must be obtained for them by 'managers'; also, the totality of nursing resources must be organised to ensure that they are used to maximum advantage. However, this should not detract from the key position of those who are the providers of care.

Much has been written about the role of the nurse and it is still a subject of debate. It does not lend itself to precise definition because it has many dimensions. It is a role which is still evolving as the image of the nurse as the 'handmaiden of the doctor' fades into the past.

In the absence of precise definition I would express my conviction that there is a unique nursing role complimentary to, but not subordinate to, that of the doctor. I believe that the nursing role, in the sphere of clinical practice can be and should be extended, but as a **nursing** role and not as that of 'the physician's assistant'.

The nursing profession must formulate policies as to the extent to which experienced nurses, with further education and training, can properly develop their role in depth and breadth, in the interests of enlarging their contribution to health care; this cannot be done unilaterally. Health care involves a team of professionals and a team only functions effectively on the basis of mutual understanding and mutual respect. In such a setting conflict is a disintegrating influence.

I am saddened when I learn of instances of apparent conflict between doctors and
nurses as nurses have sought to identify their unique function, based on a
growing body of knowledge; I believe that traditional attitudes and role images
are largely responsible. The two professions are interdependent. Nurses, as
the evolving profession, should take the initiative in promoting increased
understanding of their aspirations and their aims and seek consensus with
doctors and other health care professions. The case they put forward must be
well argued and based on all relevant information; defensive attitudes and
emotional presentations are not conducive to conviction.

I am in no doubt that there will be a positive response provided that it can be
seen that the primary concern of nurses is to utilise to the full their
knowledge and skills in the development of patient/client care services and that
they are not motivated by professional aggrandisement.

Professional Education

Education is the corner stone on which developments in nursing must be built,
and professional education should be seen as a continuum. The system of nursing
education differs from country to country, in some countries it has moved into
the university setting or into the general education system, in others it
remains largely within a separate structure, closely linked with, or part of,
the health service structure.

The system itself is not of prime importance, it is the means to an end; the end
is to produce the type of nurse who is required within the health care system in
these closing decades of the 20th century and looking ahead to the 21st.
However, I would pose some questions about "the system":-

(i)   Does it produce true professionals with the requisite knowledge to inform
       practice, with appropriate attitudes, with developed communications skills
       and with a real appreciation of the art as well as of the science of
       nursing?

(ii)   Do its 'products' have an analytical, problem solving approach to the
       practice of nursing, and an ability to respond to changing health care
       needs? Do they have a real appreciation of the importance of continuing
       education to maintain competence and of further education to prepare for
       new and extended roles; are they capable of self-initiated and self-
       directed learning?

(iii) Is the system geared, primarily, to producing a competent worker in an
       institutional setting with an emphasis on functioning in the area of acute
       care, one who lacks the educational base required readily to respond to
       changing needs, to absorb and apply new knowledge and to utilise
       technological developments?

I have identified extremes in order to highlight what I believe to be a key
issue namely that, in the context of social change, of demographic projections,
of limited resources in money and manpower and of a changing emphasis in health
care needs, it is crucially important that we satisfy ourselves as to the
adequacy and relevance of our particular system of professional education; and
that we initiate change if this is seen to be necessary. If we fail to do this
then I fear that, as we move towards the 21st century, the nursing profession
will find itself ill equipped to respond to the demands made upon it.

Another vital dimension to this issue is the people who have prime
responsibility for making the system work - the nurse educators. If the system
is such that they are frustrated in their aim to produce the type of nurses they
know to be required, they will either become a rapidly changing population

moving elsewhere for professional fulfilment, or they will stay and become a disillusioned group rather than an inspired and dynamic one. Neither outcome is conducive to maintaining an educational environment supportive of the nursing students who will become the professional practitioners of the future.

Changes in the system of nursing education have far reaching implications. This is particularly so in those countries where, traditionally, nursing students have formed a significant part of the health service labour force. Plans must be made in the light of all relevant information; different models need to be examined before the blue print is decided upon. Although change may have to be effected by a process of evolution, goals and timescales are essential in order to maintain momentum.

As computers become more widely used by government departments, within the health service system and in the sphere of general education, the information required to make sound plans for changes in nursing education will become increasingly available. Furthermore the use of computers as an educational tool may well facilitate some of the changes required.

The Management of a Professional Service

A professional service, such as nursing, must be managed by fellow professionals with the knowledge, ability and experience to speak authoratively on behalf of the profession and to secure, and manage, the resources required to provide a quality professional service. This implies that funds and facilities must be made available to provide the requisite further education to equip potential top nurse managers for their key roles; desirably this preparation should be within the university system or within Business Schools, and it should be multi-disciplinary. Nurse managers must be capable of functioning, on the basis of equality, alongside managers of other disciplines, of utilising new knowledge and of applying new techonology in promoting the effectiveness and efficiency of the professional service they manage.

Nevertheless I believe that posts in nursing management should be kept to the minimum necessary to facilitate the effective delivery of care. Furthermore, nursing management should not be the only avenue through which a nurse may progress to reach a professional pinnacle, in career terms. Key clinical posts, with wide ranging responsibilities, would allow the able and committed practitioner to realise her professional potential while continuing to fulfil a role in the direct care delivery system.

The contribution which computers may make in providing management information and in carrying out important tasks which currently take up a great deal of time, may well facilitate this change in the nursing service structure. There will also need to be a change in concepts and attitudes which cannot be achieved by a computer.

Research

Nursing must become a research based profession. Many of the issues to which I have referred previously will only be satisfactorily resolved as a result of relevant research. Over the last quarter of a century there has been significant progress in nursing research. In the United Kingdom this has been well supported by the relevant government departments. Much of the early work related to 'nurses'; I would describe it as sociological research. While this was, and will continue to be, an important sphere of research activity, I believe research needs to be developed into **nursing**, supportive of the clinical role of the nurse, as this serves to deepen nursing knowledge on a scientific base.

The development of computer technology has been a great facilitator of research.
I do not need to elaborate on this statement to a forum of experts, but a
question which has to be asked is - are we producing a sufficient number of
potential nurse researchers? I fear that in many countries the answer is 'No'.
This brings us back to the system of nursing education. Unless the importance
of research is appreciated by nursing students there will continue to be a
dearth of nurse researchers. Education and research should go hand in hand, in
the School of Nursing as in the University. This has implications not only for
the system but also for the preparation of nurse educators and for their
teaching load.

Another key issue is the funding of nursing research, particularly in those
countries where the national economy is causing governments to cut back on
programmes previously funded. Nurse researchers must be of a calibre to compete
with researchers of other disciplines to obtain funds from any available source.
They must be able to convince grant making bodies that research in nursing is no
less important than in other disciplines to which it has long been recognised as
integral, and that the aim of nursing research is improved standards of nursing
care.

Conclusion

In identifying various key issues in nursing I have indicated my view that
computer science may well be able to contribute to their resolution. If that be
so then the application of computer science certainly has a part to play in
facilitating and supporting developments in nursing.

In spite of my very limited knowledge and experience in the computer sphere, one
thing I do know, namely that however sophisticated the hardware may be the
effectiveness of the computer is determined by the input. And so the extent to
which computer science may assist in the development of nursing, will be in
direct proportion to the expertise which nurses can acquire in the preparation
of relevant programs assisted, of course, by appropriate technical staff.

In all scientific and technical developments man is, and must remain, the
master. Man must never become the minion because his birthright is that of an
intellectual being. It is he who must solve the problems, and identify the
implications of the technological marvels of this and every age, and it is he
who must make the moral judgements as to their usage. As nurses it is for us to
determine how we can use computer science, appropriately and effectively, in
facilitating the contribution of our profession to the provision of health care.

Health for all by the year 2000; this is a goal towards which we should all be
striving. In support of this goal the nursing profession must play its part in
promoting the most effective use of available money and manpower in the
provision of health care in each and every country. At the same time the
nursing profession, world wide, must endeavour to improve the standards of the
service it provides and to increase its contribution within the health care
systems. In order to do this we must be prepared fully to utilise the growing
body of nursing knowledge and relevant technology.

CHAPTER 3

COMPUTER TECHNOLOGY IN HEALTH CARE

This section of the book provides a framework for placing some of the concepts, developed in later chapters, in the context of computer technology and what it has to offer in terms of its capabilities and limitations when applied to nursing needs. It includes an overview of available computer facilities. Some of the themes expounded here are developed in the Nursing Management Section, Chapters 13-15.

The Impact of Computers on Nursing
M. Scholes, Y. Bryant and B. Barber (eds.)
Elsevier Science Publishers B.V. (North-Holland)
© IFIP-IMIA, 1983

3.1.

GETTING STARTED

Richard Turner

1. Types of Computer

For many people a computer is something they read about or hear about but do not have the opportunity to use themselves. However the situation is changing as the price of computer equipment falls, and this paper discusses factors which should be taken into account by potential users. The three main types of computer are the Mainframe, the Mini and the Micro, and each has a number of characteristics as far as the user is concerned which are independent of the actual power (in computing terms) of the machine involved.

1.1. The Mainframe (£50,000 - £1m and over)

This is the kind of computer most used in the National Health Service at the present time, and is to be found particularly in Regional Health Authorities or District Health Authorities (Teaching) although it is used in a different way in these two situations. In the Health Authorities it is used for batch processing, and the usual arrangement is that the users fill in batches of pre-printed forms using a pen (whether these be payslips, Hospital Activity Analysis (HAA) forms, Equipment returns, or whatever) and the computer summarises them and produces output either on striped paper or in the form of printed payslips etc. which are sent out from the computer centre in the post. In the Hospitals the Mainframe computer usually has a lot of terminals connected to it and users input data and receive output via these, although printed copies can be obtained through the post if required (or be produced on a local printer attached to the terminals).

The characteristics of Mainframes are:-

1. They are expensive, which means that only large organisations can afford them, although smaller organisations occasionally get together to purchase one.

2. They are usually programmed by professional computer programmers who set the machine up to do whatever the users want it to do and who are employed by the purchasing organisations.

3. They can process large files efficiently, and usually have facilities for sorting and analysing data which are not found on smaller machines.

A professional service based on a Mainframe can offer a number of advantages in that programs can be tailored to the users requirements and altered to suit any changes in these requirements **without** extra money having to be found every time an alteration is required. If errors or problems occur the programmer is on hand to put it right, and the programs can be rewritten or adapted to take account of any improvements to (or replacement of) the computer itself.

In a well-run computer section each program is documented so that newly appointed programmers can quickly take over when staff leave, and most computer sections also employ systems analysts who are available to discuss ways of using computers with potential users, and who can also discuss how the user might change the way in which he or she works in order to make the best use of the machine.

The other advantages of the Mainframe approach is that if part of the machine breaks down (for example a terminal or a Disk storage device) it is usually possible to carry on by plugging in a replacement without loss of any previously stored information and often with hardly any inconvenience to the user.

It is true, however, that the users are entirely dependent on the skills of the professional staff, and this means that they have to spell our their requirements in advance rather than adopt a trial-and-error approach. This can be a chicken and egg situation, in that the user is expected to say what he wants from a machine which he does not really understand and has no experience of. Furthermore, the professional staff are often in short supply, and there may seem to be an inordinate amount of bureaucracy involved in obtaining agreement among users who have to reach agreement in order to make the programming task easier (quite apart from the benefits of standardisation which may be very real).

A further problem is that the Mainframe computer supplied by one company is often incompatible with that supplied by another (often by design rather than by accident) so that users become "tied" to one supplier.

1.2. The Minicomputer (£20,000 - £80,000)

Minicomputers share many of the advantages of Mainframes, but they are usually much less expensive, do not require to be housed in a special building, and are usually programmed by agency staff or by the suppliers or sometimes by the users themselves rather than by professional computer people employed by the purchaser.

Minicomputer suppliers usually employ salesmen who know the capabilities of their equipment and can discuss the users requirements to a certain extent, particularly when these fall into the most commonly recognised categories such as storing and retrieving details of customers, stock control, payroll systems, and accounting systems. Any out of the ordinary requirements are likely to be expensive to commission, and expensive to alter later, but the equipment supplied is usually built to last, is easily serviced, and can usually be upgraded (by adding more terminals or more disk drives, etc.) to meet any future needs the customer might have, until the Mini has virtually the same capacity as the Mainframe. The problem of incompatibility between machines supplied by different suppliers remains, but the customer can be sure that a Minicomputer supplied by a reputable manufacturer can be made to do what he wants, although it may end up costing more than he thought originally.

1.3. The Microcomputer (£3000 - £20,000)

Microcomputers are cheap and cheerful and incredible value for money for some applications, but they are not a good substitute for Mini or Mainframe computers in many areas.

They are usually supplied 'across the counter' by shops which are frankly not interested in what they are going to be used for, and are often used to run general purpose programs such as "database management systems" or "financial modelling packages" which cannot be modified in any way by the average purchaser. They can function as an electronic card index which can be used to hold details of several thousand patients or as a calculator which can remember all the figures which are put into it, or a word processor which can also save typing out the same names and addresses each time. The Microcomputer can work wonders. However, if any component goes wrong, the whole machine is out of action and if great care is not taken to make back-up copies of files, the entire record file can be lost in a second. Taking back-up copies of large files can be time consuming and expensive in relation to the initial cost of the machine if a magnetic tape or duplicate disk drive is used, but taking such copies is even more important than with the larger machines since Microcomputers are generally not constructed as well as Mini computers or Mainframes, and their disk drives or keyboards can begin to give trouble after a year or two, by which time the model may have gone out of date.

All this may change with the generation of Microcomputers just coming on the market which are produced by Mini computer or Mainframe companies and are intended to be used as stand alone machines or can be used as terminals to larger and more powerful computers. However, the problem of writing programs which are sufficiently generalised to be of interest to a large market and thus worth the effort of writing them, but yet are sufficiently useful to the individual, will remain.

In general, exprience has shown that NHS users rapidly require more and more access to computer power once they start, and many Micro computer users would now give a lot to have access to superior facilities and reliability of the Minicomputer or Mainframe, not to mention a systems analyst or a programmer.

2.   Practical Procedures

In a professional computer unit, every aspect of computing is considered separately. The terminals are designed to be as easy to use as possible, with individual labelled keys for commonly performed functions. Each item of data entered is checked for range errors (i.e. sex must be M or F), and for incongruity where possible (so that a query is raised if the sex is female and the patient has had a prostatectomy). Cross checks are also made to ensure that all cases have been recorded and backlogs of data to be entered do not build up because there are sufficient operators to cope with peak demand. Holidays or illness do not cause a problem if there are sufficient numbers of operators, and an individual is not asked to enter the same kind of data day after day.

Back-up copies of all magnetic files are made regularly, and a journal is often kept on a separate disk of all changes made to the files so that if something happens to the main disk, a copy can be made from the back-up copy together with the journal. In a large installation, 24 hour cover can be provided by maintenance engineers, and sufficient numbers of spare devices can be kept for emergencies. Each of the above tasks becomes the responsibility of a named individual, and is thus more likely to be carried out efficiently than would be the case in an office with only a small machine where everything has to be done by one or two people. All these factors become more and more important as time goes by and increasing reliance is placed upon the computer.

Security is also important, and a copy of a single floppy disk from which an unscrupulous individual could obtain at leisure a list of prominent citizens with their diseases, for example, might have considerable commercial value. The professional bureau can afford to take proper security precautions.

3.   Introduction of the Computer

A computer is not likely to be used to maximum advantage if considerable forethought is not given to it's introduction into the workplace, and a number of books have been written on this subject. In particular, all staff (including those who will not be using it themselves) should be consulted, and a proper training (with the possibility of going back to the supplier during the period just after installation when problems are most likely to arise) should be offered to those who will use it.

The location of the machine is important if different users are to have access to it at different times, and wherever possible reliance should not be placed entirely on one machine. There is an advantage in finding out what other computer systems are in use locally, both as back-up if all else should fail on site, and in order that programs and experience can be shared.

It may be necessary to limit access to certain records (or parts of records) to particular individuals but as far as patient records are concerned, greater cooperation between members of the primary care team is likely to be achieved if all the members can see what each other have recorded.

Lastly, before the machine is introduced, it should be remembered that there is one device which has been around for a number of years which has unparalleled advantages for many applications. It can be used for letters, digits, graphs, photographs and diagrams. It can be sent through the post, requires no special training to use, is very cheap, requires no electricity, is easily portable and can be expanded indefinitely and with care, will last longer than any magnetic medium. This is paper, and its only real disadvantage is that it is difficult to cross-index the data it contains.

The Impact of Computers on Nursing
M. Scholes, Y. Bryant and B. Barber (eds.)
Elsevier Science Publishers B.V. (North-Holland)
© IFIP-IMIA, 1983

3.2.

MICROCOMPUTERS FOR NURSING: AN OVERVIEW

John Kwok

1.   Introduction

As the largest professional group in the service and as a group having the most direct involvement in the care of patients, the nurse plays a significant role in promoting improvements in health care. By providing the required information and in effectively controlling essential clinical equipment, the microcomputer will prove to be an invaluable ally to the nurse in achieving a better service to the patients.

Before we consider how microcomputers can be used for nursing, perhaps we should first consider what are microcomputers? There is a bewildering array of equipment, costing anything from £50 up to £25,000 or more which falls within the definition of a microcomputer. Some of this equipment will not be suitable for professional use. We ought, therefore, to examine certain general properties and characteristics of different types of microcomputers that are available, to provide us with the necessary perspective and a common frame of reference.

2.   What are Microcomputers?

Microcomputers are essentially small computers which use standard microelectronic integrated circuits in the form of solid-state components - the micro-chips - to perform various information processing and storage functions. Although a micro-chip is physically small, it can contain a very large number of transistors, made of semi-conductor materials, to form highly complex electronic circuits.

With the latest miniaturisation techniques, it is now possible to produce a chip containing over half a million transistors on a tiny silicon wafer a quarter square inch in size. These transistors can be arranged in groups of interconnected rudimentary circuits or "gates", to form tens of thousands of more complex individual circuits. This level of complexity, known as 'Very Large Scale Integration' (VLSI), is more than adequate to implement a conventional 32-bit Von Neumann type processor of a current mainframe computer.

There are many different kinds of chips being used in a microcomputer. Each kind of chip is designed to perform a specific function, e.g. as Processor, Memory, Input/Output, Controller, Uncommitted Logic Array, etc. From these basic 'Lego-like' building blocks mounted on 'printed circuit boards', an extensive range of increasingly versatile and powerful special-purpose and general-purpose microcomputers have been developed.

3.   Special-Purpose Microcomputers

We are all familiar with the more common examples of special-purpose microcomputers; even though, sometimes we are unaware of their crucial role when they are incorporated in a particular piece of equipment:

```
1.    TV GAMES (Purpose-built 'Amusement Arcade Games machines')
2.    TELETEXT/PRESTEL UNITS
3.    WORD PROCESSORS/'ELECTRONIC OFFICE' TERMINALS
4.    INDUSTRIAL PROCESS CONTROLLERS AND ROBOTS
5.    SELF-SERVICE PETROL PUMP CONTROLLERS
6.    SUPERMARKET POINT-OF-SALES TERMINALS
7.    '24-HOUR' CASH DISPENSERS
8.    UNDERGROUND ROUTE DISPLAYS (e.g. Euston Station)
9.    DOMESTIC EQUIPMENT CONTROLLERS (e.g. Washing Machines)
10.   COMPUTER NETWORK INTERFACE UNITS
11.   INTENSIVE CARE MONITORING EQUIPMENT
12.   BODY SCANNING EQUIPMENT
```

4.   General-Purpose Microcomputers

The general-purpose microcomputers are those computers which are suitable for data processing in the conventional manner.   In the West Midlands Regional Health Authority, we have classified general-purpose Microcomputer Systems into 6 categories:

```
Category 0   KEYBOARD-BASED VIDEOTEXT MICROCOMPUTER
Category 1   VDU-BASED MICROCOMPUTER WORK STATION
Category 2   TIME-SHARING MICROCOMPUTER SYSTEM
Category 3   HOMOGENEOUS MICROCOMPUTER NETWORK
Category 4   HETEROGENEOUS MICROCOMPUTER NETWORK
Category 5   HETEROGENEOUS INTER-NETWORK SYSTEM
```

Characteristics of General-Purpose Microcomputers:

```
        LOW COST                   USER CONTROL
        SMALL SIZE                 HIGHLY RELIABLE
        READILY AVAILABLE          INTERACTIVE PROCESSING
        EASY TO USE                MULTI-FUNCTIONAL
```

5.   Keyboard Based Videotext Microcomputer

This category encompasses a plethora of microcomputers which are primarily intended for educational establishments or for use in the home (cf. pocket camera or record player).   Such computers can sometimes be adapted and enhanced for professional purposes.   However, care must be taken in selecting a particular model to ensure that it is capable of being extended to provide the facilities which are useful in a professional context.

A typical system would comprise: (1) the computer itself, which is commonly housed within the same unit as the typewriter keyboard; (2) a standard T.V. receiver set, for displaying information produced by the computer; (3) a good quality cassette recorder for program and data storage. Beyond these, it would be desirable to attach a low-cost printer to produce the computer output on paper.   A diskette unit, although not essential, will greatly improve the efficiency of the processes of storage and retrieval of permanent files of data. A further 'refinement' is to acquire a colour T.V. set, and appropriate adapter units at the same time, for accessing VIDEOTEXT information.

An outline of potential uses of VIDEOTEXT microcomputers:

    <u>Information Access</u>   (a) Videotext: Teletext: CEEFAX
                                                                                  ORACLE
                                                       Viewdata: PRESTEL

                                      (b) Expert Systems, e.g. MYCIN

                                      (c) Public/Private Databases e.g.
                                                    BLAISE (Using 'Teletype'
                                                      Emulation program)

    <u>Training & Education</u>   (a) Computer Literacy, e.g. BBC/NEC
                                      (b) Use of computers & programs
                                      (c) Programmed learning, e.g. MICROTEXT

    <u>Information Processing</u>   (a) 'Small-scale' Record Keeping
                                      (b) Word/Text processing
                                      (c) 'Modelling' experiments, e.g. VISICALC

    <u>Entertainment</u>   (a) Computer games playing
                                        (b) Creative programming in music
                                                    graphics, animations, etc.
                                      (c) Invent other uses!

6.   V.D.U. - Based Microcomputer Work Station

For professional purposes a microcomputer in this category is required. These systems, commonly known as 'Desk-top' computers, are likely to meet the production standards of quality and reliability necessary for regular rather than occasional use. Physically, these systems can assume different forms:- A system may consist of three separate units: (1) the computer combined with mass storage facility; (2) a Visual Display Unit (VDU); (3) a printer. Alternatively, as two units: (1) the computer, the V.D.U. and mass storage; (2) a printer. There are even systems available which incorporate everything in a single integral unit.

Despite these superficial differences in engineering and design, all Microcomputer Work Stations are functionally equivalent and all use a conventional or modified VDU as the main INPUT/OUTPUT facility. They should be capable of performing a number of different operations: (1) as an independent local computer; (2) as a word processor; (3) as a communications terminal to other computers; (4) as a 'Server Unit' in a Distributed Computing System.

7.   Time-Sharing Microcomputer System

With the large-scale production of 16-bit microprocessor chips, small computers using these low-cost but powerful processor are now available. These computers are effectively microprocessor-based microcomputers sharing many characteristics of the minicomputers to the extent of using identical system software, e.g. the UNIX operating system.   Typically, a system in this category provides the facility of serving a number of terminals operating as a mult-user system.

Since for all practical purposes these systems operate as mini-computers, they are suitable for data processing tasks at present being done by minicomputers, e.g. in the Pathology Laboratories. Because of their comparatively low-cost in relation to the facilities they provide, these 16-bit microcomputers are ideal for situations where a greater processing capability or storage capacity, beyond that of the Micro Computer Work Station, is required or where a number of different tasks need to be performed concurrently.

However, in common with all 'time-sharing' computer systems, only a single central processor is available to execute the work-load of the entire system. The ability of the computer to respond to a particular user-terminal is totally dependent on the actual number of terminals requiring service at any instance in time. Unacceptable delay in response will occur if there is a large number of terminals simultaneously contending for the use of the processor.

8.   Homogeneous Microcomputer Network

The provision of purpose-designed data communications facilities to enable several microcomputers to connect to each other, and to share common resources form the basis of this category of network. They are considered homogeneous because it is necessary to use the same model of computer, or at least computers operating common system software.

A typical network consists of a microcomputer which has been designated the Master Computer and a number of microcomputers designated as User-Stations. These User-Stations are all connected via their individual network interface and transceiver hardware directly to the Master Computer or to a common network cable. The Master Computer which contains the Network Operating System software, is responsible for controlling network operations and for providing central mass storage and printing facilities. Each User-Station needs only to communicate with the Master Computer when the central facilities are required. In practice, this type of network operates in a manner similar to 'time-sharing' multi-user systems, but there is an important difference. For unlike a time-sharing terminal, each User-Station is a computer and can process its own tasks independently at high speed. Data can be transferred between User-Stations and the Master Computer very rapidly.

Since the central processor in the Master Computer is only used for communications tasks, a homogeneous microcomputer network offers better response to the users. There is no apparent contention for resources among the users, so such a network can be considered as a more satisfactory alternative to a 'time-sharing' minicomputer system.

9.   Heterogeneous Microcomputer Network

The rationale for the development of this category of network is to provide a universal communications medium to enable all types of computer: mainframe, minicomputer, microcomputer and peripheral equipment from any manufacturer, to be connected together and sharing resources distributed throughout the network.

These networks, commonly known as Local Area Networks, are designed to serve users sited at various locations within a particular establishment, e.g. a college campus or hospital complex. Special-purpose microcomputers are extensively used as Network Controller Units, Network Interface Units and Network Server Units. General-purpose microcomputers can be attached to the Network via Network Interface Units.

A truly Distributed Computing System can be implemented using this type of network. Not only all the existing computers located in various departments can be linked, but additional common resources: e.g. special-purpose processors (say, for high definition image processing), extensive storage facilities, high-speed printing and other output devices, inter-network communications server units can all be incorporated. So instead of enhancing or extending the facilities for a particular departmental computer, all resources are available to all the users.

In a hospital context, the significance of the introduction of the Distributed Computing System (D.C.S.) is the possibilities it offers in terms of information sharing, transmission and distribution. At a fundamental level, real benefits can be obtained just by making patient identification and location data more easily accessible to personnel in any department. With a D.C.S., any resource of the systems is available to every user, irrespective of where the user or the resource is physically located.

10.   Heterogeneous Inter-Network System

Both in concept and in design, the inter-network system is primarily concerned with the provision of communications facilities for the inter-connection of independently operating computer networks. Special-purpose microcomputers can be used as Network Server Units dedicated to inter-network communications.

Each Communications Server Unit is required to perform either one of the following functions:

> INTERNAL data transfer between a Homogeneous Network located in a particular department and the Local Area Network for the whole establishment;

> EXTERNAL Data transfer, using public telecommunications media, between local area networks which can be separated by vast geographical distances.

The possibility of being able to transfer data between Local Area Networks has important and 'far-reaching' implications as the implementation of inter-network systems will make the development and operation of a 'corporate information system' for a geographically distributed organisation technically feasible. It is generally recognised that the quality of decision-making depends on the availability of timely, accurate and pertinent information. The provision of inter-computer networks in the health service will enable the collation of many types of data which are at present only accessible at different locations. All the data for a District or Region, relating to patients, manpower, finance, epidemiology and community health can, in principle, be organised and presented in a meaningful form for planning, monitoring, management and research purposes. The availability of comprehensive and up-to-date corporate information should provide the basis for effective modern health care.

11.   Microcomputer Applications for Nursing

In providing computing resources where it is needed and as a means to process and convey information, the microcomputer holds immense potential for the use of nursing. The microcomputer is already being used for a number of applications and significant progress has been achieved in the development of other areas relating to nursing. Because of 'time-constraint', it is not possible to provide a detailed survey of all the existing and potential applications of microcomputers that are of interest to nursing. Therefore, only a small selection of actual or potential uses of microcomputers in areas where they are most likely to have an impact on nursing are being considered: (1) Nursing Education; (2) Nursing Administration; (3) Patient Care.

12.   Nursing Education

The microcomputer can make a useful contribution in this vital area, upon which the future of the nursing profession substantially depends. Because of its potential flexibility and comparative low-cost, a VIDEOTEXT microcomputer is ideally suitable for training and educational purposes. This type of computer can be considered as a general training facility for the School of Nursing. It can be used for at least three aspects of nursing education: (1) General Education; (2) Professional Training; (3) Extra-curricular activities.

GENERAL EDUCATION: Computers are increasingly being used as a professional tool in many occupations. The ability to use a computer effectively and a measure of computer literacy will be regarded as a pre-requisite for any profession. In its educational role, the British Broadcasting Corporation is currently producing a series of television programmes to promote computer literacy. The B.B.C. also markets a microcomputer system specifically designed for the purpose. The National Extension College in Cambridge, in conjunction with the B.B.C., is offering a short correspondence course in computer programming. The West Midlands RHA, with the same objective, is currently providing a one-week course for staff in any discipline. Familiarity with the use of computers will be an asset in preparing nurses in operating nursing station terminals in the wards.

PROFESSIONAL TRAINING: The National Physical Laboratory, the pioneers in the use of microcomputers for education and the physically-disabled, recently introduced the MICROTEXT system. In essence, MICROTEXT is a program designed for teachers to structure course material in the form of related 'instruction-frames' of text in a similar manner to the 'mechanical teaching machines'. However, MICROTEXT is more flexible and easier to use for both the tutor-author and the student.

The 'Knowledge-Based Expert System' is another important development which can be used for computer assisted instruction (CAI). In this instance, the 'data-base' of a computer contains the framework of factual data and procedures of general inference provided by a specialist in a particular field. On interrogation, the computer will interactively respond with pertinent advice according to the 'rules of judgement' programmed by the specialist concerned. MYCIN, for example, is a program developed at Stanford University to provide advice on the diagnosis and treatment of certain diseases, including indentifying the pathogen and indicating the correct dosages for treatment.

EXTRA-CURRICULAR ACTIVITIES: By the judicious use of VIDEOTEXT facilities, a nurse can be well informed of the developments in current affairs! Although the TELETEXT facilities are provided free-of-charge, it is not the case for accessing the VIEWDATA facility, i.e. PRESTEL. The telephone charges incurred by the liberal use of PRESTEL could be considerable.

The use of the computer for entertainment can be recommended, not only for the mental stimulation it offers, but as a means to vent 'harboured-frustrations'. The playing of computer games can be a palliative; unfortunately, in common with all palliatives it can sometimes be addictive!

13. Nursing Administration

Microcomputers can potentially play a significant role in assisting with the management of nursing resources. This is a field in which considerable progress has already been made; for example, the system to assist nursing officers in Staff Planning and Allocation developed by Peter Squire in Rugby.

The mainframe-based system developed by Catherine Rhys Hearn at the Health Service Research Centre in Birmingham, is pre-eminently suitable for adaptation to a microcomputer. This system is used for calculating projected nursing work-load presented by patients in a particular specialty-ward according to pre-defined standard of care.

A research team under the direction of John Yates at the Health Service Management Centre, also in Birmingham, has developed a microcomputer-based system to analyse and evaluate standard hospital statistical data to determine the comparative performance of various institutions. Graphical computer output can be displayed interactively, to illustrate comparisons in the form of graphs, pie-charts or histograms.

The microcomputer can usefully assist in many routine administrative tasks; such as Record-keeping, Statistical analyses, Inventory management, and Word Processing. For forward-planning purposes, it is possible to use a general program, e.g. VISICALC, to analyse, plan and project future requirement of resources.

In the context of clinical information, the microcomputer can be used to access central databases; for example, those provided by the British Library Automated Information Service (BLAISE), which contains extensive data on citations and references to published material relating to health care. Such a facility could assist in the development and administration of local information services.

14. Patient Care

The Nursing Station terminal for access to a hospital-based computer system is currently the usual means by which a nurse becomes familiar with computers. This terminal, with only limited facilities, has to be permanently sited at the Nursing Station or office.

A Ward-based microcomputer can perform the tasks of a nursing terminal as well as providing additional facilities, not normally available to a conventional terminal. The microcomputer can easily be transported throughout the ward on a small trolley. It only requires a standard electricity socket to operate, and can connect to the hospital computer system using an existing telephone 'jack-plug' socket sited at the bed-side.

Many microcomputer-based systems are already in operation, and more are currently being developed, in various hospital departments; viz: Accident and Emergency, Pathology, X-Ray, Pharmacy, Speech Therapy, Psychology, Cytogenetics, Endocrinology. There are, invariably, independent and un-coordinated developments, but by using the appropriate computer network technology, it is possible to integrate them into a unified system with the patient as the focus for all the available services.

A number of systems are now in operation in the community. General Practitioners are particularly active in the introduction of microcomputers to assist them in their surgeries; interestingly, it seems the 'AGE/SEX REGISTER' is almost mandatory for a G.P. System. At the Family Planning Clinic in Sandwell, a system called 'MICKIE' is providing sterling service in the field of Psycho-sexual Counselling. Microcomputers are effectively used by the Family Practitioner Committees; also in the maintenance of Child Health Records.

15. Information Technology

In its report, 'Information Technology', the Advisory Council for Applied Research and Development (ACARD) of the Cabinet Office states "Information Technology ----- which combines the technologies of computing and telecommunications ----- will perhaps be the most important area of application of microelectronics. It will eventually affect virtually every household and occupation."

It is, perhaps, fair comment to suggest that for all of us in the health service, both the goodwill and the interest are present for the acceptance of Information Technology. We are gradually coming to terms with this technology by progressively learning to harness its immense potential for, ultimately, the improvement of Patient Care.

A possible scenario for the continuing application of Information Technology in the health service would involve the development of a 'Patient Orientated Services System' (POSS). In a conceptual model of this system, the wards in a hospital would collectively constitute the 'hub' of a wheel from which 'Requests for Services' would radiate to the supporting departments, and to which the 'Delivery of Services' from the departments would converge.

There would be less handling of physical documents: whether they were test-results, meal-orders, drug prescriptions, miscellaneous requisitions, diagnostic and treatment schedules. All of them will be catered for by a hospital-based information network. The use of the telephone for communicating information would be substantially reduced, since it will be supplemented by using the microcomputer key-board and display screen. This suggestion is not really unreasonable when we consider how often it is necessary to write telephone messages in order to record them.

'Electronic Mail-Boxes' would be extensively used to convey messages and other information. Memo's and messages could be sent, simultaneously, from different sources to the same person or department. Every item of information will be stored in a 'mail-box' and despatched, each item in turn, to the person for whom they were addressed. If the person concerned is not available, then, they will be kept in the 'mail-box' until it is possible to do so. The need of having to make repeated calls because of a particular telephone being constantly engaged will be a thing of the past! In time, communications by speech would be fully reinstated when satisfactory speech recognition and synthesis equipment can be incorporated into the network. It would also be possible for high-definition images of conventional X-Ray films, and computer-generated colour images from scanning equipment to be directly displayed in the wards. Will 'the Expert Systems' by then, also be in regular use as an aid for effective diagnosis and treatment, in each G.P. surgery, in every clinical department and in all hospital wards?

It is customary to finish a paper by drawing certain general conclusions. In this instance, it is difficult to do so since there is no single conclusion upon which to rest. 'Microcomputers for Nursing' is a dynamic subject. The substance changes almost by the day. I hope my objectivity will not be too severely compromised by stating: "the advent of the microcomputer, in all its diverse forms, heralds the dawn of a new era ------ in the way we structure, communicate and process information". In terms of the future possibilities for the convergence of Information Needs with the Enabling Technologies, we are only at THE BEGINNING!

The Impact of Computers on Nursing
M. Scholes, Y. Bryant and B. Barber (eds.)
Elsevier Science Publishers B.V. (North-Holland)
© IFIP-IMIA, 1983

3.3.

COMPUTERS NEED NURSING

Barry Barber

Why bother Nurses with Computing?

The papers combined together in this book offer solid evidence that computing
will have a profound influence on nursing. Furthermore, it is too important to
leave to computer specialists. This activity needs to be approached with the
same collaborative enthusiasm as that which was achieved by the radiotherapists
and the medical physicists in their search for accurate dosage control.
Informatics is a curious word, apparently well understood by all but the
English. It is convenient because it deflects interest from the "computer"
itself to embrace the totality of the system and the mathematical analysis of
its behaviour (operational research). Nursing Informatics must be pushed higher
up in the professional consciousness of nurses. Computing is widespread and
pervasive; it offers opportunities for providing something extra - extra
information, extra insight, extra monitoring, extra control or extra time.
Systems can be fast, powerful and incredibly useful if they have been properly
designed. Clear objectives and purposeful analysis lead to useful systems.

Nurses will inevitably become more and more involved in developing computing
systems to suit their professional needs. These systems will, in due course,
provide the backbone and framework of their professional activities in caring
for patients, in educating trainees and managing staff. The design of these
systems is too important for nurses to stand aside and let others carry out
these functions unaided by the insights of practising nurses. It certainly is
not necessary for all nurses to become informaticians but it is becoming
essential that all nurses have some understanding of the systems and their use
and that some nurses obtain sufficient knowledge of informatics to enable them
to participate actively in systems selection, systems design and systems
construction. It is also essential to merge the insights of those involved in
nursing research and the development of the nursing profession to grasp the
opportunities offered by the use of computer systems and to avoid the patent
dangers that can arise from unsatisfactory systems design. Systems design
controls systems functions, systems flexibility and systems usefulness. It must
be based on desirable nursing practice and nurses must participate
knowledgeably. They must understand the systems potential, capabilities and
limitations. They must be capable of coping with the practical questions of
systems selection, purchase support, running costs and evaluation, as well as
those of analysis and time consuming systems construction. Effective
multidisciplinary symbiosis must be achieved between the professions of nursing
and informatics.

Turning to nursing management, the 27% of our health service expenditure spent
on nursing must give rise to acute interest in the effective management of this
large resource and in the way that staff spend their time looking after
patients. The basic information contained in the nursing systems described in
this book cannot but become of fundamental interest as the Health Services
attempt to control costs and allocate activities in accordance with national
plans and priorities or even simply within hospital objectives.

Nursing is too big and too important to be left free-wheeling within the system
and the more effectively nurses grasp these systems, the more effectively will
they be able to participate knowledgeably in the managerial and planning
discussions. In the same way that Health Care must be regarded as 'big
business' in the dimensions of finance, staff, equipment and management, Nursing
too must be treated as 'big business'.

These systems open the way to improvements in nursing care and to the more
detailed evaluation of nursing care. They need not stand between the nurse and
his or her patient but rather they can assist in the provision of that care.
Furthermore, the nursing record systems should readily interface with the
medical decision-support systems and provide further changes at the ever
changing interface between nursing and medical activities. Since these systems
do not have to be local, they can also offer support for isolated professionals
in rural communities where systems support can improve the effectiveness of
medical, nursing and paramedical staff operating at a distance from a major
hospital(1).

The calculator has rendered the slide rule obsolete within the last two decades
and doubtless it will itself sucumb to the future pocket computer providing
"EXPERT" professional support. The training in radiation treatment planning
that was adequate 25 years ago would be unacceptable today when extensive
treatment planning computer systems are available. The impact of computers on
nursing will be of sufficient consequence to warrent the serious attention of
the most senior and experienced nurses as well as the youngest, most able and
most enthusiastic nurses.

The Development of Interest

In preparing a paper for a conference on Hospital Information Systems in 1979,
it became clear that the nursing dimension in computing had been heavily
undervalued(M1). There have usually been some papers at medical informatics
congresses presented by nurses or on topics concerned with nursing but these
have often been squeezed in among other topics. A successful nursing workshop
at Medinfo 80 enabled I.M.I.A. to accept the proposals which led to the working
conference on which this book is based. It was designed to establish the world-
wide position and interest in nursing applications, and it was hoped that it
would initiate an international dialogue between those interested in this
developing field. This book is intended to provide basic material for training
purposes. Undoubtedly, there will be gaps in the material, references not
listed and important contributors who were not included. It is hoped that it
will provide the impetus necessary for the national and international
development of Nursing Informatics. Indeed the I.M.I.A. general assembly has
already accepted the proposal to create an international working group to assist
with this development.

Introduction of New Technology

The Health Services have an exceedingly good record in introducing new
technology in patient care. Although they operate in one of the most
emotionally charged areas of our personal lives, where we are naturally disposed
to lean towards tried and trusted remedies, our own personal mortality leads us
individually and corporately to seek solutions to desperate situations with all
the science and technology available to us. The introduction of anaesthetic
gases and antiseptic techniques made possible much that we now take as routine
and enabled surgeons to tackle much more complex procedures. These developments
involved specialised theatres and procedures and the creation of a new type of
specialist - the anaesthetist.

During Roentgen's investigation of the properties of x-rays in 1895, the first radiograph was taken of his wife's hand clearly outlining the bone structure. It was rapidly appreciated that this tool could provide a great deal of information for the care and treatment of patients and the search was on to develop effective and reliable x-ray tubes. Most hospitals now have x-ray departments together with the radiologists, the medical specialists concerned with interpreting the x-ray pictures, and radiographers who operate the machines.

It was later appreciated that much more powerful and penetrating x-ray equipment could be used to cure certain types of cancer. This development proceeded more slowly because it was discovered that an overdose of radiation could cause the breakdown of the tissue. Widespread use of x-rays for treatment had to await the cooperation between medical physicists, who developed accurate methods of dosage control, and the radiotherapists, who controlled the medical aspects of treatment. Similar collaboration led to the introduction of radium and radon treatments and then, subsequent to the availability of atomic reactors, to the use of a wide variety of radioactive isotopes for diagnosis and therapy. New professionals emerged to implement the new technologies. Antibiotics, organ transplants and CAT scanners like the other innovations discussed above started with trials in one or two centres, which then began to be adopted by most major centres and then became part of the accepted background of medical practice.

What is New Technology?

Against this background what is NEW about NEW TECHNOLOGY in the Health Services? The Health Services are very experienced in introducing new technology. The diffusion has usually been patchy, unplanned and dependent on the enthusiasm of individuals but it has always been effective. The Health Services are aware of the problems of importing new specialisms, developing new professions and expertise in handling new equipment and setting up training schemes to maintain a flow of skilled staff. However, the current situation suggests that we may be able to achieve improvements in patient care without providing extra staff. Earlier developments have tended to involve extra staffing for effective implementation. If we could be more efficient in our provision of the framework of care, this could enable us to do more at the sharp end of caring for our patients. The idea of work being a scarce commodity to be shared out seems remote from the likelihood of our lives in the Health Services - insufficient resources to carry out the caring seems more likely.

In respect of computer developments in the Health Services the most obvious feature has been that of enabling staff to cope with an increasing load of investigations, to provide a more effective and appropriate plan of treatment. Twenty five years ago, treatment planning was carried out laboriously and calculations of several hours could be needed for working out a possible plan. In these circumstances a reasonable plan has to be accepted in order to get the patient on treatment. With computer assisted treatment planning, the speed of calculation enables very many more alternative approaches to treatment to be explored and consequently it is possible to work to much more stringent limits in the calculations.

Introduction of Health Service Computer Systems

Although initially there were worries about square headed tin boxes replacing doctors, the main lines of development have been indicated in fig. 1 (M1). In the U.K., the first of the Department of Health's Experimental Projects was aimed at dealing with the medical case notes. However, the subsequent work was aimed initially at providing a basic framework in patient administration rather than in providing a record of medical care. This involved the basic information required about patients before anyone is able to tackle their strictly personal

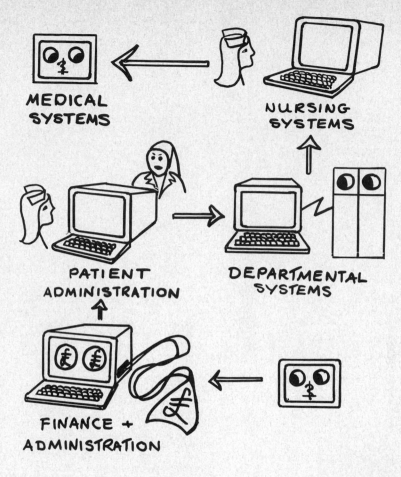

Fig. 1. Health Care Systems Development.

TABLE 1

MEDINFO 83: MAIN APPLICATION SESSIONS CATEGORISED

A.   **FINANCE & ADMINISTRATION**

      ADMINISTRATION & FINANCE (8)

      * Hospital Administrative Systems
      * Resources/Planning
      * Cost Benefit Analysis/Cost Containment
      * Accounting and Financial Systems
      * Health Insurance Systems

B.   **PATIENT ADMINISTRATION**

      HEALTH & HOSPITAL INFORMATION SYSTEMS (1)

      * Medical Records Management
      * Information Storage/Retrieval
      * Exchange of Medical Information,
        National/International
      * Problems in Patient Identification
      * Evaluation

C.   **DEPARTMENTAL SYSTEMS**

      CLINICAL LABORATORY SYSTEMS (2)

      * Haematology   * Clinical Chemistry
      * Microbiology   * Histopathology
      * Nuclear Medicine - in vitro
      * Physiological Measurements (Pulmonary/Vascular)
      * Cardiology/ECG   * EEG/EMG
      * Signal analysis   * Evaluation

      IMAGING (4)

      * Nuclear Medicine   * Ultrasound
      * Nuclear Magnetic Resonance   * Computed Tomography
      * Emission Tomography   * Digital Subtraction Radiology
      * Digital Display of Radiographic Images

      DRUG INFORMATIONS SYSTEMS (7)

      * Drug Distribution Systems   * Pharmacy - Cost Monitoring
      * Toxicology, Drug Monitoring   * Clinical Pharmacology
      * Drug Interaction

      PATIENT MONITORING/INTENSIVE CARE (9)

      * Peri - and Post-Operative Care
      * Cardiac Care Units
      * Peri - and Neonatal - Intensive Care
      * Neurosurgical/Neurological Systems
      * Closed Loop Therapy

TABLE 1 (Cont'd)

MEDINFO 83: MAIN APPLICATION SESSIONS CATEGORISED

D.   **NURSING SYSTEMS**

NURSING APPLICATIONS (6)

* Scheduling of Manpower
* Patient Management, Treatment Control
* Nursing Staff Records
* Impacts on Quality of Nursing Care
* Nursing practice protocols

E.   **MEDICAL SYSTEMS**

CLINICAL DEPARTMENTAL SYSTEMS (3)

* Surgery
* Nephrology
* Cardiology/ECG
* Endocrinology
* Haematology
* Radiology
* Rehabilitation
* Evaluation
* Obstetrics and Gynaecology
* Hypertension Clinics
* Diabetology
* Oncology
* Image Processing
* Radiotherapy
* Dental

GENERAL PRACTICE/AMBULATORY CARE (5)

* System Requirements
* Interfacing with Hospitals
* Patient Surveillance and Treatment Planning
* Experience with Products
* An Educational/Research Tool
* Implications of New Technology for General Practice
* Patient Education
* Multiphasic screening

SUPPORT OF CLINICAL DECISION MAKING (10)

* Computer-aided Diagnosis
* Artificial Intelligence for Medicine
* Knowledge of Bone Systems
* Decision Support
* Decision Analysis
* Information Analysis

EVALUATION OF HEALTH CARE (11)

* Quality Assurance
* Evaluation of Efficiency of Medical Action
* Individual Health Status Indices

NOTE

The main session numbers are listed in brackets and the subtitles indicate the anticipated scope of the session.

medical problems - i.e. the logistics of care. This deliberately low key
approach enabled the staff to gain experience of the problems of implementing
major systems in hospitals and allowed other staff to assess the potential of
the technology. In major institutions, the installation of such systems was
still a major exercise in the management of change. In parallel with hospital
wide systems, work was already in progress independently on departmental systems
to assist in clinical chemistry, haematology, and microbiological laboratories,
in radiation treatment planning, nuclear medicine, intensive care monitoring,
E.C.G. amd E.E.G. analysis. In many ways these systems presented more technical
difficulty in interfacing and programming but they were very much easier to
implement organisationally as the work was carried out for the specific needs of
a single head of department - or at least a very small group of senior staff.
At the present time the two main groups of nursing systems are those related to
patient care records and those related to nurse education and staff records.

During the last 20 years medical computing has been transformed from being the
subject of a reasonable lecture into a variety of specialities which are
difficult to encompass adequately even within a major congress. The specialists
in particular fields frequently prefer to run their own conferences devoted
entirely to their specialism rather than attending a general congress that
cannot treat their area of interest in sufficient depth. The development of
these activities is well reflected in the three-year MEDINFO congress
proceedings. (Some of these books are listed at the front of the Bibliography.)
The first congress took place in Stockholm (1974) and was followed by Toronto
(1977) and Tokyo (1980). The Call for Papers for the next congress to be held
in Amsterdam, Holland 22-27th August 1983 is already available and lists 23 main
sessions. In addition to these sessions there will be associated seminars for a
variety of professional groups to obtain a basic introduction to the application
of computers to their professional activities. If the proposed sessions on
applications systems are set against the framework of fig. 1, it is clear (table
1) how far the applications interest has moved up the heirarchy away from
administration into the medical and nursing areas.

The variety is exhausting and it involves two separate strands of activity. In
the first place, much activity is of an exploratory scientific nature where
specialists have programmed some special application and tested its
effectiveness scientifically. Secondly, there is the basically systems approach
in which scientific and technical solutions are welded into organisational
solutions to systems problems.

These might be described as the scientific and the engineering aspects of
medical computing. Within the engineering lies the component of organisational
engineering or the management of change. It is within this area that some well-
engineered systems can fail simply because the organisation has not been
adequately prepared to receive the computer system. This has been a major
preoccupation for the last decade but the increasing public acceptance of
computer systems and the wider knowledge of the care with which organisational
change has to be approached means that attention can now revert to the more
technical aspects of the systems. Furthermore, it must be remembered that as
systems are developed and the hardware becomes cheaper, today's white elephants
will become tomorrow's work horses. Furthermore, we can begin to start looking
towards the achievement of integrated health care systems based on patient care
rather than isolated systems based on individual disciplines or departments.

Towards SMART Systems

Over the years our computers and peripherals have become more versatile and they are capable of handling a number of matters themselves without the operator having to worry about some of these details - just as computer software has become more versatile and less demanding on the memory and less insistent on getting finnicky detail correct. In the case of the computer peripherals, the cleverness arises from having its own microcomputer control and in the case of software, it arises from the fact that more core storage and faster processing speeds allow more extensive software routines to be used to check, modify and retrieve problems.

At present most systems behave in concept rather like an efficient version of the old-fashioned 4-drawer filing cabinet. Information is stored and retrieved reliably and it can be presented in a useful variety of different ways. However, the systems generally do not avail themselves of possibilities inherent in the data stored by using mathematical or operational research techniques to make suggestions about more efficient ways of proceeding.

Data on waiting list patients and past admissions could be used to schedule patients more efficiently through the likely key requirements of their care. The data on the functioning of outpatient clinics can be used to improve appointment timings. Information on equipment maintenance and breakdowns can lead to suggestions for replacement and new purchasing. Information on staff sickness and absence can lead to improved staff selection and training. Information on stores requisitions can go directly into the stockkeeping and purchasing systems to provide the proposals for ordering. Many of these systems might reduce the dependence of the health service on administrative manpower. These systems could be interactively self-improving using the same sort of techniques as are used in the best chess playing programs. These systems might be called SMART or intelligent systems.

Too often someone thinks up an array of 'management information' or a set of statistics which the computer system is then programmed to provide. Too often, managers have little idea of what they might do with these reports when they arrive. A clear preoccupation with action-orientated statistics and a classification of the areas of action appropriate in different circumstances will provide more effective sets of statistical information and will pave the way for the decision-orientated or optimising systems. The general experience is that mountains of statistics serve little purpose unless they are constructively utilised in some ongoing activity. In the process of that activity the statistics are effectively checked and validated and thus become usable. Material that has not gone through this process is generally found wanting when it is first used or first used for some new purpose.

The Japanese initiative on the fifth generation of computers is, amongst other things, looking towards providing EXPERT technical assistance for specialists. Some EXPERT systems have already been devised by various artificial intelligence groups, and if one is guessing about the future(2), then it is difficult to resist the belief that suitably designed EXPERT Systems will become as commonplace as present day calculators. Whether current descriptions of EXPERT Systems and their rule-based logic will endure is a matter for conjecture but certainly professional support systems which prompt and make use of suggestions to professional staff but do not dominate or control them must be a major next stage in systems design. However, whatever the internal software structure, the external contact with professional staff will have to be practical and user-friendly. Where these developments will take us subsequently, in say two decades from now, it is difficult to predict; possibly the science fiction specialists would tackle that problem better than an applied scientist. Perhaps square-headed tin doctors will appear after all but it will only be after a great deal of solid operational research on health care systems!

Nursing Perspectives

In the context of these developments, nurses have invariably been involved with the most successful projects but their pivotal role has not often been made explicit. The current state of development of health care computing has reached the point where explicit recognition of this fact is required in order to facilitate further progress. Whether they work in hospitals or within the community the nurses provide a central link in the patients' care and they already document patient activity in their nursing notes and orders.

It is significant that:-

1.   **Data Collection**

Nurses are heavily involved in the collection of data from patients, the implementation of doctors order and the arrangements of care.

2.   **24-Hour Care**

Nurses provide the basic 24 hour framework for reporting patient care progress. Even basic patient administration systems require nursing involvement and access is required to other systems in the absence of specialist staff at night and during weekends.

3.   **Practical Involvement**

Most successful computer systems, other than purely departmental ones, have had nurses involved with the system design or implementation. Their involvement has invariably been practical and productive as they rapidly grasped the advantages and limitations of the technology. (A1, A10, A18)

4.   **Nurse Training**

The number of nurses required to run a major hospital imposes a large staff training load to ensure that new staff understand and can utilise the computer systems. In general, this load is best handled by the tutors responsible for staff induction and training.

5.   **Patient Based Nursing Systems**

The use of computer systems to handle nursing orders for patients provides a flexible basis for ward management whether on a task or patient oriented approach(C5, L7). The system provides the basis for handling ward reports when nurses review their patient care activities and hand over to the next shift. Ward activities and work load become more adequately documented both in connection with the reporting and supervision of patient care but also from the point of view of the assessment of ward staffing requirements.

6.   **Nurse Based Nursing Systems**

Schools of Nursing are becoming more stringent in their approach to the educational needs of student nurses. The process of devising suitable training courses and duty rotas needs more sophisticated means of reconciling the nurse training requirements and the service needs of hospitals. This starts with personnel and education records(J20, L8), the exploration of sickness/absence data and the effect of the training schedule on the supply of nurses for service activity(J11), nurse allocation(J12); the linkage between the education and service needs are all of fundamental importance to the efficient running of a hospital.

7. **Evaluation of Nursing Care**

The two basic nursing systems, patient based and nurse based, together open the way to the evaluation of nursing care and then lead on to the issues of medical records and medical decision making. The explosion of interest in general practice and pharmacy systems will add further support to this development. The scrutiny of key health care activities will at last allow us to examine the fundamentals of health care instead of trying to evaluate computer support for unevaluated health care systems.

Nursing Computer Systems

From this evidence, it is clear that nurses will be nursing computer systems as well as patients. However, this should not involve the acceptance of additional menial chores but rather the use of new technology to enhance the quality of the nursing care that can be offered to patients. The nursing of computers arises as nurses become knowledgeable about the technology and as they ensure that systems will be conveniently designed and simple to use. These benefits cannot be obtained without effective collaboration between nurses and informaticians in which each discipline becomes educated in the needs and possibilities of the others. System construction takes time and it cannot be handled by committees although committees can take decisions about the key features required in the systems. The effective use of computing systems requires education, knowledge and practice if solid benefits are to be achieved. However, the opportunities are there to be grasped.

In the long run, nurses will be responsible for most, non-automatic, data input about patients, hence the oversight on data entry will, except in specialist departmental activities, become a nursing function and be vital to the success and effectiveness of the system. Nurses will be in control of system development in the key interface nursing applications and all the other systems will be built with heavy nursing involvement so that they are convenient for nurses. Furthermore, nurses will also be key figures within the wider context of the design, implementation and usage of health care systems; this cannot occur without widespread nursing acceptance and involvement. The nursing systems will enable progress to be made in the understanding and measurement of nursing care - possibly by enabling incidents indicative of the lack of good nursing care to be identified. In this way nursing care, staffing and patient benefit can be related. This seems a field of endeavour that offers a great deal and is worth taking seriously. It will involve a considerable amount of operational research, as well as computer science but that will be discussed later.

REFERENCES

1. Kvamme, J. I., "Health Informations Systems in Remote Areas". Proc. MIE-81 (see bibliography) pp. 50-57
2. Townsend, H. R. A. "Expert Systems; Their Nature and Potential". Proc MIE-81 (see bibliography) pp. 898-907

The Impact of Computers on Nursing
M. Scholes, Y. Bryant and B. Barber (eds.)
Elsevier Science Publishers B.V. (North-Holland)
© IFIP-IMIA, 1983

3.4.

FROM THE COMPUTER MANAGER'S VIEWPOINT

John Rowson

1. INTRODUCTION

In its introduction, the computer can be regarded as an agent of change, and, as with any change in policy or practice in an organisation, its objectives and implementation require extensive forethought and careful planning.

This may be a statement of the 'blindingly obvious' yet, curiously enough, when it is the computer that is the agent we all tend to develop a blind-spot. As obsession with the technology itself and the procurement process obscure the more important considerations of: the organisation's information needs, its objectives, and the careful, thorough analysis of existing information systems.

Often the computer may be an entirely inappropriate mechanism for the required change; the procurement decision being influenced by the wrong, possible subconscious, motive: a showpiece, a desire not to fall behind in modern thinking and developments. As Brian Rothery observed: 'too often the whole project starts at the mythological level and stays there until the day of reckoning'.

Mindful of the inevitable (and if managed properly, desirable) march of computing into our working and personal lives, this paper considers the recommended approach to computerisation as seen from the standpoint of the chastened computer manager. The considerations apply equally whether computer specialists are employed in the project, or, as will be increasingly the case, the user himself develops or purchases his own facilities.

The emphasis of the commentary is in two parts: the essential processes prior to any purchase action, and, considerations of the characteristics of available computing facilities.

2. Preparation

2.1 Problem Identification

The application of computers could be summarised as:

THE SCIENCE OF THE POSSIBLE: THE ART OF THE IMPLEMENTABLE

There are few conceptual applications of computing that defy the capability of the technical state of the art, the potential of which has scarcely been plumbed. Failures in the implementation of computers are all too ofter foredoomed by far more mundane factors than technical shortcomings; such as inappropriate finance, inadequate planning, excessive (or sometimes insufficent) ambition, lack of objectivity, poor morale, or simply local politics. Fig. 1 expands somewhat on these factors:

Figure 1.   NON-TECHNICAL FACTORS CONTRIBUTING TO SYSTEM DISREPUTE OR FAILURE

(i)   FINANCE AND   - UNREALISTIC ESTIMATED CAPITAL AND IMPLEMENTATION
       CONTRACT   COSTS

                          - INSUFFICIENT PROVISION FOR REVENUE CONSEQUENCES
                            (DIRECT OR INDIRECT)

                          - ABSENCE OF CONTINGENCY PROVISION (e.g. FALLBACK,
                            OR DEVELOPMENT CAPABILITY)

                          - POOR CONTRACTURAL PROVISION IN PURCHASE AND
                            MAINTENANCE

(ii)   PLANNING   - FAILURE TO ACTICIPATE OR PROVIDE FOR ORGANISATIONAL
                            CHANGES

                          - FAILURE TO CONSIDER FUTURE REQUIREMENTS

                          - ABSENCE OF POLICY, OBJECTIVES

                          - INSUFFICIENT CONSIDERATION OF TRAINING AND
                            IMPLEMENTATION NEEDS

(iii) CONSULTATION   - LACK OF USER INVOLVEMENT IN SETTING OBJECTIVES
                            AND DESIGN APPROVAL

                          - LACK OF CONSULTATION WITH THOSE AFFECTED INDIRECTLY

                          - FAILURE TO PUBLICISE OBJECTIVES

                          - FAILURE TO CARRY ORGANISATION AS A WHOLE IN
                            OBJECTIVES AND IMPLEMENTATION

(iv)   AMBITION   - TOO AMBITIOUS OBJECTIVES OR OVERLARGE
                            IMPLEMENTATION STEPS

                          - IMPLEMENTATION TIMESCALE TOO SHORT

                          - LACK OF AMBITION, FAILURE TO REALISE TRUE POTENTIAL

(v)   OBJECTIVITY   - FAILURE OR USERS (OR ANALYSIS) TO FORM A DETACHED
                            OR IMPARTIAL VIEW

                          - FAILURE TO TAKE A REALISTIC VIEW OF THE DRAW-BACKS
                            AS WELL AS THE BENEFITS

                          - FAILURE TO ADEQUATELY CONSIDER THE EXTERNAL
                            PROCESSES WHICH RELATE TO THE COMPUTER SYSTEM

(vi)   LOCAL POLITICS   - FAILURE TO RECONCILE OR DIFFUSE LOCAL POLITICAL
                            POLITICAL ISSUES OR INTERESTS - ENOUGH SAID!!

The London Hospital has enjoyed a relatively successful era of computerisation
over the last two decades, thanks largely to:

i)   the vision of the original programme instigators
ii)   the unstinting commitment of the elected user representatives
iii)   the patient and the realistic attitude of the users
iv)   the continuing financial and political support from the Hospital
        management
v)   the professionalism of the computer department staff

Where reversals in the 'appliance of Science' have been suffered (however
small), these have not been attributable to computer technology, but to the
fallibility of man: an absence of realism or objectivity on the part of all
concerned: a failure to identify the true problem:

ALL TOO OFTEN A COMPUTER IN SEARCH OF THE PROBLEM

This is not to excuse the computer professional, he is as culpable as any, it is
his job to identify the problem, or at least to recognise the absence of its
diagnosis.

2.2   Systems Analysis

There is a recognised process which if pursued thoroughly should enable the
successful application of computers; the generic term is systems analysis and
design, and its logical and sequential constituents are common to most problem-
solving (including, for example, medical diagnosis). The steps are outlined
(and contrasted) below in Fig. 2.

2.3   Cautionary Reminders

If honestly followed, the described plan should produce a successful outcome.
However, there are many pitfalls and the following comments are worthy of
consideration:

(i)   The correct perception of the necessary change requires time and careful
        consideration: the prospective user must take time off from every day
        duties to stand back and carefully consider the objectives. A mistake at
        this early stage could clearly blight the whole exercise.

(ii)   The user should look beyond the current exercise to future objectives and
        requirements so that the current plan can be seen in perspective and
        decisions made will not pre-empt or prejudice predictable future
        developments.

(iii)   It should be remembered that the computer system will not exist in a
        vacuum, but is cocooned in the human activities that surround it. These
        complementary processes should be considered as part and parcel of the
        overall design; ideally, seeking the involvement of other disciplines in
        the study and revision of these tasks. It has been suggested that any
        computer system gains best chance of success if it replaces a successful
        manual/clerical system; therefore consideration should be given to a two-
        pass implementation: the first revising the clerical process; when this
        is successful, the second phase replaces manual procedures with automated
        ones.

        Even if the scale of the project, or the unavailability of staff,
        precludes the use of management science professionals, the relevant
        managers should take time to act as surrogate Management Scientists.

Figure 2(a) Computer Problem Solving – diagnosis & decision

(THE SYSTEM MALAISE)	PROBLEM SOLVING	(THE SICK PATIENT)
BY COMPUTER SOLUTION		BY MEDICAL DIAGNOSIS
Clearly define the problems	PROBLEM IDENTIFICATION	Identify and document the symptoms
Investigate current processes	DIAGNOSIS	Relate symptoms to possible diagnoses List possible diagnoses
Determine the aspects in the processes which contribute to the problem		Mount necessary investigations to confirm the diagnoses
Carry out more detailed studies to establish process objective, data flow, staff activity, and logistics. (in fact, classical: who, what, why, where, when, how)		Consider the patient prognosis
Deduce solution requirement (what facility would achieve objectives) regardless of mechanism	?ACTION/ TREATMENT	Identify appropriate treatment - consider treatment options - consider possible outcome - consider probability of success
Consider means of achieving solution		- consider costs - consider implications for patient for environment for other agencies for community?
Assess implications of possible (or at worst preferred) solution mindful of costs, logistics, staffing, ease of implementation, effects on organisation, consistency with objectives, and relevance of likely future objectives		

Figure 2(b) Computer Problem Solving - Implementation & Appraisal

(THE SYSTEM MALAISE)	PROBLEM SOLVING	(THE SICK PATIENT)
BY COMPUTER SOLUTION		BY MEDICAL DIAGNOSIS
Complete detailed system design	IMPLEMENTATION	Consult affected parties (patient, relatives, nursing, clinicians, para medics, etc.
Consult User on Implementation plan		
		Determine treatment plan
Plan development and implementation programme (including education)		Put plan into effect
Monitor programme		
Specify, program, and test		
Carry out education		
Implement		
‾‾‾‾‾‾‾‾‾‾		‾‾‾‾‾‾‾‾‾‾
Monitor effectiveness of solution	APPRAISAL	Monitor outcome of plan
Consult users		Consider success of outcome, complete or abandon

(iv) The fundamentals of the solution should be envisaged without undue regard to the mechanism to be used, which should be a later consideration. It is all too easy to become hypnotised by attractive or stimulating tools before a detached view of the requirement is formed; otherwise, therefore, the over-riding consideration becomes how to bend the processes to suit the pre-destined technology, rather than finding an appropriate solution to fit the requirement. (Rather akin to deciding on the therapy before the diagnosis is determined).

In summary, it is all too often the wrong interpretation of the requirement, which leads to an unworkable or unsuccessful conclusion; rarely is the technology itself the primary cause.

3. Future Developments

The cautionary reminder becomes all the more relevant when a forward look is taken at the next decade of computer applications.

The current volume explosion of computer applications involves a change in the role of the computer professionals. The cost of the equipment has fallen substantially, with improvements in technology and the mass production of components and assemblies in increasing numbers, to the point where the cost of designing the programming an individual system can be many times greater than the price of the equipment.

The emerging high level, 'user-friendly' software environments will ensure that the prospective user will either be able to construct his own systems or purchase a standard system that he will tailor to his own local use. The computer professional will become the consultant, adviser, policy maker, and technology evaluator. Only in the more complex applications where the logistics, technical complexity, or economy of scale are involved, will the computer specialist play his conventional role. Hence the crucial need for the user to learn the fundamental processes in the development of successful computer applications, including procurement.

4. Choice of System

4.1 General

The procurement of computer systems warrents several papers in itself covering such topics as state of the art awareness, evaluation and appraisal, contract aspects, hardware and software support; it is clearly beyond the scope of this paper to pursue all the relevant topics in detail. However by way of orientation for the aspiring computer user, the following section looks at some of the attributes, limitations and considerations attaching to the basic types of computers: micro, mini, and mainframe.

The following paragraphs attempt a generalised summary, which almost by definition will not apply in every case. So rapidly is the technology advancing that some of the observtions may be invalid by the time the paper is published.

4.2 Micro Computers

When limited, local, or discrete processing is required (eg. equipment control, single user filing systems, small business systems) micro computers are likely to be appropriate.

Data files can be supported (typically < 30 million chars in aggregate). The workload would be relatively small with a limited requirement for concurrent access by several users.

A good deal of ready-made software (facilities which can be directly used by non-specialists) is available especially with systems using the CP/M operating system, including: word processing, list scheduling, data capture and validation, simple databases, etc.   There are a variety of ready-made application packages, especially for business applications (eg. Accounting, stores).

The purchase costs of micro-processor systems are low (typically in the range £1,000 for a single user to £30,000 for a multi-user). Portability (ie. the ability to transfer applications on to differenct machines) is good, especially where CP/M is used.   Most of the popular programming languages have an implementation on some micro or other.

4.3.   The Drawbacks of Micro Computers

Since micro computers are so accessible and so attractive, it is worth setting out their key disadvantages clearly. These disadvantages include:-

a)   poor data protection against loss or corruption;

b)   limited enhanceability when applications 'run out of steam';

c)   little software and middleware support (because purchase is often through factors);

d)   limited hardware support (because cheaper hardware engineering may lead to earlier antiquity);

e)   difficulty in getting documentation on production items;

f)   incompatability within system components as supplied.

As microcomputer configurations are often intended to handle a limited throughput, there may be a reliability problem with certain of the devices typically attached (eg. cassette tapes, floppy discs) if used heavily.

Error handling and error reporting is primitive in current micro-processor software.

4.4   Minicomputers

Minicomputers offer good middle order solutions in terms of cost and capacity. Costs can range from £15,000 to £1 million dependent upon processor power, and peripheral or terminal provision. Some offer good enhanceability from low to relatively high powered machines. They can support operationally between one terminal and two hundred (or more with networking). Data capacity can be extensive and similar to that of a small to medium mainframe.

Traditionally the mini computer has been available to OEM suppliers, and supports most popular protocols. System software for supporting interactive processing and networking is arguably better than on the other two types of computers.

The system software is generally efficient providing a lower processor overhead than that on a competitive mainframe computer; hence the mini offers a good usable price/performance ratio. Most standard languages are implemented on minicomputers.

The drawbacks in minicomputer technology are in the absence of some of the refinements available on mainframes. There are usually poorer batch scheduling, system monitoring and tuning facilities hardware maintenance and software support arrangements are better than the 'depot' arrangments for micro computers but are not as comprehensive as that available with a mainframe. However care should be taken in appraising the maintenance arrangements as there are pitfalls for the unwary.

4.5 Mainframes

Mainframe computers represent the high cost, high performance (gross) end of the computer spectrum, though the generalised provisions of the system software tend significantly to affect the net processing return. Essentially general purpose, they handle batch, timesharing, and transaction processing applications with equal facility. Extensive peripheral capability can be added to a level which far exceeds most users' conceivable requirements, and there is no meaningful limit to the size of the terminal network (provided of course there is adequate processing capability). Hardware engineering organisations and diagnostic facilities are usually good. The system software is generally sophisticated and comprehensive, and is well supported by the supplier. There are extensive programming language options (including those to international standards).

Starting from an expensive 'entry point' (bottom of the processor range), there is usually an extensive enhancement path, and the customer's investment in software is usually protected in its portability to the replacement ranges of computers (eg. ICL 1900 to 2900, IBM 360 to 370 to 4300).

There is usually excellent software provided for scheduling, and monitoring computer usage and for the implementation of database applications.

Shortcomings of mainframe computers, other than price/performance, include the poor application transfer opportunities to other manufacturers' equipment, and the high cost of system upgrades. Operator costs may be high, and there is generally an assumption in the design of the manufacturer software that there will be operator attendance.

Reference:

The Myth of the Computer, Rothary, B., Page 13. Published by Business Books Ltd.

The Impact of Computers on Nursing
M. Scholes, Y. Bryant and B. Barber (eds.)
Elsevier Science Publishers B.V. (North-Holland)
© IFIP-IMIA, 1983

3.5.

THE IMPORTANCE OF NURSES' INPUT FOR THE SELECTION OF COMPUTERIZED SYSTEMS

Constance M. Berg

Introduction

Nurses must become involved in the decision making concerning the installation of computerized systems in their hospitals. Each hospital is different in it's operation, therefore it is essential that the system selected meet with the needs of the nursing department.

The Health Services are on the threshold of an exciting new era and nurses must be actively involved in it now. The nursing process, systems theory and computer technology have developed concurrently into powerful tools for nurses to use in meeting the health care needs of their patients.

Since the advent of total computerized Hospital Information Systems, nurses have had little or no input in the decision making process surrounding system selection. Then, following the decision, they are brought on board to participate in the implementation of the system because everything the system did focused around the workload at the nurses' station.

The emphasis on nurses being involved in the selection of a system for their hosptial has improved, but it is not where it should be. The evidence of a lack of nursing input is apparent in the formal questionnaires sent to vendors from hospitals. It is relatively simple to tell whether the nursing staff has been involved or not. Often these questionnaires are developed without the awareness of the nursing staff and, in the cases when they have had an opportunity to review them, they did not understand the implications of the questions.

This section describes and focuses on level three systems and their benefits and proposes a framework for the nursing staff to use as a guide to determine their needs for their system seletion process.

Nurses and Automated Systems

These views are shared with Professor Kathryn Hannah from the University of Calgary, Canada (L22):-

"The use of computers in client care will be the biggest change to confront nurses and nursing in the next decade. In the nursing profession, we are just beginning to experience the profound impact that computers will ultimately have on nursing practice and patient care. No longer is the question: "should our profession resist automation?". Given present societal, governmental and technical trends, the change to and the expansion of automation in health care agencies is inevitable.

The question now becomes: "how do we cope with the resisting forces within and among ourselves so that the result is a stable, predictable, rational approach to improving the quality of nursing practice and thus the quality of patient care?".

Many others in the nursing profession share this enthusiasm, among them June B. Somers, former nursing coordinator for data processing at Charlotte, North Carolina Memorial Hospital (D10);-

"It is the belief of most nurses, that in order to improve patient care, that care first must be evaluated. In order to evaluate it, it first must be in writing. The institution of an automated nursing care plan has made possible a process of evaluation that has resulted in an improvement of care throughout the entire hospital. The automated nursing care plan, is the tool not only of the nursing team on each unit; it also is available for use by the nursing supervisors, who constantly must evaluate the care given on the units for which they are responsible. As a result of the implementation of this system, the nurses have had to examine the nursing care they give."

Fortune Magazine has described this phenomenon: "One of the characteristics of the computer, that makes it unique among technical achievements, is that it has forced people to think about what they are doing with clarity and precision. A person cannot instruct a computer to perform usefully until she has arduously thought through what she is up to in the first place, and where she wants to go from there."

The nurses at Charlotte Memorial Hosptial, according to Miss Somers, have a most productive relationship with the computer system --- it works for them to improve the care they give. "Had they not been allowed to participate in the planning and implementaton of the system," she maintains, "the development of such a relationship would not have been possible."(D10)

If the premise that computerized medical information systems in hospitals are inevitable, is accepted, then it is important to make sure hospitals acquire ones that can meet professional and patient care needs today -- and can progress to fulfill the needs of the future.

Key Evaluation Questions

In selecting an optimal Medical Information System, the key question is "What does the system do to help me provide better patient care?" In more detail, does the system:

* automatically process physician's orders and immediately prepare and distribute complete requisitions to all hospital departments?

* automate the patient kardex files and nursing care data for each patient?

* handle even the most complicated medication and intravenous therapy reminders and reporting -- automatically?

* provide important summary reports such as: Cumulative Laboratory Test Results Summary, 24-Hour Medical Order Summary, 7-Day Medication Summary and Nursing Discharge Summary, Pre-op Summary, etc.?

* maintain up-to-the-minute status of all test results that can be retrieved in an instant?

* assist in documentation of nursing observations?

* assist in staff scheduling through a patient acuity system designed according to your department's specifications?

* automate the ordering of Central Supply items?

* ensure maximum security of Patient and Profession information?

*   assist in scheduling patients for ancillary services?

*   improve communication activities among nursing units and between ancillary
         services?

*   offer a patient data base which can be utilized for nursing research
         activities?

*   offer many other features that save clerical time and reduce frustration?

*   above all, offer nursing the opportunity to spend more time caring for
         patients?

Some medical information systems include these features for nurses, others do
not.

Error Reduction

A computerized information system should help guard against medication errors,
misinterpreted doctor's orders and overlooked treatments. George Monardo,
president of Ralph K. Davies medical Center in San Francisco, observes: "Most
mistakes made in patient hospital care come in the administration of medication,
either through omission or by mistake in transcription."(1)

These are exactly the sort of errors the hospital's Technicion Medical
Information System was designed to prevent, according to Monardo. The dedicted
system combines an IBM or plug compatible processor and software written in part
by physicians **and nurses.**

Doctors order medications or intravenous fluids with medications for their
patients, the order is entered directly into a CRT by lightpen.

These orders are processed by the computer and displayed and printed at the
appropriate nursing station and in the pharmacy, where medication is prepared.

Traditionally, a nurse would locate the patient's kardex, complete the
appropriate colour-coded medication card, send or hand carry the information to
the pharmacy, note the completion of the orders and then file the chart.

The information would then be passed along to the next shift, to a third shift
and so on throughout the patient's hospital stay. It would be constantly
manually monitored throughout the dates that it was ordered to be given and the
nurses would have to remember when it was due to be given.

The Medical Information System at Ralph K. Davies Medical Center, however,
automatically handles the information and signals nurses when to administer the
medication. It also insures that the pharmacy has prepared the medication
exactly as the physician has ordered it.

When the nurse records into the computer that she has administered a pill or
injection, they are led automatically to chart where they gave it (if
injectable) or how they gave it. The nurses do not have to chart the time nor
do they have to "sign off" each medication. The computer takes care of that
automatically. The patient is charged automatically at that moment. No charges
are made for drugs that a patient does not receive.

The key to the system is the video matrix terminal (VMT), through which a doctor
or nurse enters patient care information and calls up various displays. The
screen visually presents a list of patients, specific patient-care data, lists
of drugs, specific orders and laboratory tests.

Doctors and nurses, in turn, can use this information to send instructions to various hospital departments. Instructions for medications, for example, simultaneously go to the pharmacy and the nursing staff.

Special instructions, such as emergency orders, allergies, legal procedures for addictive drugs or special intravenous solution mixtures, are printed directly in the pharmacy on gummed labels which go directly onto the bottles, jars or tubes.

Lois Jahn, former director of nursing at Ralph K. Davies, Medical Center, records that "the MIS system keeps everything in a 'now' mode. There is no chance of a nurse administering a medication that has been discontinued or carrying out an obsolete order. Changes are made instantaneously within the system without fear of the nurse or ward clerk processing them erroneously."

Cuts Paperwork Time

How does the system affect the nurses' work schedule? Approximately 75% of a nurse's time has traditionally been spent on processing paperwork . Miss Jahn estimates that the MIS system has cut that time to less than 25%. Charting medications alone, she maintains, has been reduced by three-quaters. Furthermore, there has been **almost unanimous acceptance** of the systems by the nursing personnel and clerks in the hospital who regularly use the system and the nursing attendants who use it 'to some degree'.

"We've never met a person we couldn't teach to use it," she says. "The quality-assurance factor is the main benefit of MIS other than greater quality of care. One can write and process a page of orders in five minutes instead of 25." "You know," she says, "everything's been done that has to be done, there is no chance of a mistake, and you have more than time for actual nursing instead of clerking."(1)

The MIS system also assures that a patient will not have to remain in the hospital longer than necessary because of being poorly "prepped."

For example, if a patient gets fed at the wrong time when undergoing a fasting test, treatment can be delayed 12 hours, which is another day's stay. Where dietary orders may have been lost in transmittal before, the MIS system guards against such misplacement, saving money for both patient and the hospital. Lost or misplaced orders are a thing of the past. Communication activities are significantly improved all the way round.

Level Three System

The system described above is level three system, namely, the Technicon Data System's full Medical Information System (MIS). This type of system offers the most features and benefits for nursing and patient care. Level three system characteristics should include some of the following capabilities:

* Provide rapid response time for users who interface with the systems equipment (terminal and printer).

* Route and process messages throughout the hospital and also provide for on-line storage and rapid retrieval of data throughout a patient stay in hospital.

* Store patients' historical and clinical data, following their discharge.

* Produce most portions of the patients' medical record automatically.

* Automate nearly all manual nursing functions.

*   Provide real-time ancillary department test results such as Laboratory, Radiology, EKG, Respiratory Therapy and so forth.

*   Provide outpatient processing, as well as emergency room features for patient care activities.

*   Permit a single (one time entry) selection of comprehensive sets of orders to "explode" into detailed instructions for patient's tests and care. This is specifically helpful when many pages of orders are required for patients such as those in critical care areas.

*   Locate printers and terminals throughout the hospital in every department and in nurse stations.

*   Employ the use of a lightpen and keyboard for the purpose of entry of free-text messages. Some of the systems utilize touch screens and push buttons located on the terminals to send and receive messages.

*   Allow the professional user to interface directly with the terminal and printer, such as the physician, nurse, laboratory, radiology and other service oriented department employees. (If the physician elects to use the system directly to enter orders, it will eliminate the need for another user, such as the nurse, to enter the orders for them.)

*   Interface capabilities with other stand alone systems such as Word Processing systems, laboratory systems and Financial systems is an essential feature of a level three system.

Systems Decisions Affect Nurses

Since nurses comprise anywhere from 50% to 75% of the total number of employees of a hospital, it is to their advantage that they become part of the decision making body that determines the vendor or system selection. Because of the nature of these types of systems, the nursing workload, as it exists today, is impacted the most. It is not enough that nurses select features and functions which they would like to have someday, or attempt to delegate this responsibility to a non-nurse from the data processing department. It is important for the nurses themselves to understand, differentiate, prioritize and articulate the needs of their department, and above all have a say in the selection of a system.

Some nurses who read this paper may ask how they can become part of the decision making group; I suggest they place themselves on each and every committee they can in their hospitals and develop strategies for protecting the interests of nursing. Persuasion techniques, as well as assertiveness training may be a prerequisite, as it has been for other issues involving nursing. By participating in this decision making group, nurses must also remember that the process used for selection of a system must have the support of top level management or, very likely, nothing will happen.

The following represents an appropriate framework which nursing departments can use to measure, evaluate and differentiate level three systems.

FRAMEWORK TO DETERMINE NURSING NEEDS FOR SELECTING A SYSTEM

Step One: Establish the Nursing Component of the System Selection Committee

The leader of this committee should possess or obtain some technical or computer expertise and be fully acquainted with the present manual system that exists in this hospital. This individual should have the understanding that she or he will be acting on behalf of the nursing department. Other team members should include nursing representatives from anaesthesia recovery and any additional department that comes under the heading "Nursing". If it can be arranged, an outside expert in nursing and data systems who is entirely independent of the workings of the hospital, should be consulted.

In the summary, the focus of this component will be to determine the needs of the nursing department for the process of selecting a level three system.

Step Two: Know Your Manual System

It will be useful to document the current manual nursing information system as it exists in your hospital, for two reasons:

First; it will aid in determining a baseline for selecting a system and second; it will be a guide when it comes to the implementation of a new system. This information will be obtained from your nursing committee.

While it is not necessary to flow chart each and every function (See Diagram 1, which describes a medical order writing process), it will be helpful to at least outline in steps what the manual system is actually doing at present. It will be necessary to ask, "How many times does x occur per day, per shift, and how long does it usually take to accomplish x?" The results of these enquiries will yield many surprises as to how patient care is actually accomplished in practice.

Primary examples of these categories and activities include:

    1. The Admission of a Patient
    2. Medications Handling
    3. Patient Care Planning
    4. Nurse Care Plans

In order to carry out the analysis, the following questions are particularly revealing.

1. Admission of a Patient

* How does nursing become apprised of the new patient being admitted to their ward?

* What manual tasks must be done to admit the patient?

* How is a bed located and reserved for the incoming patient?

* Who needs to know this information?

* How does the patient admit data flow to the nursing unit?

* Has the patient been admitted to the hospital before; if so, how is the medical record obtained?

* Does the hospital perform pre-admission testing; if so how is this information communicated to the nursing unit?

* Does the hospital use a plastic or metal-type patient identification plate or card which is delivered to the nursing unit?

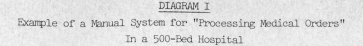

DIAGRAM I

Example of a Manual System for "Processing Medical Orders"
In a 500-Bed Hospital

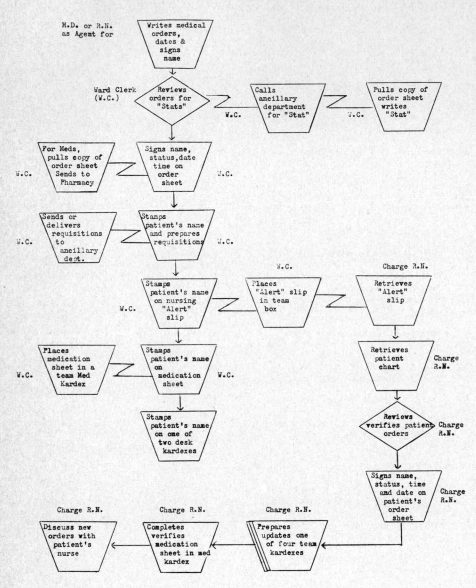

* Does the patient have an arm band which also serves as a means of identification.

* How does a nursing admission interview take place and does this information become part of the nursing care plan or patient care plan?

* How are the patients chart documents identified?

* How much time does it take to process and assemble the patient's chart and documents?

* How do the overall admission activities fit into the overall census of the hospital?

* Does the nursing staff generate a 24 hour census each night for each nursing unit?

Are there bottlenecks and problems associated with admitting patients? Examples of these types of difficulties include the delays in initiating medical orders for newly admitted patients. This is usually due to the lag time that is apparent when the addressograph plate does not arrive with the patient. When this occurs several times a week it becomes an obvious concern. An automated system should eliminate this problem.

2   Medications Handling

* Who writes the medication order?

* Is it complete - does it include the drug, the name, the amount, the route and the frequency?

* How does the order arrive in the pharmacy and how is the order filed?

* How does the nurse know there is a medication order for a patient?

* Who documents the order, the drug name, the dosage, route and frequency for the nursing staff so they will know the time when this drug is due to be administered to the patient?

* Where is this information documented?

* How is the nursing staff apprised of a patient drug allergies and is this information communicated to the pharmacy?

* How is the medication documented, as given, or not given, amount given, route, renewed or discontinued for the patient?

* How does the nursing staff know that a specific medication order is ready for renewal or cancellation?

* How are scheduled or unscheduled medications handled when, for example, lesser amounts of the medication are administered

* How is this information documented and or conveyed to the physician or other nursing staff?

* Are there occasions when a nurse must adjust the original medication order as in cases where the frequency needs to be changed?

What are the difficulties or problems encountered with the medication procedure?
One of the difficulties may be in the area of documentation. In a randomly
selected patient's record, it should be possible to review complete
documentation for the charting of medications, as "given" or "not given", to the
patient. More implicitly, would the nurse's signature and status be present
along with medication, dosage, amount, route, frequency and actual time given?

3.   Patient Care Planning

Since the term "Patient Care Planning" signifies different meanings to many
nurses, it is defined as follows for the purpose of this paper. To provide for
effective patient care, the mission of nursing is two fold, it consists of
physical care and health counselling. The documentation of the patient's
physical care activities and orders and the health counselling that care givers
provide for patients are documented on a "Patient Care Plan". This information
may be in the nurses' mind, on the physicians' order sheet, on a piece of paper
or grouped by patients' needs on a document known as rand or kardex. All these
categories of care are designed to assist the patient to recover from an illness
or to alleviate a patient's problem and ulitimately discharge him from the
hospital.

Data that can be collected here includes the following types of questions:

*   How is the patient care plan initiated for each patient?

*   How does the patients' demographic data flow from the patients' admitting
     sheet to this source document?

*   Does the nursing staff use standard terminology to plan and initiate
     patient care and how are patient care orders relayed from shift to shift?

*   How much time is spent on direct care activities as compared to the paper
     work?

*   What are the requirements for tests which indicate pre-preparation of the
     patient, such as the components of a prep for a Barium Enema?

*   How are the dietary department and the nursing staff notified that a
     patient is N.P.O.?

*   How many preps are handled by the nursing staff?

*   How does the nurse know that patients' tests are in process?

*   How are patients' tests and treatments scheduled with ancillary
     departments?

Needless to say, some of these activities involving patient care planning may
not be seen by nursing as a nursing activity per se, but, more than likely, the
nursing staff sees most of them as their responsibility.

If a hospital uses a multidisciplinary care plan in which only a portion of the
plan is the result of nursing entries, it will be helpful to determine how this
impacts nursing interventions and the "care-givers".

Other questions include:

*   How soon are physicians orders initiated and communicated to the nurse and
     ancillary departments?

*   How current is the information portrayed on a patient care plan?

* How legible is the information and is it complete; how is it updated?

What are the difficulties experienced with the development, implementation and monitoring of the patient care planning system for the nursing staff? How much time do they spend per shift accomplishing these activities?

4   Nursing Care Plans

Clearly, a computerized level three system should accomodate nursing care plans. However, the nursing department must have a clear picture of what these plans encompass.   They should be well in place in the manual system, for they represent the philosophy of the department and the quality of care that patients receive in the hospital.

To determine the nursing department's needs for the automated nursing care plans, the following areas should be addressed:

* Does the system support the areas of assessment, planning and evaluation of patient care?

* How are the patient goals for each problem documented?

* Are nursing actions or interventions documented as a part of the plan?

* Are the nursing care plans tailored to each patient?

* Are there guidelines set for the nursing staff to assist them in developing a good plan?

* Does the plan reflect short and long range goals geared to the patients' discharge?

* Is the plan current, as well as flexible?

* Does it determine the patients' progress?

* Does it provide data for other nursing personnel?

What are the common difficulties and limitations in accomplishing written nursing care plans for each patient? One area might be the time consuming change of shift reports that are shared at the end of a tour of duty and the beginning of another. Another concern will be the time that it takes to develop a care plan. Determining patients' nursing needs and prescribing nursing care takes time -- where does this time come from?

Step Three: Analyze The Data

Once the list of current manual activities have been determined, the next step is to analyze and evaluate the impact of these tasks of nursing, then prioritize and rank order them according to the needs for computerization. Areas of difficulty or concern should be addressed according to their impact on the delivery of patient care and the time spent trying to solve problems.

It is essential to the success of determining the nursing needs for computerization that a true team effort be applied since it will be helpful to have a concensus and committment to the project.

A matrix should be developed to list nursing departments' needs, (as outlined in the example Diagram II). The admission of a patient is listed as the number one priority because the patients name must be entered into the computer system before orders can be entered.

Diagram II

Matrix for Nursing Needs for Computerization

Priority	Function	Problems	Feature/Benefit
1.	Admission of a patient	a) Incorrect spelling of patient's name occurs 2 times a week on 9 nursing units/	a) eliminate use of patients addressograph plate
		b) lag time from 30 to 40 minutes occurs at least 3 times a week on 6 nursing units) when addressograph plate does not arrive with the newly admitted patient	b) generate patient identification labels to use to identify patient's documents produced by system
			c) Automatically generate patient identification data on system procedure chart documents
		c) Multiple phone calls are required to and from admitting department in effort to locate a bed for a patient.	d) Produce patient admitting document on Nurse Unit
		d) Census lists are not always current and require much time to compile - approx. 20 min. each midnight for each of 10 nursing units, seven days a week.	f) Produce electronic bed board in order to locate "beds ready" via system.

Step Four: Differentiate and Identify Level Three System Vendors

1. Demonstrate that the system works and that it is reliable. Site visits to vendor installed hospitals are highly useful for this purpose. Select a hospital which is near to your own hospital's size and type of operation and, preferably, one that is fully installed.

*   How many sucessful installations does the vendor have?

*   How long has the vendor been in operation?

*   Have they experienced unsucessful attempts to install their level three system?

*   What is their reliability record; how many hours (%) does the computer run?

*   What type of back-up system and recovery methods are available to ensure that no data is lost?

*   Verify that the system is a real live system, not a demonstration package.

2)   Demonstrate that the system consistently provides satisfactory rapid
      response to users.

*   What is the computer's cycle time? The primary function of the computer is
      the execution of instructions.   This is accomplished by reading an
      instruction from memory, interpreting its meaning, and performing the
      simple action it specifies.   This sequence of events is called the
      "execution cycle" and is repeated for each instruction executed.

*   What is the communications line speed? Often, a computer is located away
      from the devices that need access to it.   In such cases, modems or data
      sets can be used at both ends of a telephone line to connect the computer
      to a device and even to another computer.   In this fashion, a special
      telephone data link can be established with a remote data terminal and
      display terminals.   Thus, a remote hemodialysis nursing unit can have it's
      own terminal and printer far from the computer itself and not experience
      any degradation of response time.

*   What is the data rate to the terminals and speed of the printer?   The
      computer's ability to store and retrieve information would be meaningless
      unless the users could enter, alter, read and comprehend the data
      generated.   The terminals and printers are the devices used for these
      purposes.   The speed at which the user can turn a page of data in the
      system, retrieve a patient's record, print a document and generate a
      requisition in a service department, following the entry of an order, is
      of utmost importance for the user. For example, it is important to verify
      just when the nursing users will want to have their patient care documents
      printed in real-time at **their** patient's nursing stations.

*   There are many tests that can be given the vendor of the hospital who uses
      the vendor's system.   For example time the tasks for writing and entering
      a group of ten admission orders for a patient using the quickest method
      available in the system, then chart all 9:00 am.   medications for a
      nursing unit (for example 40 medications) and indicate 3 medications as
      "not given" as well as the why the reason why they were not.   Verify how
      this information gets into the patient's chart and that this will be the
      only charting activity required by nursing. Demonstrate that you are able
      to retrieve last dose times, actual amounts given and sites of infection,
      as well as receive reminder lists for "unreported medications".

*   Demonstrate that the system is "User Friendly".   Most level three systems
      employ the use of lightpens and permit the entry of free text through the
      terminal keyboard whenever required.   Others utilize a touch screen or
      selection buttons situated on the terminal. Verify just how easy it is to
      get around in these systems, change orders, discontinue and retreive
      patient orders and information without having to "sign off" the system and
      start over again between each function.

3)   Verify that the system does not have information accessible only by the
      location of the terminal.

*   This arrangement closely parallels the traditional method of keeping the
      data where it is used.   The most apparent disadvantage to this technique
      is its rigidity.   Personnel who need data on a patient, particularly float
      nurses and physicians, are not always at the location where the data may
      be accessed.   Problems may arise while patients are in the operating room
      or when they change rooms.   This also creates problems for the timely
      delivery of patients' diet trays to the patients' correct location.

4)   Demonstrate and describe the system's capability to grow and change to
        meet your hospital's future needs.

*   Growth capability -- number of terminals that can be handled.

*   Data Storage. For example, determine how long storage of the patients'
        data will be available in the system and if it is on-line real-time.
        Also, will the system allow for storage of patient demographic data and
        certain clinical types of information such as blood type. This type of
        feature is especially useful when patients are readmitted to hospital
        since access to this stored data can be very rapid.

        The key to any on-line information system is the ability to store large
        amounts of data and retrieve any item of data rapidly enough to satisfy
        the waiting user.

        Retrieval of data should be variable by the category of information which
        is convenient to the users' inquiries -- there should be choices of
        chronological data or reverse chronological sequences.

5)   Demonstrate that the vendor offers a training program designed to meet
        your department's needs.

*   Use the system's on-line computerized training class. Insist on operating
        the system personally.

*   Review the training documents for each department and supplemental
        reference materials.

*   Review the variety of courses offered and their frequency.

*   Review the vendor's training philosophies and rates of success.

*   Check the availability of the on-line training data bases for user access.
        Can on-line training be offered to all shifts as well as practice time?

6)   Demonstrate and describe the system methodology to facilitate data entry
        and retrieval, while at the same time, preventing unauthorised access to
        data.

        A good system should ensure that only those personnel who have bona fide
        "need to know" can access a particular type of data. For example, in the
        U.S.A., business office personnel have no need to look at history and
        physical data on a patient and nursing personnel have no need to look at
        history and physical data on a patient, and nursing personnel have no need
        to know the status of a patient's insurance coverage or account balance.
        In the manual system, the segregation of information comes about because
        data is retained in the department where it is used.

   a)   Sign-on access controls:

        *   Individual codes - automatically generates users' name and title;
        *   System locks out unauthorised codes;
        *   Any authorized user is able to perform functions from any terminal.

   b)   Data Entry

        *   Use of fast, convenient, accurate and easy to learn entry methods,
             suitable for optional use of professionals (lightpen or other self-
             instructional technique; no codes to memorise or look up for

laboratory tests, medications, radiology procedures, etc.; use of patient names as well as case and bed number for positive identification).

* Control by type of user (physician, nurse, admission, clerk, etc.)
* Control by specific individual (e.g. Ms. A. White, R.N., Nurse Administrator.)
* "Agent for" entries -- showing both parties (verbal order, Dr. Jackson per Ms. A. White R.N., Nurse Administrator.)
* Permanent recording of who entered each item of information and when.
* Adequate confirmation of each item of information entered (check mark, confirmation listing or other techniques.)
* Opportunity to review and confirm an entire set of information (e.g. a group of medical orders) before releasing any of the information processing.

c) Data retention and retrieval

* Retention of all data even if subsequently revised or cancelled.
* Permanent retention of all data with capability to reconstruct documents for legal or other unusual requirements, and with detailed codes which facilitate precise interpretation of data such as what medication a patient received each day (drug name, form, strength, route and times of administration.)
* On-line retrieval of administrative and medical patient data from pre-admission through post-discharge.

7. Demonstrate the flexibility of tailoring the system to the hospital's unique environment.

a) Video Display formats.

* Is format flexible so that each page can be optimally designed? (or are there limits such as 20 choices per page, choices must be in columns or rows, instructions must be limited, etc.)
* Can extra words be automatically added to a video selection without requiring space on the screen? For example, if a laboratory test requires a particular prep can that prep be automatically added when the test is selected?
* Can display contents and format be readily modified? On-Line? Without a programming change? With a check-out capability that allows for an operational version and a test version of the display to simultaneously exist? (Thus permitting checkout to occur without risk to the operational system.) Does the vendor have to be on site or responsible to make these changes or can a nurse add them to the system?
* Can nurses design and use their own unique displays? Can these be revised on-line?
* Is a generalised storage and retrieval capability available? Does this allow any type of data to be stored, indexed and retrieved?
* How many different screen formats can the hospital have? (500, 1,000, 5,000 or ?)
* Is the video display easily readable (clear, large, bright)?

b) Printed documents

* Are documents printed under table control which allows the hospital to choose when, where, and how many copies each document should print? Can this be readily revised on-line, for example, Medication Administration reminder lists, patient care plans and so forth?

* Is the design of documents tailored to meet the need to either scan or thoroughly read them. This implies techniques such as two colour printing, large and small character printing, scan titles, easy-to-scan formats, trend analysis formats, etc.
* Are documents dated, time-stamped and sequentially numbered by the computer?
* Can the nurses choose their own format for documents such as the nursing care plan or is this dictated by the system?
* Are printed documents prepared by programs which function under table control so that formats are flexible, or are printed documents "hard coded".
* Are all stored data elements precisely coded so that extractions can be made to prepare reports covering a specific range of items for a specific time period?
* Can the hospital choose the frequency that each document will be printed? Do they have the option to permit selected users to request a document on demand?

8. Demonstrate that the system effectively handles complex situations, not just simple situations:

* Change a cumulative laboratory results summary for a patient who has been hospitalised for a month and has hundreds of laboratory results, including the same test repeated many times.

* Enter a complex IV order with multiple additives and several bottles. Time this task. Change the flow rate.

* Chart a medication that was given off schedule.

* Order a medication to be given Q4H, PRN, 50-100 mg. Then chart a 75 mg. dose given.

* Have a nurse enter a telephoned order for a drug which is not listed in the hospital's formulary.

* Look up the display(s) which show standard post-partum orders (prepared by the OB department). Then write the standard order set but delete 2 orders and add 2 additional orders. Time this task.

* Can the Radiology department (and other ancillary departments) store "standard normal reports" for various procedures and use them when appropriate, thus avoiding dictation and typing? Can various house physicians use their own unique versions of these normal statements? Can a normal statement be readily supplemented by additional comments?

* Which ancillary departments can enter data into the system; EKG? EEG? Nuclear Medicine? Pulmonary? others?

* Can the pharmacy retrieve the actual doses of medication received by a patient and the times? today? for any day since admission?

* Can a physician immediately add a patient to his list to appear on all future retrievals of the patient list?

* Can a physician determine which other physician wrote each specific order for the patient?

9.   Demonstrate that responsible nurses are able to develop and enter a
      specific nursing care plan for each of their patients using the system.

      Level three systems should offer real-time on-line nurse care planning
      features such as standard protocols, which can be the hospital's own.
      This system should be working and available, not just a conceptual
      framework.   Such a system offers the nursing department retrospective
      trend data as well as concurrent information for audit purposes.   Real-
      time audits can be conducted while the patient is in the hospitals; for
      example, a Quality Assurance nurse can verify whether or not a discharge
      plan has been initiated by simply going to a terminal and reviewing the
      criteria on-line from anywhere in the hospital.

What are the Disadvantages?

I have discussed level three computer systems, their uses and advantages to the
nursing practice and laid out a framework for nurses to evaluate and determine
their needs for selection of a system.   But what are the disadvantages?   After
all, on the way to automation there are pitfalls of which nurses must be aware.

First, you don't want to develop an unwarranted faith in the computer's
performance.   Nurses who use them must remember that computers are merely
machines whose capabilities are limited by the imagination of the creators of
their programs.   Therefore, in order to get the best out of computers to assist
nursing, it is important to learn the general functions and limitations of the
computer.

It is not necessary to become a computer programmer or systems engineer, but it
is important to be able to **communicate the needs of nursing** to the people who
write the programs, design the systems and build the machines.

The second pitfall is that each computer system involves a variable degree of
rigidity or capability to adapt to changing conditions.   It is necessary to be
cautious in selecting and planning for the implementation of any computerised
function.   Future needs must be anticipated and provision for flexibility for
growth and adaption to changing needs, must be made.

A further problem is the fear that automation of health care methods will
replace nurses -- that the computer will gradually assume more and more of the
functions carried out by nurses.   Perhaps this is best answered by another
quotation from Kathryn Hannah (L22):-

"If properly developed, automation will allow the nurse to have more time for
direct patient care as the computer assumes more routine clerical functions.
But the implication is that nursing will need to reassess its status and reward
system.   Presently, she maintains, a nurse gains status and financial award by
moving away from the bedside and into supervisory and managerial tasks.   If
these functions are taken over by the computer, then nursing must reappraise its
value system and reward quality of care at the bedside with prestige and money."

There are also disadvantages when nursing managers are not committed to the
project of system selection and implementation.   Very often, in these cases,
they will not know how to use the data made available to them in the area of
management tools.

Summary

In conclusion, research has demonstrated clearly that automation provides
numerous advantages for nursing practice and many improvements in the practice
of nursing.   The use of computers frees the nurses from tedious clerical chores

and provides more time for the nursing process; that is, for the assessment, planning, implementing and evaluation of patient care.

Their use in nursing places responsibility for nursing judgements with the professional nurse. This assists in defining nursing practice and helps the profession in its search for a clearly delineated identity.

If nurses anticipate the introduction of computerization, familiarize themselves with it and prepare actively to participate in the introduction of computers into the nursing environment, then they will be providing the necessary leadership and direction to ensure that computer technology in the health care profession is used to the patients' advantage - to improve the quality of the nursing practice. Otherwise, nurses could conceivably find themselves in a quandry, with computers performing their managerial tasks and non-professionals performing their medically delegated and patient care tasks.

The choice is there and the time to make the choice is now. The decision must be whether to act traditionally and have change thrust upon the profession from the outside or to anticipate this revolution in nursing practice, familiarise nurses with it, and prepare them to take an active part in the introduction of computers into the nursing community.

The necessary leadership and direction must be provided so that computer technology is used to assist nurses in improving the quality of nursing practice and thus the quality of patient care.

Many nurses can testify from experience that their lack of understanding and false expectations regarding specific computer applications has resulted in months or years of wasted time, money and effort (B34).

This paper provides a reference document to aid the nursing profession in the selection of a level three system for their hospitals to avoid such negative experiences that Zeilstorff describes(K1). While I am confident there will be additional criteria that nurses will discover and develop to assist them in the system selection process, it is of the utmost importance they are ensured of high level involvement before, during and following the introduction of the system.

Acknowledgements

I wish to acknowledge the efforts and suggestions of Mary Kiley, R.N. of Technicon Data Systems, Chicago, Illinois; Caroline Dare, R.N., Director of Nurses, University of California Davis Medical Centre, Sacramento, California, and my sister-in-law, Susan Berg of Ottawa, Ontario, Canada. Special thanks goes to Ralph Boyce Stangrams and Robert Williams of Technicon Data Systems for their important contributions.

References

1.   Computerworld Magazine, February 16, 1976.
2.   Cook, M. Hushower, G. and Mayers, M., Computerised Nursing and TMIS Advances in Automated Analysis Vol. 1, (1976)
3.   Harris, Barbara L.,   Who Needs Written Care Plans Anyway?   American Journal of Nursing 70: 2136-2138 October, 1970
4.   Jacobs, S.   Should Evaluations of HIMS's Continue? Health Care Systems Newsletter Vol. 20, No 4. August. (1981)
5.   Porterfield, J. D., - Accreditation Problems, Hospitals, February, (1973) 28

The Impact Of Computers on Nursing
M. Scholes, Y. Bryant and B. Barber (eds.)
Elsevier Science Publishers B.V. (North-Holland)
© IFIP-IMIA, 1983

3.6.

AN OVERVIEW OF THE DEVELOPMENT OF NATIONAL HEALTH SERVICE COMPUTING

Doreen T. Redmond

Introduction

In the mid 1960's, computing in the National Health Service was in its infancy. A few regions had computers to provide payroll and accountancy services; one or two were using them for statistical tasks, and applications in pathology were being pioneered by others. By 1967 there was a growing feeling in the NHS that more could and should be done to take advantage of this "new" technology. The intention was for an initial five year research period, followed by a five year development phase. The programme consisted of projects wholly financed from central funds, with three main objectives:-

- (i)   To ensure better patient care.
- (ii) To increase clinical and administrative efficiency.
- (iii) To improve management and research facilities.

These projects were by no means confined to the hospital environment. They also embraced application areas such as primary care, child health, administration systems, scientific and clinical research. This programme ran into the 1970's. Yet as it did so, it became necessary to consider the formulation of a rational, nationally acceptable, policy for the future. In 1970 a second wide-ranging review was commissioned from a firm of management consultants (McKinsey & Company), together with the Department of Health and Social Security and National Health Service members. In 1972 their report was published, "Using Computers to Improve Health Services"(3). The recommendations included the following:-

- (i)   The need for annual reviews.
- (ii) The establishment of a five year rolling plan.
- (iii) Priority rating of applications.
- (iv) Moving new applications through experimentation, development and implementation.

Thus was laid the cornerstone for the strategy that was to be followed throughout the last decade; albeit with a number of modifications from time to time.

The other policy development that had a profound effect on the way in which computing progressed was the "Standardisation Programme". In 1971 a policy was formulated that health regions should standardise their mainframe computers on the ICL 1900 series. This was intended to pave the way for the development of standard computer systems and procedures aimed at providing improved facilities for the transfer of information and economies in the use of those systems.

There was a shift of policy from about 1976 in the relationship between DHSS and the NHS generally. As a result, a report in 1977, "A Review of Computing"(4) proposed that there should be a reduction in the amount of central control over NHS computing. This in turn led to a complete re-evaluation of the way in which computing policy had been administered; and further, of how successful it had been.   As a result, a new committee structure was formed to deal with policy, research and development, technical matters and standardisation.   This allowed for a greater degree of NHS participation but was still, in essence, a centrally inspired and administered organisation.

By the end of the 1970's we had seen rapid changes in computing technology and in the range and scale of computing in the NHS. We had also seen a massive re-organisation of the NHS itself, in 1974. All these factors had a role to play in shaping the way in which computing needs would be determined and met in the 1980's.   Indeed, by 1980 it was recognised that the time was coming when yet another full scale re-appraisal of the computing strategy would be required. Growing expectations and demand from all disciplines within the NHS for more and better computer support became evident. Furthermore, at last, there appeared a relatively large number of manufacturers and software houses who had developed, or were developing, application packages that could be used by health authorities.   This phenomenon gained even more ground with the advent of mini and micro processors.   Suddenly, the existing plans were in danger of being overtaken by events and so, it was decided to dismantle the committee structure, again, and engage in a major re-thinking.

Computer Policy Committee

Towards the end of 1981, the present National Health Service Computer Policy Committee was established.   It is charged with responsibility for those aspects of computing which are best considered on a supra-regional or national basis. It is chaired by a Regional Health Authority Chairman and has its own NHS secretariat.   Apart from the chairman and vice-chairman, membership is confined to one representative from each of the main regional uni-disciplinary group, plus one DHSS representative.   Its terms of reference are:-

"To make recommendations on policy on computing in the NHS, including the promotion of the best use of standard and transferable systems in the NHS and to obtain the commitment of health authorities to specific policies and developments to achieve that end".   Within this broad remit, specific major items of concern are likely to include the following:-

(i)   the future policy of financing supra-regional or national computing activities from NHS rather than central funds.
(ii)   the identification and implementation of those systems which an analysis of regional computer plans would indicate need to be "sponsored" by the committee (by agreement with the NHS).
(iii) the management and continuous evaluation of the existing programme of applications intended for national use, i.e. the standard systems.
(iv)   purchasing policy (subject to national requirements).
(v)   technical matters relating to current applications and the implications of technicological evolution.

The committee is expected to have access to regional computing plans and to report annually.

Körner Working Group

Working concurrently with this new strategy, and indeed very much related in its sphere of operations is the Steering Group on Health Services Information. This group was set up early in 1980, under the chairmanship of Mrs Edith Körner, to look at the masses of data that flow between all levels of the health service, including the central element, i.e. DHSS.

The group's terms of reference are as follows:

(i)   To agree, implement and keep under review principles and procedures to guide the future development of health services information systems.
(ii) To identify and resolve health services information issues requiring a co-ordinated approach.
(iii) To review existing health services information systems.
(iv) To consider proposals for changes to, or developments in, health services information systems arising elsewhere and, if acceptable, to assess priorities for their development and implementation.

At the end of its task, it will produce a report which will provide a comprehensive proposal for basic data systems within the new District Health Authorities. These systems will be primarily for the user - the clinician who needs to husband the resources available to him the better to care for his patient; the manager (of whatever discipline, but clearly nurse managers are very much users of resources and planners of services) who must control and plan for the health facilities and staff entrusted to him. The systems will therefore relate in particular to districts; but will also provide the data routinely required for management at regions or DHSS. These proposals will be consciously intended to represent an acceptable minimum data set for essential purposes within districts, and at other levels, so that the vital needs of management will have been covered. Yet at the same time, each user will be in a position to have whatever additional data that may be required locally. The group plans to review its proposals in the light of the experience gained in various pilot trials and will then put forward recommendations for a general release in early 1983.

Thus, the current and future computing needs of the NHS cannot be looked at in isolation; any more than the work of the Information Steering Group can be carried on without reference to the Computer Policy Committee. The philosophy of "No man is an island unto himself" is surely most appropriate?

Major Achievements of the Experimental Computer Programme

The programme:-

(i)   Demonstrated that computers could be used effectively in hospitals.
(ii) Spread computing into new application areas in the NHS much more rapidly than would otherwise have been the case.
(iii) Tried out a wide range of computing methods and techniques.
(iv) Demonstrated that staff of all disciplines could use computers as part of their day to day work.
(v)   Helped to create a wide range of expertise in health care computing, thus providing a base for the future.

Over the last twenty years, the problems have changed from, if and how to use computers, to how to implement systems more generally and in the most economic and effective way. Technology was, and is, developing rapidly. Computers have become more powerful yet cheaper; communications have become easier and software has become more "user friendly". It is a fact of life perhaps that any computing strategy or research and development programme must, by the very substance of its subject matter be evolutionary.

Nursing Systems

Computerised Nursing Systems create the need for a systematic approach to processing nursing and patient care information/data which can be used by nurses to enable them to make decisions on the best use of resources; short and long term.

Systems which serve the needs of nurses are of two main types; those which provide nurse managers with information to assist with the utilization and deployment of nursing manpower (Nurse-Patient Dependency, Nursing Staff Records, Training Programmes, Nurse Allocation and Sickness and Absence statistics): and those which have a direct impact on clinical nursing staff by providing them with information which is accurate, legible, complete, concise and available at the correct time and place for planning and maintaining the continuity of nursing care, (Ward Nursing Records - Nursing Orders, Nursing Reports and Nursing Care Plans).

It must be remembered, however, that many other health care systems have an equally important impact on nursing management and patient care; for example, Drug Prescribing and Administration, Drug Information, Laboratory Requesting and Reporting, Patient Monitoring, In-Patient and Out-Patient Administrative systems and Manpower and Personnel systems.

General Synopsis of Nursing Applications

Computers in the National Health Service are no longer seen as objects of fear and mistrust to be ignored in the hope that they will disappear. They are recognised as tools which must be examined with care, and their performance evaluated in order to judge their value in management of the complex process of providing the most efficient and economic health care. What the new generation of computers will and will not do in the next decade is speculative, but of one aspect we can be assured; they are here to stay. It is the nursing profession's responsibility to ensure that we are involved in the planning, and control their implementation, to monitor and develop their impact of patient care and the nursing service.

Computer systems, unlike any other single item used in support of health care, affect the total health organisational process. Invariably, demand is user inspired and a major responsibility of nurse managers is to perceive what they want in terms of information systems and machines, whilst at the same time remembering that information about about health is not just the concern of the professional providing care - it is very much the concern of people and particularly of patients.

Senior nurse managers by reason of their involvement in providing a 24 hour 7 day a week service in hospitals and in the community collectively, have a unique understanding and knowledge about the information needs of the total health care environment. Computer systems can provide methods of meeting the nursing needs in ways hitherto unexplored in depth in the UK. Some progress has been made in a number of hospitals but, so far the emphasis has been to provide information covering a limited number of application areas in order to assist doctors, administrators, technicians and medical records staff in their respective specialist needs. The information needs which relate specifically to the nursing discipline have been somewhat neglected, and although extensive work has already been undertaken at a number of hospitals sites throughout the UK over the past decade both within the R & D programme and independently, we still do not have a coherent and co-ordinated NHS policy on nursing systems, nor do we have any readily available packaged systems for nurse managers.

A number of regions have set up nursing Computer Information Working Groups with representation covering all levels and grades of nursing personnel. The aims and objectives of these groups obviously differ but when combined they form a sound basis on which to work towards achieving a National Nursing Policy for computing. This policy should surely ensure that:-

(i)   Nursing applications whether of a clinical or managerial nature which
        could benefit from computer aid are examined and identified.
(ii)   The relative priorities for computer applications are assessed and agreed
        against appropriate criteria such as validity, acceptability, benefits,
        cost and time.
(iii)   Regional Management and Computer Services Officers are knowledgeable about
        nurses' needs and are therefore in a position to help those nurses achieve
        their goals.
(iv)   Where appropriate, nursing expertise should be made available to
        committees or working groups considering policy, design and implementation
        of other health care computer systems, in order to identify and harmonise
        the implications for the nursing service. Every system seems to impinge
        on nursing.
(v)   Nurse education and training in the use of computers and the impact of
        modern technology is adequately planned.

Nurse managers generally are already in the process of examining existing
nursing structures, manpower, patient care programmes and numerous other aspects
of total health care systems; they are endeavouring to carry forward the
pioneering work of the past decade to ensure that it is not dissipated in the
present climate of financial stringency; and they are building on the lessons
learned to secure an informed professional nursing input and participation in
NHS computing, which our 21st century colleagues will undoubtedly expect to have
been done.

Examples of Existing and Proposed Nursing Systems

(a)   Nurse Managers:-

        Financial Accounting, Manpower, and Personnel Records
        Nurse Allocation,Deployment,Absence,Training and Sickness
        Schools of Nursing links with the U.K. Central Council for Nurses and
        Midwives and the four National Boards.

(b)   Clinical Nurses:-

        Nursing Process, Statistical Analysis, Nursing Records and Patient
        Monitoring
        Housekeeping in wards and departments linked to other major
        Hospital administration systems, and Regional bureaux.

(c)   Community Nursing Services:-

        Surveillance and Prevention, Health Visitors, District Nurses
        School Nurse and Psychiatric (CPNs) Records

All these systems are of immense import to nurses, and because they deal with
complex subjects and provide essential statistics for patient care and nurse
management, it is doubtful whether the information required for these purposes
could be provided or utilized without some computer aid. The major benefit of
the systems will enable nurse managers to establish a base from which to manage
work, to forecast trends and identify problem areas to organise recruitment and
training and make the best use of all the resources which are available to
provide improved patient care and planning.

In summary, computer systems should be designed to the users' specification and
needs and the objectives are manyfold; they can relieve nurses of much clerical
work in both the clinical and managerial areas. The quality, clarity,
availability and timeliness of the information provided will enable nursing
staff to plan more accurately for the increasing demands on manpower utilization
and the changing patterns of patient management.

Achievements And Lessons Learned

We now have a very active nursing force involved in most aspects of computer policy, management, design and implementation. Nurses in the UK have worked diligently to achieve systems which enable them to provide better patient care and nurse management. Nevertheless, computing in nursing has not matched or expanded in line with computing in other areas in the NHS. In hospitals, experiments have proved that nurse managers and clinical nurses have had considerable success in creating and in using computer systems for resource management and direct patient care. Nurses continue to explore areas of potential use but general geographical expansion has been slow. Community Nursing Services (with some exceptions) so far have had little support in finding areas in which computers can be of benefit. This area with its vital need for information resources needs to be examined.

In general, limiting factors have been:

(a)   Lack of awareness by nurses of the feasibilities, and by computer staff of the need, in the early part of the last decade when the R & D Computer Programme was launched,

(b)   Disruption following the implementation of the Salmon(1) and Mayston(2) reports as well as the 1974 and 1982 NHS re-organisations,

(c)   Latterly, a dearth of computer expertise and/or manpower within Regions to meet nursing demands. Some imaginative approaches have been stifled due to lack of funds or the unrecognised need to invest in areas which would in the long term achieve savings.

It has been an up-hill struggle for nurses in the NHS; and whilst they are rightly proud of their achievements to-date they recognise that even though developments are now moving quickly, much more has to be done if they are to achieve a more efficient and effective nursing service.

At Appendix 1 is a paper containing the 'collated views' from papers submitted by individual members of the **Computer Project Nurses' Group** to the Computer Research and Development Committee in 1978. The lessons learned therein are still relevant in 1982. Success or failure of computer based nursing and patient care systems depends to a large extent on the degree of nursing management, participation and involvement in the planning, co-ordination and maintenance of such systems.

Communication

Effective and precise communications between health care professionals, patients and people in general, help to minimise the possibility of error in the prescribing and provision of care. All those involved in computer systems design, and implementation, need to be aware of the vital importance of good communication and understanding. The computer can effectively act as a catalyst for change. It is important to remember that as the health care programme expands and clinical practices change, computer technology is evolving at a revolutionary pace. Few managers really appreciate the pace of change. We must ensure that the present organisation, management and materials are thoroughly examined and, where necessary, changed prior to or during the course of developing systems. It is worth noting the similarities that exist between the design and management of computer systems and the design and management of a capital building programme. For such reasons the management of Capital Building Programmes should include consideration of the use and accommodation of computers during the feasibility study. Nurse Planners and Commissioners of health buildings must have expert guidance and help to enable them to advise and pursue realistic goals for the efficient use of resources in the total health care plan.

Conclusions

Future success will depend on the promotion of a greater awareness and understanding of the advantages and the disadvantages of using computer technology in health care. Nurses should aim to co-ordinate this philosophy amongst themselves and co-operate with other disciplines, especially computer scientists, in order to achieve an effective and acceptable total care plan. Evaluation and training programmes for nurses should acknowledge and respond to developments in computer technology so as to enable them to maximise their skills with understanding and prudence.

Senior nurse managers in the NHS hold responsibility for very large budgets and they are accountable with others to ensure that due regard is given to all **financial** aspects of health care developments. The NHS already has a considerable amount of computer power and there is much evidence of future growth, which will inevitably require a greater degree of expert co-ordination and monitoring. Any technology development must be scientifically sound, adaptable and financially viable. It must be reliable and moreover, acceptable to those who are going to use it.

Computer technology is rapidly becoming more acceptable to health care professionals and nurses will need to assume a major role in all aspects of its planning, development, implementation and evaluation. It is difficult to envisage any area of health care where it would not be beneficial to have some computer aid in order to enhance patient care and to promote the economy and efficiency of the service. The use of computers will compel nurse managers and others who provide health care to seek help on aspects of organisational planning which they had not hitherto envisaged. The complexities that flow from these matters require computer specialist expertise. Only by working together will the way forward be found.

Acknowledgements

I wish to acknowledge the support I have received from colleagues in Management Support and Computers and Nursing Division, of DHSS who have helped in producing this paper.

REFERENCES

1. The Mayston Report - "DHSS Working Party on the Management Structure in the Local Authority Nursing Services Report" DHSS 1969.
2. The Salmon Report - "Ministry of Health Committee on Senior Nursing Staff Structure Report " HMSO 1966.
3. "Using Computers to Improve Health Services - A Review for the NHS" DHSS 1971.
4. "A Review of NHS Computing Needs" DHSS - HC77(11) 1977.
5. "Management and Provision of Computing Services" DHSS - HC82(9) 1982.

APPENDIX 1

THE COMPUTER PROJECT NURSES' GROUP

In 1974 the majority of hospital computer projects had a senior nursing officer or nurse analyst working as members of multi-disciplinary project teams. They provided the nursing advice, guidance and a very specialised and practical input at operations level. It was decided that it would be beneficial if there was some forum whereby these project nurses could meet together to acquire and exchange information, ideas and experience on all aspects of nursing management and patient care. The Computer Project Nurses' Group was formed and membership also included nursing officers from the Department of Health and Social Security. The Group have met regularly since 1974.

SUBMISSION TO THE RESEARCH & DEVELOPMENT COMMITTEE FROM THE COMPUTER PROJECTS NURSES' GROUP THE EXPERIMENTAL COMPUTER PROGRAMME LESSONS LEARNED - MARCH 1978

The lessons learned by nurses, from the experimental computer programme may be described under the following headings:-

1. NURSING AND COMPUTERS

1. A fundamental problem underlying many of the lessons learned by nurses, stems from a lack of understanding of the work which forms a part of the nursing function, over and above the clinical role.
2. For example, in a ward, it is the nursing staff who take the action required to ensure that treatment and investigatory procedures prescribed by medical staff are carried out. In so doing nurses become the focal point of complex communication network; they receive co-ordinate and transmit messages from a number of different and differing disciplines, about the clinical and administrative aspects of patient care.
3. If computer-based hospital systems are to be properly integrated into the routine work of the organisation, this communication function of nurses must be clearly understood from the outset. Nurses should not be expected to make a case for their involvement in the work of developing computer systems.
4. In the future, much time and effort will be saved if nurses participate in the development of health care computing, when it is known that a system interfaces with nursing activity.
5. With a few exceptions in the scientific and clinical field, the majority of hospital, primary health care, and management information systems have a direct impact on nurses. They are involved in the collection of data to update computer systems and use information produced by computer systems in their day-to-day work.
6. Hence a most important lesson learned is that of identifying the nursing role from the outset in respect of any new computer application in health care.

2. PROJECT ORGANISATION AND MANAGEMENT

1. Hospitals function 7 days per week and 24 hours per day, therefore computer units should effectively operate to produce maximum efficiency.
2. Changing objectives once a project has started can have disastrous consequences. Modifying or only partly meeting original objectives can be costly both in cash terms and staff morale.
3. In commissioning a new hospital, computer systems should be considered, linked to manual hospital and community systems, and not superimposed later.

4. Timescales should be known, agreed, and monitored. There should be clearly defined procedures for transfer of financial responsibility to the appropriate departmental head.

5. Buying computers on the basis of unproven software has led to considerable delays.

6. Key members of staff have been lost due to increasingly higher salaries outside the National Health Service. Loss also occurs when the future of a project in uncertain.

7. Operational research Organisation & Management techniques and feasibility studies are invaluable in determining whether a more refined manual system or a computer system is warranted to satisfy the needs of a specific department.

8. The computer should not be used as a disciplinary tool, to impose rules in computer systems that have not been agreed or found practical in manual systems.

9. Users, having agreed a systems specification, should not be allowed to change it unless absolutely necessary. An essential criterion for acceptability must be that all changes and developments should be as a direct result of user interface. Continuous information on progress and timescales should be communicated to users.

10. Concentrate staff of systems to be implemented first - do not have staff working on too many applications at same time. This can delay time scales which in turn demoralises computer staff causing them to leave, and also reduces user interest, involvement and support.

11. The effort needed to maintain and modify "working" systems once implemented should not be underestimated.

12. Reliability of equipment is essential, particularly in the ward situation. Visual Display Unit response times should be two seconds or less, to ensure continued user acceptance. Printers should be quiet and fast.

13. Practically all the computer systems introduced into a hosptial will affect the nursing staff. It is therefore essential to have nurse representation from the start of the project.

3. ROLE OF NURSE AND COMPUTER EDUCATION

1. Regional, Area and District Nursing Officers must take an active interest in the development of computer nursing systems.

2. A nurse who is seconded to, or employed by, a computer department must retain close liaison with all levels of nursing personnel. Such a project nurse must have continuity of senior nursing administration and nurse education support. This is vital to successful implemetation and computer education. It can be achieved by ensuring that a senior nurse is a member of multidisciplinary group steering a project, and by a nursing advisory committee which comprises nurse managers, tutors, community, ward and departmental nurses.

3. The experience gained by a project nurse who may also become a system analyst and/or programmer should be considered as an important contribution to her career. Project nurses develop skills especially suited to problem definition and problem solving. They have an in-depth knowledge of hospital communications and a detailed understanding of the complex nature of the information flows essential for the managements and scheduling of patient care. They have also become skilled at "selling "and implementing systems (whether computer or manual).

4. If a comprehensive computer system is introduced into a hospital, an extensive educational programme and the necessary finance for this is also needed. Many of the staff will be nurses, and because of the high turnover and great variety of training programmes, this will be an on going problem. The aim should be for computing to be part of the normal educational and training programmes and be taught by tutorial staff or administrative heads of departments.

5. Tape/slide sets prepared by a computer department have been found to be helpful in assisting the tutor or head of department. The use of VDUs in the Schools of Nursing is recommended.

6. Training of nurses in using Visual Display Units should be given shortly before implementation. In practice, it has been found that nurses have little or no difficulties in using this equipment, and associated tree-branching techniques.

7. Regular visits by computer staff to wards and departments have been found helpful in re-inforcing education or helping new members of staff. Ward clerks may need re-assuring that they are using the system correctly. Often this is the only way that a doctor receives information as he may miss an education day or be too busy to go to the computer department.

8. Computer staff need to be prepared to talk to all hospital staff to avoid problems - including union representatives. Benefits should be advertised.

9. The value of visits to other projects and the sharing of information should not be underestimated. Money should be available for this activity.

4. DESIGNING COMPUTER SYSTEMS

General

1. Begin by designing patient administration systems as a sound and broad basis for other services.

2. Plan the introduction of systems so that different groups of users gain advantage. It is unreasonable to ask any one group of users to keep implementing systems that do not directly benefit them or obviously improve patient care.

3. Implement simple systems - these give users most of their desired benefits earlier; and help to overcome any inbuilt fears about computers. These should save time, or at least take no longer than manual systems.

4. Printing facilities should be available in both wards and departments and should be silent if near patients.

5. Demonstration programmes including a "fictional" group of patients should be built into the system.

6. Emphasis should be placed upon the importance of capturing accurate initial data. This will be constantly reproduced and used, and the acceptability of a system may be judged by it.

7. All ward based systems should conform to standard design, eg function keys. This reduces training time, and aids user acceptance.

5. NURSING SYSTEMS

1. Flexibility of design in nursing systems is necessary to cater for different ward layouts, variations of staffing levels, variations of workload, and changes in requirements of specialties.

2. Although each nurse will have basic computer education, systems and screens should be largely self explanatory. Design should be flexible enough to allow short cuts which avoid displaying some intermediary screens.

3. Computer systems should not formally require nurses to undertake non-nursing duties even if these have sometimes previously been undertaken informally.

4. Nursing record systems can be phased, a nursing order system implemented prior to a nursing report system.

5. Interface between nurse user groups and systems analysts has focused upon nursing activities and problems, producing benefits in nursing systems whether subsequently computerised or not.

6. Computer nursing order systems prompt learner nurses to plan individual patient care. The subsequent computer printed record is more complete than the present manual kardex record.

7. Computer nursing systems provide data, and analyses that are useful for nurse education, nurse management and nursing research.

6. EVALUATION OF COMPUTER SYSTEMS AND BENEFITS NOTED BY THE PROJECT NURSES

1. Improvement of accuracy, completeness, presentation and legibility of information.
2. Reduction of transit times for reports. Also less transcription from telephone calls.
3. Saving of staff, particularly nursing staff time in handling queries and obtaining information.
4. Greater benefits cost wise from implementing in-patient before out-patient systems.
5. Sickness and absence systems are used as management tools.
6. Nurse allocation and other system are already of assistance to both nurse education and nurse managers.
7. Bedstates help emergency staff, nurse managers and others and save ward clerical time.
8. Operating theatre statistics enables better scheduling of theatre staff.
9. Pharmacy information provides an effective and direct method of obtaining drug information.
10. Computer nursing records aid individual patient care plans and help learners to plan care.
11. Nursing procedures are always up-to-date and can be printed on request.
12. Transferring applications between hospitals has produced considerable savings in design effort.
13. Computer aided nurse manpower and deployment systems have great potential but the benefits have yet to be realised.

The Impact of Computers on Nursing
M. Scholes, Y. Bryant and B. Barber (eds.)
Elsevier Science Publishers B.V. (North-Holland)
© IFIP-IMIA, 1983

3.7.

COMPUTER TECHNOLOGY IN HEALTH CARE

Discussion

Analysis of information needs

Systems analysis was noted as a major requirement for meeting the information needs of nurses. It involves the analysis of information use and the relationship between data capture and data processing. This was recognised as a complex procedure as any one individual does not always see how another might use such data. For example, the management uses of nursing data are not always obvious to the ward or community nurse. The need for capturing data accurately and completely at the time it becomes available was emphasised - only then can it be used for multiple purposes. Planning systems are now available from a variety of sources including consultants and vendors which will assist in the determination of information needs and the selection of information systems. It was apparent that nurses examining their systems requirements need to employ direct communication strategies to orient less knowledgeable users. Inevitably nursing education must set out to give all nurses an appreciation of nursing informatics. Costing of both the clerical and computer aspects of a system are essential when selecting systems or before commencing the development of a computer system.

Standardised Flexibility

The need for constructive standardisation of both information systems and data was identified. The benefits of standardisation of both hardware and software appear to be those of cost saving and quality of implementation. However, users want systems that meet their own needs and this encourages their use. Thus standardisation is an overall concept and yet these standard systems have to be flexible enough to be changed in different but important ways to meet nurses' needs. Vendors in particular have emphasised that standardising the overall structure of their systems not only helps in sharing development costs but also aids computer processing, output and maintenance. Different systems have different degrees of flexibility built into them to meet users' needs. Those that are likely to be most helpful to users, have built in techniques for changing the data content and output specification in a flexible way. There were still reservations about standardisation policies and it was felt that more research was needed into nursing requirements and nursing activity.

Terminal Requirements

When determining the number of terminals (VDU's and printers) required, it is important to analyse who will be using the system (will it include doctors, medical students, learner nurses as well as other professional users), the volume of data to be input and retrieved, where the terminals will be located (good access is necessary), the speed of the terminals and the structure of nursing stations. A suggested ratio was one VDU and one printer to 10 beds in general wards with one VDU and one printer to 2 beds in the intensive care unit.

Limitations of Microcomputers

Concern was expressed that many micro-computers are being purchased without the requirements and problems being adequately identified. These computers have no built-in database integrity and difficulties arise when attempting to transfer a system developed on one type of micro computer to another due to lack of compatible standards (such as the size and data format of floppy discs). Nurses need to be able to determine whether and when small systems will meet their information and management needs.

Reinventing Systems

Nurses should not waste time reinventing or redeveloping systems already available. Established systems should form the basis for further enhancements and should, where feasible, be capable of transferring to different sites and computer hardware. The successs and failures of systems need to be shared through national and inter-national organisations and conferences.

CHAPTER 4

CONFIDENTIALITY

This topic is included as a separate item within the book in recognition of the public and professional concern for proper safeguards for individual records of a personal nature. Clearly any work attempting to present an overview of the use of computers in health care would be deficient if it did not recognise social, political and medical implications of accessing such records.

The Impact of Computers on Nursing
M. Scholes, Y. Bryant and B. Barber (eds.)
Elsevier Science Publishers B.V. (North-Holland)
© IFIP-IMIA, 1983

4.1.

IS NURSING CONFIDENTIAL?

Josephine A. Plant

Introduction

The purpose of the paper is to explore the issue of the confidentiality of
nursing records and the duty imposed upon nurses to ensure that any personal
information they receive in the course of their work will be adequately safeguarded having special regard to the legislative situation in the UK. The
general picture is well described by the monograph produced by the IMIA working
group(1). Nursing records concerning patients or in the case of Health Visitors
'clients' will contain information and opinion imparted by the patient or client
in confidence. They may also contain private information obtained from third
parties, spouses, relatives and friends, and from other professionals, this
information may be either factual or judgemental in character. Nurses working
in management posts and in personnel departments will also compile and have
access to employee personal records which contain factual information such as
identity, qualifications, sickness and absence records, salary and incremental
points, but will also contain nurse managers' opinions concerning past
performance, projected career prospects and references submitted at the time of
application for new jobs.

For some time now, there has been concern about the potential threat to the
individual's privacy. With the rapid increase in the use of computers for
storing personal data this concern is growing. People are realising that the
computer storage of data facilitates swift processing and collation, and that it
is now possible to link data collected for one purpose to data collected for
quite a different purpose. For example if postal codes are routinely recorded
in a computerised system of personnel records, it becomes possible to link these
data with the Acorn(2) system, which is available commercially, in order to
study potential employee or existing staff behaviour and thus arrive at a useful
aid to improved recruitment and staff retention policies. The linkage   of
health, employment and socio-economic parameters with the information already
held on computer by credit rating agencies is now technically possible and
represents a major threat to individual privacy.

The Background

As long ago as 1961 a Bill was introduced into the House of Lords with the
objective of protecting a person from any unjustifiable publication relating to
his private affairs, and in the event of such publication to give him the right
of redress through the law courts.(3) During the 1960s further Bills were
introduced in both Houses but did not reach the statute book. In 1972 a private
members Bill was introduced to control both computerised and manual data banks
but suffered the same fate as the Bills of the 1960s(4). However in 1970 in the
course of a debate on Mr. Brian Walden's Bill(5), the then Home Secretary, the
Rt. Hon. James Callaghan, announced that the Government would appoint an
official committee to examine problems of privacy and that it would be chaired
by the Rt. Hon. Kenneth Younger. The terms of reference for this committee
confined its work to the private sector despite requests by the committee that
it be allowed to extend its area of enquiry to Government Departments and public
agencies.

The Younger Committee in considering the collection and handling of personal information and its possible misuse in the private sector said that most of the problems in this area were 'common to all data banks whether computerised or not' (A22) however at that time, they concluded that computers did not present a threat to individual privacy though they recognised that for the future, individual privacy could be put at risk. In the recognition of this potential threat, they directed attention to the establishment of appropriate safeguards, setting out ten principles for the handling of personal information which they recommended for immediate voluntary adoption by all computer users. These ten principles (Table 1) were subsequently incorporated into a Government White Paper entitled 'Computers and Privacy'(A21) which covered both the Report of the Younger Committee and a report arising from a parallel Government review of categories of information held or likely to be held in the computer systems of Government Departments together with information from other parts of the public sector(6).

TABLE 1

THE YOUNGER COMMITTEE'S PRINCIPLES

5012 Para 592-599

1.   Information should be regarded as held for a specific purpose and not be used, without appropriate authorisation for other purposes.

2.   Access to information should be confined to those authorised to have it for the purpose for which it was supplied.

3.   The amount of information collected and held should be the minimum necessary for the achievement of a specified purpose.

4.   In computerised systems handling information for statistical purposes, adequate provision should be made in their design and programmes for separating identities from the rest of the data.

5.   There should be arrangements whereby the subject could be told about the information held concerning him.

6.   The level of security to be achieved by a system should be specified in advance by the user and should include precautions against the deliberate abuse or misuse of information.

7.   A monitoring system should be provided to facilitate the detection of any violation of the security system.

8.   In the design of information systems, periods should be specified beyond which the information should not be retained.

9.   Data held should be accurate, there should be machinery for the correction of inaccuracy.

10. Care should be taken in coding value judgements.

In this White Paper(A21) the Government accepted the Younger Committee's recommendation that machinery was needed 'not only to keep the situation under review, but also to seek to secure that all existing and future computer systems in which personal information is held, in both the private sector and public sector, are operated with appropriate safeguards for the privacy of the subject of that information'.

Such machinery would be set up to avoid the principle dangers, whether arising accidentally or intentionally, of:-

1)   the information stored being inaccurate, incomplete or irrelevant;
2)   unauthorised access to the stored information;
3)   the use of that information for purposes other than those for which it is collected.

In view of the conclusion that the level of protection of data which can be implemented is limited only by the expense of installing and maintaining the security safeguards, and that the expense of providing the highest level of security for all personal data systems would be prohibitive, it is stated that 'the need is only to provide protection proportionate to the degree of sensitivity of the information within the system'(6), but that it is in the public interest now to take out of the hands of those using computers for the storage of personal information to the responsibility for determining the adequacy of the safeguards on privacy. Legislation is therefore proposed with the dual objectives, first to establish a set of objectives and standards based on the ten principles recommended by the Younger Committee governing the use of computers that handle personal information and second to establish a permanent statutory agency to oversee the use of such computers in both the public and private sectors. During the interim period pending enactment of the legislation, a non-statutory body - the Data Protection Committee - was set up with the function of preparing the way for legislation. This Committee under the Chairmanship of Sir Norman Lindop reported in December 1978(A12) and devoted the whole of Chapter 7 to NHS records - the kind of information recorded and the uses to which it is put - and then in a very short chapter, Chapter 24, discussed the question of patient or client access to medical and social work records. It is here that a curiously dual standard approach is outlined. Whereas computerised social work information should be available to the client and thus social work agencies are exhorted to ensure that recorded data are reliable, fair and accurate, and that subjective judgements are clearly labelled as such; medical records would be treated differently. It is recommended that factual data in the medical record such as blood group and medical history should, on request, be made known to the patient. However judgemental and speculative medical opinion need be disclosed only at the doctor's discretion. There is no specific consideration of nursing, midwifery or health visitor records, nor are the records of the professions supplementary to medicine mentioned.

In April 1982 the latest White Paper containing the Government's proposals for legislation on Data Protection was published (A20). Unfortunately this document did not receive very wide publicity and the period allowed for comment on such an important issue was very short-ending on 31st May 1982. The reason for such haste is to be found in the second paragraph of the White Paper and appears to have more to do with the protection of international commercial interest than with the protection of individual privacy. The Council of Europe has prepared a Convention on Data Protection and the Organisation for Economic co-operation and Development has prepared guidelines on privacy protection and transborder data flows. The former was signed by the United Kingdom in January 1981 and the latter endorsed in September 1981.

At the time of publication of the White Paper, no member state of the EEC had ratified the Convention which does not become enforceable until five states have ratified it. The United Kingdom will no doubt ratify the Convention as soon as it meets the precondition of having legislation in force. In the White Paper, a two year time scale is mentioned though the Convention will confer the right of countries with data protection legislation to refuse to allow personal information to be sent to other countries which do not have comparable safeguards.

The White Paper proposals for legislation are based on the report of the Younger Committee, the text of the Convention, the two White papers published in 1975 (A21 and A6) and the report of the Lindop Committee(A12). The publication of the White Paper(A20) occurred after Mrs. Korner's Steering group on Health Services Information had set up its own working group on Confidentiality. As one of many agencies, this group has been given the opportunity to make comments to the Home Office on the Government proposals for legislation which is particularly welcomed as it is felt that in the White Paper there is little sensitivity displayed towards the specialised needs of the Health Service or indeed about the individualised health information held by many other agencies such as that held in employment files, industrial occupational health services, insurance companies etc.

There are many issues in the White Paper which will be of concern to all disciplines working in the National Health Service but as this paper is directed to a nursing audience, comment will be made on the perceived nursing interests.

Data to be Covered by the Legislation

There are difficulties of definition in relation to health service data which are inadequately stated in the Government's proposals. Apart from health information contained therein, recorded personal information is probably adequately covered until it is noted that though the Council of Europe Convention covers data processing carried out in whole or in part by automated means the Government's proposals appear to be limited to automated data processing only. It seems likely whether the subject is personnel records or health records that manual recording will never be totally eliminated. It is therefore to be hoped that the eventual legislation will apply equally to both systems of recording as a health or personnel record should be regarded as indivisible.

The content of the health record is particularly difficult to define as perusal of most medical and nursing records quickly demonstrates that very different kinds of information are recorded, ranging from that which is factual which can be either proved or disproved by independent investigation and testing, such as date of birth, height, weight, blood counts at a certain point of time; and information which consists of opinions and may well concern matters other than those which first brought the individual to the attention of the nurse. The Royal College of Nursing in its booklet of guidelines and discussion points(7) highlighted this issue in stating that in part because of the fiduciary relationship which exists between a nurse and her patient/client, she is in a position to help people with personal problems arising from any area of that person's life. "No nurse would dispute that helping a patient/client to find relief for any problem that may be affecting his wellbeing is a vital part of nursing. The counselling role, with the emphasis on 'listening', in caring for the patient/client, is an essential part of nursing but information gained in this way puts a responsibility on the nurse", especially in modern methods of health care delivery when so many more people from many different agencies may be involved in the health care system. For the purpose of legislation, it might be well to modify the words 'affecting his wellbeing' to indicate a timescale of past, present or future and to define 'wellbeing' as including mental or physical conditions.

Nurses have expressed concern about the lack of confidentiality in the National Health Service in support of which they have cited:

(a)   the uses to which records are put
       -    education of health care professionals
       -    research
       -    litigation
       -    compilation of statistics for planning purposes resulting in the need for access by a very wide range of people.

(b)   Communication systems for transfer of written information between different parts of the hospital or between hospital and community staff. These may include notes, letters, files, diagnostic investigation reports which may or may not be sealed in an envelope and may or may not be transmitted by the most direct route.

(c)   The staffing of wards at night by nursing auxiliaries and the use of ward clerks during the day - all of whom have access to patients records. Nursing auxiliaries and ward clerks do not necessarily adhere to a nursing code of ethics and perhaps the sensitive area of confidentiality of patient records should be explicitly stated in their contracts of employment.

(d)   The use of computers where terminals are not ideally placed to protect confidentiality and where the required codes for accessing the data are widely known - it has been reported that these codes have been seen pinned to the wall above the terminal!.

(e)   Verbal reports and changes of shift which are conducted in locations where they could be overheard.

In the light of such concern, the Royal College of Nursing advises its members 'to record only such information as the patient/client would willingly share with any proper professional person; it may be inappropriate for a record to be made of information which is of a confidential or intimate nature' (7). However, this advice must severely defeat one of the main objectives in keeping records which is to enable medical and nursing staff to provide each person with a consistent and continuing level of care to the highest attainable professional standards. Such advice if followed will surely lead to a dual system of records - one 'public' and one 'confidential' or secret which cannot but rebound to the detriment of patient and nurse alike.

Access to Information by the Data Subject

The danger mentioned above of the establishment of dual systems of recording becomes highlighted again in the general principles which it is proposed to incorporate into the legislation (A20). 'The data subject shall have access to information held about him and be entitled to its correction or erasure where the legal provisions safeguarding personal data have not been complied with'. This principle needs clarification and considerable thought in relation to National Health Service Records. It is not stated whether the information disclosed to the subject shall be the whole record or only part of it. It is however noted that the medical and nursing professions in their evidence to the Lindop Committee(A12) have made known their views which, as far as medical records are concerned were generally accepted by the Lindop Committee. Namely that factual data could at the discretion of the doctor, be disclosed but that, without prejudice to the future, value-laden information would be withheld at the present time. However no such discretion was recommended in respect of social work records. The question for nurses is - will their records be treated like medical or like social work records? It may be suggested that in content, nursing records follow a continuum from mainly factual data in the hospital acute sector to mainly social and judgemental information recorded by a Health Visitor. It may be that the physical location of the record - being relatively easy to ascertain - will be a determining factor. Thus nursing records filed with medical case notes become 'medical'. However the question then arises concerning the status of a social report produced on medical request and filed in the medical case notes!

Discretion of the Originator of the Record in Relation to Disclosure to the Subject of the Record

There is a strong lobby from the medical and nursing professions to obtain legislation which will recognise the peculiar difficulties of the Health Service and the view that it may not always be in the best interests of patients that the subject of the record has access to the whole record. A particularly sensitive issue concerns medical and nursing records generated by employer funded occupational health schemes, should either the client or the employer necessarily have a right of access to them?

The question then arises as to who will have the right to deny subject access to the whole record. If one considers areas of Health Service activity such as Mental Handicap, Child Abuse and long term physical or mental disability, it will be recalled that the authorship of contributions to the care records of those individuals covers a multitude of agencies and people. In all that has so far been written, there is an implicit (and sometimes explicit) assumption that the final arbiter to disclose or not to disclose the record will be a medically qualified practitioner. If his decision is required to be based on the answer to the question 'will disclosure of the information contained in this record be harmful to this individual?' perhaps a medically qualified practitioner is the person who would be accorded the widest degree of acceptance in this role. However, if this decision is reached without reference to the authors of the record who may feel that their future relationship with the subject may be jeopardised to the detriment of the possible future wellbeing of that subject, then it is suggested that the advice of the Royal College to its members (stated earlier) will become widespread accepted practice. All official health service records will be made in the light of possible future disclosures to the subject and will contain only factual data. In a sense this situation is already extant in that there is no legal immunity from disclosure of the health record in a Court of Law, but this proposed legislation would appear to make the likelihood of such a disclosure a more frequent occurrence.

In legal practice the situation is different, confidences and instructions from the client to a solicitor enjoy absolute privilege. A solicitor could never be called upon, even by the highest judge, to reveal or give evidence based on information passed to him by a client. This degree of confidentiality is not legitimated even for the clergy, still less for the medical profession whose members can be ordered under subpoena to give evidence about their parishioners or patients.

Disclosure of Information to People other than the Subject

Although there are guidelines and codes of ethics extant in most professions in the public sector governing the disclosure of information to friends and relatives, professional colleagues, the press and other media, the topic of confidentiality is not specifically mentioned in the general training syllabus of the General Nursing Council but it is generally covered under standards of ethical practice. For the midwives, Rule No 8 is headed 'Duty to Regard Information as Confidential' and in the guide to the syllabus for Health Visitors Training, the Council for the Education and Training of Health Visitors recommend that issues of confidentiality of records and disclosure of

information be covered under the general topic of Principles and Practice of
Health Visiting.

The Royal College of Nursing guidelines(7) explore these issues at some length
but can be broadly summarised as follows:

Wherever possible obtain the patient/client's consent and permit disclosure of
information only according to the wishes of that person. Where patient/client
consent for some reason is not readily obtainable, the appropriate medical
consent may be sought. However there are occasions when the patient's right to
confidentiality may be modified or overruled, and these include situations where
the patient's life, or the lives and safety of others may be at risk.

This leads us into the arena of the disclosure of information, to the police.
Most nurses working in Accident and Emergency Departments and in the psychiatric
field are well aware of police enquiries and the well accepted advice to refer
such enquiries to the responsible medical practitioner. However, there is
considerable cause for concern in this respect in the White Paper (A20). It is
here suggested that in the interests of:

a)   protecting state security, public safety, the monetary interests of the
      state or the suppression of criminal offences,
b)   protecting the data subject or the rights and freedoms of others,

together with some data required by the police for the **prevention** or detection
of crime - that 'data users who make information available to the authorities in
connection with these matters will not be required to register such disclosures
of information'. Thus information recorded by nurses and others in good faith
that it would be safeguarded and kept confidential - may reach police files, or
the files of others engaged in national security work without either the data
subject or the author being any the wiser. Perhaps it must be reiterated that
all information concerning individuals which can be individually identified
whether held in manual or automated systems must be kept confidential between
the data subject and the team of people concerned with the past, present or
future wellbeing of that individual. There are occasions when nurses outside
that immediate clinical team also need access - for example in the interest of
nurse education or during the investigation of accidents, untoward occurrences
or complaints. This access should be incorporated into local rules and
procedures and should be available only after those responsible for the
management of the service have satisfied themselves that their staff fully
understand and are committed to the concept of individual privacy. It surely
goes without saying that those occupying management positions in the National
Health Service must have access as of right to the personnel records of the
staff for whom they are managerially accountable. It seems that we are poised
in a position of trying to judge in which direction is the greatest good. On
the one hand to devise data protection systems including access rules which
restrict custodianship and control greatly so that the majority of the staff
feel alienated from the system though all might agree the system to be very
secure. The alternative might be to devise a system whereby professional
responsibility and integrity are highlighted. It is suggested that such a
system may well be less secure to the determined individual who wishes to breach
confidentiality but may well result in more appropriate care for the individual
patient/client by virtue of more complete records being kept which will include
tentative opinions and hypotheses appropriately labelled as such but recorded in
the knowledge that the record could be confidentially used as a medium of
communication between professions and agencies caring for an individual who
would not, except in a court of law, gain access to those very soft and, at the
time of recording, unreliable, untested data.

In summary, there is no absolute or 'natural' morality of confidentiality: the ethics of nursing records vary with time and geography, they have constantly to be adjusted to the requirements of technology and the ultimate protection of the interest of the individual patient.

In her 'Notes on Nursing' Miss Nightingale stressed the need for confidentiality when she wrote 'and remember every nurse should be one who is to be depended upon, in other words, capable of being a 'confidential' nurse .....she must be no gossip, no vain talker, she should never answer questions about her sick except to those who have a right to ask them....'

REFERENCES

1.   Data Protection in Health Information System, Griesser, G.G. et al., North Holland Publishing Co. 1980, pp 217.
2.   ACORN - A Classification of Related Neighbourhoods.   This system was primarily designed for market research purposes, and by analysis of postal codes gives a fairly accurate view of socio-economic status in different locations.
3.   Lord Mancroft's Bill: Hansard, 14 February 1961.
4.   Mr Leslie Huckfield's Bill: Hansard, 8 February 1972.
5.   Mr. Brian Walden's Bill: Hansard, 26 November 1969.
6.   Cmnd 6354 - Computers: Safeguards for Privacy, Government White Paper 1975.
7.   Guidelines on Confidentiality in Nursing - Royal College of Nursing of the United Kingdom, London 1980.

The Impact of Computers on Nursing
M. Scholes, Y. Bryant and B. Barber (eds.)
Elsevier Science Publishers B.V. (North-Holland)
© IFIP-IMIA, 1983

4.2.

CONFIDENTIALITY

Discussion

Misuse of information

Privacy and confidentiality are controversial issues although many computer systems have greater security than those of written records. It is impossible to make either a paper or computer system completely confidential for many users. Patients, however, must be certain that no harm will come to them from the possible misuse of information they give to nurses and other health care specialists. This applies to written and other types of information systems which are now used, but more so to computerised information which is more manipulative and has the possibility of being correlated with other kinds of data. In Sweden, correlation of information from two sources (or registers) is only permitted under the Swedish Data Protection Act by a Registration Board. Since record linking is technically feasible, nurses should be aware that it may become possible for data to be accessed by other persons for whom it was not intended. Furthermore, data released for nursing research may be at risk by a third party. However, it must be recognised that for a nursing management information system to be fully successful, data will have to be matched and compared with data from different sources.

Security Systems

Modern systems have many sophisticated ways of ensuring confidentiality by the use of passwords, badges and encryption. Of these, passwords were the preferred option within a hospital environment as badges could easily be mislaid or lost. Eventually the inconvenience of present security systems is likely to be handled by systems that recognise the voices or fingerprint of individuals.

Patient Access to Records

It was noted that many international organisations are now asking that patients be able to access their clinical data to check its accuracy and validity either directly or through an agent. The implications of this particularly with regard to nursing records needs to be considered by nursing management.

CHAPTER 5

NURSING RECORDS

Documentation of individual patient nursing care is essential to ensure the delivery and continuity of this care. This section describes computer systems for planning and recording nursing care which have been developed in the USA and UK.

The first paper is based on Margo Cook's Nursing Times Lecture, and it is interesting to note that the following paper shows how the same system has been implemented in different hospitals. Reference is also made to this system in the Computer Technology Chapter 3 in respect to selecting an appropriate computer system. An overview of UK systems is included as well as fuller descriptions of individual systems.

Valuable indications are given to ways in which the computer can assist with implementing the nursing process.

The Impact of Computers on Nursing
M. Scholes, Y. Bryant and B. Barber (eds.)
Elsevier Science Publishers B.V. (North-Holland)
© IFIP-IMIA, 1983

5.1.

USING COMPUTERS TO ENHANCE PROFESSIONAL PRACTICE

(Nursing Times Lecture)

Margo Cook

Introduction

Are you in tune with current technology? Have you adapted to the benefits it offers? If I asked you the time would you consult a digital watch? That is an every day example of current applied science.

We benefit constantly as we use the tools modern technology has made available to us, but let us not forget that if they are unsuited to our need or misapplied, they may exacerbate the problems we are trying to solve. The digital watch gives an accurate answer to the question, "What time is it?" It is ineffectual for counting a pulse.

When the technology of computers is applied to health care problems, nursing may benefit greatly. It may be seriously handicapped if the system chosen has not been designed and selected with the total information needs of nursing as a primary consideration.

The subject of computers in nursing is broad and multifaceted. In this paper we will consider only the application of computer science to hospital-based patient care information systems as it affects professional nursing practice. I want to focus particularly on nurse care planning and demonstrate how the computer can be the key to unlock the door to consistent, current care planning in a hospital.

Unfortunately, the nurse is handicapped in addressing the tasks unique to nursing by underlying problems which monopolise the available time, energy, and funds. If we can successfully apply the computer system to these problems, the nurse will be freed for the professional functions for which she is trained. Of course, either the wrong computer or a wrong application can make matters worse.

Let us consider how a computer system can affect three of these basic problems which confront the nurse in today's hospital: (a) proliferating paperwork; (b) increasing volume and complexity of information to be dealt with; and (c) escalating costs in every area.

Proliferating Paperwork

Nurses are faced by the ever greater demand to write down in extensive detail all they want done and all they have done for the patient. In addition, others on the health team expect the nurse to function as their scribe, since the nurse has the most ready access to the patient charts.

Studies have shown that more than 30% of a nurse's time is spent doing paperwork. What can a computerized system do to reduce this?

It can eliminate duplicate entries. By the traditional system the nurse manually transcribes a medical order to her "Kardex," to the requisition, and to the administration sheet or card. A computer can do all this with one action.

It can keep track of recorded information. Time and effort are consumed when a lost or misplaced requisition must be tracked down. It can also make data available in several locations, not just on the chart.

On the other hand, if the system has been selected to meet the needs of someone else in the hospital, if it is not designed to take care of time consuming details or is improperly implemented, it may give the nurse multiple copies of data which must be reviewed just to check its importance. It may produce data useful to someone else but irrelevant to nurses. It may spew out data in such a random fashion that tracking down the needed items becomes a time consuming nightmare.

If nurses are to function as professionals in the care of the patient, they have the right to expect that the technology will relieve them of routine paperwork which keeps them from the more important tasks. Too often nurses have accepted a version of technology which has been inadequate to meet their needs.

Increasing Volume and Complexity of Information

What can a computerized patient care information system do to relieve the pressure of the increasing volume and complexity of information? It can store a large body of data so that it is instantly available. For example a data base of care planning information. It can provide formats to organise and sort data for ease of use. These formats can then become "checklists" for complex data gathering and assessment tasks.

On the other hand, a system may make the necessary data so difficult to find or interpret that it is, of necessity, ignored. It may require data to be entered and retrieved in ways foreign to the nurses' thinking about their work and their patients.

Escalating Costs

What can a computer patient care information system do about the cost of nursing care?

It can reduce the cost per patient per day as it frees the nurse from being buried in paperwork and swamped by the volume of information, or it may increase the cost by increasing the nurse's workload. The cost is increased when the wrong system is used or when a system is overlaid on the existing manual system. When the right system is integrated carefully with the manual system, cost is reduced.

Philosophical Issues

The philosophical issues do much to determine whether a system will be a benefit or a detriment in a given setting.

1. The first involves the interactive function of the nursing role. How does the information system provide for interaction between nursing and the other health care departments?

    Is it set up as separate units with little or no attention to nursing, which moves back and forth trying to relate to each and all of these? See figure 1.
    This situation will usually produce and/or increase the problems discussed above.

Figure 1

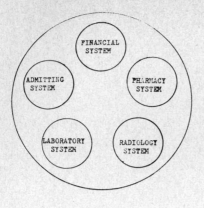

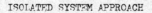

ISOLATED SYSTEM APPROACH

Figure 2

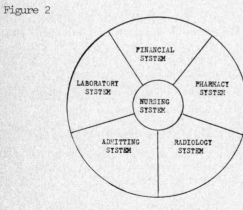

INTEGRATED SYSTEM APPROACH

Or is it designed as a whole with each component an adjacent piece of the same pie and nursing at the hub. See figure 2.

This set-up usually leads to an efficient system where nursing can function at its best.

2. The second issue involves determining if the right tool has been chosen. Has the job been properly defined by the organisation in order to find the right tool. Equally important, is the organisation prepared to spend the resources to get the right tool now?

If the answers are affirmative, we can be sure that the resulting patient care information system can do a great deal to enhance the professional practice of nursing.

We have pointed out the general effect on nursing of the great amount of paperwork which burdens each nurse. Part of this comes as the nurse acts as scribe for other members of the team. Let us consider in detail the transcription of doctors' orders.

If the computerized information system can reduce this cumbersome process to a few simple selection in the computer, the time spent can be decreased by almost 100%. Better yet, if the doctor can write the order directly into the computer, the transcription process is eliminated.

The Technicon System

In the Technicon system, in use at a number of hospitals, the doctor can sign-on to the computer. He is presented with a list of his patients wherever they are located in the hospital. He uses the light pen to select the patient he wants to write orders for, confirms the patient's name in a second selection (safety factor), and then begins the order from the "Master Guide". To enter orders for a stat blood culture and Ampicillin 500mg. IV stat, and then $\bar{q}$ 6 hrs x 3 days would require him to select "Lab Tests" and with five subsequent selections he would have the blood culture order written. Returning to the "Master Guide" (one selection), he selects "Pharmacy" and with ten selections writes the medication order. This process will take his at the most as much time as it would take to write the order by hand. However, once he has "reviewed" and "entered" these two orders into the computer, requisitions automatically print in the Laboratory and Pharmacy; the nurses' "Kardex" is updated; the nurse gets notification to give the stat medication. She will be notified of each $\bar{q}$ hr dose on a "Meds Due List" every six hours for the next three days at which time the order will automatically be discontinued.

In other words, nobody has to do anything to transcribe or transmit these orders once the doctor has put them in. The only thing required is to carry them out.

In addition, the order for the culture will stay on the "Kardex" automatically flagged "in process" each time the nurse gets a fresh copy of the "Kardex" (at least three times a day) until the results of the culture are entered into the computer. At that point the order is complete and the result in on the patient's chart.

The responsibility for insuring that the doctor's order gets to the laboratory and the results get back to the patient's chart is transferred to the computer. When the doctor questions a delay in the process, he can determine directly from the computer the progress of the order. He can then address the problem at the source. An "in process" culture is the responsibility of the Lab and the doctor will question them directly as to the reasons for the delay.

Designing Complete Systems

When the computerized information system is designed to do every phase in a given information process, it closes the information loop. The resultant reduction in time spent in paperwork and the simplification of the process is of enormous benefit to nursing.

There are other systems which also carry out the order transcription well, but there are those systems that are designed only to provide a part of the process. This results from designing a system to meet the needs of a department rather than the needs of nursing. One such system allows the nurse to transcribe the order into the computer for Pharmacy. However, it does not create a computer "Kardex," schedule the drug, or provide a "Meds Due List." Therefore, the nurse merely has a different kind of requisition. This is no help in reducing paperwork.

In another system, the order to Lab is not verified as "in process" nor is the result linked to the order. The nurse must still track down the lost requisition and bear the brunt of the complaints caused by the delay.

Partial systems have the information loop open. Each break in the loop has a high potential for lost information. The measures developed to prevent such loss multiply both computer and manual paperwork. At the same time, the process becomes more complex.

Planning Nursing Care

Thus, an ordering system designed with nursing or preferably the physician in mind can free the nurse to give patient care.

With time available, the nurse can now document her plan of care. Here a computer can provide exciting assistance. There is so much to write in a care plan and it changes so rapidly and is then so quickly erased that the tendency is sidestep writing out the care plan.

In the Technicon system is stored a data base of common patient problems, appropriate patient goals, and the necessary nursing actions. Once the nurse has mentally constructed her plan, she can sign-on to the computer. She selects her patient, then with ten light pen selections she records the patient's problem of pain, the goal of reasonable comfort, and the nursing actions necessary to make the patient comfortable.

Using the same sequence she continues to work from a list of common problems to construct the individualised nurse care plan. Once constructed, the care plan is printed and along with the doctor's orders it becomes a worksheet for the nurse. She can write on it, cross things out, and make notes because it is the individual nurse's own copy. When the next shift comes on, each nurse will get an updated copy of each patient's nursing care plan.

Updating the care plan is also easy. A few light pen selections allow the nurse the remove a problem that has been resolved or to delete a planned nursing action and replace it with a more suitable one.

At any time during the patient's stay the nurse works with a care plan that presents only current data. However, a complete record of the care planning showing the sequence of events is retrievable at any time at a computer terminal and is printed at discharge as a permanent part of the patient's chart.

If a nurse is presented with a patient whose usual care is unfamiliar to her, she has access to "standard care plan." She can identify a diagnosis and review the problems most likely to occur with that condition. This is an aid in assessment as well as planning.

At El Camino Hospital on any day of the year the norm is to find 85-90% of the patients with current, complete care plan. This is not entirely the result of the computerized system. Originally the nurses from the top nursing administrator through the entire nursing management team were required to define their care planning format and content and to make a commitment to care planning. With this support of the manual system there were current, complete care plans for 25-30% of the patients on any day.

With the computer system, the large volume of complex information is easily managed. As a result, studies showed it takes less time to achieve the 85% mark than it took to achieve the 25%.

The nurse care planning process is one of the nursing information handling tasks that is relatively easy to computerize. Thus, there are a number of computerized nurse care planning systems on the market. Many are excellent. Nurses, in an attempt to facilitate professional practice often begin by implementing these systems. Yet, they seldom have the desired results. Why? Because the nurse is still hampered by the time consuming paperwork. At the same time, integrating a computerized nurse care plan and a manual Kardex is usually a cumbersome process.

There are also computerized care planning systems available which can hinder the process. One such, provided the care plan, but rather than provide only current information, it provided all the information, flagging the inactive data. That might be acceptable if the patient's problems are relatively simple and the length of stay short. On the other hand, imagine the problems of dealing with all the care planning information for a patient whose care was complex and whose length of stay was three months. For such a patient at El Camino, the current care plan was three pages long. The complete care plan was twenty pages long.

Even for the relatively simple system of care planning, the design of the system must be carefully thought out or the system will add time, complexity and cost to the nursing process.

Recording Nursing Care

After the care planning comes another aspect of professional practice – recording nursing actions and patient results. What nurse is there that wouldn't like to reduce the time necessary to get her charting done? The nurses at El Camino spend so much less time in charting that most would find it a hardship to work in another setting. The routine charting of medications given takes seconds. Three of four light pen selections per medication and the job is done. Requirements like recording the injection site are built into the process. Should the nurse forget to chart, she is reminded by a notice before her shift if complete.

Charting the initial nurse's interview and patient assessment follows a carefully thought out structure. This ensures that recorded content of the admit note is consistently complete. The nurse enters the data using several techniques. The light pen is used to check off an item or build sentences from phrases. She may also use the keyboard to type information to describe clearly the specifics of her assessment. When this information is entered into the computer, her nurse's note is recorded. At the same time, all information pertinent to the nurse care plan is automatically recorded on the care plan as well. It is this kind of ability to use the computer to take information once

and use it in many varied ways that provides the most significant benefit to
nursing.   Nurses notes recorded throughout the patients' hospitalization are
handled the same way.

If the computer system is to enhance professional practice, in other words
facilitate the planning, executing and recording of patient care, nursing must
be provided with a suitable, comprehensive system.   Anything less may seem to be
in tune with the times, but will not benefit the professional nurse.

Conclusion

The application of computer technology can be of real benefit to nurses in the
practice of their profession only if the computer system in use has been
designed and chosen specifically to meet the needs of nursing and if the system
has been properly implemented.   The system can solve underlying problems such as
proliferating paperwork, increasing volume and complexity of information, and
escalating costs.   These monopolise time, energy and funds and keep the nurse
from the more important functions of nursing.   Once the nurse has help in these
areas, an appropriate computer system can be the key to open the door to
consistent, current care planning.   Experience has shown how a suitable computer
information system can facilitate the planning, execution and recording of
patient care, thus enhancing professional practice.

The Impact Of Computers on Nursing
M. Scholes, Y. Bryant and B. Barber (eds.)
Elsevier Science Publishers B.V. (North-Holland)
© IFIP-IMIA, 1983

5.2.

COMPUTERS IN SUPPORT OF PATIENT CARE

Shirley Hughes

Introduction

Computers have been in existence for over 3500 years. Hospitals have been utilizing computer systems for over twenty years. A recent article proclaims "The Nursing System - A Computer challenge of the 80's!"(P5). Why is it that just now a computerized nursing system is recognized as a need? Perhaps it is because Nurses are just now realizing the potential advantages of using computers to assist in patient care. Perhaps it is that sufficient numbers of nursing representatives and data processing representatives are learning to communicate with each other. Having bridged the language barrier between computerese and nursing, it has become possible for us to be aware of the possibilities and recognize the needs for computerization in support of patient care.

Various computerized systems have been created to support the hospital's information handling needs, one of these is the Technicon MATRIX MIS System. The Technicon Data Systems' (TDS) MATRIX Medical Information System (MATRIX MIS) originated over 10 years ago. Its primary purpose even then was to support patient care. Not only did the original developers take into consideration the hospital's financial data processing requirements, but, with the help of health care professionals (doctors, nurses, and technologists), they developed a system uniquely designed to support those professionals in the care of their patients. Every department in the hospital was included in the design along with the physician ordering process and the nursing process. Over 30 hospitals now use the MATRIX MIS. The nursing departments of those hospitals have been actively involved in development of their computerized nursing systems. TDS software allows each hospital to design its own CRT input screens and reports. This allows for each hospital to tailor its computer system to support its method of patient care. Therefore, the system I will be describing is not one system but many systems. The best way to illustrate how MATRIX MIS assists the nurse in caring for her patients is to describe how it supports each phase of the nursing process.

The nursing process as defined by Yura and Walsh (1) is an orderly, systematic manner of determining the client's problems, making plans to solve them, initiating the plan or assigning others to implement it, and evaluating the extent to which the plan was effective in resolving the problems identified.

Simply stated, the nursing process includes the elements of assessment, planning, implementation and evaluation.

Assessment

An effective assessment tool must include the following criteria:

1. not duplicative of investigations already available from other sources,
2. seek only information that will be used in nursing,
3. allow for discretion in collection of data,
4. be realistic - actually practiced or practicable(2).

Because the nursing system is a part of the totally integrated MATRIX MIS patient information system, data already obtained on the patient, such as demographic, pre-admission testing, outpatient/emergency visits, etc., is available to the nurse via the computer terminal and/or on printouts. This information is available even before the patient arrives at the nursing unit. Data collection efforts are not duplicated.

Programs supporting nursing assessment documentation allow for complete flexibility in defining the data elements. The components of a nursing history, the intitial patient assessment, for one hospital may be completely different to another. Even within a hospital the nursing history often differs from one service to another (i.e., pediatrics, orthopedics, obstetrics, etc.). During the process of implementing a computer system, the nursing department defines the components of the nursing history. The CRT screens are designed accordingly. By using the CRT terminals equipped with lightpens, used to make selections of words and phrases from the previously designed screens, and typewriter keyboards to allow for free text additions, the patient history is documented. Typically the screens are designed to display the various history components with lists of common responses for lightpen selection. Words and phrases may also be selected in order to compose the appropriate responses. Prompts reminding the nurse of history elements, but allowing her the freedom to type her response, are also used. Alert conditions, such as potential for skin breakdown, etc., are often flagged on subsequent patient reports as a result of the nurses's response to the history components. Thus, the computer has enabled the nurse to pass on important precautionary information to all care providers as a natural by-product of her documentation.

Screens for assessment of body systems, patient conditions, are also utilized by making lightpen selections or typing individualized statements. Programs allow the display of educational information to enhance the nurse's knowledge of conditions being assessed.

All data documented via the computerized assessment tool is stored along with the other patient information in the patient's data base. This information is available not only to nursing, but also to other care providers. It is legible, complete and was accomplished in a minimum amount of time.

Planning

Patient care planning via computer is, like the nursing history, a matter of first defining the criteria, the necessary components, and then the specific data elements. Several different approaches are used at the various TDS hospitals. In some, standard care plans are displayed on CRT screens indexed by categories of diagnosis or conditions. Common problems for the diagnosis or conditions selected are displayed, as well as appropriate expected outcomes and nursing interventions. Schedules for progress checks and dates for outcomes are also included. Most hospitals allow the nurse to lightpen select those problems, expected outcomes and nursing interventions appropriate for her patient. Type-ins are also available. This allows for optimum individualization of the patient's plan of care, yet provides the nurse with the information and guidance offered by standards of care. The nurse can even be "led" by the screens through certain pathways of information when care planning, to ensure that all aspects of the care plan are included.

The utilization of standard care plans increases and becomes more efficient when they are incorporated in the planning process as opposed to stored, unused, in books and kardex files (3).

Alpha listings of problems (nursing diagnosis) are another often used feature of TDS computerized care planning. Again, expected outcomes with target dates and nursing interventions with progress check scheduling may be associated with each selected and/or typed-in problem. A standardized terminology for nursing diagnoses is a realized benefit of this computer application.

Nursing orders unassociated with problems or nursing diagnosis are often used to enhance or further define physician orders. An example of this might be a nursing order of "walk patient in room for 5 minutes TID today", when the physician's order reads "Ambulate as tolerated".

Hospitals utilizing the TDS Patient Care Plan system have been able to achieve a very positive impact on their abilities to plan and affect quality, and continuity of patient care as a result. The care plans are more complete, utilize more consistent, and therefore understandable, terminology and are more legible. All of this has been accomplished utilizing less of the nurses' time than the previous manual systems. And more importantly, the Care Plans are readily available and are regularly utilized to care for the patient.

As in the case of the nursing history, Nurse Care Planning information may be made available by CRT retrieval and/or printouts to other health care professionals. Some hospitals have pursued the care planning capabilities of the systems to allow an integrated approach. In other words, health care professionals in other departments may add comments, interventions or problems to the care plan. The identification of the originator on each care planning entry has proven to be a great communication tool, thus ensuring a team approach toward the goal of patient wellness.

When appropriate, the care plan is easily revised by retrieving the patient's current care planning entries and modifying them directly on-line.

Implementation

With the Patient Assessment and Care Planning documented in MATRIX MIS along with the Physician orders, implementation of the patient's care is totally supported.

At the beginning of each shift and/or when changes are made, a Patient Care Plan is printed at the nursing station. This computer printout includes all the information needed by the nurse to deliver care to the patient. Pertinent information from the Nursing history, all Care Planning and nursing orders, as well as all current medical orders are included. Tests to be performed along with the appropriate test preparation instructions are also a part of this working care plan.

In addition, medication due lists automatically print just prior to the scheduled administration time prompting the nurse to give the appropriate medications for that time. This is a great tool in reduction of medication administration errors. Medications are charted via the CRT by retrieving an identical list of medications on-line and lightpen selecting "given" or "not given" along with injection sites, and other pertinent administration and/or observation information.

Documentation of care given and the patient's response, may also be accomplished with MATRIX MIS. Screens designed in the same manner as those used to enter care planning data have been extremely effective in achieving documentation of care given as it reflects the care planned.

Information presented to the nurse on charting screens reminds her to chart required data and to make appropriate observations. As a result the charting is more complete and of a better quality. Communication between health care professionals is greatly enhanced by the improved, legible and accessible charting. Accuracy and continuity of patient care are the end results.

Evaluate

Health care professionals can more readily evaluate the patient's response to his care when observations and data are made available to them in an appropriate format. For instance, the significance of test results are better evaluated when displayed in a cumulative fashion. TDS hospitals utilize many such cumulative reports. An example is that of laboratory test results presented in cumulative fashion with abnormal values highlighted in red. The appropriate normal ranges are also included for reference.

Fluid balance trends are equally important to display in a cumulative fashion. Many TDS hospitals utilize a 7-Day fluid intake and output summary. This summary also includes the patient's daily weight.

Real time audits to impact the quality of patient care at the time it is happening is another important feature of a nursing system. Hourly reminders of undocumented medications are utilized in many hospitals to avoid missed doses. A shift end report is also effective for making sure all medications are charted before the staff leaves. Alert bulletins may also be printed for pre-defined conditions. As the nurse documents the condition, a printout is printed in the Risk Management/Quality Assurance office. Tracking of that patient's care can begin immediately.

Because all of the patient's assessment, care planning and the implementation of that plan is documented in MATRIX MIS, a complete data base is available for research and/or audit. All data input is captured. The effectiveness and quality of patient care can be measured objectively. Alterations in nursing practice can be made based on the study of actual nursing actions and results.

Conclusion

The nursing process is supported by the computer systems I have described. The assessment, planning, implementation, and evaluation processes are performed by the nurse. The computer system ensures a better quality of care as well as faster and easier documentation and communication of the impact of that care to other professionals.

Many hours of effort in planning, designing, and sometimes negotiating, have been required of the nursing department in those hospitals who chose to utilize the computer in support of patient care. These pioneers have shared and learned from each other and yet made sure their own hospitals' unique needs were incorporated. There have been few attempts as successful as theirs, however, now that their accomplishments have been achieved and proven beneficial, more will follow.

REFERENCES

1. Yura, Helen and Walsh, Mary, The Nursing Process. Assessing, Planning, Implementing, Evaluating. Ed. 2., Meredity Corp, New York, 1973.
2. Stevens, Barbara J., Fist-Line Patient Care Management, Contemporary Publishing, Inc. Wakefield, Mass., 1976.
3. Barstow, Ruth E., and Nichols, Elizabeth G., "Do Nurses Really Use Standard Care Plans?", The Journal of Nursing Administration, Vol. 10, (1980). 27-31.

The Impact Of Computers on Nursing
M. Scholes, Y. Bryant and B. Barber (eds.)
Elsevier Science Publishers B.V. (North-Holland)
© IFIP-IMIA, 1983

5.3.

DEVELOPING A PATIENT CARE PROGRAM

Anne N. Gebhardt

1. Introduction

For many years it seemed as though the application of computer technology for
patient care information programs was an impossible dream. However, outstanding
advances had been made in a small number of locations, but the general promotion
and/or acceptance has been negligible. In contrast, clinical applications,
computerized monitoring and interpretation of clinical patient data have been
developing in many areas. Nurses have accepted and incorporated those systems
into the clinical aspect of patient care. However, electronic hospital
information systems have continued to be confined mostly to management
information systems with possibly ADT (Admission, Discharge, Transfer) and
laboratory programs available at the nursing unit. It is difficult to determine
whether nursing service has been reluctant to forge ahead in a "foreign field",
lacked encouragement for such an endeavour, or simply was not considered as a
user of such technology. Computer technology in the development of patient care
programs, designed by nurses, to be used by nurses is no longer a dream.
Computers have simplified work and improved communications for other professions
and industries and can have practical applications in patient care. Some of our
ideas may be futuristic but, for those ideas to become reality, the time for
development and utilisation of computers for patient care programs is here and
now.

2. Planning

In the ideal situation nursing administration should be as much involved in the
planning for and selection of the computer system for the institution as any
other potential user. In order to make a knowledgeable and valuable
contribution to the selection process, nursing administrators should become
familiar with the various types of computer systems, hardware, software,
options, etc. Special focus should be on how this would impact nursing on the
patient care unit, and potential value of computerised patient care information
to nursing staff as well as ancillary staff, and the inclusion of a nursing
management information system. More often than not the computer system is
already in place for a hospital or management information system. Nursing must
then evaluate how to capitalise on available programs and develop new programs
within the constraints of the existing hardware and software.

3. Options for Patient Care Plans

There are a variety of options available for computerised patient care plans.
These run the gamut of general care plans or instructions to highly
individualised patient programs which can process, delete, update and print out
information and even produce patient charges automatically. In the first
instance, care plans and patient teaching plans for specific disease entities
are stored in the computer and can be printed out as needed. The individual
patient needs are checked off as a guide for administering care. This can be a
very satisfactory reminder of important factors when assessing patient needs and
also for documentation purposes. Many patients, however, have multiple

diagnoses and one plan might not be sufficient. In the second instance, the individualised care plan can be developed by type-in or light pen selection and the information is part of the patient's active on-line file. This method facilitates incorporating the needs of the patient with multiple problems into one care plan.

4.   Brigham and Women's Hospital Computer System

The Brigham and Women's Hospital already had an IBM computer system for ADT and Fiscal and Management Information Programs with CICS (Customer Information Communication Systems) monitoring the software programs. The user hardware consists of a CRT (cathode-ray tube), keyboard, light pen and a printer where hard copy is needed. Entry into the system is accomplished by a combination of simple, typed commands and light pen action. Response time is less than one-second delay. The system allows for both the printout version of the general care plans and instructions and the on-line development of individualised care plans.

5.   The Setting

In the very early development stages of the patient care program, the hospital was comprised of three divisions in four separate geographical locations awaiting relocation into a new building. At this time only one nursing unit, a Rheumatology unit, was equipped with a CRT but without a printer. It was obvious that we were years away from physician involvement with the CRT and that it was unreasonable to expect total nursing involvement when the move into the new hospital occurred. Nonetheless, there must be a beginning in order to achieve a goal and that simple installation afforded the opportunity to evaluate the potential, the weak points and strong points and what changes might be needed to make it acceptable to nursing staff from all the divisions. In addition to nursing exploring the advantages of the systems, the pharmacy department was also beginning to develop its programs and to utilise the same patient population.

6.   The On-Line Patient Care Plan

The basic framework of the individualised patient care program was designed to allow for an integrated medical and nursing problem list, doctors' orders, care plan, medication and nutritional plans, and charting of vital signs (temperature, pulse, respiration, blood pressure with additional data typed in). The intent was not to try to develop an automated patient record at this time, but to provide information relative to patient care which could be easily communicated, was current and legible and would enhance documentation. It would indeed replace the manually produced nursing kardex, the medication record and diet information. Information could be updated or added as necessary and be available by display as well as printout for each nursing shift or whenever a major change occurred. This should improve the quality of the care plan and the shift report. It should also reduce time spent taking notes, recopying the kardex and minimise chance for error.

The ADT program is designed so that when a patient is admitted, the demographic data entered into the system establishes an on-line data base and file record. It also establishes the patient list for each nursing unit. This list can be displayed on the CRT. Using the light pen one can select a patient and display that patient's order entry system. See Figure 1.

```
--------------------------------------------------------------------------
|03/13/82              **  ORDER ENTRY SYSTEM   **              08.18.46|
|DOE, JANE                MRN= 000-000-0    ROOM= 14A141        NURS= 14A |
|                                                                        |
|                        SELECT ONE SERVICE AREA                         |
|                                                                        |
|    A/R               ADMIT            DATA-BANK          EMPLOYEE       |
|                                                                        |
|    COMPRESSED        PATIENT COND     PATIENT INFO                      |
|                                                                        |
|    LABORATORY        RADIOLOGY        PHARMACY           OP MSTR FILE   |
|                                                                        |
|    DIETARY           ORDER ENTRY      APPOINTMENTS       IP MSTR FILE   |
|                                                         GO BACK         |
|                                                                        |
--------------------------------------------------------------------------
```

Figure 1: Order Entry

Patient care programs are entered through the IP Master File (In Patient Master File). This program is protected by security code or password entry.

The IP Master File provides the patient data base: the same information that appears on the face sheet of the patient's medical record. This data is collected and entered by the admissions officer at the time of admission. This information is protected and cannot be altered on the nursing unit. On the lower portion of the screen are a number of options or files. In the early stages these files were Problem List, Doctors's Orders, Care Plan and Vital Signs (Temperature, Pulse, Respiration). Any one of these files could be selected by light pen. See Figure 2.

```
--------------------------------------------------------------------------
|06/01/80                 NURSING STATION    14A              13.40.32|
|                         INPATIENT MASTER FILE                         |
|                                                                        |
|   ROOM = 14A112    NAME = DOE, JANE              MRN = 000-000-0      |
| ADMITTED = 06/01/81    10.30 EST LOS = 000  ACT LOS = 001  BIRTH = 12/15/1913|
|  SERVICE = ORT    ADMITTING DIAG = RHEUMATOID ARTHRITIS    SEX = FEMALE |
|                    WORKING DIAG =                                       |
|  ATT DOC = 00000-0                          SPEC = ORT      AGE =       |
|  REF DOC = 00000-0                                                      |
|     COND =     ACCOM =          CARE LEVEL =          RELIG =           |
|  ADDRESS =                                            BLOOD =          |
|   STREET =                               DISCHARGED ON  =  /  /        |
|     CITY =                    STATE      ZIP = 00000                    |
| ALLERGIES =                                                            |
|     TEAM =         RES PHY =             H.O. =                         |
|  ROOM TEL = 0000   PRIMARY NURSE =                                      |
|                                                                        |
| PROBLEM LIST        DOCTORS ORDRS     CARE PLAN      VITAL SIGNS        |
|                     CHANGE                           GO BACK           |
--------------------------------------------------------------------------
```

Figure 2: Inpatient Master File

Up to this point, progression through the program moved very easily but the
nursing staff found that to leave one of these files and enter another, i.e.:
Doctors' Orders to Care Plan, was very cumbersome. A minor change (use of a
keystroke) eliminated several strokes of the light pen and initiated the
beginning of many changes and enhancements in the program.

Careful consideration must be given in the design stages to the sequence of
keystrokes, light pen action, etc. that the user will have to employ. Sequences
should be short and logical. Users should not be forced to perform steps that
are logically irrelevant to them to compensate for system design inadequacies.

7.   Display and Input Screens

When one selects a file (Doctors' Orders, Care Plan, etc.) with the light pen,
the information stored is displayed on the screen and no change in the data can
be made. All files display the date, program name, time, patient name, medical
record number and location plus the headings of POR NO (Point of Reference
number), Frequency, and File Title in the upper portion of the screen. At the
lower portion are options for action with the light pen. See Figure 3.

```
-------------------------------------------------------------------------------
|                                                                             |
|05/06/80     **  NURSING SERVICE - PROBLEMS/ORDERS/CAREPLAN **      19.05.10  |
|DOE, JANE                    MRN = 000-000-0   ROOM = 10B391   DIVISION = N5  |
|POR NO      FREQ       C A R E    P L A N                                     |
|                                                                             |
|                                                                             |
|              ADD-SELPEN     ADD-TYPEIN    LAST STATION    HISTORY   GO BACK  |
|NO DATA ON FILE                                                              |
|                                                                             |
-------------------------------------------------------------------------------
```

Figure 3: Light Pen Options

ADD-SELPEN function allows the user to select a category from the word frame
menu (list). Using the word frame, information is entered entirely by light pen
selection. Figure 4 shows a sample word frame.

```
-----------------------------------------------------------------------
|                                                                     |
|08/23/82  **  NURSING SERVICE - PROBLEMS/ORDERS/CAREPLAN  **    19.33.47 |
|DOE, JANE                MRN = 000-000-0   ROOM 10B391      DIVISION = N5 |
|POR NO    FREQ    CARE PLAN                                           |
| 21    XXX                                                           |
|                                                                     |
|  08/23/82:   DISCHARGE PLANNING        EXPECTED DATE OF DISCHARGE:__/__/__ |
|  _____     DESTINATION:                 |
|  HOME-                                 NURSING HOME I-               |
|  NURSING HOME II-                      NURSING HOME III-             |
|  NURSING HOME IV-                      OTHER: _____  |
|  TRANSPORTATION:                       FAMILY - _____    |
|  AMBULANCE-                            CHAIR CAR -                   |
|  TIME ORDERED:_____  -           PT./FAMILY INSTRUCTION:       |
|  CONFERENCE NEEDED ____ DATE _____ -  MEDICATION SCHEDULE: _____ |
|  ACTIVITIES _____ -     TREATMENTS: _____   |
|  COMMUNITY HEALTH:                     SERVICES NEEDED:              |
|  NURSING-                              PT-                           |
|  HHA-                                  HOMEMAKER-                    |
|  MEALS ON WHEELS-                      OTHER _____    |
|                                                                     |
|                                                                     |
|  _____                                 |
|                                                                     |
|  NEXT PAGE        REMOVE WORD        READY              GO BACK      |
-----------------------------------------------------------------------
```

Figure 4: Sample Word Frame

ADD-TYPIN displays a blank screen for free text typing of input. See Figure 5.
This is especially good for nursing notes and more involved explanations of care
than can be selected by light pen. In fact, some of the staff who are
comfortable with typing use this method of input almost entirely.

```
-----------------------------------------------------------------------
|                                                                     |
|05/06/80  **  NURSING SERVICE - PROBLEMS/ORDERS/CAREPLAN **    19.33.24 |
|DOE, JANE                MRN = 000-000-0  ROOM = 10B391    DIVISION = N5 |
|POR NO. FREQ    CARE PLAN                                            |
|                                                                     |
|                                                                     |
|PFK=  1-ADD/UPDATE      3-PRINT: D1    DELETE    DISCONT    GO BACK   |
|                                                                     |
-----------------------------------------------------------------------
```

Figure 5: Free Text Entry

Information can be deleted or changed by light penning the particular item of
data on the display screen. This action redisplays that data separately on an
input type screen where the information can be added to or modified by "type-in"
or the whole item deleted by light pen action. The staff appreciated the
features of the protected display screen and the special process required for
changing or deleting data. It eliminated some of their fears of "wiping out
everything in the system".

8.   The Selector-Pen Menu

The SELECTOR PEN MENU (see Figure 6) consists of a display screen with a series
of problem or category numbers (POR NO), a frequency schedule, and listing of
the categories of word frames available. These are all selected by light pen.
This process requires the user to know the appropriate POR NO for each category.
The POR NO allows all data entered relating to that number to be grouped
together for logical presentation. This will be further discussed under POR
NOs. Thus, if vital signs are ordered Q4H, one selects the POR NO 04, the Q4H
schedule and VITAL SIGNS. The word frame for VITAL SIGNS will appear and the
appropriate selection can be made. When the care plan is printed, the schedule
is translated into actual hours due.

At first the list of frames available was small (about eight). However, the
fact that data could be so easily selected for input and that word frames could
be composed of the most pertinent data, as established by the nursing staff on
each unit, brought about early expansion of the list to include more patient
needs and to correspond more completely with the manual kardex. Each category
can have several word frames (or pages).

```
---------------------------------------------------------------------------------
|                                                                               |
|05/06/80    ** NURSING SERVICE  -  PROBLEMS/ORDERS/CAREPLAN  **      14.43.05 |
|DOE, JANE            MRN = 000-000-0   ROOM = 3E1121          DIVISION = N5    |
|                                                                               |
|                           **  POR NO   **                                     |
|                                                                               |
|? 01      ? 02     ? 03     ? 04     ? 05     ? 06     ? 07     ? 08           |
|? 09      ? 10     ? 11     ? 12     ? 13     ? 14     ? 15     ? 16           |
|                                                                               |
|                         **  SCHEDULE  **                                      |
|                                                                               |
|? Q1H     ? Q2H    ? Q3H    ? Q4H    ? Q6H    ? Q8H    ? Q12H    ? XXX          |
|? PRN     ? QD     ? ST     ? BID    ? TID    ? QID    ? QOD     ? IV           |
|                                                                               |
|                        **  TREATMENT  **                                      |
|ALLERGIES             DIAGNOSIS        GOALS             VITAL SIGNS           |
|NUTRITION             ACTIVITIES       SPECIMENS         RESPIRATORY RX        |
|IV THERAPY            DRESSINGS        DRAINAGE          EQUIPMENT             |
|PROBLEM LIST          NURSING PLANS    PT. TEACHING      DISCHARGE PLANS       |
---------------------------------------------------------------------------------
```

Figure 6: Nursing Care Planning (1)

While this work was in progress, the nursing staff was developing a nursing
kardex for the new hospital. Several times the word frame list was changed,
rearranged and finally expanded to the present one to once again conform as much
as possible to what the staff is accustomed. See Figure 7.

```
-------------------------------------------------------------------------
|                                                                       |
|08/23/82      **  NURSING SERVICE - PROBLEMS/ORDERS/CAREPLAN  **     20.13.12|
|DOE, JANE                    MRN = 000-000-0  ROOM = 10B391        DIVISION = N5|
|                                                                       |
|                       **  SCHEDULE  **                                |
|                                                                       |
|? Q1H     ? Q2H    ? Q3H     ? Q4H     ? Q6H     ? Q8H     ? Q12H    ? QS|
|? QAM     ? QD     ? BID     ? TID     ? QID     ? QOD     ? MWF     ?PRN|
|? 000     ? 111    ? 222     ? 333     ? DG      ?         ?         ?   |
|                                                                       |
|                       **  SELECT A LETTER  **                         |
|                                                                       |
|     ? A     ? B     ? C     ? D     ? E     ? F     ? G     ? H        |
|     ? I     ? J     ? K     ? L     ? M     ? N     ? O     ? P        |
|                                                                       |
|                       **  SELECT ONE  **                              |
|                                                                       |
|01 ALERGIES       02 DIAGNOSIS       03 FREQ ORDERS      04 NUTRITION   |
|05 VITAL SIGNS    06 SPECIMENS       07 ADL/BASIC CARE   08 SUPP EQUIPMENT|
|09 IV THERAPY     10 TPN THERAPY     11 RESPIRATORY RX   12 PROCEDURES  |
|13 DRESSINGS      14 DRAINAGE        15 INFECTION CONT   16 RESEARCH PROT|
|17 PROBLEM LIST   18 EXP. OUTCOMES   19 NSG PLANS        20 PT TEACHING |
|21 DISCHARGE PLANS                                                     |
|                                                        GO BACK        |
-------------------------------------------------------------------------
```

Figure 7: Nursing Care Planning (2)

Another program design feature which was eliminated was the need to select the POR NO as well as the category (two light pen actions). The two are now combined (note on Figure 7) and the POR NO automatically entered when the category is light-penned. The schedule list was also expanded and an array of letters added to designate problems. (Some staff thought that the numbering system would be confused with hours of time.)

9.   POR Numbers

The POR NO (Point of Reference) allows a number designation for each category of word frame. No matter what order information is entered, if the proper POR NO is used the information will be grouped accordingly and in chronological order on displays and printouts. It follows that type-in information also must be entered with the appropriate POR NO in order to be inserted into the proper area of plan.

The sequence of the POR NO's on the list is significant to the total program. Word frames can be used in any of the files (Problem List, Doctors's Orders, Care Plan, or Vital Signs). If one is transcribing physician orders into the "Doctors' Orders" file, the first 16 word frames listed are the most likely used ones (see Figure 7). The last five are more appropriate for use in the "Care Plan" file or "Problem List" file. Since the nurse receives a printout of all the "files" for each shift, there is no need to enter care plans generated by physicians' orders again into the Care Plan file unless a detailed explanation is required. On the manual nursing kardex, there is space for many of these standing physician orders to be entered. The computerised plan using the appropriate files allows for distinction between physicians' orders and nursing orders.

10   Development of Word Frames

One of the most important features of the word frame portion of the program is
that word frames can be unique to each nursing unit. That means the staff on
each unit can develop word frames tailored to meet the needs of their particular
type of patients. Thus, the most frequently used datas can be rapidly selected
by light pen strokes. Less frequently needed data is available on later screens
of a word frame category.

The Rheumatology unit developed many word frames appropriate to their patients'
needs. "Nursing Plans" include a number of specific plans from "Care of Patient
with Rheumatoid Arthritis" to "Care of Patient with Total Hip Replacement". The
problem list was a combination of medical as well as nursing problems and
problems were entered in the "Problem List" file. The nursing plan related to
the problem was entered into the "Care Plan" file. The printout of the data
then included Dietary Information, Problem List, Doctors' Orders, and Care Plan
in that sequence. See Figure 8.

```
----------------------------------------------------------------------------
ROOM 14A111 DOE, JANE        MRN 000-000-0      AGE 082Y     DR. ALAN JOSEPH
   RES =                     H.O. = J. GREEN                 NURSE = S. SNUTA
                       DIET-> 7/8 REGULAR PUREED FOODS

   P R O B L E M   L I S T
               A        FRACTURED LEFT HIP
               B        PRE-OP LEFT HIP SURGERY
               C        POST-OP LEFT HIP SURGERY
               D        IMMOBILITY
               E        CONFUSION

   D O C T O R S   O R D E R S
               XXX      07/16/82   ALLERGIES: N.K.
               DG       FRACTURED LEFT HIP
               XXX      06/24/82   ADM TO 14A - COND. SATISFACTORY
               XXX      07/08/82   NUTRITION: PUREE REGULAR DIET
    18    22   Q4H      07/16/82   ROUTINE VITAL SIGNS
               XXX      07/16/82 - PRE/OP HIP SURG.

   C A R E   P L A N
               A        FRACTURED LEFT HIP
                        1.  POSITION PT. IN PROPER BODY ALIGNMENT
                        2.  ASSIST AS NEEDED
               B        PRE-OP LEFT HIP SURGERY
                        1.  PRE-OP TEACHING
                        2.  PHISOHEX SCRUBS AS TOLERATED
                        3.  EXPLAIN USE OF IV THERAPY AFTER SURGERY
                        4.  EXPLAIN THE IMPORTANCE OF PROPER BODY ALIGNMENT
                        5.  NPO AFTER MN 6/24
----------------------------------------------------------------------------
```

Figure 8: Sample Printout of Care Plan

11.   Expansion

Most of the word frames developed by the Rheumatology/Orthopedic nursing staff
were specific for "their patients" but some word frames, such as ALLERGIES,
NUTRITION, SPECIMENS, VITAL SIGNS, were general enough for use in many patient
areas. Some staff also reasoned that word frames should be standardised for use

in all areas (as the manual kardex). This would be helpful to "float" staff especially. A group of nurses, representative of the many clinical services and specialties, was organised to develop "generic" word frames. While the rationale for simplication by standardisation was commendable, in actuality the "generic" word frames need adjustment according to area to insure light-pen input is as explicit as possible and as time saving as intended. Therefore, the most commonly used selection in a category should be available on the first frame of that category for each patient care unit, thus necessitating variations in word frame content for different care units.

The greatest advantage of the system, however, is that it can grow or adjust to meet the changing needs of nursing. The nursing profession is beginning to incorporate the use of nursing diagnoses as a method of identifying patient problems within the scope of nursing. The Brigham and Women's Hospital nursing staff is developing standards of nursing care using nursing diagnosis/problems, expected outcomes, and nursing plans.

Now nursing problems are entered into the Care Plan file (rather than the Problem List as described earlier) with appropriate outcomes and plans following. Each problem is designated by a letter and the corresponding outcomes and plans are identified by the same letter. Thus, all problems are listed, then all outcomes, then all plans. See Figure 9.

```
--------------------------------------------------------------------------------
|                                                                               |
|08/18/82      **  NURSING SERVICE - PROBLEMS/ORDERS/CAREPLAN   **    12.18.54 |
|BROWN, JOHN                   MRN = 000-000-0   ROOM = 09B312     DIVISION = N5|
|POR NO    FREQ        CARE PLAN                                                 |
|                                                                               |
|  17      A          08/18/82:  NURSING PROBLEM:                                |
|                     KNOWLEDGE DEFICIT RELATED TO:                              |
|                     -TRANSPLANT SURGERY                                        |
|                     -PREPARATION FOR SURGERY                                   |
|                     REVIEWED/EVAL.  / /  . RESOLVED  / /  .                   |
|  18      A          08/18/82: EXPECTED OUTCOMES:  THE PATIENT WILL            |
|                     STATE GENERAL OPERATIVE INFO.                              |
|  19      A          07/17/82:  NURSING PLAN:                                   |
|                     ASSESS PT'S READINESS TO LEARN:                            |
|                     START INDIV.  TEACHING PLAN EARLY,                         |
|                     USE T.U. TEACHING PROTOCOL                                 |
|                     EVAL. PT. PROGRESS: USE PRE-OP AND                         |
|                     DISCHARGE TEACHING CHECKLIST                               |
|                                                                               |
|   ADD-SELPEN        ADD-TYPEIN       LAST STATION       HISTORY    GO BACK |
|RECORD HAS BEEN UPDATED.                                                        |
--------------------------------------------------------------------------------
```

Figure 9: Nursing Care Planning (3)

Here again, the need for system design change becomes evident. Future enhancements of this portion of the program would allow for better grouping of all the information related to a problem. Design changes will incorporate the use of subcategories, available by light pen, and complete follow through from nursing diagnosis or problem to nursing plan.

12.   Addition of Notes

Brief notes regarding medical history, social history, and nursing notes had
always been included in the manual kardex and the staff still felt the need for
this type of information to make the "computer" kardex complete. By specifying
POR NO's for each type of note, the note section can be well organised and
maintained in chronological order.

An advantage to this design is that the nursing notes, as well as the Problems,
Expected Outcomes, and Nursing Plans, can be printed out separately and added to
the patient's permanent record for completed and legible documentation of
nursing interventions.

13.   Conclusions

The potential of the on-line patient care program as a nursing communication
tool and as a method of nursing documentation is beginning to be appreciated and
accepted. While the development of the system described has produced a program
that presently includes a means of entering all the data usually available in
the manual kardex, it should by no means be considered complete. Enhancements,
simplification of design, and other additions or improvements continue to take
place. As computer technology increases and applications in nursing become an
expectation, program designs will become simpler for the user and the
information processing more sophisticated. In any system the output is
dependent on the input. For the computerised program for patient care
information to succeed, it must be easy to use and provide information in a
logical organised manner. However, the crucial factor is the quality and
completeness of the data that all the nurses enter into the system. The
inducement to the nurses for entering data is directly proportional to the
assistance the computer contributes to decreasing their every increasing burden
of paperwork.

The Impact Of Computers on Nursing
M. Scholes, Y. Bryant and B. Barber (eds.)
Elsevier Science Publishers B.V. (North-Holland)
© IFIP-IMIA, 1983

5.4.

CARING FOR PATIENTS WITHIN A COMPUTER ENVIRONMENT

Clare C. Ashton

1. Introduction

The potential uses of computer technology within the National Health Service were acknowledged during the late 1960's, although it was difficult to perceive at the time how these might be achieved effectively, particularly in the patient care situation. Several computer projects were established in England and Wales under the Department of Health and Social Security (DHSS) experimental research and development programme to investigate the application of computers in different aspects of health care. Other projects set up were financed from regional or individual hospital funds. Some of these applications were concerned with clinical nursing and those health care systems which require multi-disciplinary involvement including nurses. This paper discusses some of these sytems that have a direct impact on the delivery of patient care within a hospital ward or specialised unit, relating to nursing records; drug information, prescribing and administration; and patient monitoring; and considers the future strategy of computers in caring for patients.

It is not easy to imagine how we would function without computers today, and yet when these computer applications were originally suggested over a decade ago, there was considerable resistance and apprehension which, unfortunately still exist. Many nurses regarded computers as an unwanted intrusion in their working environment, either through fear resulting from ignorance; complacency; and/or sheer lack of vision. Some nurses genuinely disliked machines of any kind, whilst other were concerned that computers might dictate, at the very least, constrain them to a specific pattern of working, stifling initiative, and diverting them from their caring role.

Many of these misconceptions were overcome by computer educational programmes and involving nurses themselves in the design of their own systems from their commencement. The formation of nurse and other multi-disciplinary user groups to work with the staff of the computer departments has been a major influence in the successful outcome of these projects. The nursing contribution has been further intensified by the employment of senior nursing officers or nurse analysts working full or part-time as members of the project teams, providing nursing advice, guidance and a practical input at operational level. The need for these nurses to meet together at regular intervals, to acquire and exchange information, ideas and experiences was recognised in 1974, when a Computer Project Nurses' Group was formed. The membership included the project nurses and nursing officers from the DHSS, who have all benefited from the contact, knowledge and support provided by the Group.

2. Nursing Records

The development of computerbased nursing records within the experimental computer programme was concentrated at two centres, the Royal Devon & Exeter Hospital (Wonford), Exeter (C5,C12) and the Queen Elizabeth Hospital, Birmingham (C3). Concurrently in Scotland, a similar application was developed at Ninewells Hospital, Dundee(D4; C6) supported by a grant from the Scottish Home

and Health Department as part of the Ninewells Ward Computer Project. All three
sites owe a debt of gratitude to the pioneering work at Kings College Hospital
where one of the very early computer projects was set up. One of the most
successful applications implemented was a nursing records system (C16) operated
in two wards. Demonstrations of this system allowed nurses, particularly on
user groups, an insight into the practical use of computers in the ward.

The nursing record systems were in todays terms involved with planning care and
evolved at a time when a more individual approach to patient care was being
adopted in this country, moving away from the traditional task orientated
approach.

They have been designed independently and their development, before and after
implementation , has been influenced by local priorities, nurses acceptance to
change and the availability of computer terminals (i.e. Exeter and Dundee have
ward printers; Birmingham is introducing ward printers as an integral part of
the drugs system).

Each of these systems uses the computer for patient care planning. Nurses enter
and cancel nursing orders for each individual patient directly into the computer
using visual display units (VDU's) in the ward sister's office or at the nursing
station. Whilst assessing patient's special nursing needs and precautions on
admission and reporting on orders is only available at Exeter, all provide
various forms of printed documents to aid the implementation of care.

2.1. Entry and Cancellation of the Care Plan

The entry of nursing care is organised systematically at each hospital, although
there are differences and similarities in approach. At the Queen Elizabeth
Hospital, Birmingham, for example, nurses may select care from screens
displaying the most frequently used order's for the patient's ward. These ward
screens, usually two or three per ward and presented consecutively, display
either basic or technical care orders, grouped according to their classification
(e.g. mobility, fluids, dressings etc). They reflect the speciality of the ward
and the care provided to meet common nursing problems. Selection is achieved by
entering a date code beside the required action, indicating when the care should
begin.

A similar screen, which may be used by any ward, displays all the relevant care
for a patient with a particular condition (e.g. tracheostomy). Care is selected
in the same way, appropriate to the patient's needs. This approach resembles
the care profiles adopted for each ward at Exeter. Each care profile is made up
of orders associated with specific diagnosis or conditions, e.g. emergency
admission, radium aftercare, chemotherapy. The orders displayed are either
accepted or rejected by completing an appropriate date or 'wrong' column.

All systems classify nursing orders under the easily recognisable but
traditional headings applicable to an area of nursing activity or body system.
Each classified screen can be selected by number either from a list of the
classified nursing orders on the VDU (at QEH) or from a list attached at the
side of the VDU (at Exeter, as for the ward care profiles). Pertinent phrases
in the form of instructions and directions are displayed and the associated
number entered to build up the required nursing order. If an instruction or
direction is not available, certain freetext facilities exist on each screen
but, at Birmingham, the nurse may proceed to a freetext screen to type in the
appropriate care. If an order can only be partially selected from a classified
screen, an incomplete order may be carried over to another freetext screen for
completion. Whilst this type of screen contributes to personalising care, the
wardbased screen (care profiles and ward screens) are accessed more often as
they minimise nursing input time. An interesting development at Exeter allows

for both types of screens. From some care profiles, the nurse may be guided automatically through one or more classified screens, ensuring that all aspects of the care plan are covered.

Familiarity with the system at Exeter enables nurses to take advantage of a technique to bypass several classified screens by entering orders using the number of the appropriate screen and phrase(s). A similar but simpler approach has been adopted at Dundee where nursing orders are entered in coded form using a nursing orders dictionary applicable to the ward. Certain of these orders automatically generate instructions appertaining to recognised practices in the hospital such as those associated with the preparation of investigations and special tests. On selection of such an order, by entering the relevant alpha character at Dundee e.g. S. for Schilling test, or by number at Exeter, the appropriate instructions are displayed with dates and times automatically calculated.

The logical sequence and design of screens encourages the nurse to regularly appraise each patient's nursing care plan, provides a more individualised approach to patient care and prompts the nurse to consider the care her patients' may need. The use of care profiles and orders with associated instructions make a contribution towards minimum standards of care.

Changes to the care plan at Exeter and Birmingham can be achieved by retrieving the patient's current care plan and entering an alpha code against the appropriate order to amend, delete or terminate at the end of the day. Other features exist at Birmingham which allow for the automatic cancellation of orders to reduce the incidence of nurses physically cancelling order to a minimum. Orders which occur once only are cancelled on the day they are expected to take place e.g. Remove drain. At Dundee, a new order (except for investigations and tests) automatically supersedes an existing order of the same group whilst at Birmingham this facility only applies to those groups of orders which continually change e.g. Fluid orders. Investigations and tests at Dundee are cancelled by re-entering the same alpha code as for input and requesting deletion on the screen displayed.

2.2   The Nursing Care Plan

The nursing care plan is readily accessible on the VDU and printouts. Whilst all ward staff may have access to the nursing information on printed documents, the care plan can only be retrieved on the VDU by those authorised to do so e.g. nurses, doctors, physiotherapists and dieticians. Printed individual care plans are produced by request on printers sited in the wards at Exeter and Dundee, usually before every morning shift and when care plans are altered. Care can quickly be reviewed as these plans are placed either within the local vicinity of the patient or at the end of the patient's bed. All nursing orders are included as well as tests and investigations with their relevant preparatory instructions.

To assist with the implementation of care, it is grouped under the three broad headings of nursing orders, specimen collections and tests at Dundee whilst at Exeter more specific categories are used such as basic care, mobility, etc. which equate more closely to those used to classify orders.

The care plan at Exeter also contains information from the nursing history collected on admission of the patient. The patient's special needs and precautions e.g. Diabetes, are entered on an assessment screen and appear at the top of the care plan. Results of urine analysis and weight are also collected and printed as part of the care plan at Dundee.

A different approach was preferred by nurses at Birmingham, when the system was initially designed (in 1972), to allow the ward sister to manage patient care by task allocation or team nursing and yet still identify an individual's care plan. Furthermore, a document was required to provide an overview of the ward workload and the progress achieved in executing care. These objectives were encompassed within a nursing care list, printed for each ward on the printer in the computer room late each evening for distribution to the wards by the hospital portering service. Each care list gives the plan of care for each patient on the ward in a standard matrix with orders grouped into several columns corresponding to treatment, mobility, recordings etc., similar to those headings used on the care plans. One or more lists may be produced according to the management of care or ward sister's requirements, and either placed in a central position in the ward or taken with a nursing team as they attend their allocated patients. As the need arises, certain task-orientated lists can be printed on request at Dundee e.g. Dressings.

2.3   Reporting on Planned Care

Reporting on care given is operational at Exeter only. The patient's care plan is displayed and two slashes entered against each order completed. At Dundee, provision is made for nurses to record care when it is given on the printed care plan by initialling the appropriate time column. Orders on the nursing care list are ticked off as they are carried out. Handwritten records of detailed reports and observations are still maintained at all sites within the nursing record (Kardex).

2.4   Continuity of Planned Care

The file of nursing orders (and reports at Exeter), which is constantly being added to during the patient's inpatient episode, can be retrieved on the VDU or printout to assist with the evaluation of patient care and with the nurses' teaching programme. A cumulative history of nursing care since admission can be displayed at Birmingham in start date order with the facility to page through all orders. At Dundee, an individual printed summary of care is produced as required and on discharge, for insertion into the patient's medical records folder and for use by the community nursing service. The care is grouped in a similar manner to that used on the Exeter care plan, where a copy of the care plan on the day of discharge is forwarded, if required, to the community nurse.

2.5   Effects and Consequences of Computerised Nursing Records

As parts of the DHSS experimental programme, the nursing systems at Exeter and Birmingham have been evaluated (D6) using a predetermined set of criteria (1) covering both before and after the introduction of the computer system. This evaluation established that the main effects of computerisation are:-

-   the care plans are more accurate and complete; more precise and detailed than before,

-   the use of non-approved abbreviations has been virtually eradicated,

-   care plans are now legible, and more consistent through the use of standard terminology,

-   the identity of the author of all entries is achieved,

-   where reporting exists, a complete record of care given is provided.

As a consequence of these improvements, computerisation has:-

-       enabled nurses to assess a patient's clinical condition more easily,

-       reduced the possibility of an order being misinterpreted,

The computer system does take slightly longer to maintain and update but this is more than compensated for by the increase in the number of orders being recorded, providing a more complete record.   In fact, it does seem that the effort required to maintain handwritten care plans to the level of completeness and accuracy achieved by computerisation would be greater than that required by the systems at Exeter and Birmingham.   There is no doubt that with the improvement in the quality, quantity and availability of individualised patient information, communication, co-ordination, continuity and monitoring of care have been enhanced.   There are numerous other benefits to nurses and nurse managers which can be derived from the computerised nursing record systems and the database of nursing care orders.   In particular, they can form the basis of a nurse patient dependency or workload information system providing a means of measuring care without additional nursing input.   Each hospital has tackled this application with varying degrees of success, and this information together with other accrued advantages is discussed in more detail in other articles within this publication.

2.6   The Nursing Process and the Computer

It will be recognised from the description of these computerised nursing care systems in the United Kingdom, that they fall short in their application to the total concept of the nursing process, to which the General Nursing Council is committed.   This reflects a recent statement of Ashworth & Castledene (2) 'while good nurses have used some parts of the nursing process to some extent in the past, it has rarely if ever been used systematically, completely, explicitly and documented.'

The nursing process is seen as the systematic planning of nursing care and the various stages in this concept are described as assessment (of the patient's needs and problem), planning (of care to meet these needs and problems), implementation (of the care plan), and evaluation (of care given and the patient's response to this care).   Essentially, the computer systems do not relate care to problems or define the expected outcome with target dates.

Many nurses familiar with using computer technology believe that the computer is the obvious answer to implementing the nursing process as they demand a systematic and logical approach to data entry and should, on the basis of the computer evaluation, ensure that less time is spent on documenting the process than at the present time with the handwritten records, and resolve some of the current clerical problems.

Like other hospitals (and in the community), nurses where these systems have been developed are investigating ways of implementing the process.   It is evident that the Exeter system has developed and integrated aspects of the process with some considerable success and, as a consequence, Exeter is now currently one of 12 participating centres in the WHO medium term research programme on the Nursing Process.   A pilot scheme has been in progress since Spring 1981 to compare the different techniques employed in the total care approach using wards with computer facilities and wards at another hospital using conventional methods.   At Birmingham, after nearly five years, the computerised nursing system is now being used as a back up to the nurses endeavours in implementing and understanding the principles of the nursing process and introducing patient assignment.   Meanwhile, as an aid to the educational programme for the nursing process, it is proposed to provide a list of problems indexed from activities of living. On selection of a problem, suggestions for nursing action and expected outcome will be displayed. Nurses will have access to this information on the VDU in the School of Nursing and wards.   These screens may then provide the framework of any future computerisation of the nursing process. Further research will take place at Dundee to investigate ways in which the computer might effectively be used in the implementaiton of the nursing process.

3.   Drug Information, Prescribing and Administration

Various approaches have been developed at Birmingham, Exeter and at the London Hospital within the experimental programme in which computers have been used to provide information on drugs to avoid patients receiving inappropriate, inaccurate or potentially dangerous drugs. Drug information systems have been implemented at Exeter and Birmingham (3).   Selection is achieved from an alphabetical index of approved and proprietary drug names and/or an index based on the British National Formulary which lists drugs according to their therapeutic use and pharmacological action. For each drug in the system, information displayed may include indications and action, contraindications, side effects, interactions, dose range and administration, available preparations, storage, and advice to patients on discharge.   At The London Hospital, drugs may be checked for known incompatibilities.   If incompatibilities exist for the two drugs selected, appropriate warnings are displayed.   Both these features have been integrated into a system for drug prescribing developed over a number of years in Birmingham which provides facilities for drug administration and pharmacy dispensing. (It is documented in some considerable detail within this publication.) Facilities were provided by the Dundee computer project where a feasibility study to facilitate drug handling in a medical ward took place about 7 years ago (F6). The system designed involved the ward pharmacist entering the prescription into a VDU replicating the prescription handwritten by the doctor on the usual prescription sheet.   In the pharmacy department, tabulations were produced to allow the preparation of a trolley of drugs packed in unit doses in a separate box for each patient. These tabulations were also produced before each drug round to permit the ward pharmacist to 'top up' the trolley stock. Before each round, the nurse received a drug round list and recorded the administration of the drug by affixing, in the space provided, an adhesive label from the unit pack. 'As required' drugs were printed once a day on a separate list. The ward pharmacist was responsible for recording drugs given on the handwritten prescription sheet.

A trial period of 6 months, showed that the system was a practical method of handling drugs in the ward, indicating that such benefits as a reduction in nurse workload and an improvement in the accuracy of administration could be expected.   However, deficiencies in response time and transcription errors were highlighted.

3.1   Prescribing

The Birmingham system attempts to improve the quality of prescribing by ensuring that the doctor has as much information as possible about the patient and proposed drug treatment at the time of prescribing and to reduce errors in drug administration by the provision of a clearly printed administration document.

As the doctor prescribes for his patients using the VDU in the ward sister's office, information about the drug is automatically displayed. The drug is then checked for contraindications and interactions. After each prescribing episode, a new prescription list is printed on the ward printer. Messages are printed in the pharmacy department when dispensing is required and prescription warnings are overridden.   The printed prescription list is used by nurses to give and

record the administration of drugs. A pilot trial of this prescribing system
took place during the summer of 1981 for 5 weeks in one medical ward.

When a doctor first prescribes he completes a drug questionnaire to collect
specific data about the patient which may effect subsequent drug therapy e.g.
hypersensitivities. The required drug is chosen using the same BNF index used
for the drug information system or from a list of drugs commonly used on the
patient's ward. 'An important information' screen is then displayed including
any relevant current clinical chemistry of haematology values from the
laboratory files so that an immediate comparison can be made between the warning
and the most up-to-date information about the patient. If the doctor continues
to prescribe the selected drug, it is automatically checked against the
patient's age, answers to the drug questionnaire, the patient's laboratory data
for contraindications and the patient's current drug treatment for interactions.
If any contra-indications are found these are displayed and the doctor is also
warned if the patient is receiving the same drug with the same or another
route/formulation. Prompted by the information and warnings the doctor may
decide to prescribe a different drug, but he may continue if he so wishes - no
restrictions are applied by the computer!

The prescription is completed by selecting, by number, details of dose and
frequency and any directions from a dose screen. If any details required are
not available, the doctor may proceed to a freetext screen. (Specialised
screens have been designed to allow doctors to prescribe cytotoxics,
increasing/decreasing doses of steroids, and insulin). Another facility exists
to enable doctors to prescribe drugs not in the system. When prescribing single
doses, one of several directions must be selected from the dose screen e.g. at
once, otherwise a single dose questionnaire is displayed on which the doctor
must choose an appropriate direction e.g. specific time. This is to assist
nurses in administration. Regular drugs are automatically scheduled by the
computer to the drug round times for the patient's ward according to the
frequency chosen e.g. 12H could be 0830 & 1700 hours. It was agreed that the
drug round times should more accurately reflect the times at which these occur
in practice except where drugs must be given at specific time intervals.

If the prescription is approved, the doctor may continue prescribing other drugs
or carry out other prescribing functions such as cancelling and amending
prescriptions, prescribing drugs to take out (TTO's) and represcribing. When a
dose is changed, the drug is rechecked as if it were a new prescription and the
new dose may be compared with the old to check for an excessive dose increment
or insufficient interval between increments. When prescribing TTO's or
represcribing all drugs are rechecked for contra-indications.

3.2. Administration

A new prescription list is printed when all changes to a patient's treatment
have been made, replacing any previous list in use. Controlled drugs are
printed once when first prescribed, on a separate list. Even though the doctor
may prescribe for a patient from another ward, the prescription list is always
printed in the patient's ward. The prescription list is similar to that used in
many hospitals and is familiar to ward staff at the Queen Elizabeth Hospital;
even the same colour as the handwritten sheet has been used so that it is easily
recognisable. Each prescription list is identified with the patient's details,
list number and date and time of printing, and any hypersensitivites are printed
at the top of the first page. As the list may continue over more than one page,
the page number is given together with a message at the bottom of each page.
Prescriptions include those for single doses 'as required' drugs, regular drugs,
drugs with frequent dose changes and discharge drugs. Cancelled drugs are
printed only on the list produced after cancellation.

Before each drug round, the nurse collects any new prescription lists from the printer and places them on the drugs trolley. Lists of more than one page are stapled together. On the pilot ward, prescription lists were held on a clipboard at the end of the patient's bed. It was agreed that this should continue when the computer system was introduced. During the drug round, the nurse initials drugs given in the boxes provided. Boxes are blanked out with 'X's to indicate to the nurse when the prescription is to start/or finish if appropriate. The date, time and dose is printed in the boxes for increasing/decreasing doses and some cytotoxic regimes. The number of boxes for controlled drugs is restricted to the number of doses specified and each dose is numbered.

If the patient has a new prescription list, the nurse first checks the old sheet to ensure that all drugs were given on the previous round and to ascertain when the last 'as required' drug was given. The old sheet is then placed inside a clear plastic pocket folder on top of any previous sheets. Drugs checked and given are signed for and the new sheet placed outside but on top of the plastic folder which are then put back onto the clipboard. If any confusion should arise as to which is the current list, information on the most up-to-date list is available on the VDU.

The printing of messages in the pharmacy department ensures that no prescription list leaves the ward and provides an additional safeguard when drugs are prescribed partly or completely in freetext or when the doctor has overridden warning messages to prescribe the drug.

Approval was given by the Home Office to allow the doctor to use his log-in code or password as his signature, as in hospital, he writes an order to nursing staff to supply to the patient. This does not apply when prescribing drugs to take out as the order is written to a pharmacist. Therefore, local procedures were agreed to test out during the pilot trial.

3.3. Advantages and Disadvantages of Computerbased Prescribing

As with the nursing systems, the drugs system was evaluated after the trial involving medical, nursing and pharmacy staff. Nurses and pharmacists were generally pleased with the system whilst medical staff were concerned with certain aspects. The main effects of computerisation would appear to be as follows:-

- the prescription lists are clear and well laid out,
- prescriptions are legible and complete with specific administration times applicable to the ward drug round times.
- represcribing and prescribing TTO's are easier to accomplish
- it is a useful education tool,
- the warning messages assist in deciding the appropriate drug,
- prescribing is said to be safer.

The disadvantages are considered to be as follows:-

- prescribing is more time consuming and takes place away from the patient (routine practice in many surgical wards),
- the printers operate too slowly (a system constraint) to allow the doctor's to check the prescription list,
- important information and warnings need to be more selective (particularly for more experienced medical staff),
- the computer system is not available 24 hours, and is sometimes unreliable and prescribing cannot take place in the Accident/Emergency department.

Although these problems are recognised and some have already been resolved, this trial has demonstrated that a computerised drug prescribing system is viable. It is planned to extend the trial into other wards, in particular a surgical ward, so that prescribing of post operative drugs using the VDU's in the operating theatres can be assessed. Further evaluation studies will prove whether it is acceptable throughout the hospital and establish whether using a real-time system, the clinician can be adequately influenced to modify his choice of drug, dose and route of administration before the prescription is finalised.

4. Patient Monitoring and Other Systems

Several computer systems have been introduced into specialist units caring for the critically ill patient although the approach used has varied as in other spheres of the health service. Most have been developed elsewhere in other countries and modified to the U.K. users requirements and/or are available as commercial packages.

Typical of these systems are those at the Coronary Care Unit, Burton Road Hospital, Burton-on-Trent(E15) and the Cardio-thoracic Unit at Killingbeck Hospital, Leeds, where they use computerised monitors. The latter generates alarms to alert staff to significant or abnormal ventricular arrhythmia by using colour codes on the monitor.

At Killingbeck Hospital, the Oxford Medical Computerised Patient Monitoring system is being evaluated and compared with the standard 'Kontron' monitor. The monitors use the following facilities; ECG, measurement of blood pressure, one other selected pressure and cardiac output, and display of two temperatures. VDU's at the central station can display information from the bedside monitors and give 8 hour trends. A wide range of alarm conditions may be generated which are indicated by a flashing message on the command module at the bedside and at the central station. There are also optional audio alarms. When specific values fall outside set limits, e.g. heart rate, these will also flash on the command module and at the central station. The evaluation seeks to determine if ccomputers can provide a more comprehensive and reliable form of monitoring. Future studies include assessing closed-loop therapy.

Many hospitals in the U.K. now use automatic data processing within their laboratories to process requests as quickly and efficiently as possible with a high degree of accuracy. Laboratory results, essential to the ward team to assist them in decision making and evaluating care may be printed individually in a standard format. At several of the hospitals in the experimental programme with a real-time information systems these results are communicated faster, and displayed and printed in cumulative form so that significant trends in a patient's condition can be easily recognised. Abnormal results may be highlighted, with standard deviations according to sex and age and confidence limits provided. X-ray reports are also displayed at The London Hospital.

Other information, like drug information, which can be readily updated and easily retrieved on a VDU and/or printout, can assist nurses and other staff in their delivery of care such as nursing procedures (Exeter & Birmingham) and various laboratory and X-ray tests and investigations.

5. The Future

Progress in the development of computer systems to aid nurses with giving patient care within hospital has been slow. There are many reasons for this but probably one of the most important is finance and will continue to be so in the foreseeable future. The nursing systems were mostly developed on costly mainframe computers as an integral part of a hospital information system, but with the advent of cheaper small mainframes, minis and microcomputers, development and maintenance should be less expensive. Another factor is that resources in terms of systems and programming staff have often been delayed due to the priority given to other systems such as laboratories. Whilst as a general philosophy patient administration systems should be implemented first to provide patient identification, they have taken so long to develop in the past that other systems have suffered. Furthermore, with systems directly involved with patient care, particularly drug prescribing and administration, the amount of time required to design, program and then test the system should not be underestimated. Testing must be extremely thorough to ensure that patient lives are not in danger as a consequence of the computer system.

Computers can create additional problems when introduced into the ward situation. Training and supporting staff in the effective use of the systems can be time-consuming particularly when learner nurses are continually changing hospitals in which only one hospital has computing facilities. Unreliability and non-availability of the computer hardware can be very frustrating particularly as machines wear out and the necessary paper back up can cause confusion and irritation.

Whilst recognising these problems this should not prevent us from progressing further. In the present economic climate this is obviously not going to be easy. The original experimental programme was discontinued in the late 70's with responsibility for computing devolved to the Regions. A NHS Computer Policy Committee is now established to oversee national computing projects, although it does have funds at its disposal for further research and development.

It is envisaged that with the introduction of patient administration systems into District Health Authorities in the next few years, the possibility of extending further computer systems into the wards becomes a reality providing nurses grasp this opportunity. Other but cheaper solutions on microcomputers may well be developed by innovative nurse managers co-operating with computer specialists.

6.   Conclusion

Computers can aid nurses in the delivery of care. Nurses must work together to ensure, that as a profession, computer technology is developed to its full potential to the benefit of both patients and nurses. There is a need to critically examine current nursing practice and determine which patient care functions can be assisted with computers. It is the nursing profession's responsibility to ensure that it is involved in the planning, direction and control of future nursing systems.

Furthermore, it should be possible for experiences gained from the three U.K. nursing record systems to be incorporated into a standardised nursing record system enabling nurses to use the computer as an aid to the nursing process.

References

1.   D.H.S.S. (CR3C) London, Performance Criteria Project Report, March 1978,
2.   Ashworth P.M., & Castledine G., Nursing - Using the Nursing Process, Medical Teacher, vol 3 No 3 1981
3.   Beeley L., A real-time drug information system to assist prescribing - Computer aid to drug therapy and drug monitoring, 1978, 261-268. IFIP North Holland Publishing Company.

The Impact of Computers on Nursing
M. Scholes, Y. Bryant and B. Barber (eds.)
Elsevier Science Publishers B.V. (North-Holland)
© IFIP-IMIA, 1983

5.5.

PLANNING AND CONTROLLING PATIENT CARE WITH THE EXETER SYSTEM

Alison E. Head

1.   Introduction

The role of a nurse is to care for patients and systems designed to assist her must ensure that the majority of her time is still spent with the patients. For the care to be appropriate and effective, it must be planned using information received from the patient, from other nurses, doctors and others in the Health Care team. This information will be either verbal or from the Nursing Record and this requires that the Nursing Record must be an effective means of communication.

Methods of maintaining the Nursing Record have been the subject of continuous discussion during the last decade. In 1970 the Department of Health and Social Security accepted a proposal to computerise the Nursing Record as a part of the Exeter Community Health Services computer project, which covered not only Hospital but General Practitioner systems. These systems have proved so successful that all the parts of them are now running on replacement computers which should ensure their availability in the late eighties.

2.   Approach

With an on-line interactive computer system covering the patient's record from GP, through hospital administration to the ward, a strict password system was an essential prerequisite. This led to the concept of individual passwords each with their unique identity number, users initials and individually set access rights.

It was recognised that the use of the computer by nurses was only a means of achieving a clearer and fuller Nursing Record. Consequently, great emphasis was placed on designing a system which is largely self-teaching. It does not rely on nurses remembering codes, but nevertheless it allows short cuts if their familiarity with the system enables them to use these. The problems inherent in training nurses, both trained staff and learners, to use a computer system, while respecting the confidentiality of patient information, led to a completely fictitious training ward being available to anyone entering the training password of 100000.

Nursing care plans are patient oriented and printed copies, requested via ward visual display units, are produced on locally situated printers (one patient per page). Lists for night reports, diets and IV's are also available on request. Since nursing records can be required for legal purposes all input has the nurse's identity and initials automatically generated from the nurse's password. The system enables nurses to use predetermined, ward specific, profiles of care such as the care in fig 1 as well as to set up specific detailed care selected from screens of the type shown in fig 2.

FIGURE 1: Emergency Admission Screen

```
------------------------------------------------------------------------
| 81 Emergency Admission                                                |
|                                                                       |
|                                                                       |
| Accept orders below from        Today, Tomorrow   or Date    WRONG    |
|                                                                       |
| INTRAVENOUS FLUIDS AS                                                 |
| PRESCRIPTION SHEET.............   (  )      (  )    ( .01.82)   (  )   |
| FLUID CHART FOR BALANCE........   (  )      (  )    ( .01.82)   (  )   |
| RECORD TEMPERATURE, PULSE,                                            |
| BLOOD PRESSURE 4 x DAILY.......   (  )      (  )    ( .01.82)   (  )   |
| RECORD PULSE HOURLY............   (  )      (  )    ( .01.82)   (  )   |
| RECORD WEIGHT..................   (  )      (  )    ( .01.82)   (  )   |
| ROUTINE URINE TEST............    (  )      (  )    ( .01.82)   (  )   |
| MIDSTREAM SPECIMEN OF URINE....   (  )      (  )    ( .01.82)   (  )   |
| PASS NASO-GASTRIC TUBE,?.......   (  )      (  )    ( .01.82)   (  )   |
| CHECK CONSENT FORM.............   (  )      (  )    ( .01.82)   (  )   |
| SHAVE.........................    (  )      (  )    ( .01.82)   (  )   |
| PREMEDICATION.................    (  )      (  )    ( .01.82)   (  )   |
| NOTHING BY MOUTH, TILL SEEN BY                                        |
| DR............................    (  )      (  )    ( .01.82)   (  )   |
| PREPARE FOR THEATRE............   (  )      (  )    ( .01.82)   (  )   |
| INFORM RELATIVES OF PROCEDURE..   (  )      (  )    ( .01.82)   (  )   |
| *<<GENERAL HYGIENE>>...........   (  )      (  )    ( .01.82)   (  )   |
| *<<FACIAL HYGIENE>>............   (  )      (  )    ( .01.82)   (  )   |
| *<<PRESSURE AREA & SORE CARE>>.   (  )      (  )    ( .01.82)   (  )   |
------------------------------------------------------------------------
```

FIGURE 2: Ward Test Screen

```
------------------------------------------------------------------------
| )BILL J JONES           URINE TESTS (WARDS)                          |
|                                                                      |
|                              :19 2 x weekly on [day 1, day 2]        |
|                              :20 weekly on [day]                     |
|             1. ROUTINE       :30 daily                               |
|             2. FOR BILIRUBIN :31 2 x daily                           |
|             3. FOR BLOOD     :32 before meals                        |
|             4. FOR PROTEIN   :33 [?]-hourly                          |
| URINE       5. FOR SALICYLATES :34 Teach patient                    |
| TEST        6. FOR SUGAR & KETONE :35 Teach relative                |
|                BODIES        :36 If positive test with ferric        |
|             7. FOR UROBILINOGEN    chloride                          |
|             8. FOR SPECIFIC GRAVITY :37 At [?]-hours                 |
|             9. FOR PROTEIN (ESBACHS) :38 Every specimen             |
|            11. FOR KETONES   :39 At night                            |
|            12. FOR ACID/ALKALINITY (pH) :40 At [?,?,?,?,?,?]-hours   |
|            13. FOR SUGAR     :41 At 0600- hours                      |
| 10. FILTER ALL URINE         :42 At Nappy Changes                    |
|                              :43 If possible, blood glucose          |
|                                  estimations                         |
|                              :44 Refer to insulin sliding            |
|                                  scale                               |
| 50 SERIES OF URINE SPECIMENS FOR COMPARISON                          |
| 51 24-HOUR COLLECTION FROM [?]-HOURS, IN PLAIN BOTTLE, FOR VOLUME,   |
|    DAILY                                                             |
|                                                                      |
| List additions (6,38                 )NO ADDITIONS()                 |
------------------------------------------------------------------------
```

3.   Current Position

Papers have already been published describing the Ward based nursing systems currently used in the 14 wards of the district general hospital in Exeter(C5,C12). These papers give outlines of the systems for admission and transfer, and examples of the systems for selection and amendment of nursing instructions (Orders) and for reporting that orders were carried out. The patient movement system provides a display of the ward layout which reflects the actual bed location and incidentally the number of vacant male, female or childrens beds. The discharge system automatically gives a discharge summary print containing current information. The handling of deleted information is also described.

The use of the admission, patient movement and discharge systems enables the system to produce daily bedstates without further nursing input.

The order and report systems enable the nurses to maintain up to date complete and legible records of all instructions on care to be given and confirmatory reporting that the care has been given. A basic virtue of the computer system is that it enables the current records of orders for one day to be carried over to the following day without the nurses needing to copy it across. Reporting times are reset each night after the current day's record of instructions and reporting has been written away for later writing to microfiche.

The nurse keeps the record up to date simply by adding new statements, by changing existing ones or by "deleting directly" or by "terminating tonight" any statements no longer required. In the last three cases, the statement no longer wanted in the "current" record is passed into the "deleted" record together with the initials and identity of the nurse deleting them and the time and date.

This continuing record with its reporting not only gives the team of nurses better control of their current activities, but provides a long term document which can be used to study the effectiveness of care and to help plan future care more effectively. The management uses of the system, for example obtaining workload information, are described in the paper by Jean Jarvis in Chapter 14. Some aspects of the system have been evaluated and have been described by Kimpel & Davis(D6).

4.   Future

Already more than half the wards using the nursing systems are looking at methods of documenting the care of patients in the manner now known widely as the nursing process.

Since a computer can so readily recall stored information, for instance the profiles of care which each ward compiled for their particular needs, we are now looking at the idea of each specialty and ward having their own libraries of problem orientated care appropriate to certain treatments and conditions. In order to discover the feasibility of this approach, a ward sister, the computer-liaison nurse, a tutor and the systems designer worked together to extract the problems, aims and care from some existing profiles, (for a dental extraction). It became clear that the care given could be separated into that which is common to General Anaesthesia (fig 3) and that which is particular to the dental extraction (fig 4). Currently we are looking at ways of presenting this information both ·as a teaching aid and for inclusion in the patients specific care plans. Figures 3 and 4 show tentative screen designs from which nurses might select the phrases appropriate for a particular patients care plan.

FIGURE 3: Sample Screen for Anaesthesia

```
--------------------------------------------------------------------------------
!                                                                              !
!                          General Anaesthesia                                 !
!                                                                              !
! P-FEAR, APPREHENSION            A-reduce tension & pain                       !
! ( ) EXPLAIN PROCEDURE                                                        !
! ( ) INFORM RELATIVES OF PROCEDURE                                            !
! ( ) PREMEDICATION AT [?]-HOURS                                               !
!                                                                              !
! P-IDENTIFICATION, LEGAL CONSENT, PHYSICAL SAFETY ETC                         !
!                              A-perform reasonable checks                      !
!                                                                              !
! ( ) COMPLETE PRE-OP CHECK LIST (Identiband, consent form, prostheses,        !
!     false teeth)                                                             !
!                                                                              !
! P-SAFETY DURING & POST-OP     A-reduce danger of vomiting, avoid             !
!                               excessive period of starvation.                !
!                                                                              !
! ( ) NOTHING BY MOUTH FROM [?]-HOURS                                          !
!     Premedication as above                                                   !
!                                                                              !
! P-AIRWAY MAINTENANCE          A-ensure availability of suction and           !
!                               oxygen.                                        !
! ( ) CHECK SUCTION & OXYGEN                                                   !
!                                                                              !
! P-CHANGE IN PATIENT'S CONDITION                                              !
! ( ) RECORD TEMPERATURE, PULSE, BLOOD PRESSURE [?]-HOURLY                      !
!                                                                              !
--------------------------------------------------------------------------------
```

FIGURE 4: Sample Screen for Dental Extraction

```
--------------------------------------------------------------------------------
!                          Dental Extraction                                   !
! P-BLEEDING                    A-observe for signs of bleeding, reduce inherent !
!                               danger                                         !
!                                                                              !
! ( ) OBSERVE CHEEK PACK ON RETURN & [?]-HOURLY                                !
!                                                                              !
! ( ) OBSERVE FOR BLEEDING FROM GUMS [?]-HOURLY                                !
!                                                                              !
! ( ) OBSERVE FOR EXCESSIVE SWALLOWING [?]-HOURLY                              !
!                                                                              !
!                                                                              !
! P-MOUTH DISCOMFORT            A-relieve discomfort                            !
! ( ) ICE TO SUCK                                                              !
! ( ) SIPS OF WATER                                                            !
!                                                                              !
! P-PAIN                        A-relieve/control                              !
! ( ) SOLUBLE ASPIRIN AND OMNOPON AS REQUIRED                                  !
!                                                                              !
--------------------------------------------------------------------------------
```

5.   Conclusion

The system currently running at The Royal Devon & Exeter Hospital (Wonford), Exeter was designed before there was widespread discussion of the "nursing process". Our patient orientated care plan of Nursing Orders was even viewed with scepticism because the task sheet for all patients was still the norm in many hospitals. Despite its early design, the Exeter system is proving remarkably flexible in use with the nursing process. The idea of a problem orientated patient care plan which was first mooted in 1979 by a forward looking nursing officer is at last under general review, the subject having this time been raised by the ward nurses themselves. This shows very clearly what so many research nurses are now discovering - the enormous time span needed to bring about first, acceptance that change is needed, and then discussion of concrete proposals in a constructive atmosphere.

Researchers have voiced the opinion that such a radical new approach as the nursing process is going to take a decade or more to be accepted. We suggest that the move from Kardex to a computer aided nursing system presented a similarly radical change. Once established, however, it is clear that such systems have considerable potential for helping nurses in the process of identifying problems, establishing aims, formulating care plans and enabling total evaluation from the complete record (including all changes and amendments). It can also minimise the purely clerical difficulties which those using manual systems of recording are currently encountering.

The Impact of Computers on Nursing
M. Scholes, Y. Bryant and B. Barber (eds.)
Elsevier Science Publishers B.V. (North-Holland)
© IFIP-IMIA, 1983

5.6.

THE COMPUTER AS AN AID TO IMPROVING PATIENT CARE

Margaret Griffiths

1.   Introduction

Virginia Henderson, Research Association Emenities, Yale University School of Nursing has encapsulated the unique role of the nurse as follows:-

'This function is to help persons sick or well from birth to death with those activities of daily living that they would perform unaided if they had the strength, the will and the knowledge. At the same time and throughout this relationship nurses help people gain or regain their independance, when independance is impossible, to cope with handicaps and irreversible disease and finally to help others die with dignity when death is inevitable.'

In order to help nurses perform this function, technology has a part to play by freeing them from some repetitive tasks so that they can spend more time in the actual planning, giving and evaluation of our nursing care.

Some hospital staff, including some nurses, feel that to nurse patients with the aid of a computer somehow detracts from a patient's care or that the computer is directing the nurse how to work. This is not borne out by the practical experience of a ward sister in charge of a 30 bed ear, nose and throat (ENT) and ward at the Queen Elizabeth Hospital, Birmingham, U.K.

As well as ENT and oral surgery cases, a large proportion of the patients admitted have head and neck cancer, needing a combination of treatments; surgery, radiotherapy and chemotherapy. The ward is highly specialised and the patient turnover high (between thirty and forty patients per week). The computer is an efficient tool with certain limitations but it can be of considerable assistance.

The ward sister's main responsibility is to ensure that the patients receive the best possible care with the resources available. In order to achieve this the nurses, especially the learners, need some form of guidance in the planning of the appropriate care(1,2). The computerised nursing system at the Queen Elizabeth Hospital assists by providing an up-to-date, daily, legible nursing care plan.

2.   Queen Elizabeth Medical Centre Computer Project

This project was established in 1969 and by the end of 1973 the first system - patient and administration - was implemented, providing a basic framework for all subsequent systems.

The computer system provides a service for those hospitals within the Central Birmingham District Health Authority although the facilities are concentrated at the Queen Elizabeth Hospital. The real-time system uses visual display units (VDU's) and printers linked to a Univac 418 - 111 currently operational from 05.00 - 23.00 hours. At the Queen Elizabeth Hospital, VDU's are located in each ward in the sister's office and most other departments. There is one VDU for 30 beds.

Printers can be found in the medical records department for documentation purposes.

3.   Nursing Orders System

3.1   System Development

In 1969/70 research was done on the ways in which nursing records were kept. It was found that there were various work books, sheets, a variety of charts and odd slips of paper which together with the Kardex formed the nursing records system for the patient's stay in hospital.

As a result of these investigations, it was recognised that the recording system was in need of improvement and that these improvements could be made by using a computer. As the experimental computer project was already established and the patient administration system operational, a nurse user group comprising representatives of nursing and computer staff was established to design a 'real-time' nursing record system whose major objective was to improve the recording procedure. This was to be done by producing a daily nursing care list for each ward. It would be printed each evening from the line printer in the computer room for distribution to the wards by the evening portering staff. This would provide a framework for the nurse to work within whilst encouraging her to plan and give total care. It would also help to standardise the documentation - thus would be of special benefit to the learners when changing wards.

A colleague was a member of the Nurse User Group (NUG) and thus the ENT ward was 'volunteered' to take part in a three ward pilot scheme, which started in October 1977. The immediate reaction was one of scepticism and after being shown how to use the nursing system not all this scepticism had vanished! However, the trial was agreed.

Obviously in order for the system to be useful it needed to be speedy, efficient and flexible. It also had to be quicker than previous methods.

The design of the system was based on several fundamental principles which were common to all ward-based systems and helped in achieving those aims:

-       a tree-branching system was used so it was unnecessary to learn and memorise codes or tables.

-       typing ability was not necessary as, except for typing numbers and leaving spaces, little typing was actually done.

-       instructions were given at the bottom of each screen as to how to proceed or, if an error has been made, how to correct it.

-       there was a confirmation screen display so that you could check any information you were entering or deleting from the system.

3.2   Nursing Orders Entry

In order to produce the plan, the nursing system is updated at least daily e.g. after doctors' rounds, operating lists or in the afternoon to review all the patients' care.

To operate the system the nurse, like any other user of the real-time system, types her personal 'log-in' code of six characters. This code controls the use the nurse can make of the system, ensures confidentiality and automatically associates the nurse's name with every record she enters.

The ward list of patients is first brought up to date, any discharges are recorded and new patients allocated their bed number, so that the nursing care list is printed in bed rather than alphabetical order.

The patient in the first bed space is selected, his orders are checked and amended if necessary. The orders, from which the nurse can choose, are either on a series of ward screens which contain all the most frequently used orders; or classified screens, which contain a collection of all types of orders available. If the order is not exactly as the nurse requires, e.g. a complicated dressing, there is a free-text screen on which she can type in the exact order needed. The confirmation screen is then shown and the order confirmed or cancelled as desired. By typing the appropriate number, the next patient is selected and so on for all the patients in the ward.

3.3   Training

The staff had already received training in using the visual display units prior to the implementation of the patient administration system. As the nursing system was designed based on the same tree-branching system, training for this was only needed for the extra screens.

3.4   Benefits

The trial started and once everyone got used to using the system its benefits became apparent - there was produced a clear, easily read, plan of care for each patient which provided up-to-date information on the patients' basic and specialised care. It made the learner consider the patients total care and was more explanatory than a handwritten plan. It provided terminology in full, using only recognised abbreviations and was quicker to provide than a handwritten plan(3).

During the introduction of the system, the computer unit staff were always available if there were any problems and were very willing to listen to any comments on how the system could be improved e.g. the sequence of screens was altered, additional orders were automatically cancelled to reduce the time spent at the VDU.

The computer printout replaced all other lists and books in the ward and together with the Nursing Kardex was the only record used thus decreasing duplication and saving time for the nurse.

As well as the production of the care plan, the nursing orders system can be used as a teaching tool. If, after a clinical session; the nurse is asked to use the computer to plan a patients care the effectiveness or otherwise of the teaching can be measured!(C3,D6).

4.   Information Systems

Information systems are included as part of the hospital system and provide structured pages of up-to-date information. These are of value as an aide memoire to nurses and other staff on the ward.

The drug information presented includes available strengths, form and recommended doses, contraindications, interactions, adverse effects and instructions for special circumstances. These screens are especially useful when preparing learners for their drug assessments.

The clinical chemistry information system provides a comprehensive reference manual which includes normal reference values, guidance on result interpretation, instructions on procedures etc.

Bacteriology gives the latest information on isolated organisms and the related antibiotic sensitivities as well as various procedures.

Histopathology and psychiatric information is also available.

All laboratory procedures are particularly useful when nurses have not carried them out before or do so infrequently.

Ward and unit profile information gives details about the general activities of wards and provides some indication of ward and unit workload. It has proved useful to new personnel joining the ward staff, particularly learners.

The nursing procedure manual is now available on the system.

5. Patient Administration Procedures

5.1 Patient Enquiry

Registration information is available to all authorised users. This is of benefit to ward staff in answering questions from relatives at visiting time or handling telephone enquiries.

5.2 Requesting of Labels

Labels are a time saving facility produced automatically for all registered inpatients and outpatients. Further supplies of labels can be requested via the ward VDU.

5.3 Waiting List

A simple waiting list system is available for the ENT consultants. This is a batch system, although now they are using it, would much prefer it to be in real-time. One of our new consultants is very anxious to buy a mini computer for the department in order to computerise his head and neck cancer statistics and use them in research.

6. Future Developments

From the point of view of a ward sister, the next most useful development would be:-

- the provision of individual problem orientated nursing care plans

- a nursing discharge summary for use by the community nurse and/or to be filed in the medical records folder

- information on nursing workload

- an off-duty system

6.1 Nursing Workload

The need for efficient nursing dependency studies is essential. It is strange that in 1982 there is no uniformally accepted formula for working out staffing levels for each ward. There is no totally acceptable scientific data to uphold a sister or nursing managers opinion as to the

correct workload staff ratio.   At QE, some work has already been done
concerning nursing dependency using nursing orders and timings to attempt
to produce some workload figures.

If, by producing a dependency system, each wards' daily workload could be
measured and the off-duty was also available on the VDU, then any
abnormalities could be identified and corrected straight away, e.g. at the
start of the morning shift, the allocation of an emergency pool could be
carried out by the nursing officers with the information on the system
plus the up-to-date information given by the night sisters.   A more
scientific basis could then be used for staff allocation.

6.2   Off-duty System

It would seem prudent to produce a computerised off-duty system eg. as
used in Fairview Hospital, Cleveland, Ohio.   This would assist in staff
allocation and perhaps reduce some of the anomalies which occur with
present rota systems. It may be doubted whether any computer system can
successfully come to terms with the intricacies of a nurse's social life
but as nurses become more expensive to employ, a more efficient method of
off-duty planning is needed.   It   should improve their job satisfaction
and provide a better staff-patient ratio.   Although weekly or monthly
amendment of a masterplan may be needed, managers need to give the
learners and qualified staff more realistic duty rotas.

6.3   Statistics

The production of statistics on which Miss Nightingale laid so much stress
is far easier to produce using a computer.

One wonders if she would have been as reticent as some of our present
nurse managers in using this form of technology.

6.4   Ordering

The ordering of supplies, menus etc. could be done by means of the VDU at
ward level.   This should cut down on cost in the long term and improve
delivery time.

7.   **Disadvantages**

As with any other system the computer does have its drawbacks, one of which is
the response time which can vary depending on the time of day.

Obviously maintenance work has to be carried out on the hardware but wards are
notified in advance and a back-up system is provided.

As the real time sytem is not available twenty four hours a day there is some
delay in the registration of emergency admissions between 9 p.m. and 9 a.m.
hence some duplication of documentation at ward level exists.

8.   **Conclusion**

The Computer has now become very much part of the day to day management of the
ward.   It saves time for both nurses and doctors by the production of up-to-date
information in an easily available format.

Five years use of the computer based nursing system has dispelled the initial
reservations and it is now clear that computers have a great part to play in
nursing both now and in the future.

However, the unique role of the nurse can never be substituted by any kind of machinery be it computer or otherwise. The nurse should treat them as useful tools, never as a replacement for her art!

REFERENCES

1. Brown, W; (1965) What is work? Glacier project papers, Heinemann.
2. Pembrey, S; (1980) The ward sister-key to nursing; RCN.
3. Davis, A; Williams, R;   Evaluation of the Queen Elizabeth Computer Project: The Nursing Orders System Computer Evaluation Team (November 1980)

The Impact of Computers on Nursing
M. Scholes, Y. Bryant and B. Barber (eds.)
Elsevier Science Publishers B.V. (North-Holland)
© IFIP-IMIA, 1983

5.7.

INFORMATICS AND CLINICAL NURSING RECORDS

John Anderson

Introduction

There have been significant developments in clinical nursing records during the past two decades, not only in relation to changes in input content and methods but also in the usefulness of the output for assessing the many aspects of the effectiveness of patient care. Nursing records have always had an administrative basis with a record being kept of patient admission and discharge from the beds in a ward. The KARDEX System has been the main part of the clinical record. It has had several changes over the years but has proved its worth. Indeed nursing documentation in many hospitals was included with the medical record for archiving, as a support for what happened if there were subsequent medicolegal problems.

The nursing record has had a variable relationship to the medical record. There have been significant differences in the nursing record on both sides of the Atlantic in that so-called doctors orders and procedures for transferring requests for investigation and treatment have had a different emphasis. There has been much more emphasis on the ward team in the United Kingdom, especially in the care of the elderly, where the clinical problems are both complex and involved decisions about priorities as well as improved communication between the team, family, relatives and friends.

For many years patient communication and education has been by word of mouth. Only recently has greater emphasis been put on patient participation - a very necessary development as this encourages patient needs to be expressed and some attempt has then to be made to meet them. Nurses have been more involved in this than doctors because of their 24 hour contact. Unfortunately, not always has the team been well orchestrated in this direction. Thus the stresses and strains on the verbal system are becoming more apparent with the shorter working week. Thus verbal and written methods of communication between professionals and the patient are necessary. Also better methods of allowing patients to participate and play an anticipatory role in care can be made by means of patient diaries. The potential of such improvements and change has yet to be fully realised but relates to the nursing record as well as to the medical record.

Assisting Nursing Clinical Record Computerisation

One of the important features of any record is the degree of acceptance of formalisation to ensure that the view of the record and its contents is the same for those who create and use it. In nursing because of the need for 24 hour cover, 7 days a week, there has always been a much greater effort at formalisation than with the medical record. This relates not only to the number of users but because nursing needs an established and recognised set of procedures if optimal care is to be given. The weakest area has been the transfer of data and activities from the medical to the nursing record for execution. While documentation has improved, the medical record has not necessarily been well designed from the view-point of transferability of data.

Furthermore, documentation has had to be improved especially in the important field of the patient's therapy.

Undoubtedly better documentation has both improved the efficiency and effectiveness of care and also has carried with it the implication of better training. The investigation of the purposes and activities of nursing have become a subject of interest. The resultant enquiry has lead to the present attention to the nursing process and outcome of care. The evaluation of patient care involves investigating the structures, process and outcome of those things that effect the care process. The use of the already developed techniques of systems analysis and design have a bearing here and have given some frameworks for the exploration of these important areas which affect patient care.

There have been significant shifts in the structures involved in nursing and the managerial responsibilities of the nurse in the past half century. The ward sister's role has changed from that of being 'king in her own castle' and complete 'ward manager' to that of having some of her managerial roles taken by hospital and nursing administrators and some of her supervisory tasks changed. This process has been gradual but has had its effects on the nursing record and its relationships to the medical record and to the ward team. While the training of the nursing sister in the past was more 'on the job' than in the classroom the tendency has been to reverse this balance. There have been concomitant changes in the relationships of the senior nurses to the medical team and the medical record.

Also other paramedical staff have come increasingly to take over certain tasks such as physiotherapy, occupational therapy, social work and there also have been house-keeping assistants and clerks, changing the responsibility of some of the people who carry out such tasks on the ward. In this way nursing has been more able to concentrate on the clinical aspects of care and its management. This has increased interest in developing formalisation of both procedures and the nursing record. Inevitably these factors must relate to standardisation on a larger scale. The General Nursing Council has at least helped in this as well as the World Health Organisation. Evaluation will not be accomplished easily or effectively and at reasonable cost unless some standardisation is achieved.

A major factor for the change in nursing records has been the acceptance of nursing activities in response to new challenges. All are conscious of the new extent of the difficulties of reaching a high standard of nursing and in evaluating outcomes. Thus changes that might improve this have been welcomed. There has also been a feeling that technology has not necessarily been distasteful and many willingly accepted the challenge of change. In comparison with the difficulties reported in relation to the medical record, the nursing record has rightly pursued a different path. Because of this there is a tendency to load all possible data onto the nursing system for administrative and other purposes. This is not necessarily appropriate to the development of nursing records in the future. It is important to go on asking questions and to ensure that the spirit of inquiry persists. Better research effort into nursing records will certainly help to resolve these potential difficulties.

Finally the need for better communication between nurses in their performance of their many-sided tasks cannot be underestimated. The traditional handover can be a difficult task if there are many complicated patients. Thus the availability of written support for procedures and tests to be done and a record of what has been done is vital to this process. Clinical observations are also important and need to be made available to medical staff and the medical record through nursing record. As there are several steps in such communication processes, the possibility for error is always present. Techniques which can reduce this and highlight potential error situations are both useful and supportive. In this role informatics can help.

Finally, now that computer systems are being implemented it is possible to store references to standard procedures and tasks, so that junior nurses can refurbish their memories if necessary. Thus junior nurses with informatic support could transfer between different areas of nursing and use the system to support different tasks and procedures as necessary. The development of knowledge bases and expert systems has, as yet, had little impact on nursing. However, this is likely to be a temporary phenomenon and related to research effort.

Development of Nursing Informatics Record Systems

It is nearly two decades ago that computerised records of nursing tasks began. The first approach considered was that of formal documentation with data being recorded into a computer in batch mode for access later. To a certain extent this was due to the limitations of the then available computer hardware and software systems. Many difficulties have been overcome with the development of real time, online access sytems. Such interactive systems are essential for medical and nursing records. They are advantageous in that the health care personnel, who both enter and use data, have the system to guide them by means of its data flows and also the system can be programmed for error checks on the data that is entered. These factors have, in addition to well designed terminal interaction, encouraged nursing staff to enter data rapidly and accurately. It is important to ensure that the recorded data is accurate for subsequent analysis, otherwise only obvious conclusions can be drawn.

The first systems were designed to deal with the problems of ward administration including patient admission, discharge, movement about the ward and ward transfers. The next development was to allow nursing tasks to be initiated by sisters and staff nurses in charge of the ward for execution by the nursing team. These tasks could be carried out in different ways and different types of output were designed to meet the different care patterns, whether by job activity or nursing team activity. In this way the output was shown to be flexible and it could be adjusted to meet nursing and patient care needs. It also enabled the nursing staff to have an overall view of patient care on the ward. It was useful support for verbal handover procedures helping staff to concentrate on critical areas.

The Tunbridge Committee declared(1) that the nursing record should reflect the care given to each patient during their stay in hospital together with data about the progress and response to treatment. This recognised the previous status of nursing records which had long been kept with the medical record to deal with medico-legal problems. A systems analysis of the purposes and usage of the nursing record highlighted the many problems associated with written records. It also was important to design backup systems for later entry to the computer system so that there would be a comprehensive record which would be both reliable and effective. It became obvious that pen and paper techniques have their limitations, certainly in other systems the notes made on scraps of paper and many forms are unreliable. In order to achieve both accuracy and speed of analysis which will effect the on-going course of nursing care computerised records are necessary. It was certain at that time that few knew about the errors involved in the transfer of data and that the more transfers of data that took place the more likely was the chance of error. This may have been recognised unconciously by the supplementation of the KARDEX record with work books and sheets for fluid balance and urinary output, temperature charts and many other charts devised to meet different needs in different speciality areas of medicine.

The place of the verbal report in duty transfer is essential but its direction and content can be very different as well as its accuracy if there is appropriate informatics support. This fact not only reduces content in relation to objectives but means that time for the performance of patient care is increased. In practice systems analysts discovered that it was not always possible for all nurses to receive a detailed verbal report about all patients in their care before being called to give help to patients. Thus a new form of nursing record was essential to meet this problem. It was essential that the nurse should be able to interact with it usefully. It should always be up to date and accurate at any one time when it was accessed. In the early days, such information would be presented with job orientation view as a task to be allocated to a nurse or nursing team, depending on circumstances in a particular ward. Changes in the nursing process have brought about changes in the presentation of such information.

If the nursing record was to be kept up to date, be accessed and available quickly, then online interactive systems were essential. This means that the facilities provided by the information system had to change. The nursing record system implemented at Kings College Hospital in 1970 was the first of its kind in the UK (C3,C8,C16) and it showed that these techniques were at that time much more acceptable to nurses than they were to doctors. Unfortunately, this nursing system was taken down when DHSS support for the project was withdrawn. Much of the systems software written for this project was subsequently utilised for some very successful systems elsewhere.

The problems of interacting with a visual display unit created far less difficulties in relation to nursing than they did for the doctors with medical records. This may have been due to better system design and the already formalised nature of the nursing record. Also the interaction with computer systems undoubtedly captured the nurses' imagination and the system could be shown to have its advantages with speed of interaction resulting in improved nursing care, removing some of the previous major difficulties. These benefits were more easily recognisable in nursing than they were in medicine.

Output and the acknowledgement of tasks which have been completed does create some difficulties. At first, task acknowledgement was accepted by the nurses to enable better communication amongst the nursing team but many administrators tended to interfere with this facility using the information at levels, at which it was unimportant and at which problems could not be properly dealt with. It has been recognised that nursing staff are over-achievers, especially in relation to planning patient care. At King's College Hospital it appeared that only about 70-80% of tasks were fully implemented on the wards even when it was thought that the nursing complement was correct and appropriate. Medically it might be doubted if this concept of a full nursing complement is entirely valid. Under severe pressures, due to staff absence and illness, the number of tasks completed fell to just below a half of those ordered. For the medical staff this proved to be an interesting and direct method of determining nursing load. To others it appeared as inefficiency and poor ward nursing management. It created problems for the ward because of this attitude. However, this appears to be a universal problem in nursing. The same kind of result has been found, not only in the United Kingdom, but in the United States as well.

It is not necessary to explain menu systems for describing nursing tasks (see C5) except to highlight the necessity of adapting these to different areas in specialised nursing. Specialist nursing areas should be able to have their own special procedures and tasks and appropriate informatics support. Special procedures with the vital support, which computer systems can give, will render nursing applications more flexible. Considerable vision is required and some on the job training. Systems can be adapted to give advice and are undoubtedly very helpful in the more complicated areas of medicine, especially those in relation to care of the elderly.

Output, was at first not sophisticated nor tailored to the particular needs of individual patients, ward nurses, nursing sisters or administrators. It was not surprising originally, as the bulk of this had been done by clinical impression without job performance methodologies. This is now changing and there is emphasis and experience for appropriate, specialised, output to be used at many levels. Indeed with the progress on the nursing record, it is now out of phase with the medical record. For the medical record there will have to be a considerable catching up period.

What has also helped the acceptance of nursing informatics has been the continuing education of health service staff in computing. Using the experience at The London Hospital as an example(A3), the responsibility for nurse training, when the system was first implemented, was handled by the computer staff. However, with appropriate nurse training and teaching, this responsibility has with advantage been moved to nurse training. It has also enabled them not only to train new entrants but also to offer a service to those who have to catch up on the system who come to the hospital from other areas. Nursing staff are very mobile and a continuing education system is absolutely essential. This relies on different training responsibilites and appropriately places the responsibility on nurse training staff. These changes have been possible not only by creating the necesssary nursing links but also trying to meet the real needs of staff. Planning of the change has also been appropriate and this depends on the output of appropriate trained staff who can undertake such teaching.

The Development and Implementation of the Nursing Process

The resurgence of interest in nursing activities and in the nursing record, is a new emphasis on the elements of the nursing process. This changing emphasis has had an effect not only on nursing staff but nurse training. To some extent the changes have come about by questioning whether the nurse has become too distant from the patient, whether nursing has lost sight, by being too academic, of carrying out details of every day care and whether perhaps it takes less responsibility for hygiene and the physical and emotional comforts of the patient. It has been questioned by some that there may be a more academic approach to patient nursing, taking nurses away from the previous task orientated training approach. All this emphasizes the need for evaluation to determine the direction and the extent of change. The nursing process sets out to identify the individual patient problems and relate these to organisation and management difficulties. Both these areas have an effect on nursing services and the kind of care given. Thus the collection of patient data is a key issue and relates not only to the specific components of patient care but also to patients, their families and relatives, medical staff and administration.

Given appropriate data collection and recording of what has been done, it is then possible to review the specific components of nursing performance. Hopefully such data will be linked to indicators or indices of components of nursing performance which can be derived to improve the successful outcome of the patient care. This involves both standardised procedures and records. It is then possible to access the care of different patients and patient groups in relation to outcome. In this way a sample of care in different wards can be determined over time. By these means care can be evaluated and with it the achievement of different members of the nursing care team.

In the care of the elderly(D7), the nursing load tends to be both physically and psychologicaly heavy and where families, relatives and friends are intimately involved not only in data collection and co-ordination but in possible outcomes, especially the psychological and social components. Also it is more difficult because of the diverse problems. It is vital to encompass the necessary standardisation of vocabulary to convey all the physical, psychological and social aspects, the patient and his illness and also the relationships he has with his immediate friends and relatives and the community. This is very relevant data not only for the actual care of the patient on a day to day basis but for his return to the community. If it is possible, when the patient returns to the community, summaries of the hospital situation should be created so that the nursing team in the community can review and continue nursing care there.

In the care of the elderly the development of appropriate nursing care plans is complex but an important step. It is often possible for the appropriate care interventions to be planned before admission but if this is not possible it has to be done within the first 24 hours. The nursing record has not only to embrace the physical but also the psychological and social dimensions of the problems. First there must be links with doctors, physiotherapists and social workers who cover essential parts of the team activity so that a global therapeutic plan can evolve. It is also important to ensure that the patient can have a say in his treatment and that data will be made available to him and his relatives so that they can use it. For example, patients should be told of the patient care plan by means of a patient diary as soon as possible after admission.

Key issues need to be checked individually to see that they meet special patient needs and information has to be given to the patient's general practitioner, the practice nurse as well as relatives and friends of the patient. Social information may also be collected prior to admission which will guide the team in advising about the special features needing attention when the patient goes home. Psychological needs and the mental state of the patient must be assessed as well as physical care needs. This involves some formalisation of care which relates to the whole nursing care team involving doctors, physiotherapists, social workers etc. The standard vocabulary helps to ensure that problems are not overlooked.

It is also important to ensure that care needs are met by the care that is given. Certainly the better organisation of care given by a computer system helps in this direction. Nursing care decisions can be assisted by different types of expert program but the care plan must not be overloaded by trying to meet other people's needs. The advantage of having care plans is that they can be made available to the whole team and can be adapted to the changes in the patients condition. This is especially true in the psychological and social aspects which do change while care is being given. It is also important to ensure that the dementing patient is understood and his memory problems recognised so that repeated processes of support are undertaken.

Nursing communication must cover the feedback from the tasks undertaken in the care of patients and also must deal not only with the groups of professionals around the patient, but with relatives and friends. Records have to be kept of what the patient and the relatives have been told, especially in relation to prognosis and return to the community. In this way there may be an easier perception of patient need which enables it to be reconciled with the care given. Even for the elderly patient it is important to have their participation and the patient diary system is helpful. This is all the more useful in patients whose memories may be impaired. Also, it is necessary to chart fully the patient's mobility and continence through the day and night so that a total picture of their detailed abilities can be created. There is no doubt that patient encouragement by means of patient diaries is useful in creating the necessary motivation for recovery. The nursing discharge plan then becomes important to ensure the continuation of care after discharge. It also sets in motion an assessment of what has been achieved which can be derived from the patient's medical and nursing records.

Nursing performance and review are a check on the effectiveness of the care plan and can be related to the outcome for the patient. Adjustment of care plans to changing patient progress, is an essential part of the review of clinical care and vital to patient progress. Measurements of performance relative to the different aspects of care are especially important in the care of the elderly. Determination of nursing workload also has relevance and has to be related to nursing procedures undertaken by the care team.

A version of the care plan is presented to the patient by means of the patient diary, so that his day is described to him and also his therapy. This improves nurse/patient communication. It also allows the patient to be aware of what is happening to him and encourages communication about procedures. It also promotes good relations with family, relatives and friends, to see that the patient is interested in his progress. This provides excellent motivation in the elderly and gives them a useful source for reference in relation to clinical progress.

Future Developments

Nursing records will increase in coverage and depth and also the detailed analysis of nursing care performance will improve. The nursing interest in the nursing process has encouraged planning to develop more appropriately and the diffusion of such interest throughout all units and will become important in the future. In some areas, especially in the United States, the nursing record has been regarded as a total clinical record, specially being designed to meet administrative as well as nursing needs. Nursing records, however, take time to create and if they are overloaded, this advantage will be lost. They have also been more successful than computerised medical records. So far this seems to have been due partly to increased interest in evaluation and planning by nurses, partly by the formalisation of nursing procedures.

Undoubtedly, assistance from EXPERT systems in the process of planning care implementation will take place as knowledge develops. Also it is important to keep reviewing patients total needs especially those for self-fulfilment. It is now being recognised that the patient must actively participate if care is to be worth while and on an optimal path. The patient diary we suggest is one tool, enabling both patient and nurse maintain appropriate communication about day to day management and therapy.

Nursing records also promote better communication between the different members of the care team. These teams differ with the different types of care given but the team nature has to be underlined. Also standardisation would be appropriate in many areas of nursing and different support programs should be designed to encompass this. There is no doubt that nursing care has moved forward considerably and taken advantage of new ideas from informatics. New horizons have opened up and it is clear that this progress will continue as nurses utilise new information systems to improve their provision, and recording, of patient care.

REFERENCES

1.   The Standardisation of Hospital Records (Tunbridge Report) 1965. Central Health Services Council HMSO London.
2.   Anderson, J. (1974) Criteria for Health Care Computer Systems. pp. 47-64. International Congress on Health Systems. Systems ORSA Editor Collen, M.
3.   Anderson J. Kings College Hospital Computer System (London), Chapter 16 pp 457-516 in Hospital Computer Systems ed. Collen, M. F. 1974. J. Wiley & Sons, New York.

The Impact of Computers on Nursing
M. Scholes, Y. Bryant and B. Barber (eds.)
Elsevier Science Publishers B.V. (North-Holland)
© IFIP-IMIA, 1983

5.8.

NURSING RECORDS

Discussion

Computers and the Nursing Process

Computers are acknowledged as useful tools for exploring the nursing process, assessing the patient's problems, planning and implementing of patient care, assessing the progress of the delivery of patient care and evaluating the outcomes of the plan of care.

History-taking via the VDU

At the present time, nurses are required to enter the patient's nursing history into the computer after she has interviewed the patient. It was suggested that this duplication of effort might be overcome by encouraging the patient's themselves to enter their own history details via a VDU. However, experiments in the USA have shown that self-history taking presents problems. It was felt that history-taking directly from the patient provided a valuable contact between patient and nurse, enabling the nurse to gain knowledge about the patient as an individual. Further experiments are underway in the USA to use computer terminals at the bedside which will simplify and enhance the recording of a patient's history. Some patients are admitted to hospital at frequent intervals. It was suggested that their basic history data could be captured on a micro chip to eliminate the need to record this data each time the patient visited a health care facility. More research into this use of technology was advocated.

Approaches to entering Nursing Care Plans

Different approaches to entering the nursing care plan were identified - by nursing problem (potential and real), nursing diagnosis (in USA), medical diagnosis or frequent orders. These raised several comments emphasising the need for defining and formalising the role of the nurse and the nursing model to be followed. Concern was expressed that in using the nursing process, nurses were moving away from the concept of medical diagnosis which cannot be disregarded as the illness affects the patient and enables potential complications to be defined.

Research into Care Planning

The need for research into various aspects of care planning was recognised such as analysing nursing care given in specific situations, evaluating the content and presentation of information on patient care plans, establishing the value of care plans in delivering care, testing the validity of standard or established care plans and determining the usefulness of standard or non standard care plans in various situations.

Some computerised nursing record systems include reporting on care given (either reporting on all care given or exception reporting) and also progress notes. Where either are handwritten, some time wasting duplication is inevitable. The nursing care plans are usually used during the shift handover procedure.

Investigation is required into which data are used from the plan in communicating the needs of the patient and whether this method is timesaving.

Caution

It was noted, that the computer does not always, or automatically, alleviate problems existing before implementation such as queueing to update care plans. Care is required in systems design to ensure that any new problems that are introduced are understood and acceptable in comparison with the other advantages being offered by the system.

CHAPTER 6

MEASUREMENT OF CARE

Considerable interest has been shown in developing methods for measuring patient care. A well validated manual system is described in this section which is currently being examined for computerisation.

Whilst computers have been used to process patient data collected manually and to calculate workload, few systems exist which utilise a computerised nursing records database. An example of this type of system is referred to in this section and also with a paper in Chapter 14, Resource Management.

The Impact of Computers on Nursing
M. Scholes, Y. Bryant and B. Barber (eds.)
Elsevier Science Publishers B.V. (North-Holland)
© IFIP-IMIA, 1983

6.1.

PLANNING AND MEASURING NURSING CARE: AN INTEGRATED APPROACH

Charles Tilquin, Diane Saulnier, Pierre Lambert, and Jocelyne Carle

1. NURSING CARE PLAN AND NURSING PROCESS

The care plan is an instrument of written communication supporting the nurses' structured method of working, which is commonly called "the nursing process". The latter concept will not be discussed here. It has received many interpretations with the different conceptual models of nursing. But what is important to remember, is that the nursing process, whatever its form or modes, aims at each patient receiving the individualized care he requires. To do this, the nursing team is required to justify each of its interventions a priori and then to evaluate their results a posteriori.

Recognition of the relevance of written care planning arises from the hypothesis that every scientific or systematic approach is inconcievable without the support of a formal record - of a written plan. The need for memorizing is obvious. One cannot in fact claim to ensure the continuity, coherence and relevance of something that cannot be remembered, nor a fortiori to evaluate what cannot be remembered. The question is rather to know whether this memory has to be formalized i.e. made explicit in a standard format. For advocates of the care plan this is obvious, given the context in which nurses practice their profession: (a) intervention of the team with several patients each with special needs; (b) intervention of several members of the team with the same patient. Furthermore, the usefulness of the care plan is even greater when the state of health, the condition, the needs and the patient's problems are more complex.

In short, formalization of the nursing process memory guarantees its uniqueness. The care plan is the nursing team's unique collective record. Existence of such a record is a condition which is necessary if not sufficient to ensure the relevance, coherence and continuity of care; and particularly to allow for its evaluation.

It will be noted that there are no restrictions made on the medium to be used to "preserve" the care plan: paper (KARDEX) or computer. The debate with regard to the appropriate medium takes place on another level - which is less fundamental from the nursing viewpoint. It is more a question of easy access to data, of the ease with which it can be updated, of security, confidentiality and reliability, etc.

2. MEASUREMENT OF THE WORK LOAD AND MANAGEMENT OF NURSING RESOURCES

A system of measuring work load in each ward at each shift is a **management tool** which supports the process of decision making and evaluation of the nursing administration with respect to resource allocation in terms of hospital nursing staff.

The assumption is made that the nursing administration, within the context of budgetary constraints, wants to balance overall supply and demand(1) in each ward at each shift. Concretely, such an objective may be measured in terms of three broad sub-objectives:

1.   by ensuring the presence of **all** nursing staff required to fulfill the patients needs.

2.   by ensuring the presence **only** of nursing staff required to meet the patient's needs.

3.   by not exceeding the budget.

The second sub-objective is economic in nature - to avoid wastage by not allocating more staff than necessary. The first sub-objective refers more to the quality of care from the structural viewpoint. The presence of staff required to satisfy patient's needs must be ensured, as this is considered as being a condition which is necessary, if not sufficient, to assure the quality of the care process. The latter is itself considered necessary for attaining the ultimate objective of the quality of care **outcomes**.

The two objectives, economic and qualitative, are contradictory. The closer one tends to approach one, the further one is from the other. They can only be attained simultaneously, when a perfect balance is reached between supply and demand. Such an equilibrium is difficult to obtain because of the complexity of the phenomenon of building nursing care supply (supply in a given shift results from a series of decisions taken over the long, mid, short and very short term), and of the little control that the nursing administration may exercise over the demand for care. As a result, there is an unstable balance in the wards between supply and demand, supply being higher than demand at certain shifts and vice versa. The indicators mentioned above measure these fluctuations.

In order to be able to correct such fluctuations it is necessary to explain them. This is the role of management evaluation. From the time one is able to identify decisions that resulted in the breaking up of the balance at a particular time or during a given period, and the part played by each decision in explaining the imbalance, then the decision processes involved can be reviewed to obtain a greater equilibrium of supply and demand. This diagnostic process is relatively complex and requires the use of a computer. However, it will not be discussed further as it is not related to the present paper.

In the same way as the implementation of the nursing process requires the support of a basic tool (the care plan) so the scientific allocation of nursing resources cannot be achieved without certain instruments - the first being a system of measuring work load at each shift in each ward. In fact one cannot claim to balance the unknown. If measurement of care supply never poses problems (it suffices to account for staff presence) the same cannot be said for the measurement of the work load imposed by patients (demands).

Nursing workload is in fact a vague and uncertain entity. The times of nursing actions vary from one place to another, and one patient to another. Much depends also on the person carrying out the intervention. There is in addition, very often, a rather large margin between **care given** to a patient, particularly the time which is devoted to him, and the **care required** by this same patient, especially the time to be devoted with regard to the requirements of a qualitatively acceptable care practice. Finally, one would normally wish to measure the work load in advance (at least one shift ahead), if this measurement is to have impact on the process of resource allocation. If measurement of the work load is only available at the end of the shift, it will allow for evaluating the quality of resource allocation, but it will be too late to correct this allocation.

Measurement of the work load is therefore essential for the manager because it supplies him with the indicators needed for deciding on and evaluating the way in which he manages the rare and costly resources at his disposal.

3.   THE CARE PLAN AND MEASUREMENT OF THE WORK LOAD

The two proceding sections analyzed separately the ground for existence and usefulness of the two tools: the care plan and the measurement system for the work load. If these two tools are dealt with in this text, it is not by chance. One of the unique features of the research studies in these two fields consists of integrating the measurement of work load into the care planning process.

There are numerous systems of measuring work load. Their common denominator is the fact that to obtain an estimate of the overall work load, they measure, firstly the **care required by each of the patients individually** and secondly, the load imposed on nursing staff by activities other than individual care, for example, administrative or maintenance duties concerning the entire ward. This paper is concerned only with measuring care required by patients individually; this is the most difficult part of the workload to measure and also it represents most of this load (approximately 80%).

It is not necessary to discuss the way in which existing systems proceed to make this measurement. It is sufficient that they are criticized about measuring **care given** to patients rather than care required by the latter, about being unable (by construction and their method of operating) to really individualize measurement of care required, about not being or barely being transferable, being specialized, and about not being insufficiently validated. An attempt has been made to resolve these problems by constructing a system of measuring care required by the individual patient integrated into the care planning process, and hence, into the nursing process. This system is known as the PRN system(2).

3.1   The care plan design

The objective pursued in developing the PRN care plan (Figure 1) was to equip nurses with an instrument containing all the elements of the nursing process (as applied to one particular patient) which must be memorized to ensure the relevance, coherence and continuity of care. Moreover, this tool should be compatible with any conceptual model of nursing care, utilizable in all types of wards, and easy to use.

Several attempts have been made in Quebec hospitals to use a multitude of careplan forms and often without much success. Nurses are reluctant to devote their time to writing up the care plan under the pretext that it is more appropriate to use this time for giving care, and that in any case, they already have a great deal of writing to do whether it be in the patient record or in other forms. The primary concern therefore was firstly to eliminate all additional forms by designing the care plan in such a way that it can collect all the information related to patient care.

Besides, from the viewpoint of the nursing process interpreted strictly and theoretically the care plan design should be very simple; one sheet of paper divided into three columns entitled respectively:

    1.   Needs - problems - objectives
    2.   Nursing actions
    3.   Results

NURSING CARE PLAN

Allergies		☐ Supervision	
☐ Isolation technique			
		☐ V.S.: B.P.-PLS.-R.-T°	
Particularities		☐ N.S.	
		☐ C.V.P.	
		☐ F.H.- U. cont.	
		Pace-Maker - Monitor	

Hygiène	Confort	Feeding and hydration	Elimination	Respiration
Bath	Self care	Diet		☐ 02
☐ Self care	Up c̄ help	☐ Self feed	Self care	☐ Humidifier
☐ Partial		☐ c̄ help	Bathroom c̄ help	☐ Resp. exerc.
☐ Complete	☐ Walk c help	☐ Complete		
☐ Bath tub		☐ Hydration	☐ Urinal	
		☐ Bottle feeding, baby food,	Bedpan	
S-M-T-W-T-F-S	In bed	mat. feed		☐ Tracheostomy care
☐ Hydrotherapy	☐ Skin care and posit.		☐ Diapers	
			Incontinence	☐ Intubation care
			☐	
	☐ Musc. exerc.	☐ Naso gastric tube	Condom	☐ Respirator
☐ Oral hygiene		☐ Gavage	☐ Uretheral cath.	
	☐ Restraints			
☐ Beard shave				☐ Aerosol
	☐ Tranction, prosthesis,			
☐ Hair wash	stockings, bandage,	☐ Intake - Output	☐ Ostomy	☐ Suction of secretions
	corset			
S-M-T-W-T-F-S				

☐ Communication   ☐ Teaching

Date	Problems/objectives	Nursing actions	Evaluation
			Verso

FIGURE 1. PRN CARE PLAN.

In the first column, according to the conceptual model that guides its approach, the nursing team write up the patient's needs and/or problems which it identifies consequently and/or the objectives that have to be pursued as a result of these problems. These objectives will normally be expressed in terms of "behaviours" expected from the patient. In the second column, the nursing team write up the proposed interventions it plans in order to fulfill the needs/problems/objectives identified in the first stage. Finally, the third column serves to evaluate care results, essentially in terms of the patient's "behaviours".

This method of care planning is however only simple at first glance. (These forms are large and difficult to reproduce effectively in a book - see Figs 1 & 2). The large majority of nurses find it very difficult to define and formulate needs, problems and objectives. Moreover, for certain very "obvious" needs/problems, or very "common-current" ones, this procedure may appear unnecessarily cumbersome. Thence, even if care planning in terms of and according to the nursing process model is theoretically ideal in practice, certain compromises are necessary. What was done in the PRN care plan, was to complement the section designed according to the nursing process by a more traditional section aimed essentially at collecting data on **nursing actions** planned for the patient. What constitutes the originality of this section, is the fact that it is structured according to themes and sub-themes (categories of needs/nursing actions) for each of which a work space, with a particular design, has been reserved. These themes and sub-themes are as follows:

1.   Identifying the Institution
2.   Identifying the Patient
3.   Special data (allergies, isolation...)
4.   Surveillance elements
5.   Basic care:
     5.1   Hygiene
     5.2   Comfort
     5.3   Feeding and hydration
     5.4   Elimination
     5.5   Respiration
6.   Communications and Teaching
7.   Therapy
     7.1   Medication
     7.2   Treatments
     7.3   Intravenous therapy
8.   Diagnostic Methods
     8.1   Weighting and Measuring
     8.2   Collection - specimen - simple analysis
     8.3   Blood bank
     8.4   Examinations - RX
9.   Consultations
10. Clinical and Social profile

The work space intended for each theme or sub-theme is itself structured and certain key terms are precoded: the nurse therefore has to circle them or check them off according to the patient's needs.

Thus, in the first section of the care plan, designed according to the principles of the nursing process, little support is offered to the nurse for care planning but, on the other hand, she is not constrained by an a priori structuring of needs/interventions nor by work spaces of predetermined size and shape. From the theoretical and professional viewpoint, this is ideal. The nurse can order her care priorities as appropriate and develop features that appear most important to her. Nothing limits her in the format (structure, space) of the care plan. The second section is more restrictive because care planning here is more preorganized: specific spaces reserved for one category or another of nursing actions, precoding of nursing actions, etc. On the other hand, for the nurse who feels less at ease with the care planning process, this framework is reassuring, it serves as a guide and reminder, it simplifies her task: precoding, preorganization of the planning "text". Consultation of the care plan is also facilitated, as the same data is always repeated in the same place.

The advantage of this approach is that nurses, according to their familiarity with the nursing process, can utilize one or another section of the form, and eventually both, during the transition period in which the team goes progressively from the traditional planning method (limited to the drawing of nursing actions) to the method proposed by the nursing process (where the elaboration of nursing actions falls within their a priori justification and their a posteriori evaluation). In use, it appears that the existence of the two "concurrent" sections in the care plan form not only allows teams to go progressively from one method to another, but also that the **mixed** planning remained relevant even when nurses had mastered planning according to the principles of the nursing process. This is easily appreciated when one realizes that the care plan essentially fulfills **two functions** and that each of the above mentioned sections corresponds respectively to the needs of one or the other of these functions. The first function is one of care **systematization**, integration, unification, verification, justification and evaluation. It is the "nursing process" section of the careplan that supports this function. It is true that nursing actions developed within the framework of the nursing process are written into this section. However, not all nursing actions will be included in this section (only the most important, those that are most "special" to the patient) and moreover, the arrangement in which they appear in this section arises more from the needs/problems/objectives as determined by the nursing team than from the realities of care organization. Finally, this arrangement varies from one patient to another.

The care plan's second function is that of a reference tool, a memorandum that the nurse consults regularly and rapidly during the course of the day to ensure that she will do or has done what the patient requires. From this point of view, the first section is not very practical. Its presentation of nursing actions is not designed according to the needs of the nurse in her role as **care provider** but according to her needs as a **"care designer"** This is where the second section of the care plan form comes to the rescue. It is true that the parallel utilization of these two sections of the care plan implies a certain duplication of information as the nursing actions developed and written into the first section being repeated in the second section. However, this duplication hardly consumes any time given the format of the second section and it is not useless because it corresponds to a verification of the care plan.

Evaluation carried out in hospitals which are users of the PRN form arrived at the conclusion that the introduction of this form led to a considerable improvement in care planning in terms of exhaustivity, coherence and relevance.

3.2   Measurement of care required by the patient

The basic approach in the PRN method for measuring care is that of measuring the time for care required by each patient individually, by adding up the time required for each of the nursing actions scheduled (planned) for the patient.

The main advantage of this approach is that it allows for the **individualization** of the measurement (time) of care **required** (not given) as scheduled for the patient, therefore, written into his care plans. Its relationship with care planning is therefore direct. Moreover, this method of measurement has the advantage of being systematically validated on its content. This validation has

been taking place for the last eight years by a process of continuous feedback.
Finally, it was possible to make the measurement system transferable, from one
ward to another, and virtually from one hospital to another and universal i.e.
applicable in all types of wards: medicine, surgery, paediatrics, gynaecology,
post-partum, nursery, intensive care, coronary unit, long term care, nursing
home, psychiatry, (except in wards where the patient stays for less than 24
hours).

This approach however, as theoretically attractive as it may be, still has
certain problems with respect to its implementation. It is difficult to
associate a fixed time to a given nursing action, because its duration can vary,
mainly according to the patient concerned, and according to the members of staff
who carries it out, and also according to the setting (physical and
organizational). These problems have been satisfactorily resolved as follows:-

(a)   Environmental Variation
      For the sources of variation due to the **environment,** by playing on the
      definition (content) of nursing actions; for example:

      -     by not including into times for nursing actions, the travelling
            times associated with them (the time for the latter varies with the
            context)

      -     by considering in the time for nursing actions, the times for
            procedures related to this action given at the patient's bedside and
            outside the patient's room. (for example: preparing equipment). In
            fact from one place to another, the "at bedside/outside bedside"
            distribution of procedures can change considerably.

(b)   Patient Variation
      For the sources of variation due to the **patient,** by dissecting the care
      activities extremely finely. In fact the PRN form for measuring the level
      of care required (Figure 2) distinguishes 85 different categories of
      nursing actions (each corresponding to a very specific patient need) and
      within each of these categories, the nursing actions are differentiated
      further to take into account directly or indirectly the patients' special
      characteristics, which make the duration of the nursing action vary. In
      this way finally, 214 nursing actions or groups of nursing actions called
      FACTORS, have been identified with different timings   These 214 factors
      have been regrouped into the 85 previously mentioned categories. Some
      examples of these factors are the following:-

      -     for certain categories of patients (ex.:babies)

      -     that take into account the number of nursing staff members who
            participate in carrying out the same nursing action.

      -     that consider the different modes of managing the patient (support
            advice and orientation, partial and complete aid) for a given
            nursing action.

      -     which consider the intensities (for eg. constant presence), range
            (for eg. the percentage of the patient's bodily surface) and
            frequencies (for eg. 20 X a day) of the same nursing action

(c)   Staff Variation
      As far as the sources of variation due to the staff are concerned, by
      determining the duration of the nursing actions by not making reference to
      one member of the staff in particular but rather to a **normal nursing team**.

Finally, by careful construction of the measurement form and its utilization rules, the research team have ensured that the measurement tool is complete (it covers all the care thay may be required by one particular patient) and **non redundant** (one does not count the same thing twice).

From the point of view of the user, the PRN form for measuring the level of care required appears therefore as a list of 214 factors. Each factor represents one or several nursing actions qualified by certain attributes: type of patient concerned, modes of patient managements, range, intensity, frequency,...etc. Each factor has a weight (a value) expressed in points equivalent of minutes (one point = 5 minutes). This value represents the time required to carry out a certain number of times (specified explicitly or implicitly) the nursing action or actions considered by the factor during a 24 **hour period**.

The list of 214 factors is structured. As previously indicated, the factors are regrouped into 85 subsections, the latter themselves being grouped under seven themes:

- respiration
- feeding and hydration
- elimination
- hygiene and comfort
- communications and teaching
- treatments
- diagnostic procedures

These seven themes correspond to the themes of the care plan form. The two forms, at least as far as their common content is concerned, are therefore structured in the same way.

Moreover, in use, the instruments strengthen each other. It will be noted that squares appear to the left of the nursing actions in the care plan form. These squares are reserved for writing in the values of factors (relevant in the case of the patient concerned) from the form for measuring the level of care required. A space is further set aside at the bottom of the care plan form for writing up the sum of these values, which is called the **level of care required** by the patient. This level is expressed in points but one point being worth five minutes, the time for care required by the patient during the following 24 hours is in this way permanently written into the care plan. Each time the nursing team updates the care plan (in practice at least every shift), the "values" of the nursing action are also updated, as well as their sum (level of care). Thus, care measurement is automatically integrated into the process of care planning. Frequently updating (at each shift) is easily done and at almost no cost. In fact nurses learn rapidly the values of the factors and the time for measurement is then essentially that of writing the values for the factors into the appropriate spaces of the care plan form; (this means a few seconds per patient at each shift).

By associating the process of measuring the care level required to that of care planning resulted in greatly improving the latter. This is easily explained: measurement of the level of care required is not an end in itself. This measurement is utilized by the manager for resource allocation. Bedside nurses soon realized this and consider that if their care plans were incomplete, they would not measure all the care required by patients, which, at the end of the line will mean less resources allocated to care for these patients. The user hospitals noticed that with the introduction of the PRN there was a significant increase in the "quality" of care plans at least, in terms of their completeness.

CROS
Equipe de Recherche Opérationnelle en Santé

PRN SO

FORM FOR MEASURING THE LEVEL OF NURSING CARE REQUIRED

NURSING ACTIONS for health promotion, prevention of health problems, treatment, reeducation and rehabilitation.

RESPIRATION

Humidifier and/or fan		1
Respiratory exercise	guide	2
Respiratory exercise (c pr)	1-6 times	4
Respiratory exercise (c pr)	7 times or more	12
Chest physiotherapy exercise (c pr)	1-2 times	4
Chest physiotherapy exercise (c pr)	3-6 times	12
Chest physiotherapy exercise (c pr)	7 times or more	21
Chest physio and vent app (5 times or more)	Less than 3 min	3
Chest physio and vent app (5 times or more)	3 min or more	15
Aerosol	guide	3
Aerosol (c pr)		14
Suction of secretions	1-6 times	3
Suction of secretions	7-19 times	6
Suction of secretions	20-47 times	13
Suction of secretions	48 times or more	24
Administration of oxygen (catheter/mask/etc)		3
Administration of oxygen (croupette/covered tent)		6
Tracheotomised or intubated care		4
Tracheotomised or intubated care (respirator/ventilator)		8

FEEDING AND HYDRATION

Feeding infant		10
Feeding infant (c pr)		19
Feeding infant (special precautions)		40
Feeding self-care patient		2
Feeding partial help		5
Feeding complete help		15
Hydration per os		3
Milk extraction		10
Continuous gavage	24h 24h	4
Drip or syringe gavage	1-6 times	6
Drip or syringe gavage	7 times or more	10
Gavage (c pr)		14

ELIMINATION

Diapers (infant)		6
Occasional bedpan and/or incontinence		1
Urinal and bedpan		3
Bedpan (female)		5
Assist to the toilet (c pr)		6
Incontinence and/or condom		8
External care of urethral catheter and bedpan		2
Stomy care	1 stomy	6
Stomy care	2 stomies or re	15

HYGIENE AND COMFORT

Hygiene care 0-4 year old patient	1 time	3
Hygiene care 0-4 year old patient	2 times or more	6
Hygiene care self-care patient	1 time	2
Hygiene care self-care patient	2 times or more	4
Hygiene care partial help	1 time	4
Hygiene care partial help	2 times or more	7
Hygiene care complete help (c pr) (bed)	1 time	7
Hygiene care complete help (c pr) (bath)	1 time	9
Hygiene care complete help (c pr) (bed/bath)	2 times or more	16
Hygiene care and hydrotherapy burns (prep)		8
Hygiene care and hydrotherapy burns (c pr)	1 time	11
Hygiene care and hydrotherapy burns (c pr)	2 times or more	19
Formal dressing		4
Oral hygiene	4-11 times	1
Oral hygiene	12 times or more	3
Beauty care and/or beard shave		2
Hair-wash		3
Hair-wash and cut		6
Hair-wash and removal of adhesions		9
Up with help	1-2 attendants	4
Up and walk with help	1-2 attendants	6
Up and/or walk with help	3 attend or more	9
Rubbing and positioning (4 times or more)	1-2 attendants	7
Rubbing and positioning (4 times or more)	3 attend or more	16
Passive and/or active muscular exercises (c pr)		4
Structured passive and/or active muscular exercises (c pr)		10
Application of physical restraints		4

COMMUNICATION

Teaching the patient and/or his relatives	1 time	3
Teaching the patient and/or his relatives	2 times or more	7
Individual supportive communication		3
Interview with the patient and/or his relatives for data collection		3
Interview with the patient for specific data collection		9
Ind psychotherapy of physical integration	guide and direct	3
Ind psychotherapy of physical integration	partly compens	9
Ind psychotherapy of physical integration	wholly compens	17
Ind psychotherapy of psycho integration	guide and direct	3
Ind psychotherapy of psycho integration	partly compens	9
Ind psychotherapy of psycho integration	wholly compens	17
Ind psychotherapy of social integration	guide and direct	3
Ind psychotherapy of social integration	partly compens	9
Ind psychotherapy of social integration	wholly compens	17
Ind non verbal comm of bio-psycho-soc int	guide and direct	3
Ind non verbal comm of bio-psycho-soc int	partly compens	9
Ind non verbal comm of bio-psycho-soc int	wholly compens	17
Psychotherapeutic meeting with relatives	guide and direct	6
Psychotherapeutic meeting with relatives	partly compens	12
Group psychotherapeutic activity type A	1 time	3
Group psychotherapeutic activity type A	2 times or more	6
Group psychotherapeutic activity type B		5
Group occupational therapeutic activity	1-2 times	3
Group occupational therapeutic activity	3 times or more	7
Group educational therapeutic activity	1 time	4
Group educational therapeutic activity	2 times or more	9
Group socio-therapeutic outing	less than 2 hours	4
Group socio-therapeutic outing	2-3 hours	9
Group socio-therapeutic outing	more than 3 hours	17

FIGURE 2. THE MEASUREMENT OF NURSING CARE.

TREATMENTS

Medication (P.O./P.R./P.V./Ung./Drops)	1-4 times	1
Medication (P.O./P.R./P.V./Ung./Drops)	5-14 times	3
Medication (P.O./P.R./P.V./Ung./Drops)	15-24 times	4
Medication (P.O./P.R./P.V./Ung./Drops)	25 times or more	5
Medication (I.D./S.C./I.M.)	1-3 doses	1
Medication (I.D./S.C./I.M.)	4-7 doses	3
Medication (I.D./S.C./I.M.)	8 doses or more	6
Medication (I.V.)	1-3 doses	2
Medication (I.V.)	4-10 doses	5
Medication (I.V.)	11-15 doses	9
Medication (I.V.)	16-30 doses	15
Medication (I.V.)	31 doses or more	24
Intravenous (establish)	1 O.V.	4
Intravenous (establish)	2 O.V. or more	7
Intravenous short-term (monitor)		1
Intravenous permanent solution (monitor)	1 solution	4
Intravenous permanent solution (monitor)	2 solutions	8
Intravenous permanent solution (monitor)	3 solut. or more	14
Intravenous short-term (blood and deriv.)	1-2 transfusions	6
Intravenous short-term (blood and deriv.)	3 trans. or more	15
Intravenous total parenteral nutrition	24h:24h	12
Peritoneal dialysis (ambulatory)		20
Peritoneal dialysis (24h/24h)	1-17 cycles	32
Peritoneal dialysis (24h/24h)	18 cycles or more	70
Insertion tube or catheter	1-2 times	3
Insertion tube or catheter	3 times or more	6
Catheter(s) or tube(s) open/closed AND/OR insert. rectal tube		1
Free drainage	1-2 tubes	1
Free drainage	3 tubes or more	2
Drainage under water (closed circuit)	1 tube	3
Drainage under water (closed circuit)	2 tubes or more	6
Drainage continuous suction	1-2 tubes	3
Drainage continuous suction	3-4 tubes	6
Drainage continuous suction	5 tubes or more	8
Thoracic tube manipulation		3
Irrigation (all kinds)	1-2 times	2
Irrigation (all kinds)	3-6 times	4
Irrigation (all kinds)	7-12 times	6
Irrigation (all kinds)	13-19 times	8
Irrigation (all kinds)	20 times or more	14
Gastric irrigation with iced water (4000 cc's)		24
Colostomy irrigation		4
Colostomy irrigation (c pr.)		7

Shaving	1-20%	3
Shaving	21-65%	6
Shaving	66% or more	12
Aseptic skin preparation	1-20%	2
Aseptic skin preparation	21-65%	4
Aseptic skin preparation	66% or more	8
Inap. perm trac. AND/OR inst. trac./prot./stock	1-2 times	2
Inap. perm trac. AND/OR inst. trac./prot./stock	3 times or more	4
Application of ice or hot water bag	1-2 bags	2
Application of ice or hot water bag	3 bags or more	6
Application of ointment	30% or more	8
Application of ointment with covering	30% or more	17
Packing and/or dressing removal		1
Sutures or cast removal		3
Open wound cleaning and/or lamp positioning	1-8 times	2
Open wound cleaning and/or lamp positioning	9 times or more	6
Dressing dry or moist	1-2 times	2
Dressing dry or moist	3 times or more	6
Wound dressing with discharge	1-2 times	3
Wound dressing with discharge	3-6 times	9
Wound dressing with discharge	7 times or more	24
Dressing for skin regeneration	1-2 times	7
Dressing for skin regeneration	3 times or more	18
Debridement of wound		6
Open wound: rolling graft		6
Application of ointment burns	1-20%	10
Application of ointment burns	21-45%	22
Application of ointment burns	46-70%	42
Application of ointment burns	71% or more	72
Application of dressing burns	1-20%	14
Application of dressing burns	21-45%	36
Application of dressing burns	46-70%	72
Application of dressing burns	71% or more	96
Application of isolation technique		5
Application of isolation technique (sterile)		10

DIAGNOSTIC PROCEDURES

Systematic observation	1-10 times	1
Systematic observation	11-40 times	4
Systematic observation	41 times or more	12
Systematic constant observation shared	2 patients or more	38
Systematic constant observation exclusive	1 patient	76
Vital signs	1-3 times	1
Vital signs	4-14 times	3
Vital signs	15-24 times	8
Vital signs	25 times or more	18
Vital signs (B.P. s./s./1.)	1-6 times	3
Vital signs (B.P. s./s./1.)	7 times or more	7
Neurologic signs	1-11 times	2
Neurologic signs	12 times or more	6
Central venous pressure	1-11 times	3
Central venous pressure	12 times or more	6
Evaluation: foetal heart and/or uterine contraction		2
Intake and/or output record	1-19 times	1
Intake and/or output record	20-65 times	4
Intake and/or output record	66 times or more	8
Weighing and/or measuring	1 attendant	1
Weighing and/or measuring	2 attend or more	2
Collection stool and/or sputum		1
Collection urine		2
Spec. sec and/or stool and/or urine(smp anal.)	1-5 times	1
Spec. sec and/or stool and/or urine(smp anal.)	6 times or more	2
Spec. urine culture	guide	2
Spec. urine culture (complete help)	1-2 times	2
Spec. urine culture (complete help)	3 times or more	5
Specimen and implantation of ocular secretions		3
Specimen blood	1-3 times	2
Specimen blood	4-8 times	6
Specimen blood	9 times or more	13
Simple analysis on Ward	1-8 times	2
Simple analysis on Ward	9 times or more	6
Respiratory routine	1-4 times	1
Respiratory routine	5 times or more	4
Ass. examination or X-Ray (c pr.)	1-2 examinations	2
Ass. examination or X-Ray (c pr.)	3 exam. or more	4
Ass. Dr. intervention (c pr.)	1 time	8
Ass. Dr. intervention (c pr.)	2 times or more	16

EROS - PRN 80 - August 1981

FIGURE 2. (CONTINUED.)

4.   METHODOLOGICAL APPROACH

The development of the system began in 1974 and was continued under the direction of the same research team. However, this development has essentially been in the hands of the users of the system themselves.

The two main tools of the PRN were developed by committees of nurses from hospitals utilising the system. The method was essentially one of structured group discussion (nominal group method). Members of the committees have at their disposal a computerized bank of empirical data that contains at the present time, more than 6000 patients care plans collected in the wards of about 15 hospitals. Moreover, a process of continual feedback was established between users of the system and the research team. Through this process, the system is permanently validated on its content. Data supplied by feedback is compiled and organized by the research team for the committees.

The form for measuring the level and the care plan form have therefore been revised four times since 1974. Revision of the care plan form is the easiest: in general, one or two committee days are adequate for carrying out a revision process. Revision of the form for measuring the level is much more complex. During the last revision session, the committee deliberated for the equivalent of six weeks before being able to reach a consensus of opinion on all the factors of the form.

5.   COMPUTERIZATION

The question of computerizing care planning and measuring hardly arose until now in Quebec, as few hospitals had a computer terminal in each nursing station. The situation is evolving very rapidly however and in a year or two the large hospitals are likely to be suitably equipped. Work has therefore begun on an interactive system of care planning that will automatically produce a measurement of the level of care required by the patient.

In addition work has been undertaken during the last three years on a computerized data system for the nursing care manager. This system would provide assistance in decision making and of control and/or diagnosis, using a data produced by the measurement module of the work load of the PRN system.

NOTES AND REFERENCES

1   Finer or cruder definitions of supply and demand are possible: for example: supply and demand of each **category** of nursing staff at each **hour** of the day. The nursing administration's objective can be formulated in terms of a balance between supply and demand as defined in these terms. Such a balance, desirable as it may be, is more difficult to attain than the previously defined balance, and to achieve it is less easily verifiable. In this text the first definition is used because it is more easily operationalized. In general however, the approach described applies to any definition of balance between supply and demand.

2.   Tilquin et al: Measuring the level of nursing care required - PRN80, I.M.S.A., 3535 Queen Mary Suite 501, Montreal, H3V 1HB, Canada (1981). Full details of the measurement forms and instructions on their use are available from the authors.

The Impact of Computers on Nursing
M. Scholes, Y. Bryant and B. Barber (eds.)
Elsevier Science Publishers B.V. (North-Holland)
© IFIP-IMIA, 1983

6.2.

DATA CAPTURE – FROM A REAL TIME COMPUTERISED NURSING SYSTEM

Christine R. Henney and Lesley H. Stewart

1.   Introduction

This paper describes how a real-time computerised nursing system evolved, the impact it has had on the delivery of nursing care and on nurse education in that time, and to discuss future developments in the light of this experience.

A real-time computerised nursing system has been operational on six medical wards at Ninewells Hospital, Dundee, for the last six years. It comprises a patient administration system together with a nursing care system and all patient data is entered by the nurse in charge of the ward using a visual display unit linked to a Modular I computer.

The nursing care system relies on selection by the charge nurse of items from a standard precoded list of nursing orders, specimen collections and tests to allow a daily care plan for each patient to be devised. The plan, (Fig 1) is printed in the ward on A4 size paper, and placed at the foot of the patient's bed to give an immediate visual notification of required care and recording of care given.

All nursing care given to a patient can be stored on disc and recalled on a VDU or print-out as a nursing care summary when required. This summary provides a continuous record of basic and technical nursing care along with weight and urine analysis. The chronological programme is clearly documented and certified by the charge nurse. It becomes an integral part of the case record.

The system's primary aims are to improve organisation and documentation, both for basic and technical nursing care, to facilitate continuity of nursing care in hospital and on discharge, to facilitate educational programmes, and to assist general nursing administration. An additional benefit of the system is the opportunity to provide care on a patient-orientated basis(C7).

2.   Organisation and Documentation

The advantages to nurses using the computer system can be appreciated in the light of the complexity of modern diagnostic methods. For example it facilitates the planning of various nursing procedures by automatically providing a cascade of instructions appropriate to a procedure, or investigation. In addition, lists of patients who have to be fasted for diagnostic purposes at different times can be printed out from the computer memory. Thus the well-organised nursing care plan produced by the charge nurse using the computer reduces the possible timing errors that can unnecessarily extend a patient's hospital stay. Surveys of nurse users of the computer also suggest that communication between nurse and patient is improved. The adoption of patient-orientated nursing instead of nursing by task lists (also available in the system) which allows the delivery of nursing care by the same nurse of nursing team have organisational benefits leading to improvement in nurse-patient relationships.

FIGURE 1 PATIENT CARE PLAN
(excluding 4 colums for night staff & manual back up signatures)

WARD 06   PATIENT CARE PLAN   14:16   04/05/82   ADAM JOHN   2310321234   WT 56.4 KG   BAY 1

	START	AM			PM	INITIALS		
		8	10	12	2	4	6	8

NURSING ORDERS

	START
BED BATH	26/04/82
HAIR CARE	26/04/82
PRESSURE AREA CARE - 2 HOURLY	26/04/82
URINAL	26/04/82
COMMODE	26/04/82
FLUID CHART	26/04/82
SHAVING	26/04/82
LIGHT DIET	26/04/82
4 HOURLY TEMPERATURE/PULSE/ BLOOD PRESSURE	28/04/82
FEED BY SELF	28/04/82
ORAL HYGIENE - 4 HOURLY	28/04/82
UP FOR 30 MINS	28/04/82
PHYSIOTHERAPY	28/04/82
WEIGH DAILY	28/04/82

SPECIMEN COLLECTIONS
SPUTUM FOR BAC. LAB.   04/05/82 DD

TESTS
SCHILLING - DICOPAC   04/05/82 08:00
  8 AM - PATIENT VOIDS BLADDER
         COMMENCE 24 HOUR URINE COLLECTION
         ADMINISTER TWO CAPSULES TO PATIENT

  10 AM - ADMINISTER INJECTION CYANCOBALAMIN 1000 MICROGRAMS
  8 AM TO 12 MIDDAY - PATIENT CAN DRINK WATER IF DESIRED
  12 MIDDAY - PATIENT MAY TAKE SOLID FOOD

BARIUM MEAL   08/05/82 09:30
FASTING BLOODS   05/05/82 EM
  PATIENT FAST FROM MIDNIGHT TONIGHT

The well-organised and legible nursing records produced by the system are the basis of the majority of the benefits to both nurses and patients which stem from the use of the computer.

3.   Continuity of Care

In the last decade, the organisation of nursing care has changed radically, both in an administrative and an operational sense. A major organisational problem has resulted from a reduction in nursing hours and the requirements of new nursing curricula. The nurse scheduling changes caused by these developments has produced difficulties in the provision of continuity of nursing care. There has been an increase in "communication interfaces" - a nurse who takes over the care of a patient must be provided with accurate unequivocal information about the nursing care previously planned. The legible and well-organised daily care plans and summaries provided by the computer minimises communication problems is of course complemented by normal verbal reporting.

Another problem militating against continuity of care is the growth of specialisation, which results in frequent transfers of patients between wards and hospitals. The consequence of the breaks in continuity produced by such transfers can be minimised by the rapid transmission of computer-generated care summaries between wards in hospitals. If transfers of nursing data are required for community nursing services the print-out of the nursing summary can be utilised to achieve continuity.

4.   Education

In recent years, the role of the clinical tutor in nurse education has increased. However, the tutor has special difficulties when teaching on the ward - the teaching has to be opportunistic and educational and service objectives are frequently in conflict. These problems can be overcome by a co-operative ward sister, but in wards where the service pressures are great, communication between them may be difficult.

The current nursing care plan and summary generated by the computer provides a data base which allows the tutor to teach effectively without having to make unreasonable demands on the time of the charge nurse. Another important contribution to the work of the clinical tutor is the nature of the patient-orientated record which, as described above, is a by-product of the computer system. The value of such records to the in-service training of all nursing staff cannot be over-estimated.

5.   General Administration

One of the major problems in nursing administration lies in the field of nurse scheduling which can be defined as a method of achieving the optimum match of nurse staffing resources to nursing workload. The potential of the computer system has been explored in this field in the following way. The automatic data capture of the system was used to develop an index of nursing workload (Ninewells Index I) for general medical wards based on the assignment of a score to each nursing order on a 5 point scale which is summed for the individual patients on a ward to give an index of the nursing workload for that ward. The number of points assigned to each nursing procedure was based on the opinion of an experienced nurse. The number of nursing orders in the system is over 200 including tests and specimen collections. Moreover, in order to obtain some indication about the mix of grades of staff required, the nursing procedures are classified as basic or technical, the latter being defined as those carried out by trained staff. This method of assessing nursing workload has been shown to be very sensitive to workload changes(D15). Using the Ninewells Index I the relationship between basic and technical care, which has been regarded by some workers as constant(1) was investigated, as was the relationship between the allocation of nurses and the workload in the six medical wards using the computer system. The results have been reported by Henney et al(J5) and showed an absence of correlation between them. This finding is dependent upon the validity of the Ninewells Index I as an estimate of nursing workload and in order to test this assumption a survey was mounted to establish agreed ratings for standard nursing procedures by a large number of experienced charge nurses in the medical wards of teaching and district general hospitals in Scotland. A Delphi type survey(2) was carried out by a questionnaire involving 115 medical charge nurses in Scotland who graded the same procedures on a 5 point scale (Delphi Index I). Good agreement with the two indices was found. The Delphi Index I was transferred from the original ordinal scale to an interval scale (Delphi Index II) to facilitate statistical handling of data. These ratings represent the general opinion of the sisters who participated in the Delphi survey and thus it may be argued that they reflect a consensus opinion in Scotland of the relative workloads. Further evidence regarding the validity of this approach was obtained by comparing the ratings based on Delphi Index II and the timings of a representative sample of nursing procedures(3-6) and demonstrating that a strong relationship exists between those two measures of the nursing workload. The strong correlation between ratings and timings also facilitated the transformation of the Delphi II ratings to timings and the establishment of a Ninewells Index II based on time and thus potentially more useful than the other indices. A few conversions interval scale ratings to timings are shown in Table 1.

6.   Future Developments of the System

The basic principle underlying the development of the real-time computerised nursing system in medical wards was to adopt a stepwise implementation of the system which would allow it to evolve by adapting to the needs of the users. The success of this approach underlay the decision that the basic system should be introduced to other nursing areas e.g. surgery, paediatrics, obstetrics etc. and modified as appropriate. A start has been made in general surgery and the basic computer system has been introduced to one surgical ward during the past year and additional facilities developed to give for example(Fig. 2):-

1)   Dressing Lists
      The dressing list is a record of the dressings to be carried out for each patient. It is also a means of reporting and recording the condition of the patient's wound. The type of dressing used is also contained on the individual care plan and the summary.

2)   Theatre Instructions
      Production of instructions cascades on individual care plans to give details of fasting instructions and theatre preparations on the day before operation and the day of the operation have been provided. Also built into these orders is an instruction to check that the pre-medication prescription and anaesthetic form have been signed. The day after operation the signal "first post-operative day" appears automatically on the care plan and the computer continues to identify subsequent post-operative days in sequence until the patient is discharged.

It is intended to extend the system in a similar manner to the other surgical wards in the hospital, and in due course to other specialities and other hospitals.

TABLE 1

RATINGS AND TIMINGS OF INDIVIDUAL NURSING PROCEDURES

NURSING ORDERS	NINEWELLS INDEX RATINGS	INTERVAL SCALE RATINGS	TIMINGS
BED BATH	4	32	27
SHOWER WITH ASSISTANCE	3	26	16
ORAL HYGIENE - 4 HRLY	2	25	31
CATHETER INTERMITTENT	4	25	44
TUBE FEED - 2 HRLY	4	28	105
WEIGH WEEKLY	1	20	7
SPECIMEN COLLECTIONS			
BLOOD CULTURES	5	23	11
GASTRIC WASHING	4	25	15
TESTS			
RENAL BIOPSY	5	35	33
SIGMOIDOSCOPY	3	28	20

FIGURE 2

```
-----------------------------------------------------------------------
|              DRESSING LISTS AND THEATRE INSTRUCTIONS                 |
|WARD 8        DRESSING LIST                   09:14      19/05/82     |
|                                                                     |
|MILLER        1106130022          POST-OPERATIVE DAY   5              |
|ELIZABETH     AGE 68  BAY 3                                           |
|                                  DRESSING DAILY                      |
|                                  APPLY SOFRA TULLE DRESSING TO AREA  |
|                                                                     |
|DARGIE        2511040069          POST-OPRATIVE DAY    2              |
|JEMIMA        AGE 77  BAY 4                                           |
|                                  CHECK WOUND                         |
|                                  DRESSING AS REQUIRED                |
|                                  CARE OF COLOSTOMY                   |
|                                  MILTON PACK                         |
|                                  IRRIGATE WOUND TWICE DAILY          |
|                                  HALF QUANTITY PEROXIDE              |
-----------------------------------------------------------------------
```

7.   Future Research Applications of the System

The automatic data capture of current nursing workload in the medical wards
where the computerised nursing system was developed provided an opportunity to
investigate the effectiveness, and acceptability, of utilising this data-base
for nurse scheduling purposes.

It is proposed to develop this project in three phases, the first of which is
almost complete.

Phase 1
During a period of one year both nursing workload (computer captured) and nurse
allocation (manually captured) will be obtained and analysed for the six medical
wards to ascertain the matching of nurse staffing to workload achieved without
the information on nursing workload being available.

Phase 2
During a four month period the "nurse schedular" will be provided with the data
captured by the computer. The matching of staff to workload achieved by
providing the information will be compared with the equivalent four months of
the control year.

Phase 3
During this phase, which will also cover a four month period, organisational
changes such as the size of the nursing charge and the size of a reserve nursing
pool, will be added to the procedure in phase 2 and the results evaluated.

It is hoped that this approach to research in the field of nurse scheduling,
made possible by the data-capture from the computer system, may solve some of
the intractable problems associated with previous studies in this area.

Another research application which it is proposed to investigate is the
contribution which the computer might make to the implementation of the "Nursing
Process".   A first step in this development is to produce a dictionary of
"nursing problems" which will allow the production of a computer-held nursing
problem list for each patient and which when linked with the nursing solutions
to these problems (the nursing care plan) will allow evaluation of outcome to be
made and so complete the nursing process.

8.   Conclusions

The automatic data capture achieved by a real-time computerised nursing system
has been exploited to improve the organisation and documentation of both basic
and technical nursing care in six medical wards using the system. Recovery of
data from the data base and its presentation in a variety of forms has been used
to improve continuity of nursing care and to facilitate nursing educational
programmes. The data captured by the system has allowed the development of
nursing workload which can be applied to solving the problems of effective nurse
scheduling.

In conclusion future developments in computer technology such as the
availability of powerful and relatively cheap micro-computers, associated with
electronic and software advances which will allow the micro-computers to be
linked one with another or with mainframe machines (networking), will increase
the number of computer applications in nursing practice. It is hoped that this
description of the Ninewells computerised nursing system will encourage the
development of the automatic data capture systems for the benefit of both nurses
and patients.

9.   Acknowledgements

We are greatly indebted to Professor James Crooks for his assistance and advice, Miss M. E. Scholes, Chief Area Nursing Officer, Miss S. MacRae, District Nursing Officer and Miss A. Duthie, Divisional Nursing Officer, for their help and encouragement and Mr Yannis Chrissafis and the technical staff of the Ward Computer Project, Ninewells Hospital, Dundee.

REFERENCES

(1)   North Eastern Regional Hospital Board, Nursing Workload per Patient as a Basis for Staffing.   Scottish Health Service Study No. 9, Scottish Home and Health Department, Edinburgh (1969).

(2)   Dalkey Norman C., (1969)   The Delphi Method: An Experimental Study of Group Opinion RM-5888-PR, Rand Corporation, Santa Monica, Calif, June.

(3)   Collings T., (1977)   An Evaluation of the ward computer project at Ninewells Hospital H.S.O.R.U.   University of Strathclyde.

(4)   Gloucester Health District (1978)   A total care nursing dependency study of the tower block in Glucestershire Royal Hospital, April.

(5)   Grant N.,   A method for calculating nursing workload based on individualised nursing care.   University of Edinburgh.   Ph.D. Thesis (1977).

(6)   Rhys Hearn C., Private Communication.   Department of Social Medicine, University of Birmingham.

The Impact of Computers on Nursing
M. Scholes, Y. Bryant and B. Barber (eds.)
Elsevier Science Publishers B.V. (North-Holland)
© IFIP-IMIA, 1983

6.3.

MEASUREMENT OF CARE

Discussion

Measurable Care Items

There is a requirement to identify aspects of nursing care that can be measured efficiently. Once this has been clearly defined the effective use of computerised care planning in measuring the quality and quantity of care can and needs to be explored and exploited.

Accuracy and Completeness of the Nursing Data Base

An examination of the quality of the data fed into a care planning system is critical. The accuracy and completeness of the data must be measured if the data is to be used in providing and evaluating nursing care. The support of the nursing administration is crucial in developing, implementing and measuring computerised care systems.

Quality of Care Audits

Tools for measuring clinical practice (quality of care audits or quality assurance) are being developed but these do not always reflect the problems which lead to a fall in care standards. Therefore, the measures resulting from these tools should be related to the underlying nursing problem diagnosis. Evaluation obtained from these audits needs to be forwarded to the nurse managers and fed back to the nurses providing care in a timely fashion if patient care is to be improved.

Measuring Nursing Skills

Tilquin's PRN 80 system, developed on the basis of identified measures of care plans, is an example of a system designed to provide information needed for nurse staffing decisions. The problem of differences in skills among individual nurses is accepted by both Tilquin and Henney in their reports. Managers need to decide whether or not they want to accept this limitation or invest in even more complicated and expensive staffing methologies that include measures of nursing skills.

CHAPTER 7

PATIENT MONITORING

An increasing number of computer systems are being introduced into specialised units which are capable of identifying potentially serious conditions and presenting large volumes of data in a meaningful form so that significant trends can be easily identified.

Within this section, a computer system in a cardio-thoracic unit in the U.K. (originally developed in Sweden), and in a renal unit in Belgium are described which rely on hospital staff, particularly nurses, to input much of the patients' clinical data.

The Impact of Computers on Nursing
M. Scholes, Y. Bryant and B. Barber (eds.)
Elsevier Science Publishers B.V. (North-Holland)
© IFIP-IMIA, 1983

7.1.

COMPUTERS – HELP OR HINDRANCE TO THE CLINICAL NURSE?

Jill M. Martin

1.   Introduction

Computers were first introduced into British hospitals in the early 1960s, when their primary use was for administrative purposes (i.e. pay-roll). At the time there was considerable speculation as to the value of their potential contribution towards patient care. From then onwards, dramatic improvements in technology have provided a wide variety of very powerful mini and micro computers which have opened the doors to far more extensive computer usage throughout the health service.

The costs of health care services, which are met from public funds, are not only very large, but have been growing significantly faster than the United Kingdom's gross domestic product. In consequence efforts are being made to find ways of limiting the rising costs, or of obtaining greater value for money within existing budgets. It therefore appears a logical development to extend the use of automatic data processing into the field of planning and rationalising the various types of health care and services connected more directly with patient care. This extension of computer usage necessitates that the nursing profession should become much more involved than before in their use. In this paper a brief description will be set out of a computer system, that although used by a multidisciplinary group of doctors, nurses, technicians and para medical staff was very much nurse dependent for its success and further development. Certain conclusions, to be drawn from the implementation of this system, will be indicated.

2.   The Computer System

This paper is based on a real-time, patient-data system, developed at the Karolinska Hospital in Stockholm (William-Elsson et al, 1969). The system, with certain modifications, was purchased by the North-Western Regional Health Authority and was installed in March 1973 in the Wythenshawe Hospital cardio-thoracic department. It now operates in the hospital over a range of departments including the intensive therapy unit, and cardiology department, the pathology laboratory, the blood gas laboratory, and cardio thoracic theatre (1, 2, E4). The system is, in essence, a collection, storage and presentation system in which the input and output of information is extensive; facilities are available for fluid balance, blood balance, and electrolyte balance calculations.

A common problem, arising in all types of specialised units involving major medical and surgical care, is that of handling the amount of data generated during the patient's stay. Reliance is placed on ward personnel for collection, manipulation and presentation of important data.

In relation to this the care of the patient is very dependent on the medical staff having quick and easy access to all the most recent information, together with a good dependable form of communication within the relevant areas. Further, it is necessary that this information be presented in such a way that important and significant trends in a patient's condition can be easily recognisable and rapid decisions with regard to therapy be made. If all these facilities are to be met, the inter-linking of all the departments involved in the care of the patient is essential.

Manual recording and communication of data places a great amount of work on ward and laboratory staff, as well as impeding the inter-action with the patient. This can also result in errors or loss of information during transfer.

3.   The Equipment of the System

The total system consists of Censor 908 Processor (Manufactured by Stansaab Elektronik AB., Barkarby, Sweden) with 64K bytes of core store, a 2 megabyte fixed-head disc, paper tape facilities, a hard-copy printer, 10 Grafoskop visual display units, 59 push-button intercoms - used for data input and inter-departmental communications, together with all specified programs.

However, from the user point of view one is only concerned with the following equipment:

Grafoskop Terminals

Grafoskop terminals comprise of 14 inch screens and typewriter keyboards with additional special function keys. Nine of the ten visual display units are distributed throughout the Cardio-Thoracic department, one in each of the operating theatres, 4 in the Intensive Therapy Unit, 2 in the Coronary Care Unit, 1 shared between the Cardiac Investigation Unit and Respiratory Function Unit and the remaining visual display terminal is situated in the Haemotology and Bio-chemistry laboratories.

These visual display terminals all operate independently of each other and are used to display all aspects of the patients condition in graphical, tabulated and free-text forms. Trend indications are easily recognisable and facilities are available for more detailed analysis of data as required, for example - alteration to time scale and back dating of information. Although the Grafoskop is primarily used for more detailed analysis of data, it's function as an input terminal is well established. The standard displays and resulting formats are readily available and easily understood by anyone who might be attending the patient.

Intercoms

The greatest proportion of numerical data is entered via the intercom system and originates from the **patients' bedside,** as well as from operating theatres and laboratories. However, intercom sets are distributed throughout the department, in both offices and clinical areas. Of the total of 59 sets, 39 are used for input of data. These intercoms, the primary data gathering terminals for the system, function with a touch-tone push-button keyboard, containing several special function keys, in addition to digits 0 - 9. For input of data such as blood pressure, urine ouput and 108 other numerical values, including laboratory results, a 2 digit code system has been developed. To achieve an input the intercom is linked into the computer, the patients hospital number is keyed and this is followed by a code and value. Intercoms which are specific to one patient, e.g. by the bedside, become 'patient connected' once the hospital number has been keyed and it remains so for the duration of that patient's stay, thereby making it unnecessary to repeat the hospital number.

The procedure for data entry entails calling up the computer, in the same way as one would call up any other extension on an intercom communicating system and then carrying out the patient and variable identification procedures, followed by the entry of the value. For example, code for systolic pressure = 11, expired minute volume = 56, sinthrome = 96. The completion of each step of data entry at these terminals is acknowledged by a distinctive answer tone, with separate tones to identify values within the normal range, abnormal range and not acceptable range. Values of variables within the normal range, are automatically accepted by the computer, abnormal within the pre-determined abnormal limits will only be accepted if the value entry step of the data entry procedure is repeated and unacceptable values which fall outside these limits will not be accepted. The full data procedure can be carried out very quickly after a relatively short experience of the system. An average time for a nurse to become proficient in this procedure was approximately fifteen minutes.

Printer

A 120 character per second printer is situated in the Intensive Therapy Unit. Some hard-copy printouts occur automatically at pre-determined times of the day. However, there is a facility for requesting individual printouts, when appropriate, via any of the visual display units.

When patients are discharged from the clinical areas served by the computer system, a hard-copy printout summary is inserted into their hospital record and all the computer data is transferred onto punch paper tape, which is retained in the computer office. Because the procedure is associated with the erasure of the patient's record from the system, the transfer of data onto paper tape is not usually carried out until a few days after discharge from the clinical areas, in order to avoid the need to put the data back into the system - in the event of the patient requiring to be re-admitted for treatment.

The basic philosophy is that a carefully designed computer controlled real-time system can considerably reduce the task of data handling and calculation, in addition linking together all departments concerned in the care of the critically ill patient.

The computer based data handling system, at present still in operation at Wythenshawe Hospital, can effectively collect data, which is inserted manually at its' source, manipulate it as required, store and display it in a clear and concise form - and functions 24 hours per day for 365 days of the year.

4.   Implementation

Although permanent computer staff had not been envisaged for the system, the intention was to employ specialists to organise the introduction and training of the users; consequently a nursing officer with experience of Intensive Care and coronary cases and a technical adviser with a computer background were appointed and commenced post in May 1973. They were joined in January 1974 by a part-time secretary, who is still in post and responsible for the day to day management of the system. Outside emergency facilities can be called in as necessary on the event of hardware faults.

These people working together have reported to and worked under the general guidance of a hospital computer committee, which consists of representatives from the senior medical adviser from the North Western Regional Health Authority.

The initial job they (i.e. nursing officer and technical adviser) had to undertake was to identify themselves with the users and gain their confidence. They found that the initial attitude towards the Patient Data Display System, from nearly all personnel, was one of apprehension, not merely because they were going to be asked to use a computer based system, but because of a general lack

of knowledge as to what the system could do and how they would be able to use
it. A number of people were concerned that they would be the odd person who
would be unable to master the system. To overcome this apprehension and whilst
planning the training programme and phased implementation of the system, they
regularly visited all personnel for informal discussions explaining the 'raison
d'etre' of the system and correcting misconceptions about computers in general
and the place of Data Display Systems within patient care areas in particular.

These initial reactions made it imperative to take great care with the training
programme for all categories of staff, including nurses (who would prove to be
the key users, if the system was to be a success), doctors, laboratory and paramedical staff. They were all trained during their own working hours so as to
avoid inconvenience to them, and this involved working to fit in with the
staffs' convenience not their own. They were also concerned that the first
introduction to the system for all staff should be by them, so as to stop the
spread of false impressions by partly trained staff. Especially important was
the need to have an understanding of the work of the intensive therapy, coronary
care and cardiothoracic areas - the importance of employing a nurse with this
experience to implement such a system.

Staff were trained individually where possible and never more than three at a
time. Part of the training was to go to the computer room to see exactly how
the data was removed on punched paper tape, re-entered into the system as it
would be if a patient was re-admitted, and also to examine the hardware of the
computer. It was felt that it created a more meaningful use of the system and
stimulates further interest to know just where all the information is being
stored, and how it is handled in the computer room, although this is not of
direct consequence to the actual users of the system. The training which was
completed before staff were asked to use the Patient Data Display System,
enabled them to build up a useful rapport with the staff, and to gain their
confidence. They were indeed quick to point out the shortcomings of the system
and were soon telling them how they would modify it to suit their particular
needs.

The friendly and informal relationships built up whilst training the users
proved essential to reassure them that they were operating the system for their
benefit and the patients and not for the benefit of a computer department.

The initial conception of the system at Wythenshawe was that it should be
installed and operated for a period of one year without modification. They
adhered to the spirit of this but not the letter, for example it soon became
clear and indeed, the nursing staff told them in no uncertain manner, that the
printer in the Intensive Care Unit was too slow, and so after six months of
operation a faster printer was installed, and there were also a number of very
minor, but necessary changes to the system made to accommodate oversights in the
initial planning. The 'burden' of use of the system fell very much upon the
nursing staff, and it was therefore critical that difficult problems were
tackled promptly if user acceptance was to be enhanced.

Such a system they learned, although a powerful tool, will only be a success if
the users see it as making a significant contribution to the quality of care
that can be given to their patients.

During this initial period the users were able to gain experience of operating
the system as it stood, knowing that it was in a fixed state and that it would
not change while they were off duty or away on holiday. It was felt that this
was of considerable importance so that the users could gain confidence in the
use of the system. While they know it is in a stable state they are better able
to build up a general appreciation of what the system is trying to do for them
and how it is trying to help them in their work, and thus integrate it better
into their routines.

After about six months of operation they began to ask the users (mainly the nurses who are the prime users of the system) what ideas they would like to incorporate to improve the system if they were given a free hand. Ideas came much faster and freer than expected and there was no shortage of good material. Naturally many of the ideas were self-conflicting and, of course, they were not able to accommodate all ideas, but they did feel that during the period of initial running the moratorium on changes gave the users an opportunity to develop a much better idea of what they really wanted the system to do. Then when they were asked for their opinions they would give them with much better reasoning and with much more thought than they would have been able to do if asked before the system commenced operation.

There was, naturally, quite a long period of discussion between them and the computer manufacturer about the development of the new ideas, and naturally money had to be provided for their implementation. Their philosophy was that the computer manufacturer should do all the system changes, which were mainly software and they should not do any programming themselves. This again ensured that the system was in a fixed state as far as the users were concerned, and that the modifications when done by the manufacturer would be tested by him, on an in-house machine, and installed late one night at the users convenience, and so could be introduced with a minimum of inconvenience to the users. Thus the users did not have large numbers of programmers continually interrupting the operating of the system while new programs were being tested.

It had always been their intention to run the system for the convenience of its users. Hence the system changes, when completed and tested by the manufacturer, were installed during the night of a period during the holiday season, when the load of the Intensive Care Unit was at a minimum, and the theatres were not functioning except for emergency cases.

The first section of the changes which mainly comprised a completely redesigned blood and fluid balance system, again designed by the users with a little assistance, was installed during August 1974. The second part was installed at the end of March 1975, during the Easter holidays. The users were pleased to see that their ideas had in fact been used, and were delighted with the new system, which they themselves had designed. Undoubtedly much of the co-operation between the installation team and the users was due to the friendly and informal way in which they had been trained, and introduced to the system. Many ideas about the complicated nature of computers had been dispelled (in fact it was not called a computer system but a Patient Data Display System) and this helped to overcome many of the psychological barriers.

The Wythenshawe system is now running under the day-to-day guidance of a Computer System Officer, it is her job to unload patients' data when they leave the system, look after the day-to-day needs of the computer and to train new staff as they come onto the wards and laboratories.

It is necessary for the continued success of such a system that the project should evolve with active liaison between all members of staff using it, by means of meetings and informal discussions, a process now developing at Wythenshawe Hospital.

During the first few years there was a consciousness of the need to gain information in particular about:

i)   user attitudes to a real-time patient data display system
ii) whether the introduction of computers could help to relieve staff
     shortages, improve the collection and dissemination of information,
     particularly in respect of the specialist trained nurses within intensive
     therapy environments.

To this end, systematic collection of information was implemented. The
informtion so gained may well be useful when considering the essential need to
involve nursing staff in the future use and development of computer systems
within the clinical environment.

With two years experience, a study was carried out in the Spring of 1975(3) into
user attitudes, and information was collected by questionnaire from a
representative body of some 200 staff who had used the system. There was a 100%
response to the questionnaire from nursing staff, which demonstrated their very
great interest in the system, and therefore the potential extent to which the
nursing profession can, and should, become involved. The questionnaire sought
to ascertain views about the system from the staff actually using it, and free
comment was encouraged.

The study highlighted certain major conclusions:

i)   Nurses took longer than doctors or technicians to become confident in
     using the system. This was to be expected in that nurses needed to be
     familiar with all functions of the system for both input and retrieval of
     data, whereas doctors and technicians are concerned primarily only with
     certain aspects of the data.
ii) All groups indicated that they trusted the information generated by the
     system.
iii) The output from the system led to less need for telephonic communication
     and messenger systems, which augmented the time available to nursing staff
     for patient care.

iv) Nurses and technicians confirmed that they did not wish to return to a
     non-computerised system, however clinicians were doubtful.
v)   Recruitment of nursing staff was more difficult following the introduction
     of the system, due to the lack of computer trained nurses.

In general it appeared from the replies to the questionnaire that the degree of
confidence in the system reflected the extent of the individual's involvement in
it. In effect, the less you used it, the less you liked it.

5.   Conclusion

This paper has concentrated upon specialised patient care, but the need for
information about the average patient in a general ward environment must not be
forgotten.

Computer information about such patients is currently in use in many areas, but
if this technology is to become an accepted part of the ward environment, it
will need the active support of the nursing staff responsible for patient care.
In order to obtain such active support:

i)   Consideration must be given to nurse education in connection with computer
     developments.
ii) there must be active liaison between all staff required to participate in
     the use of the system from its conception to total implementation.

Finally, the development of computer nursing systems can only be achieved with the active support of the higher echelons of the professions. If this support is to be effective, it must be fully informed about the practical details of the implementation of computer systems.

REFERENCES

1.   William Elsson et al, 1969   - Private communication.
2.   Ashcroft, J.M., Berry, J.L. (1955) 'The Wythenshawe Hospital Patient Data Display System'. European Journal of Intensive Care Medicine 1. 49-54.
3.   Morlander, O. (1976) 'Medical Information Systems Intended Especially For Intensive Care and Surgery Departments'. British Computer Society Meeting - Guys Hospital.
4.   Bradshaw, E.G., Thompson, G.R. (1975) 'User Attitudes to a Real-Time Patient Data Display System'. Belgian Congress of Anaesthesiology. 26 suppl. 191-199

The Impact of Computers on Nursing
M. Scholes, Y. Bryant and B. Barber (eds.)
Elsevier Science Publishers B.V. (North-Holland)
© IFIP-IMIA, 1983

7.2.

NURSES' EXPERIENCE WITH A COMPUTER IN A NEPHROLOGY–HYPERTENSION DEPARTMENT

G.M. De Pooter, M.M. Elseviers, G.A. Verpooten, R.L. Lins, J.P. Van Waeleghem, J. Van Pellicom, and M.E. De Broe

1. Introduction

One of the major tasks of a department of nephrology is the treatment of patients with end-stage renal disease by peritoneal or hemodialysis. The hemodialysis patients are submitted three times a week to a rather standardized treatment. During this repetitive treatment a large number of medical, administrative and technical parameters are measured and registered, leading to an enormous amount of hardly accessible data.

For this reason the hemodialysis unit was the first to be computerized, when the department switched to electronic data processing in 1979. The aim of the introduction of the computer in the daily activities in the hemodialysis unit was threefold:

(a) **Improved patient care:** The computer should allow verification of data recording accuracy. It should produce conveniently arranged summaries of reliable patient data, so that problems are more rapidly noticed. Medical orders and nursing directions can be planned systematically and prospectively and their execution can be checked.

(b) **Administrative Efficiency:** A number of administrative tasks can be performed by the computer with less effort and more accurately.

(c) **Clinical Research:** The systematic and accessible form in which data are recorded, allows much more effective use of patient data in clinical research projects.

This computer program package, called DIALAZA, has now been used for 15 months in two hemodialysis centers. This paper describes the DIALAZA system and provides a first evaluation of its effectiveness.

2. Hardware

A Hewlett-Packard 9845B desktop computer with 60 kilobytes of random access memory and a 20 line video screen, two flexible disk drives of 2 x kilobytes (Hewlett-Packard 9885) and an external matrix printer with graphic capabilities (Hewlett-Packard 2631G) were chosen for this project. This configuration is the minimum requirement for a unit having 30 patients in hemodialysis.

3. Software

The programs are written in HP BASIC. The data base is built up as a modular system and each module is filled up sequentially. A pointer is used for each patient to keep track of the last data entry. New data can be entered easily via a typewriter keyboard, with immediate display on the screen. The information is coded as much as possible but space is provided for patient based remarks. Data output is on the video screen or as hardcopy via the printer. Data retrieval is possible by patient or on a list of all patients, per item, per module or as a periodical survey.

4.   Structure of the Data Base

The contents of each unit (called module) of the data base is as follows:-

(i)   Identity

This module contains the basic administrative data of the patient, such as name, address, birth date, social security number. The name and address of the physicians involved in the treatment are also listed.

(ii)   Diagnosis

In this module the patient's medical history and medical diagnoses are recorded. A summary of the applied treatments is also added.

(iii)   Vascular access

This module contains the reports of surgical intervention and the results of angiographic examinations of the vascular access.

(iv)   Laboratory

Contains the results of monthly and quarterly blood and urine examinations.

(v)   Hemodialysis

This module includes the information necessary to perform the actual dialysis session. It is divided in three parts

        (a)   Permanent data and orders:
               - concerning the patient: blood group, diet, warnings about allergies,
                 etc.
               - concerning the technique: type of dialyser and dialysate, optimal
                 weight, blood flow,...
        (b)   Medication:
               name of the drug, packing form, start and end date, dose, and time
               of intake.
        (c)   Dialysis data:
               blood pressure and weight pre and post dialysis, temperature, heart
               rate, complications, quantity of administered fluids and blood
               transfusions,...

(vi)   Chronic Ambulatory Peritoneal Dialysis (CAPD)

The information stored for CAPD patients is the data recorded at the monthly visit to the outpatient clinic (blood pressure, temperature, physical examination, culture of the peritoneal fluid) and data of eventual peritonitis periods (cause, symptoms, type of organism, treatment).

5.   Dialysis Forms

The input of identity, diagnosis, and laboratory results are carried out by administrative personnel under medical supervision. The input of hemodialysis related data is however under the full responsibility of the renal nurse.

A computer form for each patient is generated before the dialysis session. This form is used as well as a work sheet during dialysis and as input form after dialysis. An English translation of this form is shown in Fig. 1. The upper part of the work sheet contains general information about the patient and specific orders to perform the dialysis treatment. During the course of the

UNIT/POST :
RESP. NURSE :
TRANSPORT :

BLOOD GROUP :
ALLERGY :
HEPATITIS B Ag :
DIET :

TYPE OF TREATMENT :
TYPE OF DIALYZER :
DIALYSATE :
PRIMING :
BLOOD FLOW :
HEPARINE (ml/h) :
OPTIMAL WEIGHT :

MEDICATION DURING DIALYSIS

ALARM CONTROLS :
TEMPERATURE
ART. PRESSURE
VEN. PRESSURE
BLOOD LEAK DETECT.
AIR DETECTOR
STROKE VOLUME

DATE
HOSPITALISED (1=NO, 2=YES)
RESP. AT START
RESP. AT END

WEIGHT GAIN
U.F. COEFFICIENT

DATA FROM PRECEEDING DIALYSIS :
WEIGHT E.D. :
BLOOD VOLUME :

VASCULAR ACCESS : NUMBER OF PUNCTURES
COMPLICATIONS

1 = NONE - 2 = HEMATOMA - 3 = BLEEDING (PRE-DIAL.)
4 = BLEEDING (POST-DIAL.) - 5 = THROMBOSIS

HOUR	B.P.		WEIGHT		PRESSURES		Q.B.	VOLUME		HEPARIN	REMARKS
	SYST.	DIAST.	PROGRAMM.	EFFECT.	V.D.	D.D.		PROGRAMM.	EFFECT.		

SALINE (ml) :
HEMACEL (ml) :
BLOOD/PACKED CELLS (ml) :
COMPL. HR 1 :
2 :
3 :
4 :

1 = NONE
2 = HYPOTENSION SYMPT.
3 = HYPOTENSION A-SYMPT.
4 = HYPERTENSION
5 = CRAMPS
6 = HEADACHE
7 = VOMITING
8 = NAUSEA
9 = ANGINA
10 = HYPOGLYCEMIA

PROBLEMS

PLANNED FOR TODAY

FURTHER PLANNING

Figure 1. The Dialysis Worksheet (English Translation).

dialysis the results of periodical parameter control and the observed complications are noted in the middle part of the form. At the lower part space is provided to write down problems and appointments for special examinations and treatments. The investigations will automatically be printed out in this area, on the appropriate day. Changes in medical orders or medication are also noted in this part of the form.

After each dialysis session the most important parameters, the complications and the changes in treatment, are entered in the computer. The mean duration of the input procedure is 45 seconds per patient. The printing of the dialysis forms is strongly influenced by the slow response time of the flexible disks. For this reason a special print program able to produce the forms without direct supervision was developed.

A form presenting a summary of the last 14 dialysis sessions is updated every week (see fig. 2).

6   Discussion

Fifteen months after the introduction of the DIALAZA system in two dialysis centers, it is worthwhile to make a first evaluation of its acceptance by the staff and its impact on patient care.

Since there exist only few reports in the literature concerning computer aided patient care in hemodialysis (1,2,3), profound discussions were necessary in the development phase of this computer package. It is well known that the content and form of most medical records are not suitable for computerization. The first problem was the selection of the items to be stored in the computer.

After this selection several clinical parameters had to be transformed into a coded form. Thereafter, provisional versions of the dialysis work sheet and other forms were tested in practice. After several staff discussions the final draft was entered in the computer. During the initial run-in period of the program the main problem was the acceptance by some staff members (3); their reluctance to use the computer expressed itself as a careless use of the computer forms. However, this problem gradually solved itself, when the users became familiar with the possibilities of the DIALAZA system.

One of the main objectives of the DIALAZA system was the **improvement of patient care**. A major factor contributing to this improvement is the continuity in patient care built into the system. Through the dialysis work sheets all members of the dialysis team have direct access to the updated dialysis prescription. Human errors and misunderstandings amongst staff concerning patient treatment and care are minimized. For example a medical order or a prescription for a special pre-dialysis blood sampling will only be withdrawn if execution is confirmed. The recognition of trends in the patient's vital parameters is facilitated by the printed survey of the preceding dialysis sessions. Moreover, this survey facilitates the rapid diagnosis of pathological conditions and contributes to the decision making process in the staff meetings.

A second positive element of the DIALAZA system is the **administrative timesaving** for the nursing team. There is no need for transcription of the permanent orders, since they are printed automatically on the dialysis work sheet. Monthly reports, lists of diagnoses and laboratory results are generated by the computer. The automatic handling of physician fees, hospital accounts, transport bills and other financial data is greatly appreciated by the administrative unit.

NAME OF THE PATIENT	26/07	28/07	30/07	02/08	05/08	06/08	09/08	MEAN
BP SYST. PRE D.								
BP DIAST. PRE D.								
BP SYST. POST D.								
BP DIAST. POST D.								
WEIGHT PRE D.								
WEIGHT POST D.								
TOTAL BLOOD VOLUME								
HEPARINE								
SALINE								
HEMACEL								
BLOOD/ PACKED CELLS								
NUMBER OF PUNCTURES								
FISTULA RELATED COMPL.								
OTHER COMPLICATIONS								

VASCULAR ACCESS RELATED COMPLICATIONS

DIALYSIS RELATED COMPLICATIONS

REMARKS

LABORATORY RESULTS

PLANNING

MEDICATION SURVEY

GENERAL DATA

DIET :

LONGTERM GOAL :

HEPARINE :

OPTIMAL WEIGHT :

Fig 2: Summary Form for recent Dialysis Sessions (English Translation)

The patient data stored by this program have already found application in a few **clinical research** projects. For example, a study of vascular access survival in function of dialysis related complications has recently been conducted.

Although the DIALAZA program is still in a transitional state, we think that it already contributes substantially to the quality of the patient care in our dialysis unit.

REFERENCES

1. DEGOULET P., GOUPY F., BLAMOUTIER A., HIREL J.C., AIME F,. REACH I., JACOBS C., LEGRAIN M.   Evaluation of the DIAPHANE dialysis registry, Proc MIB 79, 1979,711-719.
2. GYSELINCK-MAMBOURG   A.M.,   RORIVE   G.,   VAN   CAUWENBERGE   H. Assistnceinformatique a la fonction medicale dans un centre d'hemodialyse. Min. Nefr., 1973, 20, 308-311.
3. STERN M., NORMAN R., BLASCO N., KANTER A.   Computer care: 20th century nursing. AANNT, 1977, 4, 177-185.

The Impact of Computers on Nursing
M. Scholes, Y. Bryant and B. Barber (eds.)
Elsevier Science Publishers B.V. (North-Holland)
© IFIP-IMIA, 1983

7.3.

PATIENT MONITORING

Discussion

Available Systems

There was surprise at the limited number of commercial or individually developed
real-time systems available in this field, particularly within renal units.
Several developments are currently known to be taking place including two
systems in the USA which are concerned with creating models to study the
optimisation of treatment.

Automatic Data Acquisition and 'Slave' Screens

At some sites, large 'slave' screens are used to echo the read-outs of
computerised monitors, displaying the information for several patients on one
screen. Although these enable nurses to spend more time at the bed side, the
effect of using these screens on both nurses and patients was unclear as was the
reaction to using computers to collect data directly on-line from the patient.
For example, if the nurse constantly watches the screen, does the patient ever
receive her total attention? Concern was expressed about the effect of false
audio alarms - when too many of these were generated, nurses tended to ignore
all alarms.

Accuracy and Effectiveness of Data

Where patient data is entered into the computer using an intercom device which
does not display the values input at the time of entry or transcribed from
handwritten documents, care must be taken to ensure that the data is accurate.
The display or printing of too much data can easily mask vital information.
Systems which highlight or select genuine anomalies can overcome these
difficulties. Again, the point was reiterated that nurses must be involved in
the design and implementation of these systems particularly with those aspects
where they will be expected to input or retrieve information.

CHAPTER 8

DRUG MANAGEMENT

A description is given in this section of computer systems for handling drugs in hospitals in the U.K. and U.S.A. involving doctors, nurses and pharmacists. Other references to this topic can also be found in papers within the chapter on Nursing Records. Each system provides for the prescribing and administration of drugs on the ward and dispensing in the pharmacy. Differences should be noted in the approach to providing information at the time of prescribing, the recording of drugs given and the dispensing procedures adopted. Other uses of computer technology such as pharmacy stock control and financial accounting, drug dosage calculations and formulation of intravenous feeding solutions are not included.

The Impact of Computers on Nursing
M. Scholes, Y. Bryant and B. Barber (eds.)
Elsevier Science Publishers B.V. (North-Holland)
© IFIP-IMIA, 1983

8.1.

COMPUTERIZED MEDICATION SYSTEM

Margo Cook

Design Perspectives

The discussion of a computerized medication system provides the opportunity not only to review the components of such systems but also to address the issues relevant to designing any computerized patient care information system. The issues are:

1. breadth of design while allowing segmented or incremental development and implementation.
2. program development that identifies the elements common to all settings to create a framework, yet allows individualization of the variable elements.

When designing a medication system it is necessary to maintain a wide perspective. A medication system encompasses the doctor, the nurse, the pharmacist, the drug supplies and most important, the patient. It deals with data for procuring and providing medications (inventory systems) as well as the information to get the right medication in the right dose via the right route at the right time to the right patient (information systems).

The design must take all these elements into consideration. It must also address the interelationship of data for all users of both the inventory and information aspects of the system.

Development can be more selective. This paper with the focus on nursing systems describes an information system in use at one hospital. This description will be followed by an analysis of the design elements and the variables that have enabled this same system to be used in some 30 hospitals with no progressing charges.

Drug Prescribing

This system is constructed to be used in conjunction with what we call an ATD (Admission, Transfer, Discharge) system and with a basic nursing system. It begins with the physicians order. Approaching any VMT (Video Matrix Terminal) in the hospital the doctor signs on with his unique code and gets his list of patients in hospital. He selects the appropriate patient, confirms the name and moves to the master guide where he selects pharmacy. He is presented with a display which lists drugs concerning his specialty and an alphabetic access to all drugs available in the pharmacy. Selecting a drug name, (either a brand name or the genuine name, both are used in the index) he is taken to the drug screen which has several elements:

1. common orders which are pre-constructed, complete orders that are used frequently
2. list of the drugs in the dose forms available and a place for a type-in dose, and
3. common schedules.

From this screen he constructs a drug order. If he wants a special schedule, he accesses the schedule pages and selects any schedule he deems appropriate. Once he has entered the drug orders to the computer a number of actions take place.

Drug Interaction Aspects

Before proceeding to review these actions it is appropriate to consider the aspect of drug information and interaction as part of the ordering process. First, drug information - a number of options have been constructed with data built-in to give the doctor information about the drug. Experience has shown that these systems usually take longer to use and more importantly, can become very annoying to the user who must go through the same learning pathway many times a day. Instead, this system provides some drug information on request. As chart audits indicate problems with drug use, special control screens are built to educate the doctor. This approach to the use of forced information has proved to be extremely valuable and has been shown to improve practice.

Drug interaction information is not a part of this system at present because a study of 2 years of El Camino drug ordering data (taken from file tapes) revealed less than 1% significant interaction in drugs ordered. The cost of such a system and the considerable problems of maintaining the drug interaction data base made such a return seem inappropriate. They may well deserve more consideration as new results become available. Thus, using a rather straight-forward ordering system the order is placed on the patients record. Immediately two documents are produced, one for pharmacy and one for the nurse. The pharmacist gets a prescription in label format for use in dispensing the drug. The nurse gets a notification of a new medical order.

Drug Supply

Subsequently, for as many days as the order is in force, the pharmacist gets a medication supply list to enable him to dispense another 24 hour supply of the drug. This list serves as his patient medication profile. Floor stock drugs such as control substances are also noted. They are not dispensed, but they are on the profile.

Drug Administration

For the nurse, two basic documents are printed. The care plan is printed at the beginning of the shift with all the medications listed, and together with the list of hourly medications due.

These lists are used to enable the nurse to give the right drug to the right patient at the right time. The nurses skill and judgement come into play in determining the frequency for PRN drugs or in helping ensure that a patient can in fact take the drugs prescribed.

A record must be made of the fact that the patient did in fact get the drug and possibly its effect. Using the computer, with just a few light pen strokes the patient is identified and the PRN drug is recorded. Because it was PRN it is necessary to document the reason for giving the drug. If no record is made of the site of an injectable drug, the computer will give an error message.

Drug Records

Once charted, the computer stores the time given for easy retrieval when deciding or subsequent PRN doses. It is also possible (and desirable) for the nurse to record the patient's response to the drug. This is easily done later when the response has been observed. In the case of scheduled medications, the pathway is even simpler. In less than a minute, it is possible to chart all medications given at 9 a.m. to 6 or more patients.

Because the computer record is the legal record a number of by-products are derived from these few simple actions. The record is available in several formats, daily summary as well as a 7 day summary, charge per dose of the drug administered and workload data both for the nursing and pharmacy.

Transferable Systems

This system is run on a computer which two other hospitals share. They use the same programs - common elements are drugs, doses, frequency as orders on drug, dose, time for recording as well as scheduling parameters and charge and workload capture. The formularies for each hospital are different, as are their specific scheduling patterns, yet the system is both common to each and unique to each.

Last but not least it should be noted that the medication information system under normal processing took 21 steps, with the computer there are 10 steps. The time to order, dispense and record medications is reduced as well. In addition, this system is already integrated with an ATD system and the data is organised for future interface with an inventory system. Thus the medication system can be the model for other systems development.

The Impact of Computers on Nursing
M. Scholes, Y. Bryant and B. Barber (eds.)
Elsevier Science Publishers B.V. (North-Holland)
© IFIP-IMIA, 1983

8.2.

A COMPUTER SYSTEM FOR DRUG PRESCRIBING AND ITS IMPACT ON DRUG
ADMINISTRATION

Clare C. Ashton

Introduction

This paper describes a hospital computer system for drug prescribing and the
facilities it provides for drug administration and pharmacy dispensing at the
Queen Elizabeth Hospital (QEH), Birmingham. The system has been developed in
the computer department over a number of years in conjunction with doctors,
nurses and pharmacists. It forms part of an integrated hospital information
system using a Univac 418-III computer with visual display units (VDU) and
printers sited in wards and departments which, in addition, provides patient
administration, reporting of laboratory results and the ordering of nursing
care.

Inappropriate, inaccurate or potentially dangerous prescribing may occur for
many reasons, but probably results from a failure to use all the available
information about a drug and the patient and to relate these at the time of
prescribing. Drugs may be prescribed in the wrong dose or by the wrong route;
the importance of age or renal function may be ignored by or unknown to the
prescriber; and incompatible drugs may be prescribed concurrently.
Prescriptions may be ambiguous, incomplete and illegible. The combination of
these errors and the increasing use and numbers of drugs potentially increases
the risk to the patient.

The computer system was therefore designed with the following objectives:

-      to improve the quality of prescribing by ensuring that, at the time of
       prescribing, the doctors have as much information as possible about the
       patient and proposed drug treatment
-      to prevent the prescribing of inappropriate or potentially dangerous drugs
       by the use of checking procedures
-      to reduce errors in drug administration by the provision of a printed
       administration document with clear, unambiguous prescriptions
-      to provide a data base for studies of prescribing patterns and for
       detecting and monitoring adverse drug reactions.

The computerised drug prescribing system enables doctors to prescribe for their
patients using the VDU in the ward sister's office. As each prescription is
made, information about the drug is automatically displayed. The drug is then
checked by the computer for contra-indications and drug interactions. After
each prescribing episode, a new prescription list is printed on the ward
printer, adjacent to the VDU, which nurses use to give and record the
administration of drugs. Messages are printed in the pharmacy department when
dispensing is required or when prescription warnings are overridden.

A drug information system, which provides a back-up to prescribing, can be used
independently and has been available throughout the hospital since 1977. A
pilot trial of the prescribing system took place during the summer of 1981 for
five weeks in one medical ward. Following an evaluation of the system, it is
planned to extend the trial into other wards.

Development of the Drugs Project

The computer project at the Queen Elizabeth Medical Centre was established in
1969 as part of the experimental computer programme sponsored by the Department
of Health & Social Security (DHSS). Later that same year, the Drugs Project was
set up with separate DHSS funding under the medical direction of Prof. J.M.
Bishop, to investigate the role of computing to improve the efficiency and
safety of drug use.

At first, the Drugs Team (initially composed of a systems analyst, medical
registrar and pharmacist) undertook a literature search of manual and computer
systems concerned with drug handling and monitoring adverse drug reactions. The
decision was taken to exploit the computer's real-time potential to monitor drug
usage by designing a system for drug prescribing and administration rather than
pharmacy stock control.

The drug handling procedures at the hospital were studied. A structured
prescription sheet was being introduced similar to that originally designed at
the London Hospital(1), which is still in use today with some modification. The
doctors are instructed to prescribe drugs wherever possible by their approved
name and to indicate frequency by ringing the times of administration on the
sheet. One of the two nurses, required to check drugs and qualified to give
drugs, records the administration of the drug by initialling the box provided.

An assessment of the drugs used at the hospital was made by examining the
pharmacy stock control cards. A method of classifying these drugs for computer
selection was devised based on the familiar British National Formulary (BNF)
according to their therapeutic use and pharmacological action, and tested out on
several house officers using cards equivalent to VDU screens.

Outline proposals for a computerbased drug prescribing and administration system
were put forward during 1970. A simplified prescribing system based on these
proposals was recorded on a video cassette to obtain doctor's opinions. This
was followed by a demonstration system programmed to simulate the prescribing
sequence using a PDP 9 computer linked to a VDU to assess the doctors' reactions
to using 'tree-branching' techniques. Meanwhile, an analysis of drug usage was
undertaken to establish a list of the most commonly used drugs, followed by two
small surveys to establish the incidence of errors attributed to prescribing and
drug administration.

The data collection on drugs commenced in 1971 for the compilation of
information screens and for the checking procedures within prescribing. A
survey of interruptions during drug rounds at four hospitals within the Central
Birmingham District Health Authority was completed. During 1972 with the
assistance of the Department of Psychiatry, a study to determine reaction times
to the choice of type face on VDU screens indicated that the use of upper and
lower case influenced the behaviour of operators - (these results subsequently
affected the design of screens used by all ward based systems). Later that same
year, a survey of drug prescribing(2) commenced to define and measure the errors
of drug use and prescription writing, supporting the value of the project, and
to establish a base-line for future evaluation of the system (36% of all
prescriptions were found to have at least one error whilst the number of other
errors were, in fact, very small - not a great deal of scope for measurable
improvement). For the same reasons, in 1981, the prescriptions made for
approximately 600 patients during their inpatient treatment were collected
together with relevant laboratory data.

In 1973, the drugs team directed their attention towards drug administration. A
detailed survey of administration procedures highlighted some deficiencies in
the prescription sheet introduced in 1969. Proposals in 1974 (F1) provided for

drug round lists and enabled nurses to report back to the computer 'as required' drugs given and regular drugs not given (i.e exception reporting). However, several problems were identified and an alternative administration system was considered. Two further surveys were undertaken to calculate the average number of changes in a patient's drug treatment during an inpatient episode and the number of 'as required' drugs that a patient may be prescribed at any one time. Approval was then given for the system to print individual prescription lists, similar to the current manual prescription sheet, for the nurses to give and to record the administration of drugs. These new proposals were reviewed again in 1980 when all options suggested throughout the history of the drug project were considered, in particular the original suggestion in 1970 to print prescriptions on adhesive labels was re-examined in detail and compared with the proposed prescription list.

An examination of prescribing activities in operating theatres in 1976 indicated a need for VDU's for anaesthetists to prescribe to ensure the viability of the prescribing system. Consequently, a case was made for these to be purchased and installed.

Progress with the detailed design and programming of the drugs system was slow due to delays in the allocation of resources from the project. However, as these resources improved, the drugs team expanded and a drug information system was implemented in 1977 as a precursor to the prescribing system with screens of fixed data in a drugs format file and an alphabetic index of all drugs in the system by approved and proprietary names. The information was specifically designed as an aid to prescribing and includes contra-indications, important side effects, incompatible drugs and dose modifications for patients with impaired renal function. Comparative information on a group of drugs or recommendations on the way a drug or group of drugs should be used is also provided. Approximately 600 drugs in several formulations are now available and those in the QEH formulary are marked with an asterisk. For each drug, the usual range of doses used in the hospital in the available strengths and forms are displayed and only includes those regimes which are acceptable in terms of efficiency and safety. During 1978 and 1979 surveys were undertaken in a surgical and a medical ward and a specialised (renal) unit to determine the current volume of prescriptions, the peak time of prescribing and the location at which prescribing most commonly occurs. These suggested that the computer should be capable of handling the additional load when prescribing is implemented without effecting its current performance.

The very detailed design and programming of this complex system progressed steadily incorporating (as for the information system) the system design principles common to all ward based systems(3) where the user is required to operate the system as a routine function of his/her duties. The computer file structure was determined by the primary objective of maintaining a maximum response time of two seconds between screens. This has been achieved by using direct files (linked to an active patient index) for storing prescription records in start date order and including the code and decode of each item. A 'housekeeping' routine initialised via the console early each morning transfers any orders marked as 'delay cancelled' or 'cancelled' from a direct file of current and future prescriptions to a direct file of non-current prescriptions, so that current prescriptions are stored in the minimum number of blocks (on average one block; approximately 5/6 prescriptions per block). A drugs master file was set up containing all the interactions and contra-indications for each drug with appropriate messages and all the details for each option on the dose screens.

Throughout the development of the drugs project, consultation with users was achieved through a medical user group, including pharmacists, and a nurse user group. Combined meetings were held as necessary. The medical user group was particularly involved with approving the content of the information screens and other doctors were approached as necessary.

Early in the project, advice was sought from the Home Office and the DHSS about the acceptability of a log-in code as the doctor's signature. In hospital the doctor does not legally 'prescribe' but writes an order to the nursing staff to supply to the patient. For this reason, no problems were raised for inpatient prescribing. However, when prescribing drugs for the patient to take out, the same situation does not apply as the doctor prescribes an order to a pharmacist to supply to a patient. It was therefore necessary to introduce local procedures to comply with the statutory Misuse of Drug Regulations 1973. Professional organisations were also approached including the Royal College of Nursing, British Medical Association and the Pharmaceutical Society.

Implementation of Pilot Trial

Following discussions with nursing and medical staff, it was agreed to pilot the drugs system in a medical ward. As the ward chosen was due for closure for upgrading the trial took place for 5 weeks immediately before this event. It was agreed that prescribing of post-operative drugs in the operating theatre would not be introduced until the system was implemented in a surgical ward. Arrangements were made for a small matrix 80 printer to be installed in the ward sister's office and the pharmacy department and linked to the main computer.

Approximately 5 weeks prior to implementation, a parallel run took place for one week as a final check to ensure that the computer system was functioning correctly as a result of the many months of testing, simulating where possible the anticipated plan for implementation. This was carried out by the drugs team who entered each day (in the computer department) all the prescribing activities that had occurred during the previous twenty-four hours for each patient on the trial ward into a parallel database together with questionnaire answers (for new patients) and any abnormal laboratory data. Prescription lists and pharmacy messages were printed in the ward and pharmacy respectively. All the interaction and contra-indication warnings displayed were noted, and the computer records and printouts scrutinised. Any problems were logged and reviewed at the end of the parallel run.

Training of medical, pharmacy and nursing staff took place in the computer department two to three weeks before implementation. Meetings with medical records and pharmacy staff, night sisters and nursing officers were arranged. A letter together with an example of a printed prescription list was sent to appropriate personnel throughout the hospital one week before the trial started giving information about the pilot scheme and the changes to home displays (which the drugs project had brought about) affecting many authorised users.

The take-on of all the inpatients' current prescriptions took place during a weekend when the house officer was on call for emergencies and other medical wards. Assisted by members of the drugs team, half of the patients' prescriptions were entered on Saturday afternoon/evening and the remainder on Sunday. A rota system involving all members of the drugs team was operated throughout the trial to provide support for staff on the ward and in the pharmacy department and to monitor the drug prescribing system. During the first few days, a member of the drugs team accompanied the nurses on drug rounds. All doctors who had patients on the ward used the system to prescribe so that up to eleven doctors eventually took part in the trial, including those doctors providing medical cover for the house officer on the ward. Some of these prescribed for patients on the trial ward using the VDU on the ward where they normally worked.

Prescribing for an inpatient may occur at any time but in particular takes place after a patient has been admitted, during and after ward rounds, before, during and after an operation or investigation and when a patient's condition changes. Under the manual system, prescriptions are written up during the ward round. With the computer system, the house officer memorised the prescriptions agreed during the ward rounds or wrote them down in a note book and entered them into the computer afterwards. As the drugs system does not allow prescribing IV fluids or anaesthetics, IV fluid charts and anaesthetic records continued to be used as necessary. No doctor could use the prescribing system unless his log-in code had been amended to allow him to do so; the same applied to senior medical students with regard to represcribing. This assisted the drugs team in monitoring the system usage as well as meeting legal and data security requirements.

It was agreed that during this trial, all prescriptions would be printed in the pharmacy since the programs for checking non-ward stock items had not then been written. It also allowed this part of the system to be tested more thoroughly than would have otherwise been possible.

The trial was complicated by the fact that both the house officer, ward sister, one of the staff nurses and ward pharmacist took annual leave during the trial period and patients from another medical ward spent a week on the ward whilst their ward was being cleaned!

SYSTEM DESCRIPTION - PRESCRIBING

Initial Entry

To enter the real-time hospital computer system, the doctor, like any authorised user, identifies himself to the computer by his unique personal 'log-in' code of six characters on the terminal keyboard. This code, which is not displayed on the screen, controls the information the doctor may enter or retrieve and ensures confidentiality, and enables the doctor's name to be associated with every record he enters on the computer files.

After the log-in code has been checked, the computer displays the appropriate 'home display' (determined from the code) listing those activities doctors commonly use. The doctor selects by number the activity he requires and thereafter is lead through a series of screens, either completing forms or selecting a number from a list of choices, illustrated in fig 1.

In the system for drug prescribing, the doctor receives the list of patients (in alphabetical order) for the ward appropriate to the VDU's location and a list of patients for any ward in the hospital. If the doctor is prescribing for the first time, the computer responds with a patient questionnaire which the doctor must complete before he may proceed any further. If the patient is already receiving drugs, a list of the patient's current prescriptions is displayed before any prescribing activity can take place (fig 2).

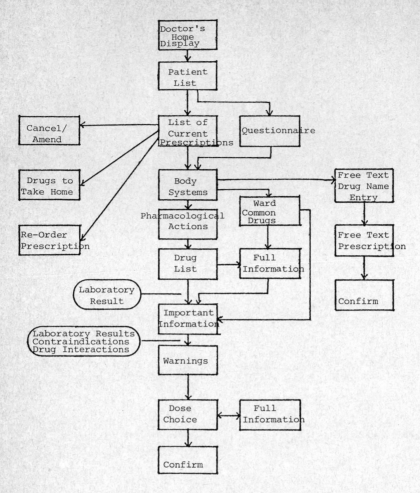

Fig 1.   Flowchart of Prescribing Sequence

```
-------------------------------------------------------------------------------
| E1A  JENKINSON SARAH  M  G999061/8    FEMALE    age 78   DR BROWN            |
|            civil state   M  rel CHURCH OF ENGLAND                            |
|          LIST OF CURRENT PRESCRIPTIONS                17.07.82              |
| Start  Cancel                                          Dr's Initials        |
| Date   Date   (to take effect at end of day)           Start  Cancel        |
| 15/07         PROCHLORPERAZINE IM 12.5mg 4H As required     LBJ             |
| 15/07  22/07 CD PAPAVERETUM IM 10mg 4H for 6 doses As required LBJ   LBJ    |
| 15/07         FERROUS SULPHATE TABLETS 200mg 8H            LBJ             |
| 15/07  22/07  ERYTHROMYCIN TABLETS 250mg 6H For 5 days     LBJ   LBJ       |
| 16/07         TEMAZEPAM CAPSULES 10mg 24H At night At 2200  NB             |
| 17/07  22/07  DIGOXIN IV 0.25mg Single dose At once        MCA   MCA       |
| 17/07         MODURETIC TABLETS 1 tablet 24H               MCA             |
|                                                                             |
|                                                                             |
| Enter ONE or MORE of the following (1-4):- 1 Cancel or amend prescriptions  |
|           2 Make new prescriptions       3 Prescribe TTO's  4 Represcribe   |
| OR enter  5 View previous prescriptions OR 6 Previous TTO's                 |
|                                                                ......... |
|                                                                             |
-------------------------------------------------------------------------------
```

Fig 2. List of Current Prescriptions

Details of the prescriptions, displayed in start date order, include start date,
drug name, route/formulation, dose and frequency, any directions, prescriber's
initials, and if appropriate any predetermined cancellation date and the
initials of the doctor cancelling the prescription. From this screen, the
doctor selects appropriate prescribing activities - cancellation/amendment of
current prescriptions, prescribing new drugs and drugs to take home (TTO's), and
represcribing. Should the doctor wish to review past treatment, either previous
prescriptions or previous TTO's, he may do so by choosing the required option
from this screen. A cumulative list of cancelled prescriptions or TTO's is
displayed with the latest cancelled prescriptions retrieved first. Facilities
exist to page through all the previous prescriptions or TTO's.

Patient Questionnaire

This questionnaire must be completed when the doctor first prescribes in order
to collect specific information about the patient which may affect subsequent
drug therapy, eg. drug hypersensitivities, pregnancy (fig 3). According to the
patient's sex, a male or female questionnaire is displayed and each question
answered by entering 'Y' (yes) or 'N' (no or not yet known). Trimester of
pregnancy is recorded by entering '1', '2' or '3'. If hypersensitivities are
present, these are indicated by typing 'Y' against the appropriate group of
drugs and/or the name of the hypersensitivity. Space is provided for an entry
in freetext, if the required item is not available on the list provided. All
the answers are presented to the doctor for his approval before the drug files
for the patient are updated.

```
--------------------------------------------------------------------------------
| E1A   JENKINSON SARAH  M   G999061/8  F  age 78   DR BROWN                    |
|                 civil state M  rel CHURCH OF ENGLAND                          |
|                                                                               |
|                          FEMALE QUESTIONNAIRE                                  |
| This must be completed as this is a new patient                               |
|                                                                               |
| SECTION 1 - Answer all parts by typing Y for Yes, N for No or Not Known       |
|             HAS THE PATIENT TAKEN A MONO-AMINE OXIDASE INHIBITOR              |
|                                    WITHIN THE LAST TWO WEEKS?                  |
|             IF THE PATIENT IS ALREADY TAKING AN ORAL CONTRACTPTIVE,           |
|             WILL SHE CONTINUE TO DO SO WHILE IN HOSPITAL?                      |
|             IS THE PATIENT PREGNANT?                                           |
|             IF THE PATIENT IS PREGNANT, INDICATE THE TRIMESTER BY             |
|             TYPING 1, 2 OR 3                                                   |
|             IS THE PATIENT HYPERSENSITIVE TO ANY DRUG OR OTHER SUBSTANCE?     |
|-------------------------------------------------------------------------------|
|                                                                               |
| SECTION 2 - Indicate any hypersensitivities by typing Y against the           |
| appropriate group, otherwise leave blank.  If not in this list, specify       |
| in freetext area.                                                             |
| . PENICILLINS       . CEPHALOSPORINS      . SULPHONAMIDES                      |
| . PHENOTHIAZINES    . ANTIHISTAMINES      . LOCAL ANAESTHETICS                 |
| . IODINE            . PHENYLBUTAZONE       . SALICYLATES                       |
| . PETHIDINE         . BARBITURATES        . OPIUM DERIVATIVE                   |
| . UNIDENTIFIED DRUG OR SUBSTANCE (Please specify when identified)             |
| Freetext..................................................                     |
| NB  THE FOLLOWING DRUGS MUST NOT BE STOPPED SUDDENLY - BETA BLOCKERS,          |
|     ANTICONVULSANTS, CORTICOSTEROIDS, OR CLONIDINE FOR HYPERTENSION            |
|                                                                               |
--------------------------------------------------------------------------------
```

Fig 3.   Female Patient Questionnaire

The doctor may amend this information if necessary during the patient's stay in hospital. It can also be inspected by nurses and pharmacists, as well as doctors, by making the appropriate selection on their own 'home display'. Any hypersensitivities recorded are printed at the top of the patient's prescription list (fig 10).

Prescribing A Drug

After confirming questionnaire answers or selecting the prescribing option on the list of current prescriptions, the doctor receives a list of Body Systems (fig 4). The required drug(s) can be chosen either via a tree-branching system using the BNF classification (Section 2), or by selecting it directly from a list of drugs most commonly used on the patient's ward (fig 5).

```
--------------------------------------------------------------------------
¦ E1A   JENKINSON SARAH  M    G999061/8                                    ¦
¦                                                                          ¦
¦       BODY SYSTEMS                                                       ¦
¦                                                                          ¦
¦    1  MOST FREQUENTLY PRESCRIBED DRUGS FOR THIS PATIENTS WARD            ¦
¦    2  ALIMENTARY SYSTEM                                                  ¦
¦    3  CARDIOVASCULAR SYSTEM AND DIURETICS                                ¦
¦    4  RESPIRATORY SYSTEM                                                 ¦
¦    5  ALLERGIC REACTIONS                                                 ¦
¦    6  NERVOUS SYSTEM                                                     ¦
¦    7  RHEUMATIC DISEASE AND GOUT                                         ¦
¦    8  INFECTIONS                                                         ¦
¦    9  ENDOCRINE SYSTEM                                                   ¦
¦   10  MALIGNANT DISEASE AND IMMUNOSUPPRESSANTS                           ¦
¦   11  NUTRITION AND BLOOD                                                ¦
¦   12  LOWER URINARY TRACT                                                ¦
¦   13  OBSTETRICS AND GYNAECOLOGY                                         ¦
¦   14  EAR, NOSE AND THROAT                                               ¦
¦   15  EYE                                                                ¦
¦   16  SKIN                                                               ¦
¦   17  VACCINES AND RELATED PRODUCTS                                      ¦
¦   18  PREMEDICATIONS                                                     ¦
¦   19  DRUGS NOT IN THE SYSTEM                                            ¦
¦                                                                          ¦
¦ Select Body System(s) required                                          ¦
¦                                                                          ¦
--------------------------------------------------------------------------
```

Fig 4. List of Body Systems

```
--------------------------------------------------------------------------
¦                                                                          ¦
¦  E1A   JENKINSON  SARAH  M    G999061/8                                  ¦
¦                                                                          ¦
¦                  MOST COMMONLY USED DRUGS ON WARD E1A                    ¦
¦                                                                          ¦
¦    1  ALUMINIUM HYDROXIDE ORAL     17  HEPARIN INJECTION                 ¦
¦    2  AMOXYCILLIN ORAL             18  HYDRALAZINE ORAL                  ¦
¦    3  ASILONE ORAL                 19  LACTULOSE (DUPHALAC) ORAL         ¦
¦    4  ASPIRIN SOLUBLE ORAL         20  METOCLOPRAMIDE ORAL               ¦
¦    5  BENDROFLUAZIDE ORAL          21  METHYLDOPA ORAL                   ¦
¦    6  CEPHALEXIN ORAL              22  MODURETIC ORAL                    ¦
¦    7  CHLORPROPAMIDE ORAL          23  OXPRENOLOL ORAL                   ¦
¦    8  CO-TRIMOXAZOLE ORAL          24  PARACETAMOL ORAL                  ¦
¦    9  DIGOXIN ORAL                 25  PHENYTOIN ORAL                    ¦
¦   10  DIHYDROCODEINE ORAL          26  POTASSIUM CHLORIDE EFFERVESCENT ORAL¦
¦   11  DISTALGESIC ORAL             27  POTASSIUM CHLORIDE SLOW RELEASE ORAL¦
¦   12  DORBANEX ORAL                28  PREDNISOLONE ORAL                 ¦
¦   13  FERROUS SULPHATE ORAL        29  PROCHLORPERAZINE INJECTION        ¦
¦   14  FRUSEMIDE ORAL               30  SALBUTAMOL METERED DOSE AEROSOL   ¦
¦   15  FRUSEMIDE INJECTION          31  SPIRONOLACTONE ORAL               ¦
¦   16  GLYCERYL TRINITRATE ORAL     32  TEMAZAPAM ORAL                    ¦
¦                                                                          ¦
¦ Select drug(s) required or drug and 83 if drug information required      ¦
¦                                      .....................               ¦
--------------------------------------------------------------------------
```

Fig 5. A List of Commonly Used Drugs on a Ward

After the doctor has selected the required drug, an 'Important' information screen is automatically presented for any drug having contraindications or cautions (fig 6). Details of these are stated as on the drug information screens - in particular, those relating to diagnosis should be noted by the doctor as this is not held within a current inpatient's data set and cannot therefore be automatically checked by the computer. If any contra-indication or caution relates to laboratory data, the patient's relevant current clinical chemistry or haematology values are displayed so that an immediate comparison can be made between the warning and the most up-to-date information available about the patient eg:-

> **Impaired renal function (serum creatinine <300 micromol/1) - dose reduction advised**
> *** THIS PATIENT'S SERUM CRETININE = 465 micromol/1 on 17/6/82**

If no value exists, 'NO RESULT THIS ADMISSION' will be output after the equals sign.

In some cases, current laboratory data is provided even though there are no specific recommendations to these values eg. serum glucose for insulin and oral hypoglycaemics; prothrombin time for anti-coagulants; white cell count, haemoglobin and platelet count for cytotoxics. This information is essentially to aid the prescriber and does not form the basis of any subsequent checking.

```
--------------------------------------------------------------------------------
|                                                                              |
| E1A  JENKINSON SARAH  M   G999061/8  F  age 78    DR BROWN                    |
|                     civil state  M   rel CHURCH OF ENGLAND                    |
|                                                                              |
| DIGOXIN, MEDIGOXIN and STROPHANTHIN G - IMPORTANT INFORMATION                 |
| CONTRA-INDICATION                                                            |
|       Hypertrophic obstructive cardiomyopathy                                |
|                                                                              |
| CAUTION IN                                                                   |
|     Electro-cardioversion - if possible withdraw 72 hours before             |
|     Incomplete heart block, recent mycardial infarction, ventricular         |
|     arrythmias                                                               |
|     Severe pulmonary disease                                                 |
|     Elderly patients - dose of digoxin should not exceed 0.25mg daily        |
|     The following conditions increase the risk of toxicity:                  |
| Renal failure (serum creatinine >150 micromol/1) - dose reduction advised    |
|                                                                              |
| * THIS PATIENT'S SERUM CREATININE = 465 micromol/1 on 17/6/82                 |
|                                                                              |
| Hypokalaemia (serum potassium <3 millimol/1)                                 |
|                                                                              |
| * THIS PATIENT'S SERUM POTASSIUM = 2.9 millimol/1 on 15/6/82                  |
|                                                                              |
| Hypercalcaemia                                                               |
| Hypomagnesaemia                                                              |
|                                                                              |
| TO CONTINUE select one of the following                                      |
| 1 Drug dose display.    2 Return to drug list   3.  Discontinue              |
| 4 Renal failure dose display (Digoxin and medigoxin oral ONLY).              |
|                                                                              |
--------------------------------------------------------------------------------
```

Fig 6. Example of an Important Information Screen

If the doctor decides to continue prescribing the selected drug, the system automatically checks this drug against the following information:-

- the patient's age
- the answers to the patient questionnaire for hypersensitivities or pregnancy
- the patient's laboratory data for contra-indications in renal failure, hypokalaemia etc.
- the patient's current drug treatment for potentially intereacting drugs.

If any contra-indications are found, further warnings are displayed (fig 7). These checks and warnings are explained in more detail in the following paragraph.

```
-------------------------------------------------------------------------------
|                                                                             |
| E1A JENKINSON SARAH M  G999001/8  FEMALE   age 78      DR BROWN             |
|                              civil state   M   rel  CHURCH OF ENGLAND       |
|                                                                             |
| PRESCRIPTION WARNING/S for:-                                                |
|      DIGOXIN TABLETS                                                        |
|                                                                             |
| THIS PATIENT IS CURRENTLY PRESCRIBED THE DRUG ABOVE BY ANOTHER ROUTE        |
|                                                                             |
| DOSE REDUCTION ADVISED - AGE > 60 years                                     |
|                                                                             |
| DOSE REDUCTION ADVISED - SERUM CREATININE >150 micromol/1                   |
|                                                                             |
| CONTRA-INDICATIONS - SERUM POTASSIUM <3 mmol/1                              |
|                                                                             |
| DRUG INTERACTION/S                                                          |
|      A   DIGOXIN ORAL                                                       |
|      B   MODURETIC TABLETS                                                  |
|      CONCURRENT USE OF (A) & (B) MAY INCREASE RISK OF DIGOXIN TOXICITY      |
|      OBSERVE PATIENT FOR INTERACTION                                        |
|                                                                             |
| TO CONTINUE select one of the following                                     |
| 1   Drug dose display   2   Return to drug list   3   Discontinue          |
| 4   Renal failure dose display                                             |
|                                                                             |
-------------------------------------------------------------------------------
```

FIG 7.   Warnings Screen

For those drugs where the starting dose and/or maintenance doses should be reduced in the elderly, a warning will be given for any patient over 60 years. All drugs contra-indicated at a serum creatinine of <150 micromol/1 are also contra-indicated in elderly patients eg.

INITIAL DOSE REDUCTION ADVISED - AGE >60 YEARS

Appropriate warnings are given if the patient is hypersensitive to the selected drug; is pregnant and the drug contraindicated or to be avoided where possible; is taking an oral contraceptive or mono-amine oxidase inhibitor which interacts with the chosen drug eg.

PATIENT IS HYPERSENSITIVE TO SALICYLATES
CAUTION - AVOID IF PRACTICABLE IN PREGNANCY 3RD TRIMESTER

If the patient's laboratory data exceeds the level at which the drug is contraindicated or a dose reduction advised, warnings will be displayed.

>   DOSE REDUCTION ADVISED - SERUM ALBUMIN <30 g/l
>   CONTRAINDICATION - SERUM URATE >550 micromol/1

The laboratory data, which may be checked, includes serum creatinine, potassium, calcium, urate and albumin, and blood pCO_2. If the chosen drug interacts with a drug the patient is already receiving, a warning message will be displayed giving the name of the two drugs, the likely consequences of the interaction and the action to be taken eg.

>   A   PHENYTOIN TABLETS
>   B   CONTRIMOXAZOLE ORAL
>   CONCURRENT USE OF (A) AND (B) INCREASES RISK OF FOLATE DEFICIENCY OBSERVE
>   PATIENT FOR INTERACTION

The synonyms, A & B, are used within the message to refer to the relevant drugs. Other examples of interaction messages are expressed as follows:-

>   EFFECT OF (A) MAY BE REDUCED BY (B) DUE TO INCREASED FLUID RETENTION
>   CAUTION - THIS PATIENT IS ALREADY RECEIVING A PHENOTHIAZINE

The severity of the possible interactions and the action to be taken is indicated by one of the following messages:-

>   AVOID THIS COMBINATION
>   CAUTION WITH THIS COMBINATION
>   OBSERVE PATIENT FOR INTERACTION

In certain cases a reference will also be made to the drug information system if more details of the interaction are given there, eg.

>   SEE DRUG INFORMATION FOR FURTHER DETAILS

Any combination of these messages may be displayed. In addition, the doctor is alerted if the same drug with the same or another formulation/route is prescribed by an appropriate warning message eg.

>   THIS PATIENT IS CURRENTLY PRESCRIBED THE DRUG AND FORMULATION/ROUTE ABOVE

The doctor may still continue to prescribe by selecting the dose screen option but if warnings have been displayed and the prescription later confirmed, a further safeguard is provided by printing the prescription, with the warnings, in the pharmacy for a pharmacist to check and discuss with the prescriber if necessary. However, the doctor prompted by the information and warnings may change his choice to another drug, or route/formulation or reduced dose.

The doctor selects details of the prescription from a dose screen. As indicated on fig 1, this is displayed from several different points within the prescribing sequence depending on the doctor's original method of drug selection (ie Drugs most commonly used on patient's ward or BNF classification), whether he chose to view drug information before continuing to prescribe, the existence of an 'important' information screen for the drug concerned and/or if warnings were identified. There are three types of dose screens:-

-      standard dose screens where the prescribing choices may be made as numeric
       selections (Fig 8).
-      non-standard dose screens where some or all details of the prescription
       are entered in freetext; used to prescribe cytotoxics and insulin

(maintenance regimes and different doses according to the patient's level of glycosuria).

dose screens where only the administration of the drug can be recorded, used for drugs given in emergency situations or where the dose is tailored to the patient's requirements e.g. adrenaline IV. There are few screens of this type which allow a patient's drug history to be completed.

```
-------------------------------------------------------------------------
 E1A  JENKINSON SARAH M    G999061/8

 DIGOXIN
   Tablets 0.0625mg, 0.125mg, 0.25mg    Elixir 0.25mg in 5ml

 1  0.062mg 24H          21 Tablets          51 At once
 2  0.125mg 24H                              52 Early morning
 3  0.25 mg 24H          27 Elixir           85 TTO 3 days
 4  0.25 mg 12H                              86 TTO 7 days
 5  0.25 mg  8H

 6  0.062mg Single dose           Free text direction
 7  0.125mg Single dose           ........................
 8  0.25 mg Single dose
 9  0.5  mg Single dose           . Number of days until start
10  0.75 mg Single dose           . Number of days since start
11     1 mg Single dose

 For each instruction select a dose, a formulation and any directions
 required
    Or 73 (Digitalisation)
    Or 79 (Renal failure dose display)
    Or 82 (Freetext dose screen) with a formulation
    Or 83 (Information)
    Or 90 (Guide to the treatment of arrhythmias)    .............
-------------------------------------------------------------------------
```

Fig 8. A Dose Screen

On the standard dose screens, details of dose and frequency route/formulation (where appropriate) and optional, qualifying directions (including a freetext entry) are selected. Unless a retrospective or prospective start date is indicated (by entering a numeric date code 1 - 9 where 1 in the appropriate field indicates yesterday or tomorrow) it is assumed the prescription will commence that day. The choices made are validated to ensure that the prescription is as complete and safe as possible; choices must be made of dose and frequency must be made; checks for incompatibility between dose and route formulation, dose and direction are carried out; a direction indicating the number of doses must be selected for a controlled drug unless the dose is a single dose. Other options are available from the dose screens for the doctor to access other prescribing screens for the same drug to allow for dose reduction in renal failure, increasing/decreasing doses or information on the specific drug or group of drugs. A freetext facility is also available for any details not offered on the dose screens.

Drugs not in the system may also be prescribed from the List of Body Systems (fig 4) using this freetext facility but checks for contra-indications etc. are not carried out. The drug required, either approved or proprietary, is checked against an alphabetic index to determine if it is already in the system. If so, the doctor is informed of the available routes/formulations. The freetext dose screen permits the prescribing of various types of prescriptions eg. single doses, prescriptions where the dose size is constant, prescriptions where the dose size is different at different times of the day etc. Comprehensive validation is carried out on all structured freetext prescriptions to ensure their completeness although, as before, a safeguard is provided by printing the prescription in the pharmacy so that the details can be checked.

When prescribing single doses from standard dose screens, one of several directions (i.e. at once, early morning, at night, in the evening) must be chosen or a single dose questionnaire is displayed. This enables the prescriber to specify as clearly as possible when the single dose is to be given to assist nurses in administration. He must either select one of four directions; to be given when instructed/one hour pre-op/on next drug round or the dose has already been given or either a specific time and/or a freetext direction.

The completed prescription is displayed for confirmation with the following details:-

-       prescription start date
-       prescription concellation date; this may be predetermined automatically by
        the computer for controlled drugs (referred to as CD's) or when specific
        directions indicating a number of days treatment are chosen
-       prescription details
-       administration times
-       a message if the drug and route/formulation is not available as ward stock
        (this check to be implemented in the future).

Administration times are either entered by the prescriber or automatically scheduled by the computer to the drug round times for the patient's ward according to the frequency chosen eg. if 6H (hourly) is chosen, four times will be scheduled, which could be 0830, 1330, 1700 and 2200. From this example it is appreciated that the scheduled times are not separated by the exact frequency chosen being constrained by the standard drug round times on the ward. Approval was given by senior nurse managers to specify the ward drug round times so that they more accurately reflect the times at which these occur rather than the very general times used on the manual prescription sheet.

However, in certain circumstances the drug prescribed will affect the scheduling, for instance with antibiotics given parenterally strict frequency is observed even though the times may fall outside the standard drug round times. Similarly, certain directions chosen will affect the scheduling eg. early morning is scheduled to 0630, in the evening to 1800 and at night to 2200. Administration times are not scheduled for 'as required' or TTO prescriptions.

If the prescription is approved the patient's computer file is updated together with any associated warning messages. The doctor is returned to the List of Current Prescriptions unless he has previously chosen to prescribe more than one drug and/or he has selected to carry out other prescribing activities, in which case, the computer will automatically process the next choice selected and so on until all choices have been completed.

Cancellation and Amendment of Prescriptions

On selecting the cancellation and amendment system, the computer displays all current prescriptions for the patient. The doctor may enter one of the following codes against a prescription:-

```
C - cancel prescription immediately
D - delay cancellation in the future
R - cancel prescription retrospectively
A - amend prescription
```

The computer processes the prescriptions in the order listed above. Any prescriptions for immediate cancellation are displayed first on an appropriate confirmation screen for approval; those for future cancellation only are displayed next against which a date code, 0-9, is entered where 1 = tomorrow etc. Prescriptions for which a number of doses have been specified eg. controlled drugs, may not be delay cancelled since these are printed once at the time of prescribing and there is no facility to inform the nursing staff of the new cancellation date. In addition, if a cancellation date was set at the time the prescription was made the new cancellation date may not exceed that date. As before, these prescriptions are presented for approval with the date codes interpreted. Prescriptions for retrospective cancellation are dealt with in a similar manner except that the date codes are restricted to 1-9.

The amendment facility applies only to dose changes. The drug is rechecked and the details selected as if it were a new prescription. However, where relevant, the new dose is compared with the old to check for an excessive dose increment or insufficient interval between increments. Warnings are displayed and printed in the pharmacy department as before eg.

CONTRA-INDICATION - MAXIMUM DOSE INCREMENT EXCEEDED
CONTRA-INDICATION - MINIMUM INTERVAL BETWEEN CHANGES NOT EXCEEDED

Both the old and the new prescriptions are displayed together so that they may be compared by the doctor before confirmation, after which the old script is cancelled immediately and the new prescription is added to the patient's drug file.

Prescribing drugs to take out (TTO's)

Some patients are discharged from hospital or for home leave on drug treatment. This can be prescribed in one of two ways. The usual prescribing sequence is used for all drugs the patient is not currently receiving or for those which are to continue but with a different dose. The doctor must select an appropriate direction, 'TTO 3 days' or 'TTO 7 days', available on all dose screens to indicate that he is prescribing a drug to take out and the number of days supply required for the pharmacy to dispense.

A facility is provided to enable doctors to prescribe discharge drugs easily if they are a continuation of inpatient treatment. The doctor receives the patient's current prescription list and enters the required number of days supply against the appropriate prescriptions. Certain drugs such as single doses and controlled drugs may not be prescribed using this facility and these are identified with an asterisk. Each drug selected is rechecked for contra-indications and warnings displayed as before. All the approved discharged drugs are printed in the pharmacy department for dispensing, together with any warning messages (fig 10).

Represcribing

This facility is used when a new prescription sheet is required for drug administration. Unlike present manual systems, a new list is produced each time a patient's treatment changes providing further administration boxes. However, when treatment remains unchanged all administration boxes become filled after 8 days and a new list has to be scheduled through represcribing.

According to local policy, senior medical students are permitted to represcribe except when a patient's treatment includes anti-coagulants. On selecting the option to represcribe, the doctor receives the list of current prescriptions. Certain drugs which may not be represcribed such as controlled drugs (where the number of doses must be specified) and single doses are indicated by an asterisk. To represcribe all those drugs without asterisks, the doctor must enter 'Y' on this screen. These drugs are then rechecked for contra-indications and any warnings displayed as before. After confirmation, the original prescriptions are cancelled, the new prescriptions are added to the patient's file, a new prescription list is printed on the ward, and any warning messages are printed in pharmacy.

As drugs are automatically rescheduled to the drug round times of the patient's ward, represcribing is used when a patient is transferred to a ward where the drug round times differ from those on the patient's previous ward. The doctor can also use this system to recheck long-standing prescriptions against more recent laboratory data.

When all the choices selected have been processed in turn, an up-dated list of current prescriptions is displayed for the doctor to review. He may choose to select further prescribing activities for this patient, prescribe for another patient, return to the Home display or leave the system by pressing the key 'log-out'.

SYSTEM DESCRIPTION - DRUG ADMINISTRATION

Prescription List

A new prescription list (fig 9) is printed on the ward printer when all changes to a patient's treatment have been made, replacing any previous list in use. Controlled drugs (except for single doses) are printed once when first prescribed, on a separate list so that a patient may have more than one list in current use. This procedure was adopted to avoid these drugs becoming open-ended (if reprinted each time the treatment altered) which would have been unacceptable as it is necessary to specify the number of doses each time they are prescribed.

The list has been designed to appear as similar as possible to the document used for handwritten prescriptions with which the ward staff are familiar - even the colour of the paper (blue) is the same so that it is easily recognisable. This similarity reduces the effect of a computerbased prescribing system in only one of several hospitals in which learner nurses within the Central Birmingham District Health Authority gain their practical experience.

Each prescription list is identified with the patient's details (name, age, sex, consultant, ward and registration number) the list number, indicating the number of lists printed during the patient's current episode; the page number, as the list may continue over more than one page; the date and time on which the doctor last changed the patient's treatment. Any hypersensitivities recorded on the patient questionnaire are always printed at the top of the first page. So that nursing staff are able to ascertain if they have all the pages of the current prescription list, including those for controlled drugs, a relevant message is printed at the bottom of each page eg.

        'NO FURTHER PRESCRIPTIONS FOR THIS PATIENT'
        'FURTHER PRESCRIPTIONS FOR THIS PATIENT ON LIST NO 1 PAGE 2'
        'Please refer to Controlled Drug sheet(s) for:-
             METHADONE TABLETS CD'

```
               PRESCRIPTION LIST NO 1    PAGE 1    AS ON 26/05/81 AT 0957
               --------------------------------
   E1A   JENKINSON SARAH M   0823456/6          F Age 049   DR ELIAS

THIS PATIENT IS HYPERSENSITIVE TO PENICILLINS

      SINGLE DOSE DRUGS
                                      .DATE .TIME.   DOSE    .SIGNATURE
      ************************************************************************
      FRUSEMIDE TABLETS                  .     .    .          .
      20mg Single dose At once           .-----.----.----------.---------------
      CHECK DOSE NOT ALREADY GIVEN
      Date to be given 26/05/81
       JGRAFFY
      ************************************************************************

      AS REQUIRED DRUGS
                                      .DATE .TIME.   DOSE    .SIGNATURE
      ************************************************************************
      PARACETAMOL TABLETS                .     .    .          .
      1G 4H As required                  .-----.----.----------.---------------
                                         .     .    .          .
      Start 26/05/81                     .-----.----.----------.---------------
       JGRAFFY                           .     .    .          .
                                         .-----.----.----------.---------------
                                         .     .    .          .
                                         .-----.----.----------.---------------
                                         .     .    .          .
                                         .-----.----.----------.---------------
                                         .     .    .          .
                                         .-----.----.----------.---------------
                                         .     .    .          .
                                         .-----.----.----------.---------------
                                         .     .    .          .
                                         .-----.----.----------.---------------
                                         .     .    .          .
                                         .-----.----.----------.---------------
                                         .     .    .          .
                                         .-----.----.----------.---------------
                                         .     .    .          .
                                         .-----.----.----------.---------------
                                         .     .    .          .
                                         .-----.----.----------.---------------
                                         .     .    .          .
                                         .-----.----.----------.---------------
      ************************************************************************


      REGULAR DRUGS
                                      MAY .26 .27 .28 .29 .30 .31 .01 .02 .
      ************************************************************************
      DIGOXIN TABLETS                   0030.    .   .   .   .   .   .   .
      0.25mg 12H                          .---.---.---.---.---.---.---.---.
                                        1700.    .   .   .   .   .   .   .
      Start 26/05/81                      .---.---.---.---.---.---.---.---.
       JGRAFFY
      ************************************************************************

PRESCRIPTION LIST NO 1    PAGE 1 -NO FURTHER PRESCRIPTIONS FOR THIS PATIENT
```

Fig. 9. Example of a Prescription List

The prescriptions are always printed in a similar order to the handwritten list as follows; single doses, 'as required' drugs, regular drugs, drugs with frequent dose changes, discharge drugs and cancelled drugs. All prescriptions contain the following information:-

-    drug name
-    route or formulation
-    dose and frequency of administration
-    any specified directions
-    the prescriber's name (originally from the log-in code)
-    the prescription start date, and cancellation date if specified.

Any represcriptions entered by a senior medical student are identified by the words 'med', in brackets to indicate 'senior medical student'. Thus any prescriptions so marked are represcriptions.

Each single dose is printed with labelled boxes in which the nurse administering the dose can record the date, time and dose and her full signature. Each prescription has the additional message 'check dose not already given' printed above the prescriber's name, since there is a remote possibility that if more than one prescription list is printed between the prescribing and the time scheduled for the administration of the dose, that it could be given more than once (hence the reason to force the doctor to select a time or direction when prescribing single doses). Because of these difficulties, single dose prescriptions are printed on all lists up to the specified day and administration time, or if a specific time is not given (eg. one hour pre-op) to the end of the day on which the drug is to be given. It is thus essential for the nurse to check that the dose has not already been given and recorded on a previous sheet. If the dose has already been given when the prescription was made, then the word 'GIVEN' is printed in the date box and the remaining boxes are blanked out with 'X's.

'As required' drugs are printed with the same administration boxes as for single doses except that provision is made to record twelve doses. Certain 'as required' drugs are included in the section for regular drugs as they may be given at a specific time eg. Temazepam 10 mg 24H at night as required.

The area for recording administration for regular drugs is identical to that on the handwritten prescription sheet. Administration boxes (for 8 days) are provided, according to the frequency of administration per day with the dates (from the date of printing) printed horizontally and the scheduled drug round times printed vertically. If the duration of the prescription is less than eight days or a future start date has been specified, appropriate boxes will be blanked out with 'X's to indicate clearly when the prescription is to start and/or finish.

Drugs with frequent dose changes occur infrequently and include those entered on the increasing/decreasing dose screen for corticosteroids and the glycosuria (sliding scale) insulin dose screens. The administration area is as for 'as required' drugs except that for increasing/decreasing doses and some cytotoxic regimes, the date, time and dose are printed in the appropriate boxes and the nurse is only required to record her signature when it has been given.

Any drugs prescribed for the patient to take out (TTO's) are printed without administration boxes under the heading of 'Discharge drugs'.

Any drugs cancelled are printed only on the list produced immediately after cancellation to inform nursing staff. Details given include the drug name and route/formulation, the date and time of cancellation and the name of the prescriber cancelling the drug.

Controlled drugs are printed with an administration area as for 'as required' drugs except that the number of boxes is restricted to the number of doses specified and each dose is numbered. Prescriptions for non-controlled drugs with the number of doses specified (referred to as pseudo - CD's) are treated in exactly the same way as controlled drugs.

Drug rounds and filing prescription lists

The ward chosen for the pilot scheme held the patient's prescription sheets on a clipboard at the bottom of each bed unlike some wards where they are held collectively within a ring binder. Although the recording of the administration of drugs on the computer printed lists is carried out exactly as before, it has been necessary to amend certain procedures. Whilst it has not yet been proven, it is probable that these procedures would also apply where the prescription lists are held in a ring binder. It was agreed that a clear plastic pocket folder (with the left hand side and bottom sealed) should be used to file previous prescription lists for the following reasons:-

- the previous sheets are separated from the current sheet, and therefore minimise the risk of using the wrong prescription sheet
- it ensures that all prescription sheets are filed in the same place for each patient
- nurses and doctors are able to view the immediately preceding sheet through the clear plastic cover.

Prior to each drug round, any new prescription lists are removed from the printer by the nurse and placed on the drugs trolley. (When present, the ward clerk may remove them from the printer and leave them for collection in a document tray sited beyond the printer). The nurse notes the names of those patients with new lists, and where a list is composed of more than one page, staples the pages together at the top left hand corner with a small stapler attached to the trolley.

During each drug round, the nurse will commence using any new printed prescription sheet for the appropriate patient. However, she may need to refer to the patient's previous prescription sheet to check that all drugs were given as scheduled during the last round (in particular, single doses) and to ascertain if necessary, when the patient was last given an 'as required' drug. The nurse replaces the previous sheet with the new prescription sheet, and places the previous sheet in the plastic pocket folder behind the current sheet on the clipboard. This procedure is adopted each time a new prescription sheet is printed, the previous sheet always being placed on top of any existing previous sheets within the plastic folder. Any current controlled drug sheet is also retained behind the new list outside the plastic folder.

When the doctor prescribes treatment which is to be administered before the next drug round (eg. single doses to be given 'at once') the nurse removes the appropriate prescription sheet from the printer and proceeds as usual.

Should nurses be uncertain as to the most up-to-date prescription sheet, they can refer to the Prescription List Information for the appropriate patient on the VDU. This gives them details of the previous and current prescription sheet numbers, and date and time of printing. Doctors and pharmacists may also view this information. Although the average number of lists per patient is approximately three, the plastic folders of long term patients can become too bulky. When this occurs, some of the earliest prescription sheets are filed in the patient's medical records.

Computer Breakdown

When there is a prolonged computer breakdown or the computer system is closed down, the familiar handwritten prescription sheet is used as a back-up document to prescribe and record administration of drugs. It is also used for emergency patients admitted when the registration department is closed. The sheet is filed on top of the current computer printed list (if present) at the patient's bedside. Thus the computer printed list and the back-up document constitute the patient's current drug treatment.

When the computer system is available, doctors enter these prescriptions as soon as possible thus generating a further prescription list which is filed according to the agreed procedures.

Pharmacy Messages

These are automatically printed in the pharmacy if:-

-       the drug prescribed requires dispensing from pharmacy stocks
-       the drug has been prescribed partly or completely in freetext
-       the doctor overrides warning messages.

These are produced immediately after the prescription list is printed on the ward and ensure that prescription lists do not leave the ward, for dispensing as in the past.

Each message (Fig 10) is identified with a message number, date and time of printing and the patient details as they appear on the prescription list. The reason for the message is printed eg. 'WARNINGS for:-' or DISPENSING - TTO's together with full details of the prescription. Any warnings including any relevant laboratory values (displayed on the Important Information screen) are printed as seen by the doctor. Only the potentially more serious drug interactions are printed (ie. those with the action to observe the patient are ignored).

```
-----------------------------------------------------------------------------
|                                                                           |
| MESSAGE NUMBER D004                    PRINTED AT 12.14 ON 29/04/81        |
|                                                                           |
| E1A    JENKINSON SARAH M    G823456/6     F Age 072    DR ELIAS           |
|                                                                           |
| DISPENSING - NOT WARD STOCK                                               |
|                                                                           |
|      GLYCERYL TRINITRATE SUBLINGUAL TABLETS                               |
|                                                                           |
|      One 500mcg tablet  As required                                       |
|                                                                           |
|      Start 29/04/81                                                       |
|      DGCLEMENTS                                                           |
-----------------------------------------------------------------------------
```

Fig. 10   Example of a Pharmacy Message

The pharmacist is required to sign and date the pharmacy message in the space provided at the bottom of the sheet when dispensing is completed and/or the warnings or prescriptions checked. Requests for reprints or any pharmacy message can be made using the VDU in the pharmacy.

All TTO's must be signed by the doctor as his log-in code is not acceptable as his signature. A reprint of the pharmacy dispensing message is taken to the patient's ward by the ward pharmacist and placed in a ring binder for the doctor to date and countersign. The signed printouts are removed for filing in the pharmacy department for an appropriate period. The same procedure is followed for TTO controlled drugs except the doctor is required to rewrite the whole prescription and sign it. These local arrangements were agreed with pharmacy and medical staff for the trial period to avoid prescription lists leaving the ward.

Evaluation of the Pilot Trial

After the five week period, the system was evaluated by two members of the West Midlands Regional Health Authority Management Services both formerly members of the QEMC Computer Evaluation Team. In view of the complexity of the drug prescribing system, structured interviews were designed in conjunction with the drugs team for all three groups of users; medical, nursing and pharmacy staff. Certain core questions were asked of all three groups.

Whilst nursing and pharmacy staff generally viewed the system favourably, the medical staff were critical of certain aspects. This was perhaps to be expected since the majority of the workload created by the computer system is the responsibility of the doctor. The main advantage to nursing staff was the clarity of the prescription lists, providing legible scripts with specific administration times. Whilst few problems were experienced with administering drugs, (particularly since the lists no longer leave the ward), some nurses reported difficulties in aligning the paper in the printer. Drugs with frequent dose changes were considered much easier to administer.

The pharmacy staff believed the system made prescribing safer. It has removed the supply function of the ward pharmacist enabling him/her to take on additional work such as patient counselling and reviewing treatments. The pharmacy messages proved satisfactory and few difficulties were experienced with dispensing TTO or non-ward stock drugs. Very few warning messages required any action from the pharmacist during the trial period. However, given a longer period in several wards, the situation might be very different.

Whilst those doctors who regularly used the system to prescribe found it was more time consuming than prescribing manually, other prescribing activities such as represcribing and prescribing TTO's were quicker to use. They considered the printers operated too slowly (a constraint imposed by the computer configuration) and the number of lists produced excessive and confusing. The facility to prescribe from any terminal and the educational role of the system were advantageous. There was concern by doctors on the pilot ward that the act of prescribing was taking place away from the patient, who served as an aide memoire, although it was noted that this was the routine practice in other wards particularly surgical wards. Whilst in principle the doctors agreed the warning screens were useful, they would be more effective if the computer was more selective.

Many users felt that for a computerised drug prescribing system to operate effectively, the computer needed to be very reliable and available 24 hours a day with a 'round the clock' registration service and a VDU for prescribing in the Accident and Emergency department. The simultaneous use of two systems created additional work for the medical staff and was held to be potentially dangerous.

Some suggestions were made by the medical staff to speed up prescribing, assist in locating the appropriate drug and to reduce freetext facilities. The suggestions included a revision of ward's commonly used drugs, the use of changes to some dose screens, additional drugs to be added or reclassified and indications where a drug can be found in the BNF classification when a drug is in the system and the freetext facilities are being used.

Since this evaluation, many of the points raised have been acted upon. Extending the availability of the real-time computer system is now a viable proposition since development work has almost ceased and there are plans to site a VDU in the Accident/Emergency department. Problems still remain in providing further registration cover since the demands on this department overnight cannot justify it.

Conclusion

The pilot trial demonstrated that a computerised drug prescribing system is a viable proposition, although it is recognised that some problems do exist. Further trials particularly in surgical wards, will determine if the system is acceptable throughout the hospital. When the system is reintroduced it is hoped to compare the incidence of prescribing errors between the computer system and the manual system, using the data collected on 600 patients (5000 prescriptions) and checking it as if the system had been used. It is hoped that this analysis together with further evaluation studies, will demonstrate that the objectives originally identified by the drugs project have been achieved.

ACKNOWLEDGEMENTS

The system was developed in the Computer Department of the Queen Elizabeth Hospital in conjunction with medical, pharmacy and nursing staff. The author would like to acknowledge the help of all concerned in particular, Dr. L. Beeley, consultant clinical pharmacologist, members of the medical and nursing user groups, staff on the ward on which the pilot trial took place, and computer staff in the drugs team at the time the author was a member, in particular Mr. M. Pinson, senior programmer now team leader, and Mr. N. Ballantine, staff pharmacist.

REFERENCES

1.   OAKES, A.F.M and WIGMORE, H.M. (1968). The London Hospital prescription sheet. J. Hosp. Pharm., July, 1968, 177-181.
2.   BEELEY, L; CLEWETT, A.J, TESH, D.E.; and WALKER, G.F. (1975) Errors of Drug Prescribing. Br.J.clin.Pharm.2,Jan,1975,403-409
3.   HILLS, P.M. (1980) Computer Systems at a U.K. Medical Centre Information Privacy vol.2 no 5. Sept, 1980, 207-211.

The Impact of Computers on Nursing
M. Scholes, Y. Bryant and B. Barber (eds.)
Elsevier Science Publishers B.V. (North-Holland)
© IFIP-IMIA, 1983

8.3.

DRUG MANAGEMENT

Discussion

Drug Information at the time of Prescribing

Several differences between the two systems described were noted. At Birmingham, the automatic display of information together with specific automatic checks when prescribing a drug is an essential feature of the system. Except where specific problems have been experienced, no drug information is given at the time of prescribing using the Technicon system. This reflects the general approach to computerised medication systems in the USA. Whilst difficulties had arisen in the USA in persuading doctors to prescribe using the computer system, further trials of the Birmingham system will prove whether this will apply in England.

Approach to recording drug administration

Recording of drugs given in the computer is an integral part of the system in the USA. Certain aspects of this were considered to be partially interesting; for example, provision is made to record the site an injection is given and the reason for a patient receiving drugs such as analgesics, to which can be added the outcome of giving these drugs.

Unit dose of ward stock system

The design of the computerised drug systems are influenced by the approach to supplying drugs to the wards. In England, this is usually based on a ward stock system whilst in the USA, unit dose systems are in operation which enable drugs to be charged to the appropriate individual account.

Nurse involvement in pharmacy stock control systems

It was noted that pharmacy stock control systems may be separate from, or a sub-system of, a total drug system. In either situation nurses must be involved in their design and implementation as for other housekeeping activities concerned with supplies and stores.

CHAPTER 9

COMMUNITY BASED CARE

With the increasing emphasis of nursing patients within the community, the need for information to manage nursing resources is even more critical than hitherto. Examples are given on how this information is being collected, collated and used based on individualised patient care or community nursing activities.

Preventive medicine is now given a high priority in many countries and this has resulted in the creation of health centres responsible for various primary care services. A computer based information system (FINSTAR) for such a health centre in Finland is described which was developed from the widely used system called Computer Stored Ambulatory Record (COSTAR). Some specific aspects of preventive medicine in the U.K. and Japan are described. The Japanese system, developed as part of the PL hospital medical screening facilities, is of particular interest since it is concerned with the growth and development of children and how this relates to the parent-child relationship.

The Impact of Computers on Nursing
M. Scholes, Y. Bryant and B. Barber (eds.)
Elsevier Science Publishers B.V. (North-Holland)
© IFIP-IMIA, 1983

9.1.

COMMUNITY NURSING INFORMATION SYSTEMS

B.E.M. Warne O.B.E.

1. Introduction

Nurse staffing has long been acknowledged as one of the most important factors in the provision of health care and preventive services. The use of the nursing workforce with its variety of skills, is subject to greater pressures of demand and open to more public scrutiny than at any time in the past. This is not surprising as better education and public awareness has increased public expectation of the service and the cost of the nursing and midwifery service in England in 1980/81 was £2,250 million, some 32% of the current spending by National Health Authorities (excluding Family Practitioner Committees)(1).

Finance is inevitably a major concern of all nurse managers. Hopefully most of them are not only involved in budgetary control but also in budget setting and therefore both know and have agreed the parameters. The good nurse manager is the one who firstly ensures that the workforce is made up of staff with the **right skill mix**, and secondly that those skills are used to best advantage by using **her budget in a flexible manner**. In order to do this she must know (a) what work the nurses are doing now? (b) what the needs of the population are both now and in the future?

Defining the type and quality of skills required is not an easy task. Traditionally the community workforce has been made up of nurses, midwives, health visitors, school nurses and a support staff of administrative and clerical officers. The picture is now more complex with the advent of community psychiatric nurses and nurses caring for the mentally handicapped at home, as well as specialists working in specific areas, e.g. those caring for the dying. The answer to the question "what are the nurses doing now?" is far from simple, but must be known to safeguard the service both now and in the future and provide information which ensures that the right number of people are trained with the appropriate skills.

Manpower planning is a useful tool in the total context of health care planning which must be carried out if the other question, "what are the population's needs?" is to be answered. Health care planning for "care groups", (such as the elderly, the pre-school child) has been developing in the U.K. and, although open to some valid criticism as to methodology, has improved in the past eight years. Planning for the future is another vital concern of nurse managers who need the information to finish the equation of "nurse/patient ratio = workload" which enables them to allocate staff now and prepare and train nurses for the future.

Nurse managers have always been, and must always be, concerned with the proper use of the nursing resource. An information system should provide accurate, timely, information for the day to day management of the community service and also provide a basis for future manpower and service planning.

2. Objectives

In March 1979 a Community Nursing Information Project was set up; it included community nurses, a personnel nurse, a management services officer and the regional statistician. The overall objective was "to produce detailed monthly information on the work of community nurses. This must be adequate to satisfy the needs of nurse managers,. provide sufficient planning and monitoring information, and supply statistics for the DHSS annual returns". This was to be achieved by:-

(a)   to provide information for the rational deployment of community nurses

(b)   collect data to show trends in nurse workload

(c)   provide information for future health care and manpower planning

(d)   supply information for DHSS returns.

In fulfilling these objectives it was agreed that the number and variety of forms used should be reduced to a minimum and that the time taken by nurses to provide the data should be kept to a minimum.

3. Background

The first step was a survey of the community nursing forms currently in use in the 10 Districts in Wessex. These numbered 173 from 7 Districts and it became evident that many had not been reviewed for many years. A survey of forms used by all community staff, not just nurses, showed that one District used 167 different forms and this was by no means an exceptional number(2).

This was followed by a national survey on methods of information collection. One computer application was already in use at Leicester and another in West Dorset, these were studied and information was also gathered on manual systems.

Work commenced on **the Leicester System** in 1971 when a feasibility study was initiated. This recommended that a computer system could be developed, aimed at providing:-

1.   A basic record for each patient, which would give the nurse up-to-date information.
2.   A daily visit schedule for each nurse.
3.   Continuity of records including a link between day and night staff.
4.   Management information(G6).

It was decided that the system would deal with nurse workload indices which would assist with the deployment of staff, manpower planning and health care planning. It was decided not to include a computerised nurse patient record system or work scheduling system, as in Leicester, on grounds of flexibility (a "batch system was not sufficiently flexible to permit updating of priorities at short notice), confidentiality and cost; the project team wished to avoid suggestions that the computer was "running" the nurses and to promote the concept of the computer as a useful tool for nurses.

4. Method

The source of the data is the nurses working in the community and they were involved with the nurse managers from the start. This consultation and discussion ensured that the nurses were committed to and understood the proposes of the project, and that they agreed data could be conveniently collected. This participative and educative approach was found particularly fruitful.

The system requirements were outlined for domiciliary nursing, domiciliary midwifery, health visiting, school nursing, and community psychiatry.

Work has been completed on the first four groups. The community psychiatric nursing system has been tried out but not completed.

Trial System for domiciliary nursing

Input
A daily record form was produced together with a detailed list of instructions for completing it. The daily record was used to avoid transcription errors and it was designed to be used as a working document and be completed after each visit to a patient - thus taking a minimal amount of time to produce.

Data
The data included information on:-
(a)   Patients Visited
        Age, sex of patient
        New patient or repeat visit - source of referral
        Place of visit
        Reason for visit and/or treatment carried out

(b)   Other work
        e.g. Clinical session
             Staff meetings
             Travel.

Output
The same basic analysis is provided as a monthly summary for each individual nurse, as a monthly summary for each nursing officer by team or grade for her unit and as a district summary for all staff. It provides an age analysis of patients seen, together with an age analysis associated with the places visited and the treatment given. It includes an average number of visits per patient and the number of ineffective visits. Liaison visits and treatment sessions are analysed together with staff time and travelling. The amount of computer output is extensive and informative, and it provides a solid basis for the examination and the management of community care.

5.   Results

The objectives were achieved with one exception: the information was not timely - the delay in receipt of outputs was too protracted to enable it to be used for short term management and deployment of staff. Additionally the cost was high because of the volume of data processing which had to be undertaken.

6.   Review

After the system had been in use in the five Districts for a period of at least one year, it became obvious that it needed review. Familiarity with the printouts had made the nurse more aware of the possible uses of better, more accurate information, in this they had been helped by the Regional Statistician who had assisted them to look at alternative formats for the outputs and given them help in interpreting data.

The high financial cost and the long time delay (approximately 4 weeks) in return of information made it imperative that alternative solutions were considered.

In 1980 an investigation into a computerized record system had been completed in the Cambridge Health District. A manual system had been introduced designed for transfer to a computer at a later date. This system was studied during the review period(4). It was based on a weekly return using an optical mark reader document. This was not adopted because the nurses wished to continue using a daily form and transport it with them during their daily work.

In August 1981, a User Group made up of nurses from the five Districts together with technical staff met to review the data collected, to reduce the revenue costs and to reduce the time taken to obtain reports from the data supplied.

Appropriateness and completeness of information

At the beginning the computing services officer undertook a series of individual visits to each participating District. He helped the nurses to define the output they required and took into account individual requests. Familiarity with the existing system enabled many of the nurses to forecast their possible requirements for the future which meant that a degree of flexibility had to be built into the programme to enable ad hoc surveys to be undertaken.

At the same time as the District visits were made the Review Group met at approximately 6 weekly intervals to decide if the data was the most appropriate for indicating workload and identifying planning needs. These meetings took place during the period that the "National Steering Group on Health Services Information" were considering, Community Information and the results of these national discussions were also taken into account.

Modification of Data and Programs

(a) Age of Patient

Wessex has an abnormally high proportion of elderly people in its population, with some variation from one District to another - in three Districts over 20% of the population are over 65 years. The older the patient the more probable they are to call on the domiciliary nursing service and the greater is their need and dependency. The elderly age group were further subdivided into age bands 65-74, 75-84, 85-94, over 95.

(b) Treatment or reason for visit

The use of the nursing process in domiciliary nursing makes task orientated treatment an inappropriate form of nursing record. Tasks of themselves such as "injection", or statements such as "general care", "surgical", do not give an idea of the patients total need and therefore the workload. It was agreed that the length of time taken to complete the visit and thus provide the necessary care was more informative and therefore "treatment" was changed to time span of visit and called **analysis by dependency:**

> less than 15 minutes
> 15 to 30 minutes
> over 30 to 60 minutes
> over 1 hour

(c) Diagnosis of patient

It was considered that the medical diagnosis of the patient, used in conjunction with the length of time needed to provide care, would give a better indication of workload than time only, and also provide valuable planning information.

The nursing diagnosis was considered and rejected as it would probably be a multiple diagnosis, and difficult to record. It was agreed that the medical diagnosis, as interpreted by the nurse, would be a useful indicator.

A simplification of the system used by the College of General
Practitioners and Office of Population Census Survey was carried out and
agreed as the classification of morbidity. The nurses would identify the
main diagnosis which contributed to the necessity of a visit.

(d)   Deaths and Discharges
       Previously, new patients were identified and the addition of this
       information enabled more accurate estimates of workload to be made.

(e)   Ad Hoc Enquiries
       Spare code numbers were included so that each District could undertake
       whatever ad hoc enquiry they required.

Output
The general format of the output had been found to be very satisfactory, that
was, by individual nurse, aggregated up to nursing unit and District total. It
was agreed that as well as a nursing unit identification a code could be
inserted, if required, to identify each general practitioner or group practice
so that allocation of staff could be better linked to meet the general
practitioners requirements, either individually or collectively.

Modification of Computer Application
Considerable thought was given to methods by which the "turn round" of the
results could be improved. The nurses, who used the system in four out of the
five Districts, decided that they wished to continue to use a daily input form
as this ensured the greatest accuracy, prevented errors in collation and kept
the time they used for paper work to a minimum. The high cost of the scheme had
already been identified as due to the amount of data processing necessary as a
result of a daily form.

7.   Proposed Solution

The suggested solution, which is now in process of adoption, was that a micro
computer based scheme, involving local data capture with onward transmission to
the Regional computer main frame (ICL 2960) should be introduced.

The daily forms would be input using the VDU of the micro computer in each
District and transmitted to the main frame at the end of each month for
processing(5).

The advantages of this approach were:-

(a)   the daily form could continue to be used.
(b)   the data could be input throughout the month, thus ensuring a minimal
       delay at the end of each month before the programme could be run.
(c)   validation of data could be built into the system at source, in the
       District, and so protracted delays would not occur at the end of the
       month.
(d)   the design of the input form on the VDU could be tailored to individual
       needs, if some data was not required it could be omitted on the display.
       Any subsequent modification which might be required would be at minimum
       cost because the software would not need to be altered.
(e)   the revenue costs, in a large District, would be at least halved. The
       capital cost, including the cost of the software to be developed by the
       Regional Computer Services Office would be minimal, approximately £8,000
       maximum.
(f)   the micro computer would have spare capacity for other applications and
       had the advantage of a direct link with the regional main frame computer.

The software package is now being developed and should be operational in one District by August 1982. It will then be available for all other Districts in the Wessex Region and it is probable that seven out of the ten Districts will introduce it in 1982/83, the three remaining Districts have yet to come to a considered opinion, including the District with the smallest population where the cost effectiveness would probably be least beneficial. The review group is continuing to meet and revise the data associated with domiciliary midwifery, health visiting and school nursing and the same system will be used to provide for their information needs.

8. Use

The main aims of the system had been identified at the outset, and had been achieved. They were to provide information for:-

(a) rational deployment of community staff - both short term, retrospective, and long term, manpower planning
(b) showing trends in workload which merit further examination as to course
(c) health care planning - this has been of greater value than previously estimated. Manpower studies linked to the percentage of each nurses time used for care of a specific age group enables detailed planning to be related to specific populations of individual District Health Authorities.
(d) D.H.S.S. returns

in additon the facility for "ad hoc" surveys has been included and it has been a useful tool in budget setting and budget managememt.

9. Conclusion

Groups of nurses, throughout the country, involved in computer applications related to community information have ensured that systems have been developed to meet their particular needs; within those needs is a common core of information applicable to all users. In a comparatively new field of computer application this is valid; innovation and trial will probably lead to the development of a system which can provide the information core required by all, with a flexibility in the programming which gives freedom to the users to obtain either additional routine data or make ad hoc enquiries. Therefore, whilst no single solution has yet been found, the work in Leicester, Wessex, East Birmingham and Cambridge has contributed to the exploration of nursing needs and community care.

Nurses are becoming more aware of oomputer technology, are gaining confidence in using the enhanced information thus made available and learning to specify their requirements in relation to their objectives in providing patient care and planning the services of the future.

One aspect of computerised information which has so far not been tried in the community is "real time" computing, which because of the geographical scatter of centres of population, and consequently of the nurses, may not be so appropriate as it is in its application to hospital nursing, but it should be constantly borne in mind as a possible option if the computer is to serve its purpose of providing cost effective, accurate, timely information.

In each instance the nurses have been the innovators and driving force but have not hesitated to ask for and have received advice and help from specialist staff which has enabled them to achieve their objectives.

REFERENCES

1. Nurse Manpower.   Department of Health and Social Security, March 1982.
    ISBNO - 902650 - 46 - 7.
2. O and M Department, Management Services Division, Wessex Regional Health
    Authority.
    First Progress Report of the Study into the Development of the Community
    Nursing Records Information System (January 1978).
3. Stillwell, Brian.   Community Nursing Information System.   BURISA 48.
    April 1981 15 - 16.
4. Community Nursing Information System. Cambridge Health District.
5. Regional Computer Division, Wessex Regional Health Authority. Community
    Information Review Group.

ACKNOWLEDGEMENTS

The author wishes to acknowledge her indebtedness to:-

Miss O. M. Bonner, lately District Nursing Officer, Cambridge Health District,
Miss D. G. Hussey, OBE, District Nursing Officer, Leicestershire Area Health
Authority, Michael Slattery, MA, MSc, Regional Statistician, Wessex RHA, Brian
Stillwell, MMS, AMBIM, Principal O and M Officer, Wessex RHA and Michael Wright,
BSc, Principal Computer Services Officer, Wessex RHA and the Community Nurses in
Wessex Region.

The Impact of Computers on Nursing
M. Scholes, Y. Bryant and B. Barber (eds.)
Elsevier Science Publishers B.V. (North-Holland)
© IFIP-IMIA, 1983

9.2.

A COMPREHENSIVE, COMPUTER-BASED SYSTEM FOR PATIENT INFORMATION IN PRIMARY HEALTH CARE

Pirjo Hynninen

1.   Background Information of Primary Health Care in Finland

Primary health care services in Finland were reorganized in 1972 through a Public Health Act. The renovation gave higher priority to preventive medicine and ambulatory care services and it was to improve the accessibility of health care services, especially in remote areas. A mechanism for centralized planning and evaluation was also introduced.

Health centres became the basic organisational units. Today they are responsible of all primary care services for 15,000-100,000 people living within a defined geographical area. Various primary care services, such as traditional general practitioners office visits, maternity care, child care, home care for elderly people, dental care, occupational health etc., were concentrated at one administrative entity. Physically the health services are often delivered in several locations depending on the population density and other local circumstances.

Especially in rural areas, the health centres are now the only source of primary care. In larger cities, private general practitioners and specialists working in group practice units deliver a significant part of ambulatory primary care services.

There are about 220 health centres in Finland. One of them, the health centre of Varkaus, acting as pilot site for the new computer-based information system of the district, was established in 1975 by three communes. The city of Varkaus is mostly industrial but the other two smaller communes are typically rural areas. The total population is about 34,000.

In each commune there are health stations for ambulatory services. There are also two small hospitals, about 100 beds altogether, for more or less chronic patients.

Currently 14 physicians, 12 dentists and 26 public health nurses are working in the health centre. The total number of employees is 222. About half are working in the hospital wards. The total number of ambulatory care visits was 210,000 in 1981. 60,000 of them were visits to the physicians which is little less than two visits per inhabitant during one year.

2.   A Project to Improve the Data Processing in Health Centre

The change of the organization of primary care brought to light many problems in handling the patient information. Some of them, for example, accessibility of the medical records, legibility and structure of the record and lack of quality control, are well known in all health care fields. However, the problems became more visible when the various branches of health care were integrated into one comprehensive system. Furthermore, the new methods of planning and evaluation on a local level and on a county level, as well as on a national level require more information in a further developed form than in the past. As a consequence, the various professional groups spend an increasing proportion of their working time for various data processing activities.

During the year 1978, a detailed analysis of the information flow, the bottlenecks and the description of individual work programmes was carried out in the health centre of Varkaus. Simultaneously, many of the existing computer-based information systems were looked into. After these preliminary studies it was decided that a computer based information system should be built up and evaluated as a pilot system in the health centre of Varkaus.

The work was carried out during the years 1979 to 1981. The project was financed by the National Board of Health and the Fund for Research and Development in Finland.

The University of Kuopio was responsible for the technical design, programming and implementation of the system, whereas the health centre was responsible for the functional specifications and systems design from the users point of view.

The co-operation between the various parties was organized fairly well. The active dialogue between the users and the programmers created an innovative and stimulating environment so that each professional group actively took part in moulding the system to fit their own needs. The provision of efficient software tools ensured that the process worked out better than on the average. The users were encouraged without limitations to present changes to the functions specified by themselves or other participants.

On the other hand, everything in the system which was specific for the health centre of Varkaus was carefully implemented as parameters in order to avoid reprogramming when the system is implemented in other health centres in Finland. One of the natural conditions for funding the project was the high portability of the system.

3.   From Costar-System to Finstar-System

During the preliminary studies in 1978, it was found out that the system, called Computer Stored Ambulatory Record (COSTAR), was clearly the most advanced for primary care. More than 100 manyears had been spent to develop the system. Most of the work had been carried out in the Laboratory of Computer Science in Massachusetts General Hospital in Boston(1).

As the system was available to the project on the basis of mutual exchange of future development, it was chosen as the basis of the work. The work would not have led to any practical or applicable comprehensive information system with the resources available for the project without the initial investment made in U.S.A.

On the other hand, the technical part of the project consisted of not just the translation of English dialogue into the Finnish language. COSTAR provided means for setting up demonstrations, but many new functions had to be generated and some of the basic COSTAR functions could not be adopted due to the different needs of the users. Approximately 15 manyears, excluding the time spent by various professional groups in the health centre to specify and test the new feature, were spent to build up the system, which was named as FINSTAR.

4.   Description of the System

4.1   Physical Environment and Principles of Operation

Interaction and communication between the user and the system mostly take place through video-terminals. Printing terminals are used only when a document on

paper is needed. Much attention has been paid to developing a simple dialogue
which can be taught to the newcomer within a couple of hours. The use of codes
has practically been eliminated. The user can address various medical items or
select between options using plain language or abbreviations known to the
medical personnel.

The system is based on the use of a local minicomputer to which all of the
terminals are connected. No-one with professional EDP training is needed to run
the system.

In Varkaus, the computer is located in the basement of the building near the
largest health station of the city of Varkaus. Twice a week, an assistant nurse
goes down to the basement and takes back-up copies of all of the disc files.
There are 27 terminals located in most health stations of the health centre.
They can be, and often are, all active simultaneously.

The FINSTAR-system has been built using the modular, top down concept. The top
levels of the pyramid, basic functions, are briefly described in the following.

4.2   Registration

The registration section enables the demographic and basic administrative data
of the clients of the health centre to be entered and up-dated. Most of the
registration data is delivered once a year on a computer tape from the National
Population Register Office in Helsinki. Only information on patients who have
recently moved to the area or who have changed their address is entered manually
to the system.

The user may define, without any programming or outside help, which additional
administrative data items he wants to keep in the system, (e.g. insurance,
policies, accounts or guarantors, employers).These additional items are usually
entered into the system during the patient's first visit.

The subsystem is needed to identify the clients and for the basic administrative
routines but, as the system contains information of the total population, it is
feasible to use the system to pull out patient lists or mailing labels for
defined age groups or risk groups for interviews or screening studies or just to
make tabulations for planning purposes.

4.3   Scheduling

Scheduling subsystem allows effective on-line scheduling of patients to any
provider or other resource in the health centre. The system may look up
possible time slots, book, cancel and display appointments and print lists for
any user or any day.

The system offers the means of maintaining weekly and daily work schedules for
each provider. The system can also be used to produce summaries of activities
for a given health station or given set of providers.

The scheduling can be centralized but there are no technical limitations in
booking time from any terminal. For instance, a physician can book time for his
patient using his own terminal with any provider in the health centre.

4.4   Medical Records

Medical Records systems was the most important subsystem in COSTAR. It causes
the biggest part of the costs and benefits of the system and also makes the
greatest changes compared with the traditional way of medical data processing.
The subsystem has been designed to meet all the record keeping needs within

primary care. However, implementation of the system may evolve over time, and individual installation can be implemented to cover only a subset of the functional capabilities.

In Varkaus the classical paper record is no longer written. Only the electrocardiograms or X-ray pictures or some other special material are stored in a traditonal way.

There are three different ways for a provider to enter data from each encounter. He or she may write down the data on a special encounter form designed for each practice. Encounter forms are collected after each day and taken to the typist's office where she enters the data to the computer system. This is a good way for a newcomer to start. He will then get familiar with the structure of the medical record.

After some experience with the system, the provider may use the dictating machine and read the encounter information in a "structured form" on to diskettes or tapes which are then transferred to the typist's office.

The third way is to enter the data directly using a personal terminal. Physicians use this method when the amount of information is small, like renewing prescriptions. However, some providers have found it to be the fastest way of entering data and they use it most of the time.

All data generated in laboratories is entered directly using the terminals located there because it is the fastest way. As soon as the result of a lab test has been entered into the system, it can be viewed through the terminal in any office in the health centre.

There are several ways of displaying the medical data. It may be viewed by visit or as a summary report for specified data sections like diagnoses, medications, laboratory results etc. A predefined follow-up report may be viewed. It is possible that a particular problem, may be specified together with the format of a follow up report for diabetes mellitus, hypertension, anticoagulant therapy etc. The data items may also be printed against a time scale. The work schedule can be stored and later the follow-up reports can be produced of any patient and any period of time. Even if there is no follow-up report stored, the user can specify items from medical records, he wants to review at the time.

Medical records can be printed on paper and this is done when a patient has been sent to a central hospital or is moving to other area.

4.5. Occupational Health

The health centres are responsible for providing occupational health services to enterprises and other employers in the area if they want to make a contract with the health centre. The larger enterprises usually have an occupational health station of their own but smaller companies with less than 400 employees usually buy these services from the health centre.

FINSTAR-system has a special subsystem for occupational health care. It uses the same basic functions for medical records, but there are additional functions for billing, reporting and handling data from enterprises and site visits.

4.6 Accounts and Billing

The extensive patient accounting subsystems were removed because the communes and state jointly cover practically all of the costs of primary care in Finland. This subsystem now functions automatically to produce bills for the extra fees payable to physicians and dentists for the work they have done outside the office hours or for the procedures or duties which have rated to produce extra fees on the top of the monthly salary.

There are also functions for the health centre to bill some other parties, like employers in the occupational health system, for its services. Some special programs have also been made for the financial inspectors of the health centre.

4.7   Management Reporting

As practically all of the information of the clients and the activities of the health centre are now in the computer system there are almost unlimited possiblities to produce reports, summaries and tabulations for various purposes.

There was a relatively easy-to-use report generator in original COSTAR system and it has now been further developed for FINSTAR. An essential feature of the system is that the user may, without any outside help, define the selection criteria, contents and outlook of listings or tabulations of the report that he is interested in. He may then store the specification in the memory of the computer system and run the report when needed, covering a period of time in which he is interested.

Many of the reports defined and used in Varkaus have replaced laborious data collection procedures. These reports are run periodically and are mostly sent to outside parties like the National Board of Health, Social Security Institution, County Office, Central Hospital. The reports are used for local administration and planning.

The user may also run one shot reports answering specific queries. The reports may take some time to be completed, especially if the computer has to look through the whole population and an overnight computer run is often convenient. Authorisation for management reports is usually given only to those few people who are directly responsible for a branch of the activities of the health centre.

4.8   System Maintenance and Other Functions

Through the functions in system maintenance, the user can change the system in order to adapt to the changes in its environment. An important function is to authorise new users and define their access restrictions and define the restrictions for each terminal.

There are several features in various subsystems which can be changed by the user without outside help. He can create a new health station, define user groups, necessary data items for registration, parameters in scheduling and outlook of displays and print outs of the medical records subsystem.

There is one huge directory in the FINSTAR-system which contains much information about the drugs, laboratory tests, diagnoses, procedures etc. Part of this directory is maintained centrally. When the National Board of Health announces new drugs to be released, a corresponding change is made to the directories of each health centre. Some divisions of the directory can be accessed locally. If a laboratory implements a new method of analysis they must be able to change the corresponding normal values of the test.

5.   Practical Experiences

5.1   Training of the Personnel

The interactive method of building up the system, during the years 1979-1981, enabled many of the users to be fairly well acquainted with the system and they needed no special training during the implementation of various subsystems. Two of the assistant nurses participated in a two-week course during which they learned in more detail some technical and functional features of the system. They were also taught to perform some tasks traditionally done by computer operators. Taking back-up copies of disc files, loading magnetic tapes and starting up the system after a break were quickly adopted. These girls have system manager's access rights.

When a new person joins the staff of the health centre, he receives a short description of the system. One of the system managers will then place the newcomer in front of a computer terminal and instruct him how to use the terminal, how to answer the questions and other prompts given by the program, and go through the basic functions. The time needed for training depends on how extensively the person will use the system. On the average a nurse learns the basic functions in three hours and a physician needs six hours. After this elementary training he or she can start working. In the beginning, he may not be as fluent with the system as the more experienced user. One of the general specifications for the system is that if the user does not know how to proceed or what to answer, he can always ask help from the computer. Within a few days, the newcomer will have the satisfactory ability to use the system.

On the other hand, if the user knows all the features of subsystems well, he can speed up his everyday work and take more advantage of the system. It is useful from time to time, either in a meeting or individually to discuss how to use the system. If a user has found a way to handle a particular situation, he may use it for long periods and may not notice an alternative way which would be more convenient and efficient.

However, the experience in Varkaus indicates that the time needed to train staff to use the computer system is considerably shorter than when the manual system was used.

5.2   Attitudes

Fairly often it has been noticed, a newcomer has a suspicious, sometimes clearly negative attitude towards the computer system. There are several reasons for this attitude. One of the reasons is probably the inadequate training of health care personnel until now. In some curricula there is still no sign of EDP and its applications in health care. In some cases, the courses for students contain obsolete information presented in incomprehensible form by computer specialists, the probable net effect being increased suspicions.

The other source of negative attitudes may have been past experiences with difficult-to-use time-sharing systems in universities, or with batch processing systems where an inexperienced user has only a slight chance to get his run succesfully done and where the main output is error listings.

Since the FINSTAR-system was designed to be used easily it has not been too difficult to overcome suspicions, at least to the extent that they do not inhibit learning and use of the system.

The best way to stimulate active interest and inhibit negative attitudes is to let the users continue the development work. Their suggestions should be tried in a practical environment and adopted in the system, if they prove to be useful. On the other hand, too many features and extended sophistication tend to make the system more complicated and difficult to use. Furthermore, it is not possible to do development work in every health centre.

As a conclusion, the best protection against negative attitudes is to build an effective interface between the user and system so that the dialogue is simple, efficient and psychologically well designed. One of the lecturers for computer science once stated, that if the users hate your system it is easier for you to change the system than to change the users. Furthermore the users are practically always right!

5.3   Changes in content of work

One of the targets of the FINSTAR-system was to reduce the time which personnel have to spend for data processing.

Before the implementation of the computer based system, a study was carried out to measure the distribution of the working time for various tasks. The study revealed that assistant nurses spent 45% of their working hours on various information handling activities, the general nurses spent 27% of their time which is about the same amount of time as they spend for nursing. It has been shown in other studies in Finland that data processing has continuously increased. Furthermore, information handling tasks are subjectively valued as secondary and not satisfying, which leads to diminished discipline in data processing and diminished reliability of data. Especially as data collection for various management reports and studies is often despised, the result being well known to those who have tried to carry out studies on the health sector.

Computer-based system has clearly reduced the time spent by staff on data processing. The system has practically eliminated the tedious data collection routines. It has been found that less time is spent by nurses, assistant nurses and also physicians searching for information. All patient data can be viewed on the computer terminal. Patient records, laboratory results and other patient data are no longer missing. This can be experienced by observing the activities around the registration area and doctors' offices in the health station. The outlook now is quiet compared with the situation a couple of years ago, when the nurses were constantly rushing between the doctors' offices, laboratories, archives and the registration area.

6   About the Quality Control of Nursing

The impact of the FINSTAR system on patient care on to the quality of nursing has not yet been systematically studied. Several methods of measuring the quality of nursing have been developed, but the application of those methods by other research groups still seems to be rather difficult.

If an over simplication is accepted, it can be stated that there are two basic reasons for difficulties for measuring the quality of care. One is the lack of clear standards or measurement criteria to control the quality of care. The second is due to the undeveloped information systems which make it very difficult to carry out larger studies. Measurement systems which are tailored for an ad hoc study usually have a negative or positive effect on the system which is being monitored.

The FINSTAR-system can certainly be a powerful measuring instrument. It is easy enough, using the report generator, to measure the compliance of a patient or the peformance of providers.

Diabetes, mellitus and hypertension are examples of diseases where relatively straight forward care plans have been accepted. The system can be programmed to give the alarm if an unacceptable contradiction occurs between the plans and the actual situation.

Another example of quality control in occupational health care is that the various risk factors associated with jobs can be programmed to trigger certain preventive examinations. The system can automatically schedule health controls, both for the employees as well as for the nurse, who is supposed to carry out the check-up. Drop outs will be picked up automatically in the next run of the report.

REFERENCE

1.   COSTAR A computer based medical information system for ambulatory care. Barnett,G. O. et al. Proc. IEEE, 67, 9, 1979.

The Impact of Computers on Nursing
M. Scholes, Y. Bryant and B. Barber (eds.)
Elsevier Science Publishers B.V. (North-Holland)
© IFIP-IMIA, 1983

9.3.

STATISTICS, COMPUTER FORMS AND HEALTH VISITOR SERVICE PLANNING

Joyce Wiseman

1.   The Need for Data on Health Visiting?

The paper describes a survey which has been carried out by the Regional Health Authority into health visiting in three Area Health Authorities in the North West Region of England and Wales.

A "**Health Visitor**" (HV) has the basic State Registered general nursing qualification together with the additional qualification of "health visitor" obtained by one year's post registration course at a College of Further Education or University, and must have some knowledge of midwifery to undertake health visitor training. She is a family visitor and an expert in child health care, concerned with the promotion of health and the prevention of ill health through giving appropriate education, advice and support.

The Regional Health Authority is interested in health visiting because it currently allocates finance to health authorities to increase health visitor establishments. Several years ago, the numbers of health visitors within North West Regional Health Authority were some 50% below the levels recommended by the Department of Health and Social Security. Currently, although some areas are still below establishment, many are at the recommended level. The survey was undertaken at the request of the Regional Nursing Officer, to find out the state of health visiting in the Region and to assess whether health visitors are receiving education and training which equips them for the current preventive health care. Two hundred and fifteen health visitors were involved; this comprises approximately 20% of the Region's health visiting workforce.

The questions asked by the Region were: What are health visitors doing? What do they think they should be doing? What are the community needs? and, are all three aspects of activity, priority perception and community need in step?

The methodology was adopted from a previous survey by the author. The model involves three aspects of health visiting; the community; the health visitors; the organisation (represented by the health visitor's managers).

The Community is recognised in terms of care group populations, or in the words of the Health Visitor Council for Education and Training, "vulnerable groups in the community." The care groups are not static and they can be adjusted according to those identified in a community. In the original study 25 care groups were recognised, but in the Regional Survey the steering committees identified a total of 33 care groups, because more detail was required in the age bands of the "Routine", "At Risk" and "Mentally and Physically Handicapped" It is clear from the list in Appendix 1 that the care groups have maintained the traditional age group form, together with a list of descriptive groups.

Once the care groups have been listed it is then necessary to **estimate** the annual client care group populations. The most reliable data sources were used to estimate the annual client membership within the different care groups. Some sources can be considered quite reliable and the estimated care group population

predictions quite accurate.   In other cases the estimations are much less
accurate as a result of unreliable data or because no precise method of
calculation is available (see Appendix 1).   Appendix 1 indicates the data
sources and reliability of the population estimates.

The most unreliable group was that of infectious diseases where it was
impossible to accept the RHA statistics produced.   Another disappointing source
was that for the handicapped over 16 years, because no register is maintained
either by Social Services themselves or the Local Authority.   The only source
available for the handicapped over 16 years is the employment exchange, and
their weakness is that they only have records of the handicapped who have
registered for employment and are subsequently known by the disablement register
officer (DRO).

The unreliability of the general practitioners' age/sex registers are well
documented and the whole exercise has demonstrated the need to improve
statistical collation so that authorities become more aware of the health care
needs in their communities.   This will assist with forward planning and the
allocation of resources.

2.   Care Group Populations

One person can be eligible for client membership of several care groups, but it
was agreed that a maximum of three care groups for any client would be adequate
for this survey.   The care group population, for this reason, is always greater
than the resident population.   The ratios of resident population to care group
populations were 1.7 for two areas and 1.6 for the third.

Mrs Brown, aged 75 years (and therefore classed as "elderly, at risk") could be
an ophthalmic patient, an orthopaedic patient and possibly a gynaecological
patient, and so she enters into several care groups.

Estimates of the care group populations in one of the Areas surveyed, are
included in the last column of Appendix 1 in order to indicate the size of the
groups involved.

3.   The Health Visitors

Two major pieces of information were required from the health visitor.   First it
was necessary to discover what health visitors believe are their priorities.
Second, it was necessary to find out what they are doing.   In this way their
activities can be compared with their stated priorities, as well as with the
apparent community need.

4.   Health Visitor Priorities

Two aspects of priority were gained from the health visitor:

        Their judgements of **care group** priorities.
        Their judgements of two leading **functions** to each care group.

Ten health visiting functions have been identified and they are listed as
follows:

Comprehensive Appraisal   Monitoring of client
Monitoring of Services   Health Education
Screening   Prophylaxis
Nursing Diagnosis   Psychological Supportive
Social Diagnosing   Liaison and Co-ordination of Services.

In order to avoid mis-understanding, guidelines on the definition of the various functions were distributed to the health visitors. These guidelines were discussed at meetings arranged so that the researcher could describe the survey to the health visitors and allow questions to be answered thus developing the common understanding of the project.

The health visitors' judgements of their priorities were obtained in the survey from a specially designed 'priority form', which the health visitors were asked to complete at one of the above meetings.

Two types of forms were designed, the first form was a stepping stone to one which could be used for direct analysis by computer. The health visitors were requested to:

place their care group priorities in rank order;
select the reason for placing care groups as the top five priorities;
select the reason for placing care groups in the lowest five priorities.

Later, members of the research team independently examined the reasons written by the health visitors; and discovered that the reasons for high and low priority care group placings broadly fell into the following categories:

Reasons stated for placing of top five care groups

Health visitor function
Prevention
Support
Screening
Vulnerable group
Health education
To develop relationships
Time of rapid change
Monitoring
Health visitor - only agency
Multiplicity of reasons

Reasons stated for placing of lowest five care groups

Not preventive work
Other agencies involved
Self-inflicted
Care group very low in number
Care group too large in number
Not notified to health visitor
Group therapy required
Not qualified
Covered by other care groups
Not health visitor's job
Will visit on request
Multiplicity of reasons

It is recommended that for any future survey the following reasons are eliminated from the computer form, because they tend to disguise facts, and they are: "health visitors function", "multiplicity of reasons", "not health visitors job" and "will visit on request". It is interesting that one Area using the computer form, with the option to use the "multiplicity of reasons", did not use it once, and so it was possible to identify that "vulnerable group" was the most common reason for placing a care group in the top five priority. The most frequent reason for low priority care group placing was given as "other agencies involved".

The health visitors indicated the two most important functions to the care groups by circling two function boxes for the respective care groups. High levels of agreement were indicated by the health visitors of the leading functions to the respective care groups, the function selections varying for the different care groups.

5. **Possible Use of the Health Visitors' Priority Selections**

Now that a priority selection form has been designed for computer analysis, it will be possible to broaden the survey across a whole region, so that the priority selections of the total health visitor workforce can be known.

Knowledge of the health visitors' priorities helps to define more clearly the work of the health visiting profession. The vagueness surrounding the health visitors' role has given rise to a great deal of debate. As a result of studies such as this the health visitors will be able to "state their case" and so help to shape their professional future.

There was high statistical significance between the health visitors on all aspects of health visiting priorities - this must be reflective of health visitor training, and will help to show where extra training is required if health visitors are to broaden their preventive health service.

The health visitor's own interest in specialisation can also be identified and hence this approach can help with career development.

6.   Health Visitor Activity

Knowledge of the health visitors activities were obtained from a self-completion computer form. It is hoped that such a form will replace the statistical return forms which are currently in use in the North West Region. It was this hope which helped to influence the health visitors' co-operation with the completing of the form.

The activity survey was carried out over an eight week period with a total of 215 health visitors, working within the three Area Health Authorities.

The activity computer form was designed by a regional community statistician, and each health visitor was supplied with "an instructions for completion form". The survey has revealed the need to educate health visitors (and, no doubt, nurses as a whole) on how to complete computer forms.

For the first two or three weeks of the survey one of the research team was fully occupied looking through the forms and following up errors and omissions. The most common error was the omission of a zero before single digits when a space for two or more numbers was allowed on the form. Quite often, messages were attached to a completed form, the health visitor perhaps saying "I went to a meeting earlier today", or a little extra like "I think this is the nearest care group".

The health visitors had to be reminded to enter the zero sign, complete the boxes just as directed, and that the computer interpreting the form could not read, nor think for itself!

7.   Data Gained from the Activity Form

The following data were obtained from the survey forms:-

- The number of household visits made by the health visitor each day.
- The client members in the household who received a health visiting function.
- The age group of the client.
- Those contacts which resulted in "no client access". In such a case the function section was not completed.
- The care group(s) (up to a maximum of three) of which the client is a member.
- The preliminary and secondary function to the client (one only of each).
- The agency which stimulated the contact.
- The place of contact.

It was expected that the majority of health visiting will be recorded for home visits. However, this section was left very much to the health visitor's discretion, because if she felt that she had carried out a "true" health visitor activity in the other five places listed, then she was encouraged to record it.

8. Value of the Activity Survey Findings

As a result of the analysis of the form it has been possible to explore the following aspects of the service:-

- The average daily household visit made by the health visitors from the three Areas.
- The approximate percentage of health visiting activities in the household, and "other places".
- Health Visitor contact by age group.
- Health Visitor contact levels to the various care groups.

"No Access" levels in percentage factors to the different client age groups and care groups. From these calculations it is estimated that approximately 17% of household contacts are "no access" visits. The age group which receives the highest "no access" is the 1-4 year age band.

The source referral calculations show that the health visitors stimulated over 75% of their own client contact in all three Areas. The source referral from the general practitioner varied between 1%, 2% and 5% for the respective Areas. The referrals from Social Services were less than 1% for all three Areas.

These results can be compared with the client care group population estimations within each of the Areas, and the health visitors and managers together can appraise their current practice of health visiting, and determine the health visitor target objectives for the forthcoming year. Policy decisions will have to be made; those care groups who receive high levels of contact, should this continue? Or should the health visitors be encouraged to direct their health visitor practice towards those care groups with which she does not apear to be in as close a contact?

The findings could have implications for the post-graduate education of the health visitor, together with a future policy for the organisation of health visiting.

Thus, the survey has provided essential information about the service, which together with a well thought out computer form, provides a mechanism for future health service planning.

Acknowledgements:

I should like to thank Mr P. Davis-Rice, NWRHA nursing officer; Mr K.M. Cottrell, statistician, NWRHA; Mrs S. Cunningham, NWRHA nursing section; the health visitors from the three areas to participated in the survey, together with their managers; Miss B.B. Anderson, district nursing officer, Blackpool Health District; Mrs G.M. Mills for her secretarial services and Mr A. Mogan, regional statistical officer, whose services were essential to the survey.

APPENDIX 1

Care Groups and Data Sources with Care Group Population Estimates from a
Specimen Area.

CARE GROUP	SOURCE	RELIABILITY OF SOURCE	CARE GROUP POPULAT'N
Routine Healthy			
0 - 1 year	Notification of births	Reliable	2760
1 - 4 years	Notification of births added up or census	Reliable	11080
5 - 15 years	Census or education source	Reliable	38000
16 - 29 years	Census or Local Authority rates Dept.	Fairly Reliable	42000
30 - 64 years	Census or Local Authority rates Dept.	Fairly Reliable	84700
65 - 74 years	G.P. age register	Fairly Reliable	18000
"At Risk"			
0 - 1 year			340
1 - 4 years			520
5 - 15 years			140
Over 75 years			10500
Mentally Handicapped			
0 - 4 years	Handicapped register - Local Authority	Reliable	80
5 - 16 years	Handicapped register - Education Committee	Reliable	150
16 - 64 years	Employment Exchange	Fairly Reliable*	370
Physically Handicapped			
0 - 4 years	Handicapped register - Local Authority	Reliable	1400
5 - 16 years	Handicapped register - Education Committee	Reliable	640
16 - 64 years	Employment Exchange	Fairly Reliable*	13600
Antenatal Mothers	Notification of births	Reliable	3400
Post Natal Mothers	Notification of births	Reliable	3400
Adolescent	Census	Fairly Reliable	12700
Problem Family	Health Visitor's own case records	Fairly Reliable	500
Accident/Injury	Hospital Records	Fairly Reliable	33000
Hospital discharge	Hospital Records	Fairly Reliable	19000
Terminally Ill	RHA Morbidity statistics	Reliable	2000
Bereaved	RHA Morbidity statistics	Reliable	2600
Tuberculosis	Notification - Hospital	Reliable	150
Other common notifiable infectious diseases	G.P. notifications	Totally unreliable	1490
Single Parent family	Census	Unreliable**	2000
Marital visits	Health Visitor's knowledge, Estimated divorce statistics	Unreliable Estimate only	600
Metabolic Disorders	International Classification Disease Code+ Hospital Activity Analysis	Fairly Reliable	380

Psychiatric Disorders	International Classification Disease Code+ Hospital Activity Analysis	Estimate only	720
Obesity	DHSS handbook - Research and Obesity	Estimate only	21000
Drug Dependents	Estimaions based on those estimated to smoke more than 20 cigarettes a day	Estimate only	30000
Ethnic Minorities			12000

----

*   No register maintained by Local Authority
** Shifting Population

The Impact of Computers on Nursing
M. Scholes, Y. Bryant and B. Barber (eds.)
Elsevier Science Publishers B.V. (North-Holland)
© IFIP-IMIA, 1983

9.4.

PL CHILD HEALTH CARE SYSTEMS

Fumiko Ohata

I   Introduction

The concept of a Computerized Total Child Health Data System, was first developed five years ago, in 1977, as a health care service to aid in achieving the desirable growth and development of children and perform research into the parent-child relationship as related to child growth and development.

In the PL Hospital, there is now a dual system operating for adults, in Tokyo and Osaka. Two health centers, both with on-line computer systems at the PL Medical Data Center, provide for early detection and prevention of diseases with follow-up consultations.

During the past five years we have been developing another system for children that is now in operation in the Osaka PL General Hospital.

The proposals were outlined by a pediatrician of PL at the WAMI Conference in France, 1978, and again at the MEDINFO 80 Conference, 1980, by the author. This paper presents detailed results on the research findings, some interesting facts from the nursing department evolving from these proposals and the outlook for future developments.

II   Concept of the System

1.   **Goals:**   The objective is to provide both health and medical support necessary for preserving and promoting health, plus investigation into the parent-child relationship.

2.   **Health Management Areas:**   Physical and mental development, nutrition, continuing social value and health education, vaccination, and disease control.

3.   **Data Flow:** Diagram A shows the flow of data from the various medical activities associated with pregnancy, childbirth and child development. The key event timings are the registration of pregnancy. hospital admission, birth, hospital discharge and periodic check-ups at two weeks, one month, one year and seven years after birth.

4.   **Time Schedule of Data Collection**   The detailed activity scheduling is shown in diagram B.

There are at present 171 participating memberships in the program: 45 with infants less than 1 year of age; 36 with children 1 year to 23 months; 34 with children from 2 years to 35 months; 40 with children from 3 years to 47 months; and 16 with children from 4 years to 59 months. Yearly, thirty to forty new participants enter the program, with continuous follow-up of growth and development on a monthly basis up to one year of age, followed by semi-annual checkups. As a rule, registrants enter the program from birth at our PL Hospital, but infants can be accepted from other institutions.

DIAGRAM A

The Data Flow of Total Child Health Care Systems

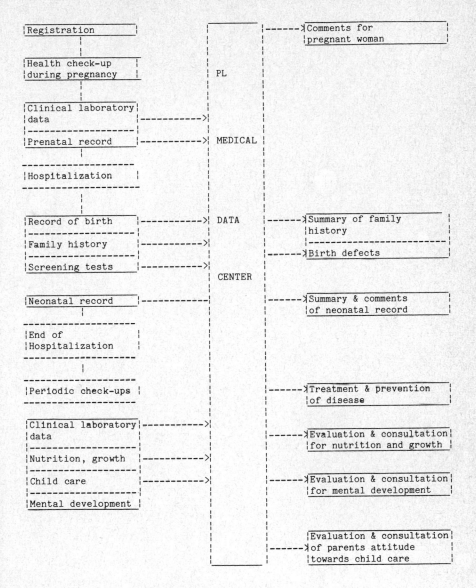

DIAGRAM B

Time Schedule of Data Collection

	P	H	B	E	2W	1M	1Y	7Y
Registration	<----->							
Prenatal record	<----------->							
Record of birth Family History			<----->					
Neo-natal record			<Daily>					

Periodic check-up
  Screening test
  Nutrition
  Mental development
  Child care
					Monthly_____		*Biannually	

A course for child care	<----------->			Monthly------->				
Consultation	<---------Appointment system---------------->							

Code: P: Pregnancy
      H: Hospitalization
      B: Birth
      E: End of hospitalization
    2W: Two weeks after birth
    1M: One month after birth
    1Y: One year after birth
    7Y: Seven years after birth

III   Explanation of Activities

The various activities in health care and health education are briefly outlined as follows:-

a.   Health Care

Monthly checkups on a regular basis, for physical growth, nutrition, mental development, and mother's attitudes, to provide both evaluation and consultation. These are based on pre-prepared, printed forms which list the optimums for monthly development. One week after the actual appointment a questionnaire is mailed for the mother to complete, to provide supplementary information with regard to the mother's attitude, and additional data concerning the child. In all, 130 items are covered by the actual checkup and the questionnaire. In cases of children who are one year or more old essentially the same system is used, but there are areas of difference due to individual age changes.

b.   Educational Activities

Doctors, psychologists, dieticians, and nurses conduct consultations on health, nutrition, feeding routines, and child's diet. These are conducted in both group lectures, and individual conferences. During group sessions mothers are instructed on a monthly basis covering the following subjects: 1. Parent's influence on children's characteristics; 2. Child care during pregnancy; 3. Research into children's abilities; 4. Development of child's independence; 5. Development of a broad sense of awareness in the child; 6. Development of pride and a sense of self-respect; 7. Development of adaptability; 8. Mental development; 9. Weaning infants; 10. Children's diseases; 11. Disease prevention; 12 Individual characteristics awareness.

By means of these lectures and citing of concrete examples, the doctors, psychologists, dieticians, and nurses assist the mothers in gaining the complete knowledge of their roles.

An example of individual counselling stemming from a mother's becoming aware of a possible solution to a problem while attending group sessions occurred as follows: The child was a second-born, 10 month boy; the problem was abnormal thumb-sucking, manifested by insertion of additional fingers into the mouth, until all five fingers were being inserted at one time. This behaviour continued until the child was inducing vomiting by deep insertion of the entire hand. At that time the mother requested an individual conference. During consultation it was found that the communication between the parents had deteriorated to such an extent as to become almost non-existent. The counsellor advised increased discussion between the parents with regard to the child's development and problems. That evening, for the first time in a long period the couple held a discussion of their child's problems and development that continued for several hours. The next day the child's abnormal behaviour suddenly stopped, apparently due to the reopening of parental communication. It is evidenced that the range of communication, parent-child, plus parent-parent, has great influence on child behaviour, and development.

The records show cases of night-crying and bed-wetting attributable to many causes, and the staff are at present engaged in examining through the use of computers, the cause and effect relationships, since these data can be mathematically formulated.

IV   Research Presentations

Yearly presentations of the project development have been made at the Japan
Child Health Congress as follows:-

**First Year (1978): Introduction of the PL Computerized Total Child Health Care
System.** Early detection and treatment of children's diseases, plus the added
advantages of prevention, not usually found in hospital care, and the detection
of abnormalities in the growth and development of children. This entire
presentation was developed and compiled by a PL team of pediatricians,
psychologists, nurses, computer technologists, dieticians, and kindergarten
teachers.

**Second Year (1979): Computerized determination of relationships between
pregnancy conditions and baby height and weight.** Birth weight is greater under
the following circumstances: First, during term the expectant mother eats a
wide variety of foods, encouraged by the husband. Second, rest habits do not
change, daily activities and physical actions remain the same as prior to
pregnancy. Third, mothers have the time and opportunity to maintain a good
personal appearance, which leads to composure. Fourth, they maintain a good
mood, and do not become irritated. Last, they maintain a calm, easy life, but
without laziness.

**Third year (1980): Exponents of birth weight, infant feeding methods, and
mental development.** Using the Tsumori-Inage testing method monthly we evaluate
mental development. This testing method has five areas which are understanding
and language learning, motor ability, eating manner and habit, social relation,
and exploratory behaviour and manipulation. Results of such testing indicate
that greater birth weight is an exponent of higher mental development,
specifically understanding and language learning, and motor ability areas.

**Fourth Year (1981): Relationships among mother's prenatal conditions, exponent
of mental development, feeding methods, teething time and illness tendencies.**
Babies whose mental development is higher have proven to be offspring of parents
who communicate well; both parents are active and have a relationship that is
natural, that is, with disputes as well as agreements. Mothers whose babies
teethe early are calm persons with gentle manner, and have a well-adjusted
relationship with their husbands. Mothers who tend to worry and be overly
concerned with problems usually bottle feed the child; breast feeding is not
common in these cases. The relationship of illness tendency in the child and
prenatal conditions, while expected to be significant, has proven to be without
basis.

Presentations have also been made to the Annual Convention of the Early
Childfood Education Association of Japan, the studies on the Parent-Child
Relationship and Mental Development.

**First Year (1978): Exponents of Parent Characteristics and Children's Mental
Development.** MPI testing conducted with 32 couples showed that children with
parents who are extroverts tend to have higher mental development. Considering
nervous tendencies tests indicate that, $N_o > N^- > N^+$ apply as an exponent of higher
mental development.

**Fifth Year (1982): Exponents of parent characteristics and children's mental
development.** Utilizing the Tsumori-Inage testing method of parent
characteristics applied to child mental development, data from monthly testing
of the child was collected at three month intervals from 6 months to 2 years and
analyses made.

It was ascertained that maternal extroversions influenced higher mental development during each analysis. A significant coefficient on the plus side appeared in the areas of development as follows: At 6 months: eating manner and habit; at 9 months; understanding and language learning and eating manner and habit; at 1 year: motor abilities and understanding and language learning; at 1 year and 3 months: eating manner and habit and a composite improvement in all five tested areas; at 1 year and 9 months: social relations, eating manner and habit and a composite improvement; at 2 years: social relations, and eating manner and habit.

Mental Development in Relation to Father's Extroversion. At 9 months: motor abilities, exploratory behaviour and manipulation, eating manner and habit, understanding and language learning, a composite improvement on the plus side; at 1 year: Effect of the Father's nervous tendency to the exponents: eating manner and habit and understanding and language learning showed significant improvements; in the cases of the fathers who attempted falsification of personality during testing, eating manner and habit and understanding and language learning, showed a minus exponent.

It was found that characteristics in the father had a significant impact at 9 months and at 1 year, but no significant effect at other tested times; such little impact was displayed that no factor could be reached. On the other hand, mother's characteristic influence was apparent throughout, after many case studies.

With the exception of two children who suffered congenital heart disease all of the case studies showed normal growth development; the disease histories show that some needed treatment and hospitalization, some had long term treatment in clinics. Since there are only 171 participants in the program it was difficult to isolate any particular diseases, or gain usable data. We are considering entering families from our Premature Baby Department into this program in order to increase membership. In order to establish counselling for disease prevention we must first study normal parent-child relationships.

Next, I wish to speak about how this information we gather is handled by the computers.

V   Method of Development of our System

The object was to construct a system for health care, education, and research as mentioned before. INTER-LISP computer language, an artificial intelligence language, was used to program the system, since it is a highly flexible database. This program was introduced at MEDIS '78 by a team from the Medical Data Center.

Using present day data-base softwares it is necessary to determine how the program will be written and what the program will accomplish prior to running it. When a program is running new sections cannot be introduced, and thus the program must be complete prior to use. Therefore, it was decided to use INTER-LISP with Japanese character output, developed jointly by Upsala University Data Center and the PL Medical Data Center, working in cooperation. Daily life revolves around Japanese characters, which necessitate a good computer language to use, furthermore the information input includes human behaviour and complicated information, so the decision was made to use the LISP database system. The merits of the system are:

1. Ease of construction.
2. The database system is able to cope with changes in specifications, and these changes are made in a short time, and at low cost.
3. A partial system is operable before the system has been fully specified.

4. Accumulated data transfer through the temporary partial system to the final database can be made with no loss of data.
5. Data and file structures obtained through the temporary system can be utilized in the final system.

The third point is very valuable as information is gathered from many areas; pregnancy history, family history, records of regular check-ups, and these data are used in counselling on health, education, and character points. There is much information collected, but only from a limited number of patients, so this, too, led to the selection of PDDL, a data base system developed by PL Medical Data Center utilizing INTER-LISP.

First stage of data input comes from questionnaires having to do with pregnancy history contained 77 questions inquiring into the history of the mother's condition (physical, mental, and social). This questionnaire was developed for the purpose of determining the mother's mental state and social condition as related to the physical, and the status of the child in growth and mental development. Eight areas are covered in the questionnaire:

1.   Physical changes; sleeping habits, medicine ingestion, and work habits.
2.   Emotional condition.
3.   Economical condition.
4.   Self-concept of physical activity and psychological changes.
5.   Eating habit changes.
6.   Mutual relationship with spouse.
7.   Positive extrovertive actions directed toward the foetus.
8.   Maternal loneliness and return-to-home feeling.

Each section has approximately ten sub-divisions. Section 6 covers the husband-wife relationship influence on growth and development of the foetus; question 1 deals with arguments between the couple, with possible answers: a. Oral with quick settlement, b. Unable to orally express and contention continues, c. Shouting, d. Physical violence, e. Other. In Section 7: Have you taken any actions to induce a calming effect on yourself and the foetus? Possible answer are: a. None, b. Yes...What did you do? More research must be undertaken into methods of collecting information and types of data on these subjects.

Since it is time consuming and difficult to research children's growth and development on a case-by-case basis, generally up to now case studies have not been conducted, but using the INTER-LISP system it is possible to explore the linkage between the mother in pregnancy (foetus-environment) and child's growth and development after birth.

Turning now to the analysis of the information used to establish a proper database. Multiple regression analysis is used to reach the correlation of multi-phasic quantities of variable data. For example, from the answers to some questions in the questionnaire (history of pregnancy) it was found that predictions could be made of the height and weight at birth. Because of this result the data were re-examined and significant items were retained and others were rejected as insignificant. To sum up, there are many aspects of the parent-child relationship, such as expectant mothers and postpartum mothers, and so forth. Much investigation has been done on the theory of child development, but much more research is required in an effort to learn the significance of parent-child relationships through the system.

VI   System Contributions to Pediatric Nursing Department

The system of nursing in Japan is to classify the children by disease, but presently this is beginning to change to the American style of classifying by age and development. Thus, nursing care of children is also falling within this framework. Nursing is aimed toward humans who have problems with health; the goal is to aid them in overcoming these. That is true in pediatric nursing as well. Full understanding of the relationship between parents and child as the most important factor in the child's environment will lead to the best care and consultation. When one of the children whose parents are in this membership is hospitalized, the summary of his development is available on the ward instantly on a computer display, and this is very convenient for the nurse. This also provides the nurse with knowledge of the parent-child relationship gained from the mother. Thus the nurse has this data available to her from the outset of hospitalization. Moreover, this will aid in reaching a speedy recovery for the child.

In the system mothers must learn their role through association and feeding the child. The theory behind our system is that the couple relationship and mother-child relationship, plus the parent-child environment has much influence on the child's growth and development. Through mathematical theory as well, the correlation between the parent factor and the child's growth and development is visible and this aids us to reach the proper nursing care methods. Computer use is vital in collating this type of information which enables us to determine the code and result of parent/child relationship in each case. Finally, the objective is to devise a method, utilizing information provided by parent-child relationships whereby disease prone children and their parents can be given more nursing care and advice.

References

1. Hannah, K. J., The Role of Nursing in Medical informatics, MEDINFO '80, Tokyo, Japan, September, 1980.
2. Roy, S.C., Introduction to Nursing: An Adapatation Model, (Prentice-Hall Inc. Englewood Cliffs, New Jersey, U.S.A. 1976).
3. Murakami, K., Uezaki, T., Hongu, U., Yasaka, T., Total Child Health Care System, WAMI, France, April, 1978.
4. Yasaka, T., Mizunuma, T., Shibata, M., Nakamura, M., Appel K., Schneider, W., Implemental and Application of INTERSISP-MIMER in Japanese (Kanji-Kana) environment, MEDIS '78, Osaka, Japan, October, 1978.
5. Klaus, H.M., and Kennell, H.J., Maternal-infant Bonding. The impact of Early Separation or Loss on Family Development, (The C.V. Mosby Company, St. Louis, Missouri, U.S.A., 1979.
6. Hayashi, S., The Development of Medical Informatics and Nursing, The Nursing 12 (1980) 50-68.
7. Whaley, F.L., and Wong, L.D,, Nursing Care of Infant and Children, (The C.V. Mosby Company, St. Louis, U.S.A. 1979).

The Impact of Computers on Nursing
M. Scholes, Y. Bryant and B. Barber (eds.)
Elsevier Science Publishers B.V. (North-Holland)
© IFIP-IMIA, 1983

9.5.

NURSES IN THE COMMUNITY — PREVENTIVE MEDICINE AND THE COMPUTER

M.G. Sheldon

Introduction

Practical experience of using computers in primary care over 10 years provides a basis for a critical examination of opportunities and dangers. Enthusiasm for the technology must not obscure the needs of the patient. The prevention of disease and illness whenever possible is a major objective of the health service. The nurse in the community is one of the most important and least regarded members of the health professions. At the present time developments in primary care systems, especially in nursing systems in primary care, are just at the beginning.

Apart from all the trauma involved, the advent of the computer has one great advantage. The changes envisaged are so great and the effects so far-reaching that the health professions are being forced completely to rethink their roles, relationships, activities and attitudes. Everyone will be affected by the technology revolution. Information is the source of all power, and information technology is perhaps the most powerful technology in history so far. With access to the right information and a few basic skills almost anyone can be a general practitioner - or even a dictator. Information technology has not only a tremendous potential for good - but also for harm.

In some ways the slow progress so far made in introducing computers into primary care is helpful. It provides the necessary time to think through all the benefits and dangers of computer use. However, computers will come - and the care professions should be more urgently examining the ways in which they can make the primary care services more efficient and effective.

Looking into the future it seems certain that computers will enable the health care professions to extend their roles, making possible tasks which at present are difficult or impossible. Before discussing the role of the computer in the community, it is worth examining the mine-field into which it is to be placed.

Community Nurses

There is, of course, no such thing as a community nurse, but it is a useful umbrella under which to include district nurses, nursing auxiliaries, health visitors, specialist health visitors, community nurses in psychiatry, midwives and any other nurse sensible enough to leave the hospital to care in some way for the patient in his own environment.

The fact still has to dawn on many members of the medical professions and also on society as a whole, that most patients who are ill never enter hospitals. Even when they do, the hospital stay contributes only a small part of the total episode of illness. Furthermore, the amount of nursing care needed outside the hospital is greater than that needed within. Coping with illness requires either adapting the environment to suit the needs of the patient, or enabling the patient to adapt to the needs of his environment. Both activities can only be achieved with good nursing care. Likewise, many patients need not enter the hospital if good nursing care could be provided in the community.

Health Services in the Community

For the patient the community consists of home, work, and social life. The health services play little or no part in these until illness occurs, whereupon the health care workers need to enter and influence each of these areas to return the patient to normal, to adapt the environment or to help the patient adapt to his environment. The secondary care services are less flexible and need the cushion of primary care to function effectively.

Many of the hospital based services enter the community, especially those concerned with obstetrics, paediatrics and psychiatry. All of these services are mainly concerned with individual care in the acute illness episode. The value and importance of preventive care is subservient to the immediate needs of patients. The community medicine services have an overall view of the communities' problems and should play an important role in co-ordinating our activities and encouraging and facilitating prevention.

The Primary Health Care Team

Different people have widely different views as to what this team is, what it is meant to do, and even whether it exists at all. The team concept is a difficult one to sustain. Usually it is a ragged collection of individuals, all acknowledging different managers, trained by different coaches, aiming at different goals and paying heed to neither captain nor referee. Some people still call that a team! The only factors that really link them is that they are all on the field at the same time and they all recognise that the patient is the ball. However, most people accept that preventive care will only work if all of the health professionals co-operate. It might be nice if everyone concerned were managed under the same administration and shared in a common training programme, but this is not likely in the foreseeable future nor is it a prerequisite for effective co-operation. The following rules can act as a basis for such co-operation:

1. **Mutual understanding** is vital and it presupposes a common language and knowledge of the different training, capabilities, responsibilities, skills and potential of the various health professions. This has to start in the medical and nursing schools and continue in the vocational training programmes for doctors, nurses and social workers.

2. **A common core of objectives** must be shared by all primary care workers, supplementing those individual objectives which are uniquely related to each profession.

3. **Regular policy discussions** are required to examine the working of these objectives in any particular community. These discussions will involve doctors, nurses and social workers in primary care, administrators, community physicians, occupational health services, Accident & Emergency departments, and certain hospital specialists. It might even be a good idea to include a few patients!

4. **Information must be shared** about patients both informally and formally on a daily basis and perhaps more formally on a weekly basis.

5. **Access to a common record system** is required reflecting both the needs of the individual and the needs of the community. This is where the computer comes in. But in my view the first four steps must happen first before the computer's technology can be used successfully as part of a team effort seeking to prevent illness.

The central question is: "Are we in fact ready for computers in this area yet?" Their introduction today could cause chaos. Where can the stimulus come from to weld the preventive and community services together so that the appropriate technology can be introduced to make prevention a possibility?

The Royal College of General Practitioners has given much thought to this area and there are an increasing number of general practitioners who are open to changes in. this direction but resistance seems to come from other quarters. What of the nursing profession, especially its administrators and the many hospital-based pressure groups of various sorts? Perhaps now is the time to start a series of activities between all the interested parties to plan ways in which the health care team can become a reality.

Prevention and Surveillance

There are several distinct activities hidden beneath this title.

1.   **Primary Prevention of Disease**

Many doctors are unenthusiastic about this concept, feeling that if one disease is prevented, then another (even worse) will come to take its place. If they are a bit more optimistic they will admit that it would be worthwhile preventing disease if, as in the past, it was simply a matter of sewage and clean water. But today it requires the individuals to do something themselves, such as give up smoking or take more exercise. The returns seem to be small for a major outlay of effort. But major efforts have been made and are effective - for example:

-    primary immunization of small children
-    effective family planning
-    health education of school children
-    antenatal care
-    health education in the consultation
-    encouraging self-help and independence in the elderly.

2.   **Secondary Prevention - Early Detection of Disease**

There is much more agreement that this is a worthwhile exercise for certain conditions, notably cancer. The earlier they can be detected the better should be the prognosis. Thus there is a mushrooming of breast cancer clinics, cervical cytology, and well-women clinics.

Each general practitioner is encouraged to detect any asymptomatic diabetics and hypertensives as early effective treatment will limit complications. Likewise, we all spend a lot of time with development surveillance in the young to detect one or two serious, but rare conditions.

3.   **Tertiary Prevention - Surveillance of Chronic Diseases**

Patients with chronic conditions need to be monitored to minimise complications and make sure that effective treatment is being provided.

It is difficult to undertake all of these preventive tasks and computer systems are needed to make the task possible with the staff and time available.

At present these preventive and surveillance measures are covered in part by virtually every member of the medical profession whether in general practice, the hospital or community medicine. Health education is mainly in the hands of teachers, health visitors and lay people. About the only member of the health care team who does not do preventive medicine is the main community nurse - the district nurse. If we really mean to be effective the tasks will have to be allocated to the appropriate group and they will then have to be provided with the necessary facilities.

How can Computers Help?

There are at least four important ways in which computers can help by collecting, analysing and making data available. These aspects are indicated briefly below:-

1. **Common Record System**

   This is a basic essential in my view. At present there are numerous records about the same patient, none of which are complete, and useful information is kept from other medical professionals. The record consists of three distinct parts:-

   a. **An open record** - that is open to all health care professionals caring for the patient in any way, and also open to the patient. This will contain a summary of important medical and life events, prescriptions issued and allergies noted. An assessment of the individual risk factors for serious disease and a plan of action for the future.

      Entries to this record would be made by the general practitioners, hospital specialists involved, and all community nursing services. The patient is a part of this team and must, of course, be given the right to opt out if he so wishes.

   b. **A record accessible only to doctors** looking after the patient. Hopefully, this part of the record would be small, but there are occasions when entries need to be made which are only significant to other doctors and may be misinterpreted by others.

   c. **A record accessible only to the present personal doctor.** This is a sort of scribbling pad on which notes and ideas can be entered, many of these later proving incorrect, at which stage they may be erased.

It should be expected that each of the other health professionals would also prefer a part of their records likewise to be confined to themselves. With computer technology it should be possible to provide access to this record for all health care workers whilst also allowing for security and confidentiality.

2. **Collection of Risk Factors**

   A lot is now known of the important risk factors for serious disease. If these were collected in the community it would be possible to institute a more efficient and effective screening programme - a **CONTINUOUS SELECTIVE SCREENING PROCESS** - in which the high risk groups are regularly screened and the low risk groups left alone.

3. **Monitoring with Protocols**

   If outlines of patient management could be agreed for chronic diseases then all health workers could participate in monitoring care using protocols contained in the computer. Various studies have indicated that most health workers are capable of following-up the patient if suitable protocols and guidelines are presented. The computer could also improve follow-up by reminding the health care professionals of tasks not performed.

4.   **Information Provision**

A common access to large central data bases of medical information and local collections of information or resources available will assist everyone to manage the work more effectively.

Problems with Computers

There are a lot of problems which have so far prevented anyone from achieving very much in this field. The biggest problem is that many people are scared of computers. Putting explicit information into an easily legible form and storing it permanently in a computer for subsequent inspection is, of course, professionally worrying. Furthermore patients too are afraid that information contained in the medical record is incomplete, inaccurate or just plain wrong.

Another problem is to decide who owns the computer into which information is put. This argument has never been settled for medical records, so why should an instant solution to the computer problem be available? With the advent of networking microcomputers there is a real hope that all professionals can have their own computer which can communicate easily with all other systems allowing us a system of individuality linked with standardisation of communication.

Confidentiality is so obvious, it is not necessary to discuss it other than to say that it has to work.

What Progress has been made?

For some time now many general practitioners have been using simple computer techniques (originally in batch mode) to assist themselves and their team in caring for their patients. The Oxford and Exeter Community Health Projects have been doing this daily for some ten years or more.

With the British system of registering patients it has been possible to build up accurate registers with details of age, sex, address, occupation, social class and risk factors about every patient in the practice.

By sharing lists of patients most at-risk for various problems with the Health Visitor and District Nurse it has been possible to keep and eye on the patients most in need. Recall registers have been easy to set up and selective screening programmes have been undertaken.

The Way Forward

At the present time the first step is to encourage every general practitioner to take on a computer to hold the following essential systems:-

    Age/sex register
    At risk register
    Recall registers

These should then be shared with their attached staff.

Next, these practice computers should be linked to the Family Practitioner Committee indexes and the District Authority systems. Thereafter, the systems need to expand to hold most of the medical record. This stepwise approach allows the development to occur and problems to be sorted out in an orderly fashion.

Despite the recent initiative of the UK Department of Industry, this process will still take some 20 years to achieve, not because the technology is not available but rather because these major changes in general practice and primary care work patterns and attitudes will only happen slowly.

This process can be facilitated as follows:-

1.   Cooperative research in nursing studies, prevention studies and primary care will provide insights into desirable primary care system requirements.

2.   The human interface between the members of the health care team is more important than training the team as computer specialists.

3.   In order to make medicine work the patient must be actively involved.

The Impact of Computers on Nursing
M. Scholes, Y. Bryant and B. Barber (eds.)
Elsevier Science Publishers B.V. (North-Holland)
© IFIP-IMIA, 1983

9.6.

COMMUNITY BASED CARE

Discussion

The Scarcity of Community Systems

Information systems for community care, be they medical or nursing oriented, are in their infancy in comparison to the variety of systems available for hospital care and administration.

One comprehensive system which has been implemented is Finstar in Finland, developed from the Costar system which is used in the USA. These provide comprehensive, real-time community systems dealing with medical and nursing care planning and patient schedules and also provide vital management information. In the U.K., in addition to those systems mentioned in the papers within this section, systems for patient-based costing of community health services for the elderly are being developed as part of a Financial Information Project in the West Midlands. These comprise a series of linked activity systems which will provide data for costing. Two of the activity systems (for home nursing records and the loan of nursing equipment records system) have been implemented in pilot form. User specifications have been developed for record systems for geriatric health visitors, domicilary incontinence service (laundry) and clinics.

Screening programmes for children have been developed in Japan, but are only relevant to the multiscreening style of prevention used in that country. The vaccination and immunisation scheduling system, which includes additional information such as notification of births, and is part of the British National Standard System, is currently being developed as a real time system in Birmingham, U.K.

The Need for Improved Information Systems

In Great Britain where the domicilitory nursing service is mostly in the hands of trained nurses, the interaction of nurse/patient and health visitor/client is on a one to one basis in any single span of time. It is probable, because of the preponderance of trained staff, and because the working situation has been perceived as a one to one relationship, that these nurses' work has been taken for granted and they are seen as able to meet the total needs of the community. Four factors are now emerging which show this perceived view to be erroneous and highlight the need for better information systems; they are:

- The emergence of the 'nursing process' and individual care plans with the need to evaluate that care.
- The escalating cost of providing a nursing service at a time of financial stringency, which brings with it the need to assess value for the money and skills employed, as never before.
- The increasing emergence of preventive services related to care groups and 'at risk' populations and the need to evaluate their effectiveness.
- The development of health care planning for total populations, in a health district or geographical area, for which little other than demographic data currently exists.

Guidelines for Community Systems

A concerted effort to develop community care systems is required but the drive and initiative is likely to come from small groups of nurses and/or general practices at local level. If these efforts are to have a practical outcome it would seem essential that some guidelines are followed. Integrated Systems suited to all potential users should be developed with a common record base - the patient - being adopted. Systems should be introduced only where there is a perceived need by the users and hence commitment on their part. Educating potential users to see the value of these systems is probably one of the most important steps toward any development. A committed user group and steering committee is essential to success. Once the initial needs have been met, the value of information systems and computer applications will probably be accepted and this opens the way to further investigations of information needs. The results of these investigations should be used to undertake cost benefit analyses. The costs, in time and money of existing systems being related to the savings, in time and money, as well as to improved quality of performance of the system. Evaluation of systems after implementation is an important part of development work and it should be possible to undertake this provided satisfactory analysis is carried out as a prerequisite of every systems implementation.

Home Computers: towards a healthy population

With the advent of the home computer, information about health care and prevention could be disseminated more easily particularly in remote areas of the community. More research into the feasibility of this approach to providing care was needed.

CHAPTER 10

IMPLICATIONS FOR NURSE EDUCATION

With computers becoming part of everyday life, including general education, they will eventually become more widespread in nursing education. This, however, has implications for both tutors, students and the development of education and training programmes, in order to ensure that a humanistic philosophic approach to patient care is maintained.

This section of the book explores these implications but recognises that there are no specific right or wrong answers as these are peculiar to given educational establishments. It is hoped that these papers will encourage some of the key principles outlined to be applied in developing the use of computers within the nursing educational field.

The Impact of Computers on Nursing
M. Scholes, Y. Bryant and B. Barber (eds.)
Elsevier Science Publishers B.V. (North-Holland)
© IFIP-IMIA, 1983

10.1.

COMPUTERS AND NURSING EDUCATION: CHANGE AND CHALLENGES

Mary Anne Sweeney

Educational Changes Stemming from the Utilization of Technology

The recent advent of low-cost microcomputers has begun to dramatically change many of the traditional aspects of the teaching-learning process. Although computers have been on the scene in some form or other since the 1940's, they have been utilized in educational settings for only the past twenty years. They have come away with mixed reviews. Many reasons have been put forth for the conditional acceptance of computers in education, but most boil down to two overriding factors: the considerable expense of the equipment or hardware, and the lack of well-designed software or programs. Considerable progress has been made in the past few years in solving hardware problems which should stimulate development of a variety of educational software in the very near future.

Large scale efforts to get the ball rolling with computers in nursing education helped to demonstrate the wonderous power and unique capabilities of computers, but never really attained the widespread use their proponents expected. Computer-assisted instruction in the United States in the 1970's was dominated by two large projects which had support from both government and industry: PLATO (Programmed Logic for Automated Teaching Operations) at the University of Illinois, later handled by Control Data Corporation, and Ticcit at the Mitre Corporation(1). Studies showed that students were able to learn course material by using PLATO computers as well or better than with conventional teaching methods, and in one-third to one-half of the time(I2). Numerous programs were developed for PLATO, but the considerable expense involved in using the system was one of the main reasons for its limited use. The technological progress of the 1970's helped to stimulate educators to continue to look for ways of using computers in their courses.

The microcomputer (the "personal", "home", or "desktop" computer) has opened the door to a whole new world of technology since its arrival on the scene in the late 1970's. Expensive acquisitions and applications no longer need to be justified since these portable marvels represent only a fraction of the costs of the large scale computers. The "stand alone" or independent functioning of this type of computer eliminates the frustration of "down time" and the expenses involved in running cables or underwriting telephone connections to mainframe devices. Microcomputers will have such an impact on society in the next decade that they will stimulate a large scale reassessment of the entire gamut of educational programs from the kindergarden level to post-doctoral study. The National Centre for Educational Statistics calculates that (as of October 1980) 52,000 microcomputers and terminals were available to pupils for instructional purposes in American schools, with one third more microcomputers in use than terminals(2). In a 1980 study of the projected growth of microcomputers in the marketplace, SRI (the Menlo Park, California research firm) predicted that sales of personal computers would reach 175,000 units in 1981. The actual figure was twice that number. Market forecasting has been a difficult problem with mircocomputers and their associated products. They have "caught on" with people much quicker than even the most optimistic predictors suspected. SRI also predicted that the biggest upswing between 1980-1990 would be in the home use market, and that the slowest growth would occur with educational uses (defined by formal or classroom education)(3). Projections by other researchers indicate that by 1985, more than 10 million microcomputers will be in use(4).

Software development is becoming a main thrust of the computer industry. A 1981 survey revealed that 21% of the sales in computer-related retail outlets were for software. The growth in this area of sales is predicted to reach 30 percent by 1985, and to level off at 50 percent thereafter. Accounting, word processing, and inventory control packages currently have the biggest market. In addition, the clientele at retail outlets has changed significantly in the past few years. The proportion of hobbyists has decreased while the business and professional customers make up roughly 66 percent of the buyers(5).

Technological and structural developments in microcomputers are rapidly changing the picture of computer use patterns. The networking of microcomputers will take over much of the work normally done by a mainframe computer and its attached terminals. The convergence of computers, telephone cables, television sets, videodisc players, and home computers will soon enable educators to explore new and unimagined worlds in the realm of learning. The overall effect on nursing education will be substantial. Some of the most important changes that will take place in the next few years will most likely be in the areas described in the following sections of this paper.

Structure of Programs

The traditional nursing program with its prescribed number of semesters will be replaced by a more flexible and imaginative system. Learners truly will be able to work at their own pace and schedule. Writers who chronicle the coming changes in society as a result of this new wave of industrialization predict that most of the future learning will take place while using a computer, and that the computer will be located in the home. Nursing schools will be equipped with computerized media centers where faculty can supervise activities such as evaluation exercises and certification tests. Some of the more affluent programs will assign a microcomputer to core groups of 6 to 8 students to use during the semester. Assignments and projects will be contained on diskettes that have been prepared from the nursing education data base. Libraries will do a brisk business in checking out all types of diskettes since programs will be available to cover everything from learning pharmacology to reviewing for licensing and certification exams. As a result, the time frame of professional educational preparation will be drastically altered as this truly individualized learning takes place. The traditional academic semesters may become remnant of the past. The newly accredited "non-traditional" external degree programs of today that feature individual pacing and challenge exams(6) will become old-fashioned in their methodology, but may become the normal structural pattern of basic baccalaureate programs in the computer age. Graduates will be moving into work settings that utilise computers in conjunction with everyday patient care.

Faculty members will not be replaced by computers, but they will find their role considerably revised. When computers are newly introduced in any setting, history has generally shown that rather than requiring less workers, the situation changes most by altering the main focus of work for the people involved. Faculty will have more time to do what they claim to like best. They can spend the bulk of their time consulting with and teaching students in individual sessions and in small groups. Much of the time formerly spent in correcting assignments, keeping up with gradebooks, and preparing tests will be computer-managed. Time formerly devoted to giving lectures will now be free to develop relationships with students and to closely monitor their clinical performance.

One of the leading figures in the United States who works to educate public school teachers and administrators about computers is David Moursund.   He clearly points out that the entire approach to teaching must change.   Teachers need to weed out unimportant functions and steps in the learning process while placing greater emphasis on experiences that encourage thinking and greater depth of understanding.   He worries that our educational system and the people who run it may not understand many of the important aspects of this computer influence at all.   While noting that no other aspect of education has turned on people nearly as much as computers, Moursund strikes a note of optimism in pointing out that the educator's task is just beginning.   He states that, "The whole idea of how computers will change what we want people to learn as well as how they learn it is still relatively new"(7).   We need to be both adventuresome and cautious at the same time.   A realistic plan needs to be drawn up to provide direction to the computer movement in nursing, and it needs to be carefully implemented.   One public school educator projects that by 1985, there will be enough microcomputer software available to provide organized computerized classes in writing and reading skills in primary and secondary schools(8).   Do we have a comparable computer strategy mapped out for nursing?

Instructional Uses for Computers

Instructional Medium

There are three general categories in which the computer can be used as an instructional medium to convey nursing knowledge to the user.   The three categories include tutorials, games, and simulations.   The most significant and exciting impact on nursing education will undoubtedly result from the development of simulations.

In constructing simulations, educators build models to simulate real systems or situations.   These replicas are especially important in reconstructing events that are impossible, inconvenient, or too expensive to study directly.   While extolling the advantages of clever computer simulations for such important functions as pilot practice for flight training, Nievergelt(9) points out that they need to be used with a "critical" capacity.   No matter how well designed the program may be, educators need to insure that simulations are accompanied by guided, well-grounded experiences in reality.

The early ventures in simulation clearly showed how the interactive nature of the computer dialogue was a fantastic interest catcher.   The most widely known simulation was the ELIZA program developed by Joseph Weizenbaum at Massachusetts Institute of Technology(10).   People became engrossed in the conversational interchange with the "therapist" despite the fact that they knew they were "talking" with a machine, and despite their own limitations with typing skills. It is not surprising that much of the recent publicity in the computer field has been focused on the development of sophisticated game-type simulations.

Simulations have been used quite extensively in the training of workers in space technology, engineering, and various airline-related fields.   In the health care field, several well-known examples have been developed.   McMaster University Medical School in Ontario, Canada developed a series of simulation models of human physiology that have been used in the education of medical students in schools around the world.   MACMAN was orginally written in Fortran and was available to anyone who could type with one finger on a minicomputer terminal. It has since been translated into BASIC for microcomputer use.   The authors explain the educational benefits as follows:

These simulation models have added a new dimension to medical education and research. Not only have they saved many animal experiments, but the students can now perform a virtualy unlimited number of experiments, repeat them several times, try a different treatment each time (or withold treatment and study the natural course of events)(11).

The nursing literature contains some examples of the development of quite simplistic simulations(I24,H4). The development of a simulation is a lengthy, and sometimes tedious process that often has more to do with content definition and test construction than computer expertise. Nursing educators now have a powerful tool available for simulating realistic patient interactions involving both communication with patients and application of manual skills. The utilization of soundly designed microcomputer programs that incorporate text, graphics, sound, animation, and colour will enable faculty to expand the student's knowledge base in ways that are not utilized at present. Computers will not, and should not, be used to replace clinical experiences, but to increase the depth of preparation for them.

Instructional Tools

Computers can also be used as educational tools to accomplish a specific task for the user. Several special purpose software packages have already been developed for assisting educators in dealing with their paperwork. This type of program is designed to save educators time by keeping track of such things as class assignments, test scores, progress reports and course averages.

Computers can also be used as general purpose tools for a whole range of nursing applications. When utilized for database management, word processing, graphic display, or authoring systems, computers can be of great assistance to instructors in a variety of ways.

Combining Computers with Other Technology

The future is difficult to predict because of all of the creative possibilities that will result from combining microcomputers with other types of technology. The videotex that will process information by combining computers, telephone lines, home television sets, and home computers will open up all kinds of possibilities. The videotex market is expected to involve 15-20 million homes in the United States by 1990(12). Educators will be able to utilize some of the audio-visual equipment that is now available in most university settings to add "special effects" to computer-assisted instruction. The most exciting development on today's horizon in interactive video.

Interactive Video

The most promising innovation in nursing education is the availability of interactive video course materials to teach clinical nursing skills. Utilization of this newly combined technology promises to provide a radical departure from traditional ways of teaching students. Such innovative instructional tools may be particularly valuable in nursing since the training process requires close supervision of applied skills in real-life work environments. The instructional material is delivered by a system that combines the special features of a microcomputer and an optical-laser videodisc player. Thus, the interactive features of computer-assisted instruction (CAI) will be enhanced by the audio-visual impact of videodisc materials.

The joining of videotaped images with the interactive computer capabilities will expand and alter the instructional capabilities of both types of media. Although students will still be able to take advantage of the capabilities of computer-assisted instruction, they will be able to use the microcomputer in a more powerful way - to "drive" the videodisc. Thus, the TV screen can reach far beyond the limits set by computer dialogue and graphic display. It will broadcast technically precise video images in the form of still frames or motion sequences. As many as 54,000 separate frames containing both pictures and stereo sound effects can be located on a single videodisc, and transmitted to the screen in a matter of seconds by the microcomputer program.

A baccalaureate nursing curriculum offers a unique set of higher education problems. Utilization of this computer technology may provide a partial solution to the problems of a) campus "clinical practice" facilities lacking the amount and type of equipment available in hospitals, b) insufficient funding to provide faculty to staff campus labs to provide for sufficient student practice time, and c) lack of congruity between exercises in practice labs and real-life hospital experiences. Nursing students must learn theoretical material that lends itself to the types of lessons that have been the proving grounds for much of the CAI available at this time. Nursing theory can be taught very efficiently (and cost-effectively) to large groups of students by combining traditional lecture methods with today's technology. On the other hand, nurses must also learn the clinical skills that are necessary to effectively care for sick patients. The teaching of clinical skills (including manual skills, professional assessments and judgements, and the application of theoretical principles to patient-related situations) is an extremely expensive and time-consuming process. One faculty member can safely supervise only 8 to 10 students each day in a hospital-based clinical setting. Students have limited clinical supervision time during a semester because of this faculty-student ratio. Therefore, if students do not have access to a practice setting that closely replicates the hospital situation in which they must perform the clinical skills, valuable learning experiences are lost.

The rate of learning to practice nursing skills is highly individualistic, and does not always relate to cognitive acumen. The new interactive video technology provides an opportunity to learn clinical nursing skills at a self-paced rate, and to practice them in a realistic fashion, as many times as necessary, before arriving at a hospital to care for a real patient. Thus, premium clinical supervision time can be utilized by nursing faculty to "fine-tune" the student's developing skills in the actual health care settings.

The potential applications for the use of this type of combined technology in a nursing program were first visualized during the course of an eighteen month Special Project grant awarded to Boston College from 1978-1980 by the Division of Nursing, of the Department of Health and Human Services. The project, entitled "Development of a Nursing Curriculum Evaluation Model" (1 D10 Nu21004), led to the development of several experimental patient-care simulations in a variety of different instructional mediums. The method of presenting material that had the most appeal to students was the microcomputer program. The microcomputer program simulated a patient, Mr. Robert Malone, who was designed to be in cardiac distress while located in the hospital emergency room. Numerous students were "assigned" to his care by reporting to the learning resource center in the School of Nursing Library. Mr. Malone was an experimental "case", housed on a diskette, who became active when played on a Apple microcomputer. Even though the design of this program was quite simplistic, the enthusiastic response from learners encouraged us to explore this area further. Although the Malone simulation showed great promise as a teaching and an evaluative tool, we were often bemoaning the fact that the television screen could be better utilized to enhance the student's learning experience.

Computer graphics can surely add to the quality of instructional materials, but a life-like image of this patient was notably lacking. If we could have included a visual sequence in which the nurse administered medicine to

Mr. Malone, or placed the leads of an electrocardiograph machine on his body, we would have had a much more powerful teaching device. We wanted to splice in a brief segment in which the nurse talked to Mr. Malone about his pain symptoms and current physical distress. Then learners could have used observational skills just as they would during a real clinical interaction. What did Mr. Malone's skin color look like? Did he exhibit signs of respiratory distress? Did he give any clues that he was anxious? Visual impact provides a crucial step in the process of teaching students how to assess the status of patients. Simulated cases must include direct observation of patients if they seek to provide realistic, work-oriented experiences. However, they must be more than movies, slides, or videotapes if active student participation is sought.

The latest developments in technology that would combine laser videodiscs and microcomputers would permit students to do any of the following: watch while a procedure is performed on Mr. Malone in real-time, in slow motion, with or without sound. A second audio channel could be used to give a running commentary on the action by a nursing instructor (or perhaps by the patient). The learner could stop the motion if desired, and study one single frame of action as long as desired. On the other hand, the student could use the reverse control to watch the action repeated over and over as many times as desired. Students could be instructed to "perform" the procedure on the patient during the simulation, and he could chat with them (in a fairly realistic fashion) while they are carrying out the steps of the process. Nursing instructors who supervise students while they practice procedures on simulated patients (the far-from-life-like Mrs. Chase mannequins) in the Campus Practice Laboratory know that actual hospital conditions are vastly different. The patient and his environment will provide all kinds of diversions and interruptions. The interactive videodisc can create an illusion of these conditions, and thus, a more life-like practice setting. Students would "interview" Mr. Malone, hear his response, and observe his reaction to various procedures in addition to reading printed words or numbers on the computer monitor.

The technology for permitting these simulated activities has just become available. Although magnetic video recording tape made its formal television debut 25 years ago, the availability of Laser optical video disks is a recent phenomonen(13). The disks provide the rapid access to the specific scene (no winding through reels full of videotape) that is required in interactive video. The picture quality is outstanding - particularly in slow motion and still frames.

Many educators feel that people learn better at their own pace and that they explore and retain material that is visually stimulating. Studies have also shown that when you increase the fidelity of automated images, you strengthen the transfer of learning. The fidelity of the videodisc exceeds the quality of the audio-visual media available in the past. A number of interesting videodiscs have been created that demonstrate the wide range of capabilities and subjects:(14)

1. "How to Watch Pro Football" produced by the National Football League for O.P.A. (Optical Programming Associates, a consortium of MCA, Phillips and Pioneer set up to demonstrate the possible uses for videodiscs.)
   Two audio channels are available for alternate descriptions of the same football play. Quizzes are built in using one audio channel for questions and the other for answers.

2. First National Kidisc produced by B. Green and Co. for O.P.A. It is a collection of 22 games and activities that invites the child to play with it - each chapter demands that the child use the videodisc in a different way.

3.   "Tank/Gunnery Trainer" a game-like simulator designed by Perceptronics of
       Woodland Hills, CA. for the U.S. Department of Defense.
       The simulator is used to train soldiers by utilizing realistic film
       segments and computer graphics to depict views from inside the tank.   It
       graphically shows the results of hits from the firing of shells.

4.   A "movie map" or visual   tour of Aspen, Colorado, produced by the
       Massachusetts Institute of Technology Architecture Machine Group.   By
       viewing the "movie map" you can drive down a street, turn corners, or
       enter a public building.   Among other features, you can fly over Aspen by
       means of a computer simulation.

The Apple II microcomputer, introduced in 1977 as the first fully assembled
programmable personal computer, is an excellent companion in the laser system.
Late 1981 brought about the interface which is responsible for allowing the two
devices to work in tandem(15).

A prototype of the type of computer program that would be used for this purpose
has been explained in detail in an article in Creative Computing.   The article
describes the programming of "Rollercoaster", a computer/videodisc adventure
simulation(16).   The combination of a videodisc covering some aspect of health
care, and a lively microcomputer program would truly present new vistas in
learning clinical skills.

The Challenges for Nurse Educators

The following five challenges will provide nurse educators with an opportunity
to incorporate computers into their own professional work, and to enrich the
learning experience of their students.   The technology necessary to carry out
computer-related educational activities is definitely available and is
constantly being enhanced.   The directions of future programs in nursing will be
greatly influenced by our attitudes and resourcefulness in meeting the following
challenges.

1.   Engage in creative exploration.   Open up imaginations and willingly try
       something new.   It is hard to envision all the ways we can use computers
       to enrich learning because there has been so little opportunity until now.
       Computers are not that difficult to learn about.   Inservice programs for
       faculty on topics like instructional design and computer use will be the
       real key to successful utilization of computers in nursing education.

2.   Define the right things to learn about computers.   Efforts to promote
       "computer literacy" need to be carefully planned.   Experts cite the
       constantly changing nature of computer technology.   If too much attention
       is focused on learning higher level languages, educators may be taking
       unnecessary risks.   In a recent article, Olds(17) points out that computer
       languages are being constantly replaced by newer languages that can be
       used with greater ease and diversity (superpilot, for instance).   He
       suggests that time could be more productively used for developing skills
       in using the general-purpose functional languages (commands) required for
       using the computer as a database manager, financial planner or word
       processor.

3.   Utilize the power.   Constantly monitor the purpose of the computer in the
       learning activity.   Do not utilize it for tasks that could be accomplished
       just as well by more traditional means.   Many writers decry the early
       utilization of computers in educational activities as mere "electronic
       page turners".   The computer will be received best and will be most
       economical when it is performing functions that would be next to
       impossible to do by counting on fingers or using an abacus.   Be sure that
       it is not a fancy new version of programmed instruction.

4. Integrate computers into sound educational designs. Try to strike an ideal relationship between software, print material, teaching experiences and clinical laboratories. Student's should have many opportunities to experience the concepts that have been selected by faculty. The computer simply provides a great variety of instructional forms in which to do this.

5. Acquire (or develop) high quality software, that is technically polished and educationally sound. The software should use all possible modes to present content such as text, graphics, sound, pictures, movement, and color. Remember that software can also be designed to engage two or more students in collaborative learning ventures.

REFERENCES

1. Nievergelt, J., A pragmatic introduction to courseware design, Computer 13 (1980) 7-21.
2. Prentice, L., Educational computing - the giant awakes, Microcomputing. 5 (September 1981) 86-89
3. Think tanks differ in thoughts about future of micros, Infoworld. 4 (June 28, 1982) 14-15.
4. NY research firm predicts over-the-counter computer sales, Infoworld. (June 28, 1982) 34.
5. NY research firm predicts over-the-counter computer sales, Infoworld. 4 (June 28, 1982) 34.
6. American Journal of Nursing. 82 (June 1982) 893, 904-905.
7. Hager, T., David Moursund: educating the educators, Microcomputing. 5 (September 1981) 56-58.
8. Nilson, J., Classroom of the future, Microcomputing. 5 (September 1981) 36-34.
9. Nievergelt, J., A pragmatic introduction to courseware design, Computer. 13 (1980) 7-21.
10. Weizenbaum, J., Computer power and human reason. (W.H. Freeman and Co., San Francisco, 1976).
11, Ahmed, K. and Sweeney, G., Medical simulations, Creative Computing. 6 (July 1980) 112-115.
12. Micronetworks, Infoworld. 4 (June 28, 1982) 32.
13. Kellner, C., V is for videodisc, Creative Computing. 8 (January 1982) 104-105.
14. Onosko, T., Vision of the future, Creative Computing. 8 (January 1982) 84-94.
15. Ahl, D., Aurora systems videodisc controller, Creative Computing. 8 (January 1982) 56-57.
16. Lubar, D., Rollercoaster: a computer/videodisc adventure, Creative Computing. 8 (January 1982) 60-70.
17. Olds, H., Through a new looking glass, Microcomputing. 5 (September 1981) 62-74.

The Impact of Computers on Nursing
M. Scholes, Y. Bryant and B. Barber (eds.)
Elsevier Science Publishers B.V. (North-Holland)
© IFIP-IMIA, 1983

10.2.

EDUCATING NURSING STUDENTS ABOUT COMPUTERS

Judith S. Ronald

Introduction

A growing number of nurses are becoming interested in the potential impact of the computer on nursing. This increasing awareness and interest in computers is not unique to nursing. It is occurring in society as reflected in the schools where computer courses are often part of the curriculum, in the home where personal computers are becoming more and more common, and in magazines and newspapers where articles about various computer applications appear frequently. Soon students entering Schools of Nursing will be computer literate. They will expect to use computers as part of their educational process and to learn about the application of computers to nursing practices. If this is true, then nursing education must consider the development of curricula which include computer concepts as they relate to nursing.

This paper will explore the education of nursing students with respect to computers. To achieve this goal it will be divided into three parts: first, a review of relevant educational programs reported in the literature; second, a description of an introductory computer literacy course offered to nursing students at the State University of New York at Buffalo, USA; and third, general curriculum goal, approaches and learning activities for a computer literacy program for nursing educators. The material discussed will be primarily from the nursing literature of the United States. The author recognizes that because of differing cultures, health care systems, and nursing education and practice, the programs described may not be transferable to other countries. However, it is hoped that specific aspects of them will be relevant and able to be adapted to diverse settings.

Overview of Computer Education in Nursing

In an earlier age, the student interested in a career in nursing did not even consider the study of computers as part of her nursing curriculum. However, it will be increasingly difficult for anyone to qualify as a competent nurse in the future without having at least some introduction to the computer and its application to nursing practice, education, administration and research. This idea is supported by many of the articles which have appeared in the literature describing various uses of the computer in nursing. In spite of the expressed need for educating nurses about computers, educational programs for nurses which have been reported are limited. Most of them are primarily related to specific computer systems installed in hospitals or community health settings. Articles which describe specific information systems usually include a paragraph or two about the way in which personnel were prepared to work with that system.

In 1976, Zielstorff described a general progam designed to teach hospital personnel how to use computer systems. She emphasized the importance of careful planning prior to the introduction of an automated system not only because any major change is often perceived as threatening, but also because computers may prompt negative feelings or unrealistic expectations from staff. The main focus in any hospital orientation program is on how to use the equipment and the program. The specific objectives and content of the program depend upon the particular system, the environment and the circumstances under which it is being introduced.

Zielstorff raises the question about whether or not such a program should attempt to modify staff attitudes about the proposed system in addition to presenting the knowledge required to effectively use the system. She comments that if nursing administrators ignore the affective components of an introduction to automated systems, they may be bypassing an important adjunct to orientation(K18). The importance of this aspect of orientation was supported by Octo Barnett when he stated that "the successful application of technology to clinical medicine often depends on the resolution of problems concerned with the interface of the technology and the human being"(1).

In addition to general guidelines for an institutional orientation program, specific programs have been described. One of these was reported by Cook and McDowell in 1975. They indicated that they began by estimating what needed to be taught and the optimal class size for learning. Lesson plans were developed based on these estimates, tested on several staff nurse volunteers and, modified as necessary. The results were that five to six people attended five one-hour classes. The teaching consisted of two parts: the first was in the classroom and related to the use of the equipment and all of the data available from the terminal; the second was on the unit and related to changing the patient data form. In the classroom setting, each person had access to a terminal. When the system was actually implemented, data processing and knowledgeable nursing personnel were available on the unit to reinforce what had been taught and practiced in the orientation sessions and to assist the staff with unforeseen problems. This proved to be an effective approach to preparing personnel to work with the system(K6).

Gluck in discussing another hospital orientation program re-inforced the idea of both a theoretical and a practical component in these sessions when she said:

> "Initial classroom orientation is valuable as an introduction to the basic vocabulary and technical skills necessary to interact with the computer; however, this introduction must be followed by on-the-job practice under the supervision of an expert in the use of the system"(G7).

The preceeding discussion of educating nurses with respect to computers has focused on reports of inservice education classes for staff nurses in a hospital implementing a specific system; because of this the course descriptions have not been detailed in relation to content. The primary goal of these orientations has been the achievement of technical competence on the part of the learner.

Little has been written on computer courses for nurses in institutions of learning. Yet this is an environment in which future nurses could be prepared to participate in the development and implementation of computerized system in many different environments. Plans for one of the first educational programs in a school of nursing were described in 1971 in Nursing Mirror. The United Liverpool Hospital in Great Britain was involved in an experimental project on the use of computers in the hospital. Although the system was not to be installed until 1973, a decision was made to develop an educational program about computers for student nurses entering in 1971 so that they would be prepared to work with computers when they graduated. A questionnaire was constructed to ·identify what the entering students knew about computers and their attitudes toward computing in hospitals. The course was then to be developed based upon their responses(K11).

In the early 1970's, a study to identify the needs of health personnel for education in medical computing was conducted by Anderson, Grèmy and Pages under the auspices of the International Federation of Information Processing. A questionnaire was sent to health care personnel in Western developed countries who were members of the International Federation of Information Processing. The survey indicated that the respondents (physicians, nurses, hospital administrators) believed that all nurses should have a general knowledge about the computer and data processing, and that this content should be part of the curriculas of all nursing schools. Respondents also indicated that they believed that a large number of nurses should be educated to the point where they could use a computer effectively and contribute to the development of automated systems(2).

From the study, three levels of training were recommended. Levels I and II were considered to be appropriate for nurses. Level I was the most basic level and comprised 20-40 hours. Half of the time was to be spent in theory and half in practical applications. The content of the course included:

1.   data processing terminology,
2.   flow of information within the computer,
3.   functions, uses and constraints of various input and output devices,
4.   manipulation and storage of information within the machine,
5.   functions and levels of computer languages,
6.   systems analysis, algorithmic thinking and flow-charting as applied to the everyday life of the doctor, and
7.   operation of peripheral devices with sufficient skill to allow student to enter and retrieve information easily(3).

The Level II course required 150-200 hours of study. About half of the time was to be devoted to an indepth study of basic information sciences and half to health applications(4). The main objective at this level was to provide health professionals with the knowledge and skill which they needed to be able to discuss, plan and co-operate with computer scientists developing medical systems. These health professionals were to be able to analyze and design a medical system in their own area of health activity(5).

In 1981, an introductory level computer course offered at the University of Minnesota Graduate School of Public Health was described by Gatewood. It was a four credit course offered to students or practitioners in health service administration including nurses, physicians and other health professionals. The major difference between the suggestions for Anderson's Level I course and Gatewood's was that Gatewood's course introduced computer programming and the use of package programs, and thus required a knowledge of algebra and elementary statistics(A9). Anderson did not advocate teaching programming in Level I and placed no prerequisite requirements on health professionals entering the course.

Few schools of nursing in the United States have a course on computers in their curriculum. Many graduate schools, however, currently include the use of the computer for statistical analysis as part of their research requirements. In addition, the computer is often discussed in courses in administration and education. At the undergraduate level, little is being done to introduce first-level practitioners to the computer and its uses in nursing.

Description of a Computer Course for Nursing Students

In order to provide nursing students with an opportunity to learn about computers in health care, an elective course entitled, "Implications of Computer Technology for Nursing" was developed at the School of Nursing, State University of New York at Buffalo in 1977. The purpose of the course was to familiarize nursing students with the present and potential impact of computers on the health care system, the health care professional and the patient. Although the course was designed for undergraduate nursing students, graduate students and nurses from the community also enrolled in it.

The discussion which follows is a report of the author's experience with that course. The major objectives of the course were to develop the student's ability to:

1. Describe the major factors which have affected the development of computer applications in the health care system.
2. Identify the benefits and constraints of a computerized information system for both the health professional and consumer.
3. Comprehend the basic concepts of computerized information processing.
4. Described major applications for computers in the area of:
   a) patient care
   b) administration of health services
   c) health sciences education
   d) health care research.
5. Understand how professional practice could be enhanced by the acceptance and use of computers.
6. Interact with a computer through a remote terminal utilizing a CAI program in nursing.

In order to achieve these objectives, the student was introduced to five major areas related to the implications of computer technology for nursing. These areas were:

1. The importance of technology in contemporary society.
2. Basic concepts of computerized data processing.
3. Present and potential applications of computers in the health sciences.
4. The nurse as a participant in a computerized information system.
5. Social/ethical aspects of health data automation.

The specific course content was based on the work of Anderson, Gremy and Pages(3) and the author's professional experience. At the beginning of the course, the attitudes and knowledge of the students with respect to computers were assessed through the use of a questionnaire followed by group discussion. In 1977, (the first time the course was offered), negative attitudes were far more prevalent than positive attitudes. At that time students described the computer with words such as: "brain", "dehumanizing", "unreliable", "scary", "complicated", "takes people's jobs away". In 1981, the opposite was true; positive attitudes were more common and although the computer was still viewed as "scary" and "complicated", it was also seen as "interesting", "helpful", and "part of our future". The content of the course began with an exploration of the importance of technology in modern society. The areas discussed included man-machine relationships, the evolution of the computer and its applications, the capabilities and limitations of computers and the attitudes of individuals towards computers. In 1977, fears of the computer dehumanizing health care and replacing essential professional nursing functions were of great concern to the students. In 1981, students seemed much less threatened by such issues.

The technical aspects of computerized data processing were presented as the second major topic in the course. The purpose of this unit of study was to familiarize the students with some of the vocabulary of the computer/information scientist was well as to assist them in gaining a basic understanding of the way in which a computer functions. This was accomplished through a discussion of cybernetic systems, digital computers, computer hardware and computer software. Students were introduced to the techniques of flow charting and computer programming. They developed flow charts describing the flow of information in work settings which were familiar to them. The first time the course was taught, computer programming was not included since students expressed great concern that the course might be too technical or mathematical for them. However, in 1981, because of student interest, an orientation to programming was added and students learned commonly used system commands and BASIC instructions. They read, modified, wrote and ran simple BASIC programs on an interactive system using both a CRT and a teletype. The students enjoyed the experience and developed a sense of computer logic as well as real time computing from it.

After gaining some understanding of the technical aspects of computers, the students explored the present and potential applications of computers in the health sciences. Both medical and nursing applications were discussed including hospital and community information systems. The use of computers as a diagnostic tool in medicine was disussed. The concept of decision-making algorithms and their application to nursing were explored and algorithms were developed for simple nursing decisions. In order to give students an opportunity to better understand some of the impact a computer might actually have in a health care setting, they identified a simple data processing problem in a familiar health setting and then developed a flow chart of it. Following the development of the flow chart of the existing system, they introduced a computer into the system and developed another flow chart. In this way students were able to see the difference a computer might make in a specific situation.

Following the discussion of patient care applications, computer-assisted instruction (CAI) was explored with an emphasis on the actual and potential use of CAI for health science students and graduates as well as for patient education. Types of CAI, such as problem-solving and simulation were introduced. Students were assigned to do one CAI package utilizing a terminal which is in the Health Sciences Library at the State University of New York at Buffalo. Interaction with the computer proved to be the most valuable experience of the course for many students. The students indicated that the actual hands-on experience with interactive computing both in programming and CAI demystified the process of communicating with a computer. Although acceptance of the computer as a learning tool was important, far more important for the purposes of this course was the expressed change in the students' attitude toward using a terminal.

Considerable time was devoted to the nurse's specific role as a data generator especially in relation to the systematic collection of data and standardization of the content of a record. The benefits and constraints of systematic standardized assessment and recording tools were discussed and compared to the commonly used free format recording tools. Discussion focused on the three areas in relation to these two types of recording tools:

1.   the informational content of each,
2.   the time required to record on each, and
3.   the professional's perceived loss of free choice in recording on standardized forms.

The final unit of the course was related to the social and ethical issues of computerization. Confidentiality of health data was a critical issue to all of the students. In discussing the control of access to health information, the rights of the following groups were considered: the patient, the data generator (nurse, physician, social worker, etc.) and the third party payer (insurance company, governmental agency). The students discussed the nature of privacy problems posed through the use of the computer and examined the present system in terms of its safeguards. One significant fact which emerged during these discussions was that the students' basic lack of trust was not in the machine side of the man-machine interface but in the human side. This realization coupled with the students' increased understanding of computers motivated many of them to express interest in becoming actively involved in the development of computerized health information systems. They began to realize how important it was for nurses to be involved in decisions about what information was to be stored in the computer, why it was being stored and how it would be used.

At the completion of the course, students' attitudes were more positive than negative toward computers. They described their feelings about the use of the computer in health care with words such as "...will take away much paper work and leave time for quality patient care", "I'd like to try it", "I feel very positive", "They can't get into the system too soon for me". They were about to identify ways in which the computer would enhance professional nursing care rather than threaten it; how it could, if properly used, humanize rather than dehumanize health care.

The students recommended that many aspects of the course, particularly the applications, be integrated into the undergraduate curriculum for all students. Some of the major areas in the undergraduate curriculum into which selected concepts related to computers might be integrated include:(H8)

1. Clinical nursing courses
   a) data collection, recording (including standardized tools), and retrieval
   b) generation of nursing care plans
   c) availability of current and pertinent information for clinical decision-making and evaluation of patient care

2. Leadership and administration
   a) staff scheduling
   b) report generation
   c) availability of appropriate information for administrative decisions
   d) facilitation of quality assurance programs
   e) reduction in clerical tasks

3. Professional issues
   The role of the nurse in a computerized environment

4. Research
   a) information retrieval
   b) statistical analysis.

Integration of computer concepts into the nursing curriculum is a complex issue. Since curriculum decisions are made by the faculty, the first step in such a curriculum modification is the education of faculty members with respect to computers in nursing. To accomplish this, relevant curricula will have to be planned for nursing educators.

Development of Guidelines for a Computer Literacy Curriculum for Nursing Faculty

Curriculum planning and adult learning theory suggest that adult education programs are most effective when they are learner-centred. In order to develop a learner-centred curriculum for faculty, it would be necessary to assess the faculty members' knowledge, beliefs and attitudes with respect to the specific content of the curriculum to be developed(6,7,8). In light of this, a study to describe the attitudes of nursing educators toward computers and their perceptions of the need to learn about selected content related to computers was recently completed by the author. The data gathered were used to develop general guidelines for a computer literacy curriculum for faculty. The population for the study consisted of nursing faculty, with a Master's degree or above, who taught in schools of nursing within the continental United States. The potential sample included 300 educators selected at random from a list of faculty who were members of the American Nurses' Association. Of the 201 questionnaires returned, only 159 were useable for purposes of the data analysis. Thirty-eight of the respondents did not meet the criteria for inclusion in the study due to retirement, job change or teaching in an in-service setting; three questionnaires were incomplete.

Data were gathered through the use of a questionnaire. The first part of the questionnaire was a sixteen item attitude scale developed by Startsman and Robinson to measure attitudes of medical and paramedical personnel toward computers(9). The second part was a needs assessment designed by the investigator. It included statements describing specific knowledge and skills which might be included in a faculty development course on computers. Subjects were asked to rate each statement in two different ways using a Likert-type scale. The first rating was with respect to the individual's perception of his/her present level of knowledge; the second with respect to his/her ideal or desired level of knowledge. The difference between the two ratings comprised the needs score for that particular statement.

The findings of the study in relation to the respondents' attitudes towards computers indicated that the overall attitude of nursing educators was positive. Their attitudes were most positive with respect to the computer's efficiency and importance in society and least positive in relation to their willingness to use and accept the use of computers. There were no significant differences in attitude based on the type of nursing program (diploma, associate degree, baccalaureate, graduate) in which the respondents taught, their age or the number of hours of instruction they had had about computers.

The findings of the study with respect to the respondents' learning needs suggested that nursing educators had a need to learn about computers. The subjects preceived themselves as having a low level of knowledge about computers ($\underline{x}$ = 1.04 on a scale of 0 to 4) and wished to have a high level of knowledge ($\underline{x}$ = 3.06 on a scale of 0 to 4). There was a high degree of heterogeneity among the educators with respect to their learning needs as indicated by a learning need mean of 2.06 with a standard deviation of .94.

The specific areas which the educators rated with respect to their current and desired knowledge included the following:

1.   Privacy considerations in a computerized information system.

2.   Role of the nurse in the development of computer applications in nursing.

3.   Ways in which computers can be used to:
      a)   help nurses care for patients (for example, develop nursing care plans, physiological monitoring)
      b)   assist nursing administrators (for example, nurse staffing based on patient profiles)
      c)   teach students (for example, simulated clinical decision-making)
      d)   help in curriculum planning (data bank of instructional objectives, content, methods, resources and evaluation tools)
      e)   aid in statistical analysis and nursing research.

4.   Effect of the computer on:
      a)   role of the nurse
      b)   role of the educator
      c)   the quality of health care
      d)   the cost of health care
      e)   the quality of nursing education
      f)   the cost of nursing education.

5.   How a computer functions.

6.   How to write an original computer program.

7.   How to use a computer terminal including "hands-on" experience.

The means of specific items on each of the scales were very close, making the consecutive ranking difficult to interpret. Thus, only the items which clustered at the upper and lower ends of the scale were interpreted. Natural breaks were used to determine the clusters.

The learning needs which appeared to have the highest priority were related to the application of the computer in education. The two statements which formed this cluster were "use of the computer in curriculum planning" and "effect of the computer on the quality of nursing education." The learning need with the lowest priority was "how a computer functions." "How a computer functions" also ranked lowest on the desired knowledge scale. The statement which ranked lowest on the current knowledge scale was "how to write an original program." There was a significant difference in the educators' current knowledge and learning needs based on the type of program in which they taught. Educators in graduate programs had the highest level of current knowledge and the lowest learning need with respect of computers. This was probably related to the fact that over 70 percent of the graduate faculty had more than five hours of instruction about computers. In other faculty groups, less than 30 percent had more than five hours.

The findings of the study were used, in conjunction with curriculum planning theory, to develop general guidelines for a learner-centred computer literacy curriculum for faculty. These guidelines can serve as a resource for curriculum planners in specific situations. There are two overall goals for the projected curriculum plan, one in the affective domain and one in the cognitive. These goals are to assist the learner to: 1) value and accept the use of computers in nursing and 2) become knowledgeable about the application of computers to nursing. Specific objectives would be dependent upon the specific faculty and setting for which the curriculum was being developed.

Both an attitude survey and a needs assessment should be done on the faculty members who would be participating in computer-related learning activities. Then specific objectives could be developed to meet their needs and interests. Initially, such objectives should relate to the interests of the learners identified in the needs assessment. As the learners became more familiar with the specific area of their interest, they could begin to develop objectives for further computer-related learning. These objectives might relate to technical aspects of computing, patient care applications and others, depending upon the group.

In order to achieve the educational goals of the curriculum, various types of learning activities would have to be utilised. These would fall into three areas related specifically to the use of computers in nursing: personal development, specialisation and continued learning skills. The personal development of the learner would be achieved through: 1) values clarification, assessment and development, 2) specific discussion and reading about computer applications in nursing and 3) use of such applications.

Specialisation would be encouraged through independent study projects, specific readings, small group discussions, panel discussions and others. The use of various means of instruction would encourage in-depth exploration of areas of particular interest to individual educators. The fact that the learners would be self-directed adults makes activities to support specialisation especially important.

The third area toward which learning experiences should be directed is that of continued learning skills. These activities would involve the "hand-on" use of a terminal, computer-assisted instructions, program packages and computerized information retrieval systems. This would provide the faculty members with computer-related skills necessary for their continued learning.

When faculty members have developed a degree of computer literacy, they will be able to make decisions with respect of what computer-related content should be integrated into the nursing curriculum, at what levels, and how it should be organized. Until faculty have this knowledge, it is probable that most nursing curricula will not include computer concepts as they relate to nursing. If the education of faculty and students about the use of computers in nursing does not become a priority in the near future, nursing applications will be developed by computer and health care specialists outside of the nursing profession. Then, neither nurses nor patients will realise the full benefits that computerization can bring.

REFERENCES

1. Barnett, G.O., and Greenes, R.A., Interface aspects of a hospital information system, Annals of the New York Academy of Sciences. 161 (1969) 756.
2. Anderson, J., Gremy, F. and Pages, J.C. (eds.), Education in informatics of health personnel (Americal Elsevier, New York, 1974) 34.
3. Ibid., 29-34.
4. Ibid., 47.
5. Ibid., 30.
6. Rubin, L., The inservice education of teachers: trends, processes and prescriptions (Allyn and Bacon, Boston, 1978) 125-6.
7. Lindemann, E., The meaning of adult education (New Republic, New York, 1926) 8.
8. Knowles, M.S., The modern practice of adult education (Follett, Chicago, 1980).
9. Startsman, T.S. and Robinson, R.E., The attitudes of medical and paramedical personnel toward computers, Computers and Biomedical Research. 5 (1972) 218-227.

The Impact of Computers on Nursing
M. Scholes, Y. Bryant and B. Barber (eds.)
Elsevier Science Publishers B.V. (North-Holland)
© IFIP-IMIA, 1983

10.3.

NURSE EDUCATION AND COMPUTERS: TIME FOR CHANGE

Ron Hoy

Time for Change

The aim of this paper can be said to be two fold. Firstly, to give some information to those who do not have any technical knowledge about some of the considerations that must be dealt with before purchasing a machine. Secondly, the paper mentions the change emphasised in nurse education in the UK suggesting that the computer by virtue of its versatility will support and accelerate that change. It could be that the final result will be a new concept in nurse education based on mixed ability grouping, thus changing the traditional nurse tutor/learner role. The case is made for the inclusion of computer studies in the basic nurse training programme.

As an introduction to this paper it is pertinent to briefly touch upon the development of the micro-processor from the old style computer, as it is this development which has produced, and still is producing dramatic industrial, sociological and educational change. Such change being seen by G. Hubbard (1978) during his speech at the 12th annual conference of the Association for Programmed Learning and Educational Technology as a second industrial revolution. Indeed, there is much evidence to support this claim. The watch-making industry, for example, traditionally based in Switzerland, has now moved to Japan as more and more watches and clocks become electronic. This revolution will continue making the usual aspirations of school leavers obsolete as more and more mechanical processes are carried out by computer controlled machines. One effect of this could be to make the more social careers, such as nursing, more attractive to the young of the future. In the current economic crisis this switch in career emphasis can be detected, and therefore be used as a "model".

One of the earliest computers produced was the Pegasus, manufactured by Ferranti Ltd., approximately 25 years ago. It cost £50,000 to install, filled an area about the size of a large sitting room, weighed over 2 tonnes and produced an excessive amount of heat necessitating the use of expensive and complicated air conditioning systems. Like other computers of its type it required 3 hours servicing per day, with a 90% maximum possibility that it would continue to work for the remainder of that day. The same capacity can be obtained today with a machine about the size of a typewriter and costing in the region of £300. (It can be argued that cost comparisons are not valid when the change in the value of money is considered). This came about by the development of micro-circuit technology in the 1960's, whereby electronic circuits were placed on a piece of monocrystallins silicon (the so called "chip") by a process developed from photolithography and micro-photography. One electronic circuit being called a gate. In the 1960's it was possible to place 50 gates on a piece of silicon but by the mid '70's this figure had risen to 1,000 and it is estimated that it will soon be possible to have one million gates on one piece of silicon. The following graphs illustrate this.

Graph illustrating the number of gates per square millimetre of silicon chip, slotted against time.

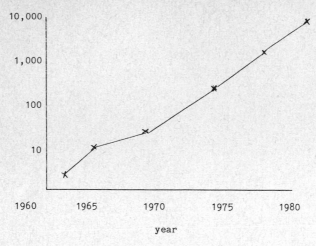

year

If the number of gates per silicon chip be plotted over time then the following obtains.

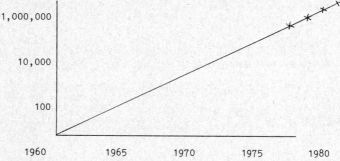

Operating times have shown the same astonishing changes. Modern gates now operate at a speed of about 10 nanoseconds. (A nanosecond being one thousandth of a millionth of a second). Some experimental gates have operated at speeds measured in fractions of a nanosecond. As circuits became faster, and more gates could be placed on a piece of silicon, costs began to fall. In 1960 one gate cost about £50, but by the 1970's one gate cost one twentieth of one penny, hence the cheapness of the modern micro-processors, bringing them within the price range not only of schools but individuals, so much so, that these machines have become part of everyday life being incorporated into cameras, watches, and toys etc. Quite a number of the latter are, in reality, simple teaching machines. This fact was recognised in 1980/1 when the Department of Education and Science allocated £19 million "to encourage secondary schools and colleges to prepare children for the electronic age"(Venner 1980).

This poses the question, of why should this affect nursing and hence nurse education and training? Industry has proved the advantages that can be gained by the use of computers that has resulted in efficiency savings. Industry has shown that some tasks can be carried out automatically under computer control, indeed, the Council for Educational Technology sees computers taking over "those functions of the human brain which operate in industry as a programmable control device". Nursing is a labour intensive industry, and therefore very expensive to run. It follows that the more nursing time used in nursing, and the more effective the nursing can be, the more cost effective is the service. Nursing has a massive information storage and retrieval problem upon which nursing care, to a large extent depends. It also has programmable control problems, as in intensive care units. It is also now possible to use computers to solve such problems as fluid replacement volumes. All this means, it is suggested, that time previously spent in retrieving information can now be reduced, and very sophisticated control systems can be used for the benefit of both the nurse and the patient. Within the field of general education computers are having their effect which is leading to the building up of a level or expertise, a level which is learning the full potential of the use of computers in education. If nurse education is to have any credence at all with the general public, and, indeed with educationalists, then, that too, must move with the times, and look to the use of the computer in the education of its learners. However, given that there is a lack of experience with computers in nurse education, the experiences gained in general education will be used as the theoretical base in this paper.

Concept of Curriculum

The concept of curriculum is now new, but as Lawton(7) points out in the past curriculum was usually taken to mean the same as content, a consideration still confusing some writers. The modern approach to curriculum stresses the total learning experience, whether that experience is gained in the school or not. "Learning which is planned and guided by the teacher"(16,7). This statement infers a different teacher/learner relationship than that regarded as the traditional one. This statement encourages a global view of teaching involving the teacher and the factors affecting that role plus all the influences acting upon the learner and the curriculum. The General Nursing Council in their policy documents would appear to be moving slowly towards this global view of education, but it must be recognised that there are certain constraints acting upon the nursing curriculum which will be discussed later.

R. Tyler (1949) suggested that four questions must be asked in connection with any curriculum:-

What educational purposes should be attained?
How can these be achieved?
How can these purposes be effectively organised?
How can we determine that these purposes have been effectively achieved?

Many models of curriculum have been suggested since Tyler published his work, but the four essential parts of the curriculum as set by Tyler still stand and therfore will be used in this paper, where necessary, but not in any order.

Resources

However well organised any curriculum is, it cannot operate unless the resources are available. The resource that this paper is concerned with is the computer, and therefore it is thought to be worth while to spend a little time considering some points that have to be borne in mind before purchasing a computer.

Technical brochures, and indeed salesman, make a lot of the central processing unit, but for all practical purposes, it is not really of importance to the operator provided that the machine does what it is intended to do. Rather more important is the ability of the machine to accept additions such as peripherals

and the like. The term interface is often used in this context. An interface
can be considered to be a plug or socket or cable (or indeed all three). It
should be clearly defined on any machine purchased. The CCITT V24 standard is
well accepted and defines very carefully the plug and socket connections. This
standard is also referred to as the EIA RS232/C. Most terminals offer the V24
standard connection.

Memory

Read Only Memory (ROM)
If the basic software must be loaded into the computer before use, then the
machine does not have ROM. This form of memory is widely used for programs that
form part of the operating system and is fixed during manufacture.

Random Access Memory (REM)
The first question to be asked is :- How much is needed?
The storage capacity of a computer is measured in "bytes", and one "byte" can be
considered to be one character, that is, one letter, one number or one space.
The standard unit of measurement being the K byte. (K = 1024). A machine
having a memory of 8K bytes will store 8,192 characters. As a general rule, all
the memory available will be used, so it will be advisable to go for the machine
with a greater memory than that actually necessary.

Programs

These are simply the instructions that tell the computer what to do, they are
written in code to which is given the name language. There are three main
languages:-

    Machine Code
    Assembler
    High level language.

For teaching purposes the high level language is used. It is so called because
it approximates to normal English. Examples of this form of language are:-

    BASIC   The Beginners All Purpose Symbolic Instructional Code.
    COBOL   Common Business Orientated Language.
    FORTRAN   Formula Translation.

Although BASIC is a very common language found to be used on most of the more
easily obtainable micro-processors, there are one or two difficulties that
should be borne in mind. No two BASICs are completely alike and can vary in :-

    Number handling
    Format of output
    File systems.

The complexity of the programs is also limited by the language.

Display

The display unit may vary from a television set connected to the computer, or it
can form part of the machine. When deciding about a computer to be used for
teaching, big is beautiful! Big means that the unit should be able to display
at least 24 lines of 80 characters. Also for teaching purposes a "graphic"
capability is necessary.

Printers

If the machine to be purchased used the CCITT V24 or EIA RS 232C interface, then any printer can be attached. Some machines have a printer incorporated into them. The advantage of a printer is that a record can be kept of the programs.

Storage

For most purposes the choice lies between cassettes or floppy discs. Cassettes load at something between 50 to 300 bytes per second. This is slow. Floppy discs operate at a much greater speeds, they have more storage capacity and therefore allow better use of the system.

It is a relatively simple exercise to buy a computer system, but the most important element must be the human one. Such question as :-

Is the computer acceptable to staff?
Who will, if anybody, control it's use?
Who will write the programs?
Who will allocate computer time in a school of nursing?

It is not possible, it is argued, to purchase any computer system unplanned and to use it with success. Any system requires a supportive organization and accommodation, which must be agreed within any given situation. Perhaps the most pressing difficulty that confronts nurse education in the United Kingdom is the lack of programming expertise amongst nurse teachers. It is possible to buy in this expertise but in that case a chance may have to be taken that the program is what is needed to suite local conditions. The use of a tutor with some interest in computing to write programs becomes a recipe for disaster. The programmer must be full time and trained.

The next resource problem to be solved is that of the number of machines needed. It has been found in the field of general education that for a group of 20 to 30 students at least 3 terminals are required in order to ensure that each student obtains the maximum computer time and hence benefit. The choice then becomes that between a number of separate machines, or a multi-terminal system. The resources requirement therefore can be summed up as follows:-

The need for tutors to be trained in computer use and programming.
Space for a computer laboratory.
Supportive organizational provision.
A number of machines.

The Computer and Teaching

The above pre-supposes a heavy financial investment, but the question remains, is it all worth it? Is there a need for such a machine? Is the computer nothing more than just a sophisticated teaching machine? (We all know what a short life those machines had). What effect can a computer be expected to have, if any, on teaching method and content?. The present system of nurse training in the United Kingdom is very clearly prescribed by the General Nursing Council, and, within a given school of nursing the standard of intake remains stable and prescribed. Does this system pre-suppose that:-

All nurse learners are expected to learn at the same rate?
All nurse learners learn in the same way?

Experience in the field of general education has proved that, with children up to 0 and A level standard these suppositions are not correct. A number of parallels can be drawn between these children and nurse learners in that they are both undergoing prescribed courses of training leading to national examinations. Work carried out at Banbury, the so called Banbury Experiment has shown that there is no difference in examination marks and academic achievement between those students taught in the traditional way and those students taught using Mixed Ability Grouping. Mixed Ability Grouping allowing the students to explore aspects of the subject matter under consideration in their own way and at their own pace. The computer, as an educational tool has a number of advantages claimed for it which include "individualisation of the learning process" which allows the learner to explore as set out above. Musgrave (1972) makes the point that those being educated do not need only to learn the given subject matter, but need to explore their world and themselves, the school providing the means whereby the possibilities of the world and the young can be tried out in safety. If this statement is slightly altered to read :- the possibilities of the nursing profession and the young nurse learner, then it can be argued that the concept of education as distinct from training becomes a reality for the nurse. This argument takes us into the realms of objectives a little. Nursing is a skill based profession and so it can be said to correct to make the objectives of any course behavioural. The question, however, must be asked :- Is a behaviouristic approach to the curriculum too limited and too limiting. Could not the flexibility that the computer brings place a greater emphasis upon "general curiosity" and a "pleasure in learning"(10). A move in fact to the expressive ojectives of Eisner?(15) The horizons of nursing are expanding at an unprecedented rate under the influence of the explosion of medical technology and the development of research in nursing requiring the broadening of the knowledge base demanded before the nurse can intelligently practice the skills of nursing. Has the computer the ability to assist in this broadening process. Consider the potential applications of computers as teaching aids in schools of nursing.

Simulation and Models

Simulations could be based upon scientific considerations (Osmosis for example), sociological, medical or pharmacological situations whilst the modelling could illustrate systems, procedures experiments or events (such as a surgical operation).

Reference Source

This is self explanatory. From a nursing viewpoint the possibilities are vast. The Data Base (for that is what, in reality is being suggested) could include :-

> Physiological norms.
> Anatomical data.
> Pathological data.

In fairness, it must be stated that building the Data Base will be a long task.

Problem Solving

Given the advent of the so called Nursing Process, which is a nursing system designing to pinpoint the patients difficulties, the use of a problem as a teaching tool would appear to be an obvious step.

The computer has the advantage of being able to :-

a)   Set the problem to be solved.
b)   Give immediate feedback to the nurse as she selects the course of action designed to deal with the problem.
c)   Give the cumulative effect, from time to time, of the nurses actions.

d)   The computer can be programmed to place the nurse under time constraints
      within which the action must be taken, thus adding realism to the
      exercise.

Demonstration

Concepts, principles and techniques can be illustrated or displayed. However it
must be argued that "doing" is a better way of learning than watching. The use
of the demonstration mode can be supported with procedures that are "private".
Also given that the computer can be programmed to be interactive with the
learner, demonstration becomes more than just passive looking.

Consolidation

Practise exercises, revision testing can be programmed relatively easily. The
advantages to the learners are :-

a)   feed back (pass or fail) is immediate and can be corrected immediately.
b)   failure does not, or need not involve another person (the tutor) as usual
      marking does.
c)   given an interactive program, the learner will be able to explore, at her
      own rate the reason for failure should it occur.

The above, it can be stated, highlights the difference between computers and the
old teaching machines, and shows the versatility that can be claimed for
computers. It also shows that if these computers are to be used there must be a
change of lesson method. Didactic teaching will not use the computer to it's
full potential. Will content be altered as a result of the computer? Consider
the development of computer systems that are directly related to patient care
and are used on the wards. These are gaining ground quite rapidly, and must
affect the educational content, if the school is to adequately prepare the
learner nurse for practise. Consideration will have to be given to including
the use of computers in the syllabus designed to prepare nurses for their
professional role, but this subject must be backed up with some knowledge of the
computer as a machine, if only to obviate the danger of a disc being wiped clean
in error. However, the humanistic approach to patient care must be emphasised
at all times.

Computers, no matter how sophisticated they become will never be able to replace
the human, the tutor, but given the potential that they offer they can greatly
increase the scope of the tutor and therein lies their major value. The use of
computers in schools of nursing must increase if nurse education is to retain
credence in the eyes of the young for the following reasons; firstly the
youngsters entering schools of nursing will have had experience of computers in
school and will therefore expect to find them in schools of nursing and secondly
various reports speak of the need for schools of nursing to liase with colleges
and universities both of which use computers regularly. Experience is growing
with the use of the Prestell and Ceefax systems which are likley to develop into
distance learning systems, so that computerized learning will be available to
all in their homes. The Open University has shown how successful distance
learning can be. Although computers in nurse education will result in a major
change in the curriculum unless they are embraced by the profession then it
could be argued that the profession will not progress educationally as fast as
it can.

REFERENCES

1. Atherton R. 1978 A computer for schools, Micro-electronics in Education pp 35 - 36
2. Brook D. & Rose P. 1978 Educational Technology in a Changing World
3. Ennals R. 1979 Historical Simulation, Practical Computing July 1979
4. Gosling W. 1979 Microcircuits Society and Education, Council for Educational Technology
5. Hennessey A, & Croft G, 1980 Carefully through a Minefield, Times Educational Supplement 7.3.1980, pp 33 - 35
6. Houghton V. 1979 How will we cope with the micro-chip? Education 18.5.1979. pp 580 - 581
7. Lawton D. 1978 Social Change. Educational Theory & Curriculum Planning, Hodder & Stoughton
8. Mee G. & Wiltshire H.1978 Structure & Performance in Adult Education, Longman
9. Roger J. 1977 Adult Learning Open University Press
10. Sledge D. 1979, Micro-computers in Education, Council for Educational Technology
11. Rahmlow H. 1978 Opportunities & Pitfalls in Computer Based Education networks, Educational Technology in a Changing World pp 317 - 322
12. Turnbull J. 1979 Computer Programmes for schools, Micro-electronics in Education pp 54 - 56
13. Venning P. 1979, The Race to train the Brains of the future, Micro-electronics in Education pp 59 - 67
14. Wright N. 1977, Progress in Education Croom Helm
15. Eisner E. W. 1967, Educational Objectives - Help or Hindrance, The School Review 1975 pp 250-260
16. Kerr J., 1968 Changing the Curriculum, University of London Press

The Impact Of Computers on Nursing
M. Scholes, Y. Bryant and B. Barber (eds.)
Elsevier Science Publishers B.V. (North-Holland)
© IFIP-IMIA, 1983

10.4.

TRAINING NURSES IN COMPUTING IN THE UNITED KINGDOM

Brian Hambleton

Introduction

It has been argued that education, like good wine, is wasted on the young - they have not got the head for it - but this is certainly not the case when it comes to computers. Young people certainly do have both the knowledge and the aptitude, coupled with an increasing emphasis on computing in our mainstream educational system, to deal with the complexities of this form of technology. The Government's programme is aimed at ensuring that every school in Britain has at least one microcomputer and for today's school children computers are becoming as much a part of the classroom furniture as desks or wall charts.

Those of us who have been in the profession for a number of years have not had the advantage of this basic familiarity with computers and have had to make the greatest effort to adopt and adapt to these technological innovations which are essentially a phenomena of the last quarter of a century.

Before embarking upon an examination of the training of nurses in computing in the United Kingdom it is perhaps valuable to consider first the question - why do we need to train nurses in computing at all? In 'Computers in Nursing', Zielstorff(1) identified 3 reasons why nurses needed to be trained in computing. They are:

a)   that computers are a valuable resource for nursing in terms of improving patient care,
b)   that computers serve as a catalyst about positive changes in the practice and profession of nursing, and
c)   that if nurses do not take a strong position in shaping automated systems that have an impact on their work, then these systems will be moulded by others who will design them to solve the problems as they perceive them.

The central theme of this paper attempts to examine three features of the training of nurses in computing in the United Kingdom, as follows:

a)   what training has been provided in the past,
b)   what training is provided at present, and
c)   what training should be provided in the future.

Past Training

In considering what training has been provided in the past the unwary might easily be lead to answer - NONE. Clearly if we examine the syllabus of any of our statutory training schemes we will find that there is a complete absence of any mention of the use of computers. Equally if we study the syllabus of any of our advanced clinical courses we will also be aware of this absence.

Management training faired only slightly better and in many instances there was still a shortage of any real grounding in the appreciation and use of computers. A survey of all English Regions and Wales which the author conducted in 1981 revealed an extremely variable picture. Of the 15 situations only about half indicated that computer appreciation featured in any way in their foundation or middle management development programmes. The situation in Scotland is also characterised by sparcity of provision although a recent survey of all senior managers including nurses, conducted by the Common Services Agency, indicated that there would be considerable interest in a computer appreciation programme. Northern Ireland also demonstrates this lack of provision with only one example being available of a local technical college responding to a request to set up training in computing for Health Service Staff. The Senior Management Development Programme, held in the five National Education Centres in England, featured and used computers rather more but still the picture was variable and a real degree of emphasis on the potential of computing was lacking in many programmes.

Nurses have gained their knowledge of computing in a spasmodic and largely unco-ordinated manner. Some through attending 'ad hoc' appreciation courses, some through the further education sector, and some through sitting next to that widely popular and much travelled lady 'Nelly'. Their motives were certainly varied, from the need to challenge the data on the computer printout of the payroll system, to the desire to become a systems analyst or to understand the workings of that funny square box in ICU. What has been lacking is an overall realization that this is a very real training need within nursing at various levels in the hierachy.

Present Training

Turning now to what training is provided at present, we see evidence of a slightly improving picture. Firstly there has been a clear realization that there is an unequivocal training need within nursing in the appreciation and use of computers. The National Staff Committee for Nurses and Midwives has been considering this issue over the past two years and the outcome of its work to date has been to adopt a two pronged approach to the problem having accepted the training need, and become aware of the extremely variable nature of the training provision. The first part of the approach has been to develop and provide, from central resources, a programme of short courses in computing open to all chief and district nursing officers in England and Wales. To date some 45 have attended these courses and three further events are scheduled for later this year. These courses have two essential themes firstly that they are related to the role of those who attend, and secondly, they provide for some 'hands-on' experience.   The principal objectives of the programme are to update participant's knowledge and awareness of the rapid developments which are taking place in computing and to consider their relevance and application in the management of the nursing function. The computer training needs of directors of nursing service and directors of nurse education have also been recognised and a centrally organised programme is about to be launched to help meet these needs. The format and nature of these events is still subject to consultation but it is likely that some attention might well be afforded to an examination of the benefits which directors of nurse education might derive from using computer assisted learning in their schools. This has considerable potential in the United Kingdom if we are persuaded by arguments that computer-based education is intended to supplement rather than supplant the teacher, and the use of a computer to present instructional information makes more effective use of both teacher and student time(I3).

The second part of the approach has been to develop advice on computer training in the senior and middle management development programmes. This advice, in both cases, hinges on the fact that 'Computers are becoming a universal component of health service activity handling many of the NHS information systems and an understanding of them, and access to them, is vital for the data analysis and presentation that is an integral part of NHS management and planning. In respect of both patient and staff orientated systems nurses are heavily involved in the collection of the basic information and it is important that they also have access to this data and know how it might be used to its greatest effect(2). In respect of the senior management development programmes pressure has mounted for an increased emphasis on computer appreciation and use within these events. The centres mounting these programmes have responded favourably to this pressure.

With regard to the advice to the National Health Service on computer training for those holding middle management posts, or what will be their equivalent in the re-structured service, a booklet containing rather more detailed recommendations is about to be published and distributed by the National Staff Committee for Nurses and Midwives. These recommendations provide advice on the content of courses which should be aimed at equiping nurses with:

a)   a basic understanding of computing concepts and language,
b)   a broad grasp of systems analysis and design,
c)   knowledge of the current variety of computing systems, and
d)   'hands-on' experience preferably with a health service system.

The training should provide insights into computing for nurse managers through an introduction to:

a)   hardware components
b)   terminals
c)   software
d)   programming and languages.

In looking at basic systems analysis and design the principles of data capture, validation, storage and destruction need to be covered. In addition the essentials of system implementation, maintenance and failure need to be examined. Important features such as user involvement and confidentiality are also signifcant.

Both Health Service systems and nursing applications should be demonstrated whilst recognising the need to translate the principles of computing into a reality which can readily be appreciated by nurses. This can be reinforced by some 'hands-on' experience using health service systems in general and nursing systems in particular. It is vital that a direct line of relevance is drawn between the principles of computing and the nurse's role for the training to be of lasting value.

Future Training Requirements

Firstly we need to accept that many, if not all, nurses coming into basic nurse training will be familiar, at least, with the principles of a computer and will recognise some of its features. Their training needs will be initially in the area of data capture and input skills which need to be linked very firmly to patient care and nursing activities. This must be recognised and incorporated into statutory training schemes and covered both in the classroom and the ward.

This knowledge is extended and deepened during post basic clinical courses in order that the skilled clinical practitioner has maximum information to make judgements about the condition of patients and choose appropriate nursing interventions(3).

Continuing education or in-service training programmes reflect the need to provide nurses with knowledge and skills to take account of rapidly changing technology. The computer has the potential to be an extremely useful tool for the organization of education in nursing both for Computer Assisted Learning and Data Management(I25).

The author would like to see identified nurse managers and educators with a Visual Display facility which allows them to interrogate programmes which contain information on the training records of all their nurses, both individual and collective. Even more important and valuable would be to have their identified and unmet training needs displayed in this manner. This facility would also contain information on specific courses which are available, their suitability, cost, and the number of nurses under that particular manager's control or field of influence who are awaiting places.

Through our management development programmes, service and education managers need to be equipped with what might be termed a computer perspective. In addition to knowledge about the fundamentals of the technology more important is an awareness of its limitations and capabilities. What is needed is the ability, backed up by knowledge, to ask salient and strategic questions in respect of computer technology.

a)   Is this particular proposal and equipment the most appropriate and cost effective in meeting our needs?
b)   What impact will it have on the organisation as a whole in addition to my particular service?
c)   What current and future applications can it handle and how long will it be before it is obsolete?

These are just some of the strategic questions with which future leaders of the nursing profession will have to grapple, both as functional heads, and members of corporate management teams. A few nurses will wish to become systems analysts especially in respect of nursing applications, and they will need encouragement and opportunity to acquire the skills which will enable them to make a significant contribution to the range of nursing programmes.

We have skated fairly quickly over three areas, what training has been provided in the past, is currently being provided and should be in the future. Current training programmes are quite costly and are likely to be even more costly in the future. The profession therefore has to decide upon the most effective approach. This revolves around the decision as to whether computer training should be integrated into existing training programmes or provided at specific intervals when the need and numbers arise; integration versus encapsulation. Whichever approach is adapted, and the author suspects it will be a combination of both, it is important first, that the training should meet the identified need and second, that it should relate to the role and functions of those attending.

The future seems likely to lead to an increased use of computer systems within the NHS in general, and in nursing in particular both in hospital and community. For nurse managers to have direct access to these systems is of prime importance. In many instances nurse managers will control their own systems having acquired mini and micro computers for the nursing service. It is important that these are used optimally and effectively and training can help ensure that this does in fact happen and that the quality of management decisions in nursing is enhanced by a more effective capture, input and use of information.

REFERENCES

1. Zielstorff R. D. Computers in Nursing, Nursing Resources, Wakefield. Mass 1980.
2. Computer Training for Nurses in Middle Management Posts. Pub. by the National Staff Committee for Nurses and Midwives England 1982 - DHSS.
3. Grier M. R. The need for Data in Making Nursing Decisions.
    (Nursing Information Systems, Werley and Grier, Springer Publishing Co.)

The Impact Of Computers on Nursing
M. Scholes, Y. Bryant and B. Barber (eds.)
Elsevier Science Publishers B.V. (North-Holland)
© IFIP-IMIA, 1983

10.5.

SOLUTION TO A DILEMMA: COMPUTER TECHNOLOGY FACILITATES NON-TRADITIONAL, POST-BASIC NURSING EDUCATION

Joan Cobin and Judith Lewis

The American Nurses' Association (ANA), an organization with over 181,000 members, is considered the professional organization for registered nurses in the United States of America. The ANA is responsible for promoting the professional and educational advancement of nurses. Toward this end, the ANA adopted an educational standard for entry to professional nursing practice, the baccalaureate of science in nursing (BSN). In an effort to meet this standard and help prepare nurses for their expanded role, nurse educators at the baccalaureate level responded by enlarging their facilities, hiring more faculty and expanding the curriculum. While these changes benefitted the programs new graduates, the practitioner already in the work force was at a disadvantage. These nurses recognized the value of earning a baccalaureate and were willing to do all that was possible toward this end, even though work and family responsibilities remained. Although efforts were made by educators and nurses alike, the working nurse still encountered multiple difficulties entering and continuing in a traditional campus baccalaureate program.

The dilemma created by the adoption of the baccalaureate as basic preparation for professional practice is a challenge to all nurse educators. Despite the ANA standard, the majority of nurses do not have a baccalaureate degree. Nursing education programs leading to registered (RN) licensure do exist in a variety of educational institutions that offer a variety of credentials. The profession has the choice of postponing the implementation of the BSN as the educational standard for entry into practice or finding ways to modify the existing system of nursing education. These two choices are self-evident: the situation can continue indefinitely with erratic periods of discussion regarding career options or a bold step forward may be taken.

Postponement, however, will be counterproductive to the goal of enhancing the quality of health care through the improved utilization of nursing knowledge and skills. The choice is clear. It is a time for action rather than rhetoric. Since mechanisms exist to systematically plan for a future nursing work force balanced with personnel prepared at appropriate educational levels, the challenge to educators is to create quality educational mobility programs which will motivate nurses to prepare themselves educationally to practice in a rapidly evolving health care system that utilizes an expanded nursing role.

The decision by the American Nurses' Association to adopt the BSN as the educational standard for professional practice has a lengthy historical background. The process was chronicled by the ANA Commission on Nursing Education in its report to the delegates of the 1982 biennial convention. The report reviewed actions taken since 1960 when the organization first agreed to "promote the baccalaureate program so that in due course it becomes the educational foundation for professional nursing". The 1982 House of Delegates was asked to vote on the motion "that the ANA move forward in the coming biennium to expedite recognition of the baccalaureate in nursing as the educational qualification for the practitioner in professional nursing practice"(1).

That nursing education belongs in institutions of higher education rather than in hospitals has been espoused in every significant study of American nursing. The National Commission for the Study of Nursing and Nursing Education in its published report, Abstract for Action, however, went beyond its mandate and made recommendations for a systematic changeover. It included national, state and local planning mechanisms for both closing and opening education programs as appropriate to the recommendation. Paramount to the successful change to high education were educational mobility opportunities for practicing nurses(2). The W.K. Kellogg Foundation, which was the primary source of support for the National Commission for the Study of Nursing and Nursing Education and which later funded the longitudinal study Towards an Unambiguous Profession(3) as a follow-up to Abstract for Action(4), has emerged as the major benefactor of the present-day quality educational mobility programs that exist across the country. The landmark-funded projects include: Sonoma State University Second Step Program(5); The Orange County/Long Beach Nursing Consortium(6); and the Southern Regional Board, Pathways to Practice(7). The first two projects demonstrated articulated approaches to educational mobility. Students in these programs are able to transfer credit earned in their basic nursing education program to the university. The third project demonstrated the relationship between education and practice levels. Most recently the Kellogg Foundation has funded the Statewide Nursing Program of the California State University Consortium. This program, like the others, is designed to meet the educational and practice needs of the employed, registered nurse who wants to earn a baccalaureate in nursing.

The California State University Consortium, one of twenty degree-granting entities in the State University system, was developed to provide an educational opportunity to students throughout the State who for various reasons could not be accommodated at a local campus. The Consortium, using the resources of the nineteen traditional campuses, has the capacity to deliver non-traditional instruction for a wide range of academic disciplines. The Statewide Nursing Program which is one of these programs evolved from the need to accommodate a significant portion of the 200,000 licensed nurses registered in the State who wish to earn a BSN in an articulated educational mobility program of study. The admission requirements are: an RN license and sufficient transferable academic credits to achieve upper division standing. Graduation requirements include: an acceptable grade point average; the demonstration of the knowledge and skill of a liberally-educated person and the attainment of required, professional-level nursing knowledge and performance skills. The program was conceived by nurse educators within the California State University system who recognised the need for a non-traditional educational program to expeditiously advance the goal of the profession for BSN-level preparation. The program was designed to articulate academically with hospital-based (diploma) or community college (ADN) nursing education programs. The curriculum and its unique delivery method evolved with the context of the following societal conditions:

1. Studies have demonstrated that the retention of nurses in the work force is negatively influenced by the lack of control nurses have over their practice(8).
2. Retention is further aggravated by the ambiguity which exists as a result of the present multiple routes to licensure and entry to practice(9).
3. Evidence exists that supports the need for multiple levels of practice in many employment settings (clinical ladder)(10,11).
4. Studies are emerging that indicate the quality of patient care improves when BSN-prepared professional nurses are accountable for the full scope of nursing practice(12).
5. The limited access for RN's into existing BSN programs is a barrier to achieving the goal of organized nursing and a frustration to the career-oriented nurse(13).
6. Articulated educational programs have been shown to be a realistic mechanism for educational and therefore career mobility(14, 15).

7.   Educational programs for nurses beyond licensure require the application of adult learner principles to their design and implementation(16).
8.   Standardized written and performance assessment mechanisms exist for nursing practice at the ADN and BSN levels(17).

The California State University, Statewise Nursing Program is designed for the RN whose lifestyle, employment status or geographic location and/or enrollment limitations are barriers to enrollment in existing on-campus baccalaureate degree nursing programs. Since students are mature individuals with a variety of life experiences and responsibilities, the program is strongly based on adult learning principles. Although adult learners are individuals, certain common characteristics are present that influence the learning process(18,19,20).

The adult learner has been described as

1)   goal directed,
2)   persistent,
3)   highly motivated,
4)   geared to success,
5)   committed to family, work and/or other responsibilities,
6)   limited in time allocated to educational activity,
7)   best able to meet education goals using their individualized learning style, and
8)   learning best when there is direct application of theoretical concepts and skills to the work situation.

With these characteristics in mind, the educator's role changes from that of omnipotent professor to that of facilitator who promotes learning in a climate of mutual respect. The Statewide Nursing Program curriculum reflects the problem-solving approach, the use of peers as consultants, experimental learning activities and opportunity for the learner to set learning goals and be self-directed.

The nurse who enrolls in the Statewide Nursing Program is offered three options to earn academic credit and to meet graduation requirements:

1)   the assessment of nursing knowledge and skill obtained from a variety of sources through written and performance tests;
2)   non-traditional course work; or
3)   a combination of testing and instruction.

Upon enrollment in the program, students are assigned a mentor who assists them in selecting the option best suited to their individual learning style, work experience and career goals, and counsels and guides them throughout their enrollment in the program. Student and mentor are paired for the entire education experience leading to graduation and acquisition of the baccalaureate degree.

The assessment option includes tests developed by the faculty of the New York Regents External Degree Nursing Program of the University of the State of New York for their own BSN candidates. The written tests are offered regularly through the American College Testing Program (ACT). The performance tests can be taken at the Western Performance Assessment Center in Long Beach, California (WPAC). The tests were developed under rigorous conditions with faculty control of the content and the construction of all test items. They are periodically updated and normed on a national sample of students enrolled in BS nursing programs(21). The instructional option consists of 53 one-unit learning modules. Nineteen of these are the pre-requisite support courses and thirty-four are nursing. Enrollees in this program are typically RN's who are associate degree graduates with 70 academic credits. A total of 132 credits is required for graduation from the Statewide Nursing Program. Instruction for all of the pre-requisite and integrated nursing courses is available at either the nurses's employment setting or at a nearby hospital or learning center and features a combination of student/faculty interactions, state-of-the-art technology, study group activities and preceptored clinical experiences.

When the Statewide Nursing Program first developed, it was anticipated that audio tapes, video tapes and accompanying workbooks would be the main mode of instruction, much as the acclaimed British Open University employs. A proposal for funding, based on this concept, was submitted to the W.K. Kellogg Foundation. The interim between proposal, submission and actual funding was a time of change. Technology was evolving to a high degree, computers were becoming more reasonable in price, a greater variety of software was available, and authoring of programs became less complex. More importantly, research indicated that although more expensive initially, computer-based instruction is cost effective in the long term and, most important of all, permits the learner to master the material at an individualized pace(22).

During this interim period a decision was made that modified some aspects of the original concept, while leaving the over-all goal intact. The goal of the Statewide Nursing Program is to greatly increase the number of BSN-prepared nurses. Movement toward this goal is influenced by these constraints:

1.   the curriculum had to be of high quality,
2.   the delivery system had to accommodate large numbers of nurses at a variety of sites,
3.   the program had to be accessible to nurses who wanted to remain in the work force,
4.   the course content had to be current and be kept current,
5.   the financial impact had to be kept to a minimum, and
6.   the components of the entire system had to meet the needs of the adult learner.

In addition, 53 learning modules had to be developed to meet the following standards:

1.   cost effectiveness,
2.   maximal use of faculty resources,
3.   easily and inexpensively updated,
4.   adaptable to evolving technology,
5.   ergonomically designed, and
6.   deliverable to a dispersed population.

The available facts made the choice clear: the logical way, the creative way to move toward the established goals was through the use of computer technology for curriculum design and delivery. This decision became a working reality when the W.K. Kellogg Foundation funded the program for $2.2 million, to be used primarily for the technological mediation of the learning modules.

Once the decision was made to use computer technology, a myriad of options had to be explored and choices made. The program required a computer that was capable of delivering computer-assisted instruction, providing learning management, was highly interactive, could be used for statewide record-keeping and communications and programmable to deliver complex concepts in the psychomotor and affective learning domains as well as the cognitive domain. In addition, the Statewide Nursing Program explored the use of interactive video instruction. This medium had not previously been used for delivering/developing nursing curriculum content. A pilot program was undertaken and the results were so satisfying that another grant proposal was written to secure funding for development of interactive video programs. A great deal of time was spent with a variety of vendors, and characteristics of their machines, costs, authoring possibilities, etc. were systemically compared. In the final analysis, no one computer was capable of providing all the functions required for this unique educational program.

A microprocessor, such as the APPLE II Plus, will be used primarily for interactive video. This type of computer, in conjunction with a video monitor and a video player provides an extremely pro-active learning environment. An interactive video program dramatizes key learning objectives which the student views on the video monitor. Expert commentary is provided to highlight salient aspects of the video tape. At intervals the microprocessor screen provides computer-generated questions, comments and responses that require the student to take an active role in the learning situation. The interactive portion of the program provides various forms of feedback depending on the student's response. Individualized remediation, as well as support through additional resources can be easily provided. The video-taped information can be retrieved through computer-generated commands, or in a more traditional linear fashion, when used in conventional television programming. Video disks will be used in the future to provide even more rapid retrieval of video information.

At this point in time, the Statewide Nursing Program chose not to be involved in purchasing communications satellite capabilities, though a computer with communication linkages throughout the State was needed. Also desired was a means of tracking student progress and keeping records of the many students involved in the program. This type of specialized computer services was available through an on-line, central computer system called PLATO, which was first developed at the University of Illinois. PLATO has a number of functions, but three specialized capabilities are particularly applicable to nursing content: simulative problem solving; animation and a touch-sensitive screen(23). Although simulations are complex to design and costly to produce, they offer a creative approach to learning through problem solving.

Each module will be presented using learning modalities appropriate to the content and learning objectives. Most often a module will consist of a workbook which is accompanied by an interactive video program and computer-assisted instruction. Other experimental activities are designed exclusively for that particular module and technological support is used where appropriate. To help decide content and format for each module, the design team relies on a systems analysis approach. This process guides the development of each module and is known as the Statewide Nursing Systems Development Review. The process begins with the creation of courseware blueprints which detail course objectives, content outlines, learning activities, learning resources and evaluation procedures. An instructional designer heads a production task force which consists of subject matter experts and computer programmers. The skills of the other members of the development team such as the media co-ordinator, the graphic artist, the word processing specialist and the instructional television staff are shared by all of the various task forces. Because there is up and down time on all productions, task forces work on several modules simultaneously. To provide a more timeless quality, content is presented as concepts; problem solving and judgment skills are emphasized. Subject matter experts are sought nationwide to provide the broadest view on a given topic. The original program is designed to easily allow up-dating; currency is of primary import in such a dynamic profession. This unique state-of-the-art approach to curriculum design is one challenge that must be met in order to increase accessibility to baccalaureate education for registered nurses.

Another challenge became evident in planning the Statewide Nursing Program: how is it possible to deliver a complex curriculum to a dispersed population of adults, using computer-assisted instruction and yet provide highly personalized human interaction? It quickly became apparent that creative energies had to go in two directions at once. Not just toward the development of an innovative, high-technology curriculum, but also toward the design and implementation of an avant-garde delivery system that is humanized and highly personalized for students.

Program delivery is administered on a regional basis through regional directors, instructors, mentors and preceptors. The director of each region is a member of the nursing faculty at one of the California State University campuses. Each regional director is responsible for delivering the program in a specified area. Regional directors have released time which is used to administer the Statewide Nursing Program, and their specific responsibilities include the identification, preparation and evaluation of instructors and mentors, as well as the initiation of student populations and follow-up counselling. Instructors are most often California State University Master's - prepared faculty who contract to teach one or more one-unit modules. The instructors agree to use only those course outlines and learning materials designated by the Statewide Nursing Program. The Program prefers to hire instructors who have a special interest in the non-traditional learner and the concept of baccalaureate education for registered nurses. While each instructor uses predeveloped course and support materials, each is encouraged to contribute his or her own teaching style, bringing a special empathy, warmth and humanity to enrich each student's learning experience and provide a more personalized touch to the learning environment. Instructors are familiar with the various aspects of the program and are able to help students with academic as well as procedural or administrative questions that might arise. In this role, instructors serve as a student-advisement resource as well as a representative for the entire program.

The mentor role carries significant importance in the Statewide Nursing Program. Each student is assigned a mentor who advises students on the various aspects of the program and who assists students in the selection of those credit options best suited to meet a student's individual learning style, work experience and career goals. In the past, external degree programs were not as successful as they might have been, due primarily to the lack of a continuing relationship with an advisor. The Statewide Nursing Program mentor provides the student with the continuing human relationship needed to maintain momentum and interest in the curriculum and to deal with individual problems that may occur. In short, the mentor is a stabilizing presence that provides constancy whether the student is taking courses with others or studying alone in preparation for an assessment examination.

The laboratory component of the program is supervised by an instructor who uses preceptors to help personalize the experimental aspects of the clinical course. Preceptors are nurses who have been selected to work with students because of their professional expertise in the practice areas. Each student develops a learning contract in consultation with his or her preceptor and instructor. Although the students are required to meet course objectives, the preparatory experiences can be highly individualized to meet student needs.

Although students have access to the libraries of their local California State University campus, a need exists to provide additional resources for participants in the program. Thus, Learning Resource Centers (LRC) were established in hospitals and other agencies that desire a great amount of participation in the program, and which are committed to bringing baccalaureate nursing education to their community. Each LRC provides a professional library as well as the audio-visual and computer hardware necessary to deliver a compentency-based curriculum. Specialized hardware includes television cameras, monitors, on-line computers, micro-processors and interactive video equipment. Each sponsoring agency assists in the purchase and maintenance of the hardware. Each Learning Resource Center is managed by an on-site co-ordinator who is assisted by a secretary. Some hospitals augment this staffing with volunteers. Staff members at the Learning Resource Center orient students to unfamiliar machinery and provide necessary assistance along the way. In addition, the on-site co-ordinator is a Master's prepared nurse who is also available to assist with student learning needs or questions about the program.

Software that is identified and/or produced by the Instructional Development Team is distributed to all of the Learning Resource Centers, and programs are readily available for student use. A future projection is that home computers will become quite common, students will be able to check out a software program to use on their home equipment.

By using this type of staffing, the human element is maintained even during high technology delivery of courseware. It could be said that the entire delivery system is designed to be ergonomic - friendly staff, user-friendly hardware.

The truths that have already emerged from years of adapting technology to learning in other disciplines are being incorporated in the evaluation/research methodology that will guide the growth of the Statewide Nursing Program, even though the scope of the Statewide Nursing Program is much broader than that of previous endeavours. The Program staff is proceeding with the knowledge that:

1)   machines do not replace faculty in technology-based learning modes - rather, they enhance faculty creativity and showcase the professor's unique interpretation of knowledge;

2)   the technology exists to simulate any experience for learning purposes, but there is a limit to the amount of fiscal and human resources an agency can or should commit to its development;

3)   finding financial resources and purchasing hardware is relatively easy compared with producing quality software that is appropriate for the money or has lasting value.

With the advent of learning technology, there is a solution to the dilemma facing the nursing profession as a whole, and nurse educators in particular. Given the potential success of the Statewide Nursing Program, quality baccalaureate nursing education can be easily accessible to registered nurses who wish to remain in the work force.

The Statewide Nursing Program has, since its inception, enrolled a significant number of students, all of them actively engaged in the profession and actively pursuing a baccalaureate degree. These students are progressing through the program at their own pace, some through assessment of previously acquired knowledge, some through non-traditional instruction, some through a combination of both of these modalities. Whatever their method for earning academic credit, these students are acquiring advanced knowledge and skills synonymous with those of students attending a traditional campus-based program. Because of commitment to the nursing profession and to high educational standards, California State University nursing leaders initiated the Statewide Nursing Program - a bold step forward.

References

1.   Commission on Nursing Education. "Education for Professional Nursing Practice", The American Nurse, May 1982.

2.   National Commission for the Study of Nursing and Nursing Education.   An
      Abstract for Action. New York: McGraw-Hill Book Co., 1970.
3.   Lysaught, Jerome P.   Action in Affirmatiion: Toward an Unambiguous
      Profession of Nursing. New York: McGraw-Hill Book Co., 1981.
4.   National Commission for the Study of Nursing and Nursing Education, 1970.
5.   Searight, Mary, Ed.   The Second Step - Baccalaureate Education for
      Registered Nurses. Philadelphia: F. A. Davis, 1976.
6.   Lysaught, Jerome P. You Can Get There From Here: The Orange County/Long
      Beach Experiment in Improved Patterns of Nursing Education. Battle Creek,
      Michigan: W. K. Kellogg Foundation, 1979.
7.   Haase, Patricia.   Types of RN Programs, Pathways to Practice, No. 2.
      Atlanta: Southern Regional Education Board, 1974.
8.   Wandelt, Mabel A., Patricia M. Pierce and Robert R Widdowson. "Why Nurses
      Leave Nursing and What Can Be Done About It".   American Journal of
      Nursing, January 1981.
9.   National Commission on Nursing.   Initial Report and Preliminary
      Recommendations.   Chicago, Illinois: The Hospital Research and
      Educational Trust, 1981.
10.   Haase, Patricia. A Proposed System for Nursing: Theoretical Framework,
      Part2, Pathways to Practice, No. 4. Atlanta: Southern Regional Education
      Board, 1976.
11.   Congress for Nursing Practice.   Nursing: A Social Policy Statement.
      American Nurses Association, 1981.
12.   National Commission on Nursing, 1981.
13.   National Commission for the Study of Nursing and Nursing Education, 1970.
14.   Searight, 1976.
15.   Cobin, Joan, Bonnie Bullough and Wilma Traber. "A Five-Level Articulated
      Program", Nursing Outlook, May 1976.
16.   Ibid.
17.   Lenburg, Carrie B. Open Learning and Career Mobility in Nursing.
      St. Louis: C. V. Mosby Co., 1975.
18.   Knowles, Malcolm S.   The Adult Learner: A Neglected Species. Houston,
      Texas: Gulf Publishing Company, 1973.
19.   Tarnow, Karen Gahan. "Working With Adult Learners", Nurse Educator, Vol.
      4, No. 5, Sept.-Oct. 1979. (pp.34-40).
20.   Knox, A. B. Adult Development and Learning. San Francisco: Jassey-Bass,
      1977.
21.   Lenburg, Carrrie B. "Emphasis on Evaluating Outcomes: The New York
      Regents External Degree Program", Peabody Journal of Education, Vol. 56,
      No. 3, 1979.
22.   Thompson, Wayne W.   Computer Based Education Is a Viable Adjunct to
      Traditional Instruction as Shown by Cost Benefit Analysis.   Unpublished
      Master's Thesis, California State University, Long Beach, 1981.
23.   de Tornyay, Rheba and Martha A. Thompson,   Strategies for Teaching
      Nursing. New York: John Wiley & Sons, 1982.

The Impact Of Computers on Nursing
M. Scholes, Y. Bryant and B. Barber (eds.)
Elsevier Science Publishers B.V. (North-Holland)
© IFIP-IMIA, 1983

10.6.

IMPLICATION FOR NURSING EDUCATION

Discussion

Role Change

The traditional role and activities of nursing educators will be affected by the introduction of computers for instructional purposes. This will occur both in the teaching and administrative areas of nursing education. First, educators will need to be involved in activities related to designing, planning and developing computer-assisted instructional materials. Second, educators will, of necessity, be challenged to develop a more facilitative relationship with learners. Thus, computer-based instruction can be expected to lead to several changes in the existing patterns of the teaching of clinical nursing practice. Several specific examples of some of the role changes may be drawn by inference from Joan Cobin's paper describing the California State University Degree Program and the materials being developed for self-directed learning. The programme has clear and significant potential for various countries.

Nursing education's administrative areas are also being affected by computer technology. Use of the computer for education's administrative purposes inclusive of planning, scheduling, and monitoring of manpower was well documented in several papers. It is evident that professional nursing educators need to become increasingly familiar with the potential for computer use in both areas.

Computer Literacy

Knowledge about and understanding of human responses to computer technology comprise essential information for the nurse educators. The level of understanding must be commensurate with an educational programme's goals and objectives for both curricular planning and curricular emplolymentation purposes. Computer technology awareness was seen as necessary to the curriculum.

Varied levels of computer literacy are necessary for faculty, administrators, and students. For example, at an introductory level for all, there is a need for knowledge about the technology and its capability of serving as an effective tool, to assist nurse education in fulfilling their specific roles. More advanced computer literacy is required when nurse educators and administrators begin to develop select or specify computer requirements for computer-based systems and materials. At this level it is essential to be sufficiently familiar with computer technology to communicate with such specialists as systems analysts/designers, programmers and computer salesmen. Without this familiarity nurse educators are severely limited in evaluating the suitability of programs, of understanding program development, and essential program documentation. This could severely reduce their capacity for making reasonable judgements and decisions.

Differing views were expressed as to how far and how many nurse educators should become competent programmers and systems analysts. However, final agreement was reached that methods for increasing nursing educators' computer awareness with continual updating opportunities must be incorporated as essential continuing education.

Computer Implementation Factors

Using computers requires flexible and creative approaches to the use of financial technological, and human resources. Joint appointments and faculty secondments are but two examples of creative resource management. Curricular planning and scheduling which takes into account time, site, distance and learning flexibility are other examples. In both instructional and administrative settings, clear and deliberate analyses must be undertaken using information from a variety of multidisciplinary sources. This can be crucial in making reasoned decisions.

Management of Change

Two additional phenomena need to be addressed: change theory and the need for research on a variety of topics including the changes accompanying introduction and use of technology and ergonomics.

Computer induced change can occur with such speed that it challenges the capability of organisations and individuals to cope with their environment. Because of inadequate research into these changes and insufficient documentation of new systems, little information sharing is occurring. Therefore, an urgent need exists: 1) to record the body of developing knowledge; and 2) to foster an understanding of, and creative approaches to using change theory.

CHAPTER 11

COMPUTER ASSISTED LEARNING

This section of the book seeks to encapsulate an examination of the development of computer assisted nursing education. The issues raised, and explored, include financial considerations, hardware and software protocols and specific applications such as the PLATO system.

Although much of this work originates in the United States, the potential is beginning to be realised elsewhere. The papers therefore serve as a source of reference for nurse educators and systems analysts in those countries wishing to embark upon this exciting development.

The Impact of Computers on Nursing
M. Scholes, Y. Bryant and B. Barber (eds.)
Elsevier Science Publishers B.V. (North-Holland)
© IFIP-IMIA, 1983

11.1.

COMPUTER ASSISTED LEARNING IN NURSING EDUCATION: A MACROSCOPIC ANALYSIS

Kathryn J. Hannah

Introduction

The use of technology in education has become extensive in the last decade. There are many reasons for this generalized phenomenon. The tremendous growth in human knowledge and the resulting increase in the amount of information to be learned is well documented and widely recognized. Educators have become much more sophisticated in identifying the learning styles of students with diverse abilities and rates of learning. The financial retrenchment in post-secondary institutions is international and has resulted in a need to maximize effective use of both human and financial resources. Advances in technology and mass production have resulted in hardware, including video playback machines and microcomputers, which is affordable by not only educational institutions but also by individual students.

In addition to the preceding general factors, there have been changes in the nature of nursing practice and in the location and type of preparation for the practice of nursing. In North America, the current trend in nursing education is to replace the earlier apprenticeship programs which trained nurses who were orientated to providing service only to patients in hospitals. The education of nurses has largely been moved to academic programs in colleges and universities. This trend is primarily a reflection of changes in the health care delivery system which now requires that nurses be capable of providing care in a highly diverse range of settings. At one extreme of this diversity lies the highly technical and largely physical nursing care required by individuals in acute care areas such as intensive care or coronary care units. At the other extreme is the more abstract and predominantly psychosocial nursing care provided to families in communities, for example family counselling, health maintenance or health promotion. Finch(18) cites two significant trends:

(a)   that the professional nurse practitioner is presumed to have greater skills in independent decision making, and

(b)   that nursing students are more critical of the quality of their education. These students are demanding help to develop skills which will continue to be useful to them when "facts" learned in school are superseded by new knowledge. The combination of the preceding general and specific factors has resulted in the need to individualize instruction in nursing education programs.

Conceptual Framework

Educational technology is a useful means of responding to the preceding changes in education generally and nursing education specifically. According to Slaughter(16), educational technology is useful in introducing new contents into, and eliminating old and obsolete contents from, the curriculum; in recording, analyzing and evaluating a particular learner's progress toward a particular objective, and in meeting society's demand for more relevant education. Educational technology permits students to be provided with course content in the medium which best accommodates their individual learning style. This might involve active or passive use of print, auditory, visual and/or kinetic stimuli. Examples of teaching strategies using educational technology either alone or in varying combinations include: programmed instruction, self paced learning modules, mechanized libraries, television, video and/or audio cassette recordings, film and/or slide-tape presentations, computer assisted learning. The latter strategy, computer assisted learning, is one of the more profound contributions of technology to education. According to Bishop(1), the fact that computers offer a technology by which, for the first time, instruction can be geared to the specific abilities, achievements and progress of individual students makes computers a potentially important, perhaps revolutionary tool. The wide range of material that can be presented by the computer, combined with a high degree of control of experimental conditions and ease of varying the course presentation, provide unusual opportunities for creating individualized instructional programs.

Unfortunately, the multiformity in the terminology used is confusing to the neophyte in the field of computer applications to education. The term Computer Assisted Instruction (CAI) has been in existence for some time. Hicks and Hunka (7) refer to CAI as that which covers a great variety of educational needs, including teaching and learning activities through the aid of digital computers. Margolin and Misch(13) define CAI as any of a wide range of educational techniques that rely on a computer to assist in the presentation of learning material. It helps to evaluate a given student's progress, and presents lessons in appropriately ordered small steps. According to Muller(15), CAI offers in its range; problem probing, simulation, information retrieval, testing, research, guidance and counselling. Bunderson(2) views CAI as a compound resulting, primarily, from a union of programmed instruction and use of time-shared, interactive computer systems. The Committee on Technology and Instruction, American Association of School Administrators regards CAI as programed learning; employing the computer's ability to store information, present questions to the learner, receive the learner's response and evaluate the pupil's responses.

In addition to the problem of authors using one term to describe different activities in the use of computers in education, Conklin(I7) points out the problem of authors using different terms to describe the same activity. According to Conklin(I7), in the literature the following terms are used interchangeably:

        Computer aided instruction
        Computer based instruction
        Computer assisted education
        Computer simulated instruction
        Computer based education
        Automated teaching
        Computerized instruction
        Computer controlled teaching device.

The conceptual framework adapted for use in this paper is one which seems to be widely accepted. Computer Assisted Learning or CAL refers to any of a wide range of educational techniques that rely on a computer to facilitate learning. CAL, is sub-divided into two related but distinct functions: Computer Assisted Instruction or CAI, and Computer Managed Instruction or CMI. Computer Assisted Instruction occurs when the teaching function of communicating new information to a learner is performed by a computer system without interaction between the student and a human instructor. Both the content material and the instructional logic are stored in the computer memory. Computer Managed Instruction, refers to an overall system for educational management in which detailed student records, complete curriculum data, and information on available learning resources are stored in the computer and integrated to develop unique programs of instruction for individual students and to facilitate optimal educational resource management.

Computer Managed Instruction

CMI carries out the educational function of monitoring a student's progress, diagnosing learning needs and then prescribing learning materials. The prescribed resource material may reside in reference books or articles, teachers, laboratories, discussion groups, or even a CAI lesson. The computer can be programmed to store test items and randomly generate unique but equivalent test forms for each student in addition to accepting, scoring and analyzing students' answers on the tests. Successful students are directed to the next unit of learning material. Students who do not demonstrate appropriate levels of achievement are directed by the computer program, according to a predetermined decision matrix, to remedial material and assignments prior to re-testing. Obviously, effective use of CMI requires establishment by the teacher - author of mastery levels for student achievement. Often this mastery requires that all test questions be answered correctly before the student earns credit for that particular instructional unit and is allowed to proceed to the next unit.

The record keeping capabilities of the computer have the potential to enhance both the rate at which research on instruction and learning can be conducted, and the accuracy of the findings. Overlaps, gaps and deficiencies in the curriculum can be identified and remedied. Similarly, strengths in the curriculum can be retained.

Finally, CMI involves the ability of the computer to facilitate complex scheduling of large numbers of students. Programmed to store class lists and time schedules, the computer can schedule instructor-student conferences, group sessions, and use of learning resources. A print-out of the computer-generated schedule can be sent to personnel in the library and learning resource centre and to faculty. This allows for efficient use of media, materials, facilities and time.

Although in nursing, computer-managed instruction finds its greatest application in the nursing faculties on academic campuses, it is branching into other nursing education settings. The expanding use of Continuing Education Units (CEU) as requirements for licensure increases the need to maintain and quickly retrieve an individual's records. It does not require large leaps in logic to imagine a scenario in which the evaluation of learning (i.e. testing) is required before CEU credit is awarded. Similarly, development of sophisticated quality assurance programs conceivably could require that health care institutions maintain records which document personnel attendance at inservice programmes and their achievement of specified learning objectives. In this latter situation, one can envision hospital accreditation requiring information which is most efficiently maintained by using a CMI system.

Computer Assisted Instruction

1.   Strategies used in Programming Nursing CAI

Meadows(H3) presents a comprehensive summary and evaluation of the range of teaching strategies used in nursing CAI. The most simplistic CAI strategy is the Page Turner program. This involves the display of information in textual or graphic form at the terminal. While it does not require user input and therefore does not involve any interaction between the user and the computer, it is effective for providing information quickly such as on a hospital information system or as supplement to other CAI teaching strategies. Used alone it is not considered an effective strategy.

Drill and Practice programs put users through repetitive drill of previously learned materials. They therefore provide reinforcement of acquired concepts, permit practice, and allow the student to gain familiarity and competence with the material. The true Drill and Practice format merely indicates to the student the accuracy or inaccuracy of responses. However, authors often incorporate into the practice sequence the opportunity for users to try the same problem two or three times with some hints and clues in response to incorrect input by the student.

The Tutorial approach involves the presentation of new material to the student. To accomplish learning, information is presented in small steps or frames and then the student is required to input information to demonstrate understanding of the concept. Depending on a student's response to a program request for input in the Tutorial lesson, the program branches to either appropriate remedial material for a wrong answer, or to positive reinforcement for a correct answer. If the response is incorrect the learner is guided by additional prompts, hints or cues to an understanding of the concept. The program's author must anticipate all possible wrong responses so that appropriate branching occurs. The Tutorial mode is similar to programmed instruction texts with the difference being that CAI requires a more active learner participation and relieves the student of the responsibility of locating the appropriate following frame.

Simultation presents the student with a "real life" situation on the computer. The CAI simulation has been found to provide an equivalent to clinical experience in facilitating the development of decision making skills within the safety of the learning laboratory. The student can identify the nursing problem of a simulated patient, make and implement a decision regarding nursing intervention, and observe the effect of her intervention. In this manner the student can identify errors in her judgement prior to clinical participation in patient care. Gaming is similar to simulation except that it usually does not represent a real life situation and there is an element of winning or losing against the computer.

Inquiry and Discovery are similar and authors appear to use the two interchangeably. These strategies are usually used within a simulation. The student requests the preprogrammed information she needs in order to solve the problem given. The student is allowed to choose any approach to a problem, but is subtly guided by the lesson program to form the best conclusions.

The most sophisticated use of the computer in CAI is the Dialogue method. The students ask questions of the computer in natural language and the computer program responds, thereby guiding students toward a logical conclusion on the basis of answers provided by the computer program to questions asked by the students. As in other CAI techniques, the author must anticipate all possible student inputs. Dialogue is therefore a very difficult type of lesson to write and must go through extensive and time consuming testing before it is ready for use.

2.   Content of Nursing CAI

Articles in the literature by nursing educators using CAI have frequently focused on reporting the content and strategies which their CAI lessons utilize. CAI has been developed by nursing educators in many content areas. Those reported in the literature include:

> Psychiatric nursing (Kamp & Burnside,I16)
> Midwifery (Naber, I22)
> Epidemiology (Donabedian, 4)
> Immobility (Hannah, I11)
> Maternity nursing (Kirchhoff & Holzemer, I17)
> Pharmacology (Kirchhoff & Holzemer, I17)
> Post-operative nursing care (Collart, I6)
> Kirkchhoff & Holzemer, I17; Conklin, 3)
> Decision making (Taylor, 17)
> Psychomotor Skills (Larson, 12).

In addition, references to nursing lessons are included in two major surveys (Kamp, 10; Wang, 18) of CAI available for use in academic programmes educating health professionals. Unfortunately it is difficult to determine the quantity of nursing CAI available. Despite the preceeding reports in the literature and in surveys, much of the information related to nursing CAI has not been formally or widely published. Simply tallying the number of lessons or programs available rather than the courseware hours underestimates the actual amount of teaching material. Conklin(3) states that larger, more complex and comprehensive CAI packages are being developed but still reported in surveys as single programs. Similarly, it is difficult to estimate the quality of available nursing CAI because there are as yet no formal mechanism for peer review publication, and distribution for lesson programs. Fortunately, it appears that access to such mechanisms is imminent (Larson, 12).

3   Nursing Education Settings Using CAI

The literature reports the use of CAI throughout virtually all facets of nursing education. Its use in basic nursing education at both the diploma and baccalaureate levels is widely reported (Bitzer & Boudreaux,(I3); Bitzer & Bitzer,(I2); Collart,(I6); Hannah,(I11); Larson,(11); Conklin,(3); Morin,(14). Several authors report use of CAI in Master's level nursing programs (Kamp & Burnside,(I16); Nabor,(I22); Donabedian,(4); Huckabay et al.,(I15); Kadner, 9). Porter(I25) and Buckholz(I5) present the use of CAI in continuing education programs while Hoffer at al.(8) describe its use in inservice education. Hospital orientation programs (Reed et al. I26) and nursing refresher programs (Levine & Weiner, I20) using CAI have also been reported in the literature.

4.   Effectiveness of CAI

The literature reveals a paucity of empirical studies which document the effectiveness of CAI in nursing. Studies or learner achievement using CAI have been conducted in undergraduate nursing education (Bitzer & Boudreaux, I3; Hannah, I11; Kirchhoff & Holzemer, I17; Larson, 11; and Conklin, 3). These studies consistently conclude that CAI is at least as effective as other teaching strategies in effecting behavioural changes in students, i.e. learning.

The effectiveness of CAI in producing learner achievement of instructional objectives in inservice education of practicing nurses is less clearly established. Valish & Boyd(I31) produced inconclusive findings in their study of learning by graduate nurses at the George Washington University Medical Centre. However, Hoffer et al.(8) demonstrated significant learning achievement by graduate nurses using CAI in a community hospital setting. The difference in findings between these two studies appears to stem from the difference in research design and the control of variables.

Substantial reductions in the amount of student time spent at learning subject matter have been demonstrated in several studies of CAI (Bitzer & Bourdreaux, I3; Hannah, I11; Conklin, 3; Larson, 11). Similarly, when CAI was compared with traditional strategies, Larson(11) found significant cost-benefit in favour of

CAI. These findings regarding the effectiveness of nursing CAI with respect to learner achievement, time savings, and cost-benefit are consistent with findings in the health professions collectively (Halverson & Bollinger, 6) and with findings in general education (Hallworth & Brebner, 5). Obviously, this meagre number of studies cannot be regarded as conclusive evidence. However, this consensus among findings from a variety of disciplines lends support to the generalization that CAI is at least as effective as other means of teaching.

Advantages and Limitations of Computer Assisted Learning

Conklin(17) identifies the following advantages of computer assisted learning in nursing education:

i.   CAL lends itself favourably to the independent study approach to learning.
ii.   CAI can facilitate student development of more creative and more flexible approaches to problem solving.
iii. CAL lends continuity of instruction to situations in which there is a shortage or rapid turnover of nursing educators.
iv.   CAI provides more effective use of instructional time and permits instructors to devote more time to individual help and to focus on teaching the psychosocial aspects of nursing. The computer easily and quickly accomplishes the tedious and time consuming tasks of testing, checking, grading and record keeping.
v.   CAI allows the student to learn more efficiently.
vi.   The program author can update a computer lesson as new nursing knowledge is identified, or as evaluative feedback from the student-learner becomes available.
vii. CAI offers excellent motivational properties due to immediate feedback provided to students.
viii. CAI is compatible with multi-media, multi-sensory approaches to learning. A learning laboratory that incorporates CAI with many other educational media represents an enriched and dynamic learning environment.
ix.   The computer is consistent, patient, fair, tolerant and approving of each and every student.

However, a note of caution is imperative. The foregoing discussion is based on a limited number of studies all of which would benefit from replication. In addition, limitations which emerge from detailed study of CAL in nursing education include:

i.   Cost Factors

The initial time investment in developing good CAI material is extensive. Perhaps 120-150 hours are required to author one hour of effective, terminal tested CAI lessons. Once instructors become more adept at CAI strategies, the time required is reduced; however extensive analyses of cost-benefit and detailed studies of the cost figures for the development and operation of nursing CAI programs are unavailable. Certainly, the cost of the hardware is decreasing consistently; however software development costs are not.

ii.   Content Control

Unless at least some nurse educators become knowledgeable in the area of CAI, there could be a tendency to abdicate to educational computer software firms the preparation of computer assisted learning for nursing. Decisions about nursing and nursing education could slip out of nursing hands. Nursing educators must monitor their own learning programs to ensure that decisions related to nursing remain in the hands of nursing content experts. Conversely, without a firm foundation, sophisticated computerized nursing curricula could emerge which could in fact become a patchwork coverage of course material.

iii.   Altered Professional Roles

Teachers who have felt secure in their role as dispensers of information may feel uncomfortable as they find their role changing to that of facilitators, moderators and coordinators.   In addition active involvement by members of faculties in computerized instruction requires that there exist a reward structure which places value on published instructional design efforts to the same extent that it values researches and other publication activities.

iv.   Technology Limitations

The lack of standardization of both computer hardware and nursing CAI lesson software complicates the sharing of CAI lessons among institutions.   Some programs are locked into a single computer language and hardware system.   The transporting of a CAI program from one software package to another may require more programming time than was required to produce the original.   This is a true impediment to wider applications of CAI in nursing.   For this reason there is probably a redundancy of CAI lessons among nursing users.   A standardized natural language authoring system is sorely needed.

The use of large central computer systems places the nurse user at the whim of the individual or group controlling the system (Hannah & Conklin, I13).   The autonomy and control provided by microcomputers appears to ameliorate this particular limitation.

v.   Deficits in the Theory of Learning

CAI is still just emerging as a learning strategy.   There is insufficient research assessing such factors as what type of person learns best by CAI, ergonomic variables active in CAI, or to compare how CAI and traditional teaching methods influence the speed, quality, retention and transfer of learning.

iv.   Lack of Formal Communication Among Users

In North America, the vast majority of information about CAL in nursing education is communicated among informal networks of nursing educators who meet at annual conferences such as the Symposium on Computer Applications in Medical Care, Association for the Development of Computer Based Instructional Systems, or the American Nurses' Association Council on Continuing Education.   One hopes that this forum on the Impact of Computers on Nursing will be the first of an ongoing series which will permit more formal and more extensive international exchange of information about the quality and quantity of available Nursing CAI.

REFERENCES

1.   Bishop, L. K. Individualizing Education Systems. New York, 1971
2.   Bunderson, C. V.   "The Computer and Instructional Design," in Holtzman, W.H. (editor), Computer Assisted Instruction. New York: Harper and Row, 1970.
3.   Conklin, Dorothy.   A Study of Computer-Assisted Instruction in Nursing Education. University of Calgary: Unpublished Masters Thesis, 1981.
4.   Donabedian, D. "Computer - taught epidemiology."   Nursing Outlook, 1976, 24 (12), 749-751.
5.   Hallworth, H. J. & Brebner, A. Computer assisted instruction in schools. Edmonton: Alberta Education, Planning and Research, 1980.
6.   Halverson, J. D. & Ballinger, M. D.   "Computer-assisted instruction in surgery."   Surgery, 1978, 80 (6), 633-640.

7.   Hicks, B. L., and Hunka, S. The Teacher and the Computer. Toronto:W. B. Saunders Company, 1972.

8.   Hoffer, E. P. "Computer-aided instruction in community hospital emergency departments: A pilot project." Journal of Medical Education, 1975, 50 (1), 84-86.

9.   Kadner 1982. "Change: Introducing CAI to a College of Nursing Faculty".Journal of Computer Based Instruction, 1982.

10. Kamp, M. Index to computerized teaching in the health sciences.San Francisco: University of California, 1975.

11. Larson, Donna E. The Use of Computer-Assisted Instruction to Teach Calculation and Regulation of Intravenous Flow Rates to Baccalaureate Nursing Students. University of Michigan: Unpublished Doctoral Dissertation, 1981a.

12. Larson, Donna E., Personal Communication, 1981b.

13. Margolin, J. B. and Misch, M. R. "An Introduction to Computer Assisted Instruction," in Margolin, J. B., and Misch M. R. (editors), Computers in the Classroom, An Interdisciplinary View of Trends and Alternatives. New York: Spartan Books, 1970.

14. Morin 1982 "A Comparative Study of Attitudes Toward Computer Assisted Instruction and Learning Styles of Nursing Students." Journal of Computer Based Instruction, 1982.

15. Muller, L. "Computers in the Classroom - Reports in Industry," in Margolin, J. B. and Misch M. R. (editors), Computers in the Classroom, An Interdisciplinary View of Trends and Alternatives. New York: Spartan Books, 1970.

16. Slaughter, R. E. "The Response of the Knowledge Industry to Society's Demand for a More Relevant Education," in Witt, P. W. (editor), Technology and the Curriculum. New York: Teachers College Press, 1967.

17. Taylor, A. "CAL - From research to practice: Computer simulations for nursing." Proceedings of the third Canadian Symposium on Instructional Technology, 1980.

18. Wang, A. C. (Ed.). Index to computer based learning (Vol. II) Milwaukee: Instructional Media Laboratory, University of Wisconsin, 1978.

The Impact of Computers on Nursing
M. Scholes, Y. Bryant and B. Barber (eds.)
Elsevier Science Publishers B.V. (North-Holland)
© IFIP-IMIA, 1983

11.2.

LEARNING NEEDS AND COMPUTERS

Mary Anne Sweeney

Introduction

Computers represent a vast change in our concept of time. The entire thrust of energy in the field is directed toward faster and more efficient ways of completing tasks. We spend a great deal of time wondering about and working on the innovations of tomorrow that will surely influence the ways in which students will learn to care for their patients. However, as educators, we need to pause for a few minutes to think about computers in relationship to the learning needs of nurses. Most of us are very conversant in the various approaches that can be taken to diagnose and treat learning needs. The purpose of this paper is to review some of the relevant points involved in the learning process when the content involves computer literacy.

The steps involved in the learning process have been set forth by a number of specialists educational theory. The following scheme has been proposed by Bloom, Madaus and Hastings(1) for teachers to utilize in enacting the instructional process:

Steps to Successful Learning

1. Identify an overall goal
2. Devise a general plan
3. Analyze a) the learner's needs
            b) the instructional process
            c) specific outcomes
4. Make instructional decisions
5. Devise a detailed plan
6. Prepare Instructional materials
7. Implement the program
8. Perform an evaluation.

The bulk of this paper will address the aspect of the third step that involves the analysis of the learner's needs.

One of the preliminary steps we need to undertake is to diagnose needs of individuals and groups of learners. Since the learner needs to be clearly identified in the initial phase, we can start by assessing personal learning needs. In this rapidly changing field, we need to be constantly developing short and long range goals for ourselves, and need to be consistently evaluating our progress in meeting them. We are all learners in this computer age. Goals will be truly individualized and may range anywhere from enrollment in a formal computer course to site visits to local health facilities for an opportunity to see varied computers in action.

When assessing learning needs of groups of nurses, it is well to remember that we have many distinct groups to work with such as: practicing nurses, nursing students, administrators and nurse educators. All of these groups have great intragroup variance, and yet they have common learner characteristics and needs that set them apart from the others. For instance, practicing nurses may need to acquire the knowledge and motor skills necessary to operate the terminal on their particular clinical unit while nursing administrators may need some knowledge of the process (without the motor skills), but may have a more pressing need for budgetary information about the same system. Ideally, all the learners should have access to classes offering a basic overview of computers and their impact on nursing. As Bloom, Madaus and Hastings (2) have pointed out, "Much evidence from research on learning demonstrates that parts are more easily grasped and remembered in relationship to each other rather than in isolation". Staff nurses (just as much as nursing students) need a framework in which to assimilate the new technological material. All groups of learners do not need exactly the same content, but a comprehensive overview of computer technology needs to be a part of each general educational plan. A needs assessment would be utilized to determine the detailed aspects of the educational plan so that programs could be tailored to specific needs.

The identification of learning needs is, of course, a complex task consisting of multiple levels of assessment. Three of the main areas of assesssment that need to be considered are the affective, psychomotor and cognitive needs of the learners.

Affective

Computers usually elicit a strong effective response in either a positive or negative direction. Very few nurses seem to be neutral toward them. Perhaps the best characterization of nurses' responses toward computers is to describe a general wariness or caution.

The educational process must first take steps to "demystify" the computer and its associated hardware and software. It usually works out best to present the classroom material with a great deal of positive commentary, a small amount of fanfare, and in a language that is as "jargon free" as possible. One can rarely be successful in "talking away" apprehensions and fears about machinery and its functions. Students need a positive encounter. If learning experiences on computers are worked out in advance to be as clear and as successful as possible, the nurse will develop a positive attitude toward the technology. This is an especially important point with nursing faculty members. It is extremely important to assist this group in the change over to technology since they have such an impact on the practice that is to come. Martellaro (3) categorizes educators into three categories: 1) those who want to keep computers out of schools because of their dehumanizing aspects, 2) those who believe computers have potential for the classroom but are a little more than frightened, and 3) enthusiasts who believe that computers are the new wave of the future and want to stock their classrooms with them right now.

Initial experiences with computers should be relatively brief (under one hour at any rate). People may learn better in this type of situation if they can be part of a small group to garner support and encouragement. Mixed age groups of learners may help since young learners may be more comfortable at first with the technology as they have been accustomed to learning from television for years(4). The author has not personally witnessed the strong negative attitude and abilities alluded to on the part of older people by some educators in the computer area. The affective response to computers often flows over to influence the other two learning domains so it is an important aspect in providing this type of learning experience.

Psychomotor

No learning exercise on computers is truly complete without a "hands-on" exercise in utilizing an actual machine. The learner must be provided with direction and supervision in this area. This aspect of a class or workshop often meets with the greatest amount of resistence. Scheduling and equipment difficulties should be worked out well in advance to permit the successful completion of this portion. The instructor needs to plan for a definite follow-up of this exercise to encourage further development of the manual skills and to check the accuracy and efficiency rate of nurses who are frequently using the machines in their everyday work. The motor exercise can truly be the most memorable aspect of a workshop or class, and can reinforce the adage that learning can be fun. Computers should be accessible outside of class time (with accurate and detailed instructions) with sufficient consultation and follow-up provided(5).

Cognitive

The key point in the delivery of theoretical material is that it should be as free from technical phrases and jargon as possible. The instructor must be carefully selected. The basic concepts surrounding the utilization of computer technology and its relationship to the health care field should be covered, but the depth of content should vary with the needs of the learners. In fact, one of the surfacing issues in this whole area in to define just what it is that nurses need to know about computers. We need to build a consensus on this area. It has often been found that the instruction of technical concepts works best if some of the examples are not related directly to nursing, but are of personal interest to the learners. This seems to help in developing a broader view toward the technology rather than a narrow picture constrained by the parameters of one's clinical specialty practice area.

The hardest lesson of all is that we will never know enough about computers in the near future, for the technology is constantly changing. Nurses need to continually modify and update their knowledge base as well as their skills. This often poses a problem for busy educators, but it is surely one that needs to be addressed. It sometimes seems that just when you get comfortable with using a computer either the equipment changes (farewell key punch machines) or the program is altered. We have to let nurses know that the exciting road to learning about computers has barely been travelled upon, and will be continually changing its appearance. The wise travellers will reach their destination with ease.

REFERENCES

1. Bloom, B., Madaus, G., and Hastings, T. Evaluation to improve learning. (McGraw Hill, New York, 1980).
2. Ibid.
3. Martellaro, H., Classroom computers and innovation theory - why don't they adopt us?, Creative Computing. 6 (September 1980) 104-105.
4. Lautsch, J., Computers and education: The genie is out of the bottle, T.H.E. Jouurnal. 8 (February 1981) 34-39.
5. Aiken, R., The golden rule and ten commandments of computer based education, T.H.E. Journal. 8 (March 1981) 39-41.

The Impact of Computers on Nursing
M. Scholes, Y. Bryant and B. Barber (eds.)
Elsevier Science Publishers B.V. (North-Holland)
© IFIP-IMIA, 1983

11.3.

MAKING THE MOST OF THE MICROCOMPUTER IN NURSING EDUCATION

Susan Mirin

Introduction

The microcomputer, with its special characteristics and capacities, is rapidly changing all aspects of our society, including the teaching/learning process. At this point in computing developments, nursing educators in both school and practice settings need to critically examine the current and potential educational uses of microcomputers as well as the issues related to software development. This paper examines the use, implications, and issues surrounding the microcomputer's interface with nursing education.

Imagine opening class discussion following a clinical experience devoted to drug administration with the following remark: "All of you charted the medication correctly, but 30 percent of you killed Mr Malone"(I24). Incredible? Not if the clinical experience was a **simulated** one in which students interacted with a microcomputer program!

The instructor speaking above was referring to her students' performance in a computer program assignment that simulated the experience of assessing and treating a patient admitted to the emergency room with a myocardial infarction. The entire experience, which allowed students to ask questions of the tireless computer "patient" (Where is the pain?) and receive responses (It feels like it's in my left chest...) took place in the nursing school library. Through this simulation the students explored the symptomology and treatment of myocardial infarction, including drug therapy, and entered the appropriate information on Mr Malone's "chart".

This simulation is just one example of how relatively low-cost microcomputers can be used in nursing education. The potential for using these personal computers to enhance educational experiences for everyone from preschoolers to post-doctoral candidates is vast; but because they were only introduced in 1972, many of the possible education applications for microcomputers have not yet been fully explored (I17). Currently, the educational literature offers more information on the computer's role in the elementary school then in higher education, and the nursing literature describes only a few instances of using computers in teaching (1,2,I2,I15,H8,I6,I25). The **potential** for using microcomputers in nursing education grows larger and clearer as mushrooming automation technology expands the capabilities of these small computers and as manufacturer's attempts to bring microprocessor prices down causes their cost to fall.

This paper provides nursing educators with background information on microcomputers, the possibilities for their effective use in higher education, and their specific potential for improving the education of nurses.

What is a Microcomputer and what can it do?

The microcomputer works much like a major computer system, but it is small. Its significance to educators lies in the combination of its substantial computer power, its relatively low cost ($600 - $10,000), and its mobility (carry it to class, to the learning laboratory, or home). Before the introduction of microcomputers, the cost and complications of implementing computer-assisted instruction (CAI) discouraged its use, although several large computer systems have been designed and implemented for educational purposes. For example, the University of Illinois PLATO system now has 1000 terminals located in schools and colleges in the USA and Canada (3). However, large computer systems require great commitment and resources from an entire school or university system and are difficult to engineer in today's resource scarce environment. With large computer systems, even the most optimistic estimates of the cost of CAI indicate that the present system of education is cheaper by a factor of ten (4).

Thus the relatively inexpensive microcomputer constitutes a major breakthrough in the use of computers in education. Nursing education faces the same demands as the rest of higher education in terms of the need to provide more education over a large portion of student life span, and more individualized instruction tailored to the specific preparation and motivation of a given student. Faculty, students, and the profession in general will benefit if nursing educators ride the crest of the wave in applying microcomputer technology to educational needs.

Basically, a microcomputer consists of a computer terminal similar in size and keyboard design to a typewriter. The keyboard prints numbers, letters, and some special symbols, allowing the user to communicate with the computer. Several systems also accept inputs from light pens or use a computer-controlled slide show to present graphic material. The computer is connected to a viewing screen such as an ordinary television set; some microcomputers have built-in screens. They can also be connected to a disk drive that translates information located on a diskette (like a 45 rpm record) into the computer. Instead of the disk drive, you can use a cassette recorder and tape cassettes for transferring information into the computer, but the recorder feeds the information in much more slowly that the disk drive. Printers and word processing equipment can also be connected to the microcomputer.

Computer Potential in Educaiton

The computer's ability to store, manipulate, and process information makes it useful for both educational administrative functions (such as record keeping) and to assist in the learning process (computer-assisted instruction) (5). This article focuses on the latter use.

With CAI, students can interact with the computer in three ways:

1) In drill and practice sessions which supplement the regular teaching process.
2) In a tutorial sense - as they would with a patient tutor - to understand a concept and develop skill using it. (For example, the student sits at the computer terminal, is given textual information to read, and is then asked questions by the computer. If he/she responds correctly the computer goes on to the next topic; if not, the computer provides the correct answer and a brief review of the subject matter.)
3) Through a simulation or dialogue in which a genuine two-way conversation between the student and the computer takes place (6). The opening illustration of the students' interaction with Mr Malone is an example of a simulation.

In reality, the student actually interacts with a CAI program (software) that is stored, monitored, and processed in the computer. Such programs are often based on a "branching" technique that moves the student to remedial or advanced work, thus fitting content to an individual student's needs. Programs that are not merely drill and practice are actually "self-teaching" systems with the computer providing the stimulation (7). Students using CAI in this sense find themselves in a give-and-take situation which they usually prefer to the passive lecture-listening one and which results in a more effective learning experience.

Granting that computer-based systems for rote learning are useful, it is very important for nursing educators to realize that the educational capabilities of computers go far beyond drill and practice, and in addition, that computer-based education is not synonymous with programmed instruction. Rather, computer-assisted instructions makes umprogrammed instruction or student-controlled learning possible by using teaching strategies that differ completely from the basic tutorial logic of most programmed instruction. For example, information may be stored in the machine in the form of simulated models of an actual system such as the human circulatory system, or, as in our opening example, the symptomology and treatment regimen for myocardial infarction. Through a set of instructions stored in the computer (algorithms), the computer is capable of calculating unique responses to different questions from students. "It is in this manner that the great computational power of a computer has been programmed to play chess with human opponents – to make appropriate moves in response to predicted behaviour"(8).

As nursing educators proceed to define the place of computers in nursing education, it is imperative that they realize that computer-assisted instruction is not merely useful for the transfer of information, but is valuable in developing critical thinking. Learning with computers has been found to be more effective than standard educational procedures in learning situations that call for judgement, interpretation of complex problems, and assessment by students of whether their solutions to problems are appropriate(9). For example, by using the computer to calculate, analyze, and display problems and possible solutions, students are relieved of some of the drudgery of problem-solving while ready visualization of options helps them to develop insight. Such use is really the "inquiry" mode of instruction, applauded for its value in developing critical thinking and intellectual comprehension. Again, the opening example illustrates such use – the student is asked to assess a patient's condition and carry out the patient's treatment. When he/she asks a question regarding the patient's condition, the computer responds with a report of the simulated patient's symptoms related to that question. If the question is not focused on a particular area of symptomology, the computer will ask him/her to make the questions more specific. (Such ability to focus questions specifically is an important skill for nurses carrying out physical assessment to learn.) As the student moves from assessment to treatment, the computer responds with a report of the expected effect of the proposed treatment on the simulated patient. Thus, carrying out such "inquiry" strategies via the computer helps students develop an investigative approach to problem-solving.

Some positive outcomes of computer-assisted instruction which Alpert and Bitzer cite and which particularly meet current needs in nursing education are:

1) Students can proceed at a pace determined by their own capacity and motiviation.
2) Provision of remedial instruction or tutorial assistance during regularly scheduled courses for students with insufficient preparation.
3) Reduction in the number of large lecture classes in favor of small instructional groups and seminars.
4) Updating skills of employee groups particularly affected by expanding technology.

5) Continuing education for professional personnel, permitting the updating of
    knowledge and skills in their own offices and on their own schedules (10).

Computer Use in the Nursing Education Curriculum

Many nursing curricula strongly stress the philosophy of self-paced and
competency-based learning.   According to del Bueno, "The most important
consideration is that we (nursing educators) treat adult learners as adults. We
must be responsive to their diversity of needs, past experiences, and goals
[11].

The preceding content on the general use of computers in education emphasized
the enormous potential of the computer for individualizing education.   These
capabilities meet the needs of nursing education in the following areas:

1.   Drill and practice:
Use of CAI may relieve nursing faculty of much of the responsibility for the
rote learning that must take place and be evaluated. For example, students must
demonstrate   a   certain   degree   of   mathematical   expertise   before   taking
pharmacology.   With CAI they are given the opportunity to skip the math module
based on demonstration of mastery on a pretest. If mastery is not demonstrated
they complete the designated computer program and takes the post-test. If the
student still doesn't demonstrate mastery, they receive a remedial computer
program, a study prescription, and a message to see a faculty member for
specific assistance. Such use of the computer eliminates the need to monitor
and grade mastery tests as well as providing students with increased assistance
and tutoring. If nursing faculty sorted out all the "rote-learning" curricular
objectives (and that could be done very efficiently by applying a computerized
data management system to the curriculum!) and developed CAI programs to achieve
them, they would have more time to spend with individual students, carrying out
more important human interaction elements of the teaching/learning process. In
addition, many of the pressing problems of the profession might be resolved if
its most highly education members, its educators, were able to delegate more
time to research and practice needs.

2.   Tutorial:
Computer programs of basically "tutorial" nature are those that offer primary
instruction in an area of knowledge and rely on coaching sequences to direct the
student to discovery of the correct answer.   At present, such information is
often presented via a classroom lecture. These computer programs are related in
theory to operant conditioning which employs reinforcement, shaping of
behaviours, and stimulus discrimination (12).   For example, Collart describes
how a CAI program on closed drainage systems of the chest was integrated into a
surgical nursing course for junior nursing students at Ohio State University
(I6).   The program was divided into six modules; first, a pretest review of the
anatomy, physiology, and physics of respiration; then four individual case
studies of patients with various respiratory conditions; and finally, a module
on the closed drainage systems available commercially. The following excerpts
show how the student interacts with the computer in such modules.

The completion question, for instance, demonstrates how the instructor must
anticipate every answer that a student might offer.

Computer: One must prevent clot occulsion of the drainage tubes by initiating
     the action of _____ the tubes every hour and prn.
     Complete this sentence.

Student: Stripping, milking, or squeezing.

Computer: Great, (learner's name), you have demonstrated the forethought of a safe practitioner (positive reinforcement).

OR

Student: Irrigated or flushed.

Computer: Oh, no! you have just given the patient a hydro-thorax! Never irrigate a chest tube! Please consider the consequences of your action and try again (corrective feedback).

This is a type of simulation that permits the student to experiment in a controlled setting and to determine the possible consequences of inaccurate intervention. If the student offers any answer not anticipated by the instructor or cannot answer the question at all, then the computer generates a series of pre-determined clues provided by the instructor to coach the learner to the correct answer. For instance:

Clue 1:   What action breaks up clots in the chest tube?

Clue 2:   Working one's fingers along the tube is called _____.

Clue 3   Don't give up! What is the act of relieving a cow of milk?

The computer will provide only the feedback that has been anticipated by the instructor and entered into the program. Obviously, this is an important element in CAI program construction.

Feedback can also be of an informative nature:

Computer: If the temperature remains constant, the pressure of a given gas varies inversely with the _____.

Student: Volume.

Computer: Good! You have just described Boyle's law. Select slide 2 for an illustration of this law.

Students may be branched to review questions as needed. The potential of the branching capability has barely begun to be realized.

Computer: Would you expect Mrs S (a chronic bronchiectasis patient with a lobectomy) to have a pneumothorax following her surgery? Yes or no?

Student: No.

Computer: A pneumothorax would be expected. Let's explore why. Is the intrapleural pressure greater or lesser than atmospheric?

Student: Lesser-

Computer: Right! Is it true or false that gases move from areas of greater to lesser pressure?

Student: True.

Computer: Right again! Can you now see how air rushes into Mrs S's chest when the surgeon makes the incision.

A ranking question enables the learner to evaluate her ability to place events in proper sequence. For example:

Computer: You are now ready to change Mr G's underwater seal bottle. Rank the following steps in order, one at a time:

    a) disconnect bottle from chest tube
    b) double-clamp chest tube
    c) prepare new seal bottle
    d) release clamps
    e) reconnect new system

Student: A.

Computer: Uh! Oh! That provides a route for air to re-enter the chest, doesn't it?

Student: C

Computer: That's better! What's your next step?

Study prescriptions can be integrated as necessary throughout a program. A final example demonstrates this point.

Computer: When suction is attached to the underwater seal bottle, what happens to the pressure inside the bottle?

Student: It builds.

Computer: No, just the opposite. Perhaps reference 2 in the course bibliography will help you better understand the physics of a vacuum. After reading this reference see your instructor to verify your understanding.

To develop optimum computerized tutorial instruction, the educator and programmer must predetermine the types of interaction that could occur and set conditions for certain feedback sequences. Two types of sequences must be specified: predictable conditions for all learners and possible conditions that depend on the data accumulated by individual students. Bundy envisioned "storing in the computer all the relevant data related to a given student, such as socioeconomic background, aptitudes, I.Q., interest profiles, vocabulary proficiency, motivation indices, and so on. The computer learning program then selects the appropriate learning sequence that best matches the entering behaviours of the student. Then, as the student works through the learning sequence, and responds actively to the materials presented, the computer "learns" more about the student and continuously modifies and improves its feedback(13)." That capability, only a vision in 1967, has now been achieved.

In addition to meeting individual students' needs, teaching via the tutorial computer program enables faculty to acquire a printout of each student's step-by-step progress, thus identifying students who need additional help in a specific area. Nursing educators can analyze their curricula to determine what objectives now met by presentation of factual content via lecture-demonstration (in which all learners must adopt the same pace and in which similar prior learning is assumed) or other methods, might be effectively met by the development of computer programs. Again, computerized data management of the entire curriculum plan will allow ease in sorting the curriculum components into appropriate teaching/learning strategies.

3.   Simulations and Gaming:

These teaching strategies enable the learner to experiment and review all the specific outcomes of an intervention.   This capability makes the computer particularly effective in health professions education because learners can experience decision-making and problem-solving situations that would be too awkward or dangerous for them to undertake in real clinical settings.   As de Tornyay stated, "Students can initially become involved with a hypothetical patient through a computerized program, identify nursing problems, test solutions, and discover the results of their interventions without involving 'real patients' with all the inherent dangers requiring close supervision and without the problems involved in the clinical areas that are scarce in the community" (H10).

As our opening illustration indicates, the capability for students to interact with a "simulated patient" through a computer that is programmed to interpret the students' input has important implications for evaluating assessment skills. For as nurses move into roles with increased responsibility and accountability, educators are concerned more and more about the development of effective decision-making and problem-solving skills.   The potential of computer simulation programs for developing and enhancing such skills, as well as making their attainment visible to faculty in an objective fashion, has great significance for the future of nursing education.

In a recent interview, Boston College Professor Peter Olivieri, chairman of the college's computer science department, who has worked with educators in the Boston College School of Nursing to develop their expertise in using computers, cited the following practical applications for computers in education.   He emphasized that computer applications in education are limited only by the creativity and imagination of the educator.   For purposes of student learning, Olivieri recommends using the computer:

1.   To review for State Board examinations (the student takes a sample test, has it scored by the computer, and gets feedback on the wrong answers).
2.   For self-paced instruction, such as a module on pharmacology.
3.   For statistical analysis of research during a student project.
4.   To "interact" with a simulated patient.
5.   To learn to evaluate electrocardiograms and other graphically represented tests results (some computers have extensive graphics capabilities).

How can nursing faculty use the computer to be more effective in their work? Olivieri suggests that faculty use the computer:

1.   To manage student records.
2.   For statistical analysis and research.
3.   For continuing education.   This capability is underway now in a major way for physicians - they have continuing education courses "played" to them on a microcomputer and interact with the content.
4.   As an audio-visual aid in the classroom.   (Not only are color graphics available, but the computer can control other devices such as a video tape recorder or a movie projector.)
5.   For its word processing potential - it greatly facilitates preparation of typewritten materials.

When asked about the impact of the microcomputer on nursing education, Olivieri noted that it has significant implications - primarily in its increased availability to all educators and the ease and diversity of its use.   Over the next few years he envisions the cost of a microcomputer falling to that of a color television or less and its "memory" (the amount of programming it can hold) increasing substantially.   He also notes that users will soon be able to

interface with microcomputers through voice communication. In addition more and
better programs will become available. Educators can only conclude that it's
time to learn to know and like computers! They may pave the way to a more
effective, satisfying professional life.

Software Development: A Critical Issue for Nursing Educators

Of course, new developments always bring with them new issues and needs. A
recent article in Classroom Computer News by Phyllis Caputo documents the rising
intensity with which computer manufacturers and educational publishers are
entering the educational computing market and warns educators that they now have
another all-important responsibility - that of playing the leading, standard-
setting role in the development of educational software for computers (14).
Nursing educators must heed this warning - as microcomputers take their place in
nursing classrooms, educators need to ensure that they, not the manufacturers,
set the pace in the development of educational computing software.

In other areas of education, the lack of initiative on the part of educators to
develop a comprehensive policy and play a directive role in software development
has created a situation characterized by lack of consistency in the quality of
available programs.   According to Caputo, about 120 software firms sell
educational packages, and although some are educationally sound, an educational
computer consortium director says, "there is so much trash out in terms of
software that it's very difficult for the teacher to buy intelligently."

Computer manufacturers predict that their emphasis on hardware will now change
to a priority in developing software that expands the educational capabilities
of microcomputers. They are joining with educational publishers to accomplish
this goal. How can educators assume the guiding role called for in this
situation? Caputo calls upon educators to form a strong, educational computing
network that will take firm control of all areas of educational computing
development and exert an educationally sound influence on it. Nursing educators
need to heed this message. With 1,360 schools and 250,385 students, nursing
education offers an enormous potential market for educational computing
software. The American Nurses' Association's Commission on Nursing Education
and other national nursing education groups should consider this issue - failure
to act quickly will result in another instance where nurses do not exert
adequate influence on developments that critically affect the profession.

Conclusion

The rapid evolution of computer capabilities, in particular the development of a
reasonably priced microcomputer of significant computer power, is
revolutionizing education. Nursing's history indicates that it spends too much
time reacting and not enough proacting. Now is the time for nursing educators
to critically examine the current and potential use of computers in education
and their specific applications to the process of preparing nurses for today's
practice.

REFERENCES

1. Davis, J. H. and Williams, D. D. Learning for mastery: individualized
    testing through computer-managed evaluation. Nurse Educator, 5(3): 9,
    May/June 1980.
2. Cheung, P. Examinations: put test questions on a computer! Nursing
    Mirror, 149: 26-8, November 1, 1979.
3. Simonsen, R. H. and Renshaw, R. S. CAI-bbon or boondoggle? Datamation,
    March, 1974, 90-102.

4.   Dorf, R. C. Computers and Man, 2nd edition. San Francisco, CA: Boyd and Fraser Publishing Company, 1977.

5.   Brunnstein, K. et. al. Computer Assisted Instruction, New York: Springer-Verlag, 1974.

6.   Dorf, R. C., 1977, p.377.

7.   Simonsen, R. H. and Renshaw, R. S., March, 1974, pp. 90-102.

8.   Alpert, D. and Bitzer, D. L. Advances in computer-based education. Science, 167: 1582-90, March 20, 1970.

9.   Alpert, D. and Bitzer, D. L., 1970, pp. 1582-90.

10. Alpert, D. and Bitzer, D. L., 1970, pp. 1582-90.

11. del Bueno, D. J. Competency-based education. Nurse Educator, 3(3): 15, May/June, 1978.

12. Resnick, L. B. Programmed instruction and the teaching of complex intellectual skills. Harvard Education Review, 33: 439-471, Fall, 1963.

13. Bundy, R. F. Computer-assisted instruction: now and for the future. Audio-visual Instruction, 12: 344-348, April, 1967.

14. Caputo, P. The Computer Industry and Education: The Issue of Responsibility, 1(1): 1,6,7, September/October, 1980.

"Portions of this paper were previously published in "The Computer's Place in Nursing Education" by Susan Mirin, Nursing and Health Care, November 1981. These portions are reprinted here with permission of the publisher."

The Impact of Computers on Nursing
M. Scholes, Y. Bryant and B. Barber (eds.)
Elsevier Science Publishers B.V. (North-Holland)
© IFIP-IMIA, 1983

11.4.

NURSING EDUCATION AND THE COMPUTER AGE IN RETROSPECT AND PROSPECT

Patricia Tymchyshyn

Introduction

"Why, this is the next best thing to going back to college," exclaims a pert grayhaired woman in a white scrub gown, as she uses a computer terminal to study a lesson on fetal monitoring. "I don't want to go on for a degree, but I like to keep learning". Another nurse, standing behind her and answering some of the questions encountered in the lesson, nods her head in agreement and contributes, "I was afraid of computers at first. I wouldn't even go into this room, but I just love it now...It's fun and it's easy...The only thing is, PLATO won't let you get by without putting in the right answer. It's much better than textbooks or lectures...I hate to read, but this is different." Yes, PLATO (Programmed Logic for Automatic Teaching Operations) and similar forms of computer-assisted instruction (CAI) are different from other modes of instruction. Nurses are using CAI on their hospital unit as part of a continuing education activity. For them it is providing an imaginative departure from traditional programs (1, I29).

Hospitals are one of the new arenas into which computer-assisted instruction (CAI) has entered. Nursing, however, has been a part of the computer age since its early years, making significant contributions in courseware development and evaluation.

The purpose of this paper is to describe CAI, its history, process, and potential contribution to the community of nurses. Although the author's experience has been primarily with the PLATO Computer System at the University of Illinois; it is hoped that the ideas and content presented here will be of use to nursing audiences at large.

IN RETROSPECT
PLATO III Nursing Study

Nursing's computer roots began with large interactive systems. Bitzer and Boudreaux (I4) published the only complete study of the role of computers in nursing education at that time. They developed twenty-two PLATO III lessons for the purpose of presenting all theoretical information in a sixteen week maternity nursing course. The teaching strategy utilized inquiry logic, an approach which gave learners the opportunity to gather data, construct relationships, and respond to questions. Bitzer contended that learning could be more efficient if the presentation of materials was in a manner that required learners to seek, sort, organize, interpret, and apply information. Encouraging the learner to take the initiative was felt to result in increased efficiency.

Learners enjoyed PLATO and generally preferred it to other instructional mediums. One commented, "You learn more if you have to search for information." Compared to traditional instructional methods of lecture and discussion, learners completed their theoretical studies in one-third to one-half the time. There was no difference in achievement according to test scores of those using PLATO as compared with those receiving traditional instruction (I2).

Evolution of PLATO IV

By 1972 most PLATO III lessons had become obsolete, as the computer system evolved into its fourth stage, PLATO IV. Its hardware was impressive, consisting of a keyset, like a typewriter, that transmitted the user's input to a large central computer; and a plasma panel display screen which could simultaneously show computer-generated graphic information along with random accessed photographic colored slides to the user. Other adjuncts included touch panels and random access audio. The response time was .2 seconds. Over 2000 characters could be displayed upon the screen, with 256 characters immediately available. The technological ingenuity far outreached the ability of authors to develop lessons using the system's capabilities. Little was known about strategies or subject matter appropriate to the delivery capabilities of the system. Authors were encouraged to experiment and develop lessons that used the computer's ability to:

(a) store, retrieve, analyze and interpret data,
(b) support drill and practice, tutorials, simultation and gaming strategies and
(c) vary presentation of information through graphics, animation and sized writing.

What PLATO couldn't do today its developers would design tomorrow. Development of creative, interactive lessons was a difficult task, one that was costly and time consuming.

PLATO IV Nursing Study

The United States Department of Health Education and Welfare (HEW) provided the economic support for a nursing project to develop and implement PLATO IV lessons into a nursing program. A study was conducted by Tymchyshyn (3) to evaluate the effects of the PLATO IV innovative program, describing events occurring during the project years, 1974 and 1977 and the factors influencing the spread of CAI prior to and following the grant period, 1968 to 1974; 1977 to 1981. Specifically, the study sought to answer the following questions:

1. In what ways did factors common to the diffusion process influence the spread of CAI in the nursing program and college?
2. What were the perceptions of students, faculty and administration during the implementation of the program?
3. What effect did the program innovations have on student learning?
4. In what ways did the courseware reflect the design contributions of the PLATO system?
5. What was the juxtaposition between instructor and computer in the nursing program?

Case study methodology was used to describe events from various perspectives. Data were gathered about expectations as well as actual events, through observations, questionnaires, interviews, and analysis of documents. The results showed that the spread of PLATO was dependent upon personal contact, advocacy, economic and administrative support, and technical expertise. Whereas students found the use of CAI to be a useful and relevant addition to their instruction, administration and faculty resisted initially, but later accepted the innovation. Faculty had difficulty in changing their role from transmitted to facilitator of information. Students preferred learning on PLATO to texts, lecture and audiovisual aids, felt it saved them time and helped them apply theory to clinical practice situations. There was no difference in achievement between those using PLATO and those receiving instruction through lecture discussion. Nursing lessons explored tutorial, drill and practice, inquiry, gaming and simulation strategies. Sized writing, colored slides, graphics and animation varied content presentation, while branching, judging and feedback provided information and promoted learner interest and interaction.

Subject matter was selected according to these guidelines:

1.   With what content in the course should each learner have practice interacting on an individual basis? What is better relegated to discussion?
2.   What cannot be taught effectively through lecture, discussion, slides, or film?
3.   What type of lesson would save the learner and instructor time?
4.   What content should be covered in class, but is not possible due to time constraints of the course?
5.   What content and interactive practice would assist in increasing learner confidence?
6.   What instructional interaction would make clinical experiences more meaningful?
7.   What content and design would promote self-direction learning?

Lessons were loosely categorized in the following manner:

INSTRUCTIONAL: In this style the major focus is on subject matter and mastery of content. The role of the computer is to provide logical sequencing of information, create a response demand environment, store and retrieve data, judge response, and present feedback. It is used with content which is well suited to convergent thinking. Drill and practice styles, although not as comprehensive as the full instructional method described, can loosely be categorized with the instructional approach. The intent here is to allow learners to test themselves.

Gaming formats are popular. The learner can play against the computer or against other student--"intraterminally". Self-assessment quizzes, because of their extensive feedback are useful to students in preparing for exams and assisting them in understanding the instructor's frame of reference in posing questions.

SIMULATION: This approach assists the learner in getting a "feel" for the clinical situations he/she will encounter. Specific patient examples are provided to enrich his/her learning environment. The computer presents information and provides opportunities for vicarious experiences. Students enjoy them because it enhances their limited clinical experiences. Instructors find them useful as a basis for discussion and promoting divergent thinking. Problems associated with this style may be oversimplification of complex patient-nurse interaction and the tendency of students to conclude that all patients are similar to examples in the lessons. Authors seem to find this approach the most conducive to presenting content in a creative manner.

AUTHOR/EDITOR SOFTWARE: One lesson was developed to allow student users to become involved in self-study by designing their own lessons. A crossword puzzle format was programmed and students made up their own puzzles, typing into the computer questions and answers. PLATO then organized the data into a puzzle. They received an additional benefit of learning that a computer is not infallible and that PLATO lessons are only as good as the content and design used by the author. Instructors used multiple-choice formats for inserting exam questions and some used a computerized grade book for record keeping of student progress. The only limitation for some students may be that the initial expansion of energy and time in learning to use the computer may outweigh the satisfaction of completing "their own PLATO lesson". It is largely dependent upon the facility the student and instructors have in working with their hand and the machines in general.

STATISTICAL ANALYSIS: Several statistical packages were written to analyze data specifically for the nursing program. They included data such as student characteristics, attitude toward the program, reaction to individual lessons, test scores and cognitive mapping results. This approach may well be thought of as labor saving and also did become the only cost effective lesson. Another benefit of the statistical packages was to provide an opportunity for the nursing faculty to conduct their own internal formative evaluation and analyze data where necessary.

Conclusions

Based on the findings of this study, it was concluded that PLATO was useful in preparing students for clinical practice, successfully replaced lecture and increased opportunities for independent study. Simulation, inquiry, and gaming were preferred strategies. Creation of quality courseware is costly and time consuming, requiring resources of commercial agencies. Diffusion of the innovation required administrative support as well as faculty advocacy.

3. IN PROSPECT

The early decades of the computer age have come to a close with educational promises of the innovation only partially realized. If computerized education is to be integrated into our activities of daily learning to the extent that informational systems are a part of our daily living, there needs to be a change in both the mechanics and philosophy of computer applications.

Experts have stated that the 1980s are a decade of promise due to the advent of personal computers and lowering of computing costs. Those who could not purchase terminals connected to large interactive systems due to high communication and computer expense apparently can budget monies for smaller "stand-alone" processing models. The remaining obstacles are lack of quality and quantity in courseware and evaluation.

Courseware Development

Pervasive in the thinking of both computer experts and manufacturers is the belief that individuals within educational institutions will produce the necessary quantity and quality of lessons. To that end, computer companies are currently funding courseware projects by supplying hardware in exchange for lessons authored by faculty. Occasionally large projects are funded involving content specialists and programmers. Independently, schools are also allocating monies for their own projects. Release Time to faculty may be given or assistantships to graduate students to author lessons. Conversely, others believe that it is the students themselves who should author lessons. Only through programming of subject matter can learning take place effectively. Support for this belief is found in projects at elementary and secondary schools where programming classes are offered to students at a variety of ages, either as part of an education program or enrichment classes after school. In this writer's opinion, it is highly unlikely that the myriad of courseware projects described above will produce the variety and quality of lessons required to meet the needs of nursing programs by the end of 1980s. Most of the projects have modest budgets that provide neither sufficient technical support nor time for novice authors to learn and apply the intricacies of computer technology to lesson development. There also appears to be no organizational plan for either identification or planning of suitable subject matter needed for substantive learning modules.

Nursing courseware developed under similar constraints has tended to underutilize computer capabilities of branching, learner interaction, and judging as well as presentation techniques through graphics, animation, color, and sound. Drill and practice and tutorial designs, rather than simulation and inquiry modes, prevail. Authors instead of learners may benefit most from the projects. Through programming and lesson design activities, they have the opportunity to enhance their problem-solving and mathematical skills. The latter involves such things as manipulation of variables, design of algorithms, and employment of conditional logic. More importantly, their level of computer literacy could rise from knowledge of hardware requisite for their needs, to understanding of learner-computer interaction and design techniques, to evaluation of published CAI lessons appropriate to their curricula. There is potential also for a pool of authors who could be hired by publishing companies for nursing courseware development. They could consult on subject matter design and evaluation separate from, or as a part of, lesson authorship.

Publishing houses have the resources and organization to develop complex and quality courseware. They would, however, have to expand their staff's capabilities in dealing with the new technology. Complex and large scale learning packages that require extensive subject matter research, employ inquiry and simulation strategies, and incorporate a large variety of presentation techniques are more suitably developed by commercial companies. Some of the most marketable products would be in the areas of critical care and occupational nursing. Faculty, faced with the task of creating their own lessons, can make efficient use of their time and energy by concentrating on lessons meeting the unique needs of their institution. Author/editor software modules offer possibilities for incorporating a variety of strategies and designs without the assistance of programmers. Authoring complex lessons can be likened to developing commercial films and videotapes. The level of sophistication reached by faculty for "in-house" audiovisual products will probably be similar to that attainable for CAI products. There are, of course, some individuals who can compose on computers and develop complex lessons independently. This is the exception rather than the rule.

Nurses involved at various levels of computer applications need to share their knowledge of appropriate computer subject matter and creative lesson formats for use on either interactive or micro-computer systems. Both systems are in evolutionary states. The former is incorporating microprocessing units, color along with video interface, and cable television to reduce costs, while the latter is increasing adjuncts, cost, and attempting interfaces with large computers for greater flexibility. A computer science director at the Medical College of Georgia has developed an author/editor that has the potential to function on both PLATO and Apple Systems. It behooves nurses to continue their involvement in the computer age despite its evolutionary status. Vital to the discipline is professional influence at the market place where policies are made as the innovation evolves. Educational values as well as efficiency need representation.

Evaluation

Protocol has been developed by some publishing companies. Minimal requirements of published PLATO lessons included lesson objectives, purpose, intended audience, and average completion time. Technical consultants reviewed each for smooth computer-learner interaction and required authors to update lesson content and make necessary programming changes. One state board of nursing felt this level of evaluation coupled with author qualifications in subject matter areas, and a brief computerized post-course quiz or attitude survey, was sufficient for the awarding of continuing education credit to registered nurses completing PLATO lessons.

There appear to be fewer requirements for lessons produced on micro-computers. Computer publishing companies solicit courseware from both experienced and novice authors; the result is an uneven quality of CAI materials, necessitating a "caveat emptor" climate. The buyer, however, cannot beware of things for which he or she has little or no experience. Evaluation of CAI lessons is different from judging textbooks or audiovisual aids for an educational program. Protocol developed by publishing companies may be thought of as base-line criteria.

The following evaluation format has been useful to this writer and is offered as a supplemental tool for those selecting CAI lessons applicable to their programs. Questions are organized around key-work phrases contained in this definition of a successful CAI lesson.

> "When successful a CAI lesson is an artful blend of organizational procedures with user and medium interaction. It combines interactive aspects of individualized instruction with some of the display capabilities of textbook, television, and computational powers of the computer. It can provide an imaginative departure from traditional methods"(2).

Each "key work" category is briefly described and contains examples of evaluation questions.

1. Blend of Organizational Procedures with User Medium Interaction. Emphasis is on judging the plan and flexibility of the lesson.

    (a) Does the format facilitate smooth passage through the lesson?
    (b) Are directions clear so that learners know what is expected of them?
    (c) Is there a consistent use of function keys throughout the lesson?
    (d) Is the lesson divided into parts or modules that can be accessed at the learner's discretion during the course of study?

2. Display Capabilities and Computation Powers. Focus is on the use the author has made of the unique capabilities of the computer to present information, initiate and judge learner responses.

    (a) Are text formats, graphics, animation, color and/or sound used to improve the presentation and clarity of content?
    (b) Do branching sequences promote data investigation and interaction between computer and learner? or
    (c) Are lessons predominately linear, resulting in electronic projections of lecture notes?
    (d) Do presentation techniques, data investigations, and computations of results save time?

3. Individualized Instruction. Questions are directed toward ways in which subject matter, designs, and strategies are used to meet the needs of individuals.

    (a) Is the presentation of information altered on the basis of learner response history as well as last response?
    (b) Are opportunities provided for internalization of concepts and facts?
    (c) Does the lesson promote self-directed learning?
    (d) Does it prepare students for discussion and/or clinical experiences?

4. Artful and Imaginative. This may be one of the most difficult areas of CAI authorship. It judges the ability of the author to match computer capabilities with appropriate subject matter to the advantage of learning.

(a)   Are techniques used to initiate and maintain interest (e.g.) personalize name, vary strategies and response sequences?
(b)   Is there a dramatic quality or an effort to make the lesson memorable?
(c)   Is it enjoyable?

Once a decision has been made about the quality of a single lesson or series of lessons, each client must decide the role CAI will play in that particular educational program. The demands of a particular setting will most likely result in variations of lesson usage. Those lessons with flexible formats, permitting reorganization or addition of lesson parts, have the best opportunity for adoption at local markets.

Closing Remarks

CAI is a unique medium, one which has surpassed earlier educational innovations: teaching machines, programmed instruction, and closed circuit television. It is assuming a predominant role in the experience of learning, acquiring status in the market place as well as educational institutions. As educational computers became integrated into activities of daily learning, illusive promisory themes of earlier years are being replaced by descriptions of its role in the educational process.

REFERENCES

1.   Buchholz-Glaeser and Tymchyshyn, "PLATO and Friends" in: Perspectives on Continuing Education in Nursing, NURSECO Inc., Ca. 1980.
2.   Steinberg, Esther. The Evolutionary Development of CAI Courseware. Urbana, Illinois, 1976.
3.   Tymchyshyn, P. "An Evolution of the Adoption of an Innovation (CAI vis PLATO IV) into a Nursing Program. Unpublished doctoral dissertation, University of Illinois at Urbana-Champaign, (June, 1982).

The Impact of Computers on Nursing
M. Scholes, Y. Bryant and B. Barber (eds.)
Elsevier Science Publishers B.V. (North-Holland)
© IFIP-IMIA, 1983

11.5.

PROTOCOLS FOR SOFTWARE SELECTION, DEVELOPMENT AND EVALUATION FOR NURSING EDUCATION

Susan J. Grobe

Introduction

There is agreement among instructional computing experts that the future success of computers in education hinges largely upon the availability of quality educational software(1). Availability is directly related to development, and influences software's continued selection. Quality, an elusive characteristic, is directly related to the outcomes of evaluative processes. Likewise, quality affects software's continued development and selection. Therefore selection development and evaluation of software for nursing education must be considered together because of their interrelation.

On the one hand some write that the development of software is as easy as 1, 2, 3(2). Others write that development is not only costly and time consuming, it is difficult. On the other hand difficulties are not limited only to development(3). This becomes apparent by examining questions posed by Kleiman for evaluating educational software. "Does the software follow good educational practices ... is it suitable for its intended users ..."and", ... does it take advantage of the capabilities of the computer?"(4). Responding to these comments about development and the questions about evaluation underscores that the selection, development and evaluation of computer software for nursing is indeed a complex challenge.

Just as software development and evaluation is costly, complex and time consuming, the selection of software should be much simpler by comparison. And yet, as in any newly developing technological arena, it is quite difficult to gather information for establishing software standards. Since a sufficient number of similar software samples are not available for comparison, the effort becomes one of making somewhat intuitive leaps using a limited data base, from "what is" to the proverbial "what should be".

Before leaping to the "what should be" however, the state of computer software development and computer technology must be taken into account. The history of audiovisual software development and distribution provides many lessons. Additionally, results from the early large, educationally based main-frame software development efforts also contribute important general information. Indeed, in analysing the present system of decentralised "programmer-developed" microcomputer based software packages, history provides a valuable perspective. In fact, few coordinated patterns of software distribution exist because only a very limited number of the major publishers have wanted to become involved in distributing educational software in these early stages of its development. Significantly, this may be used to advantage in nursing education, since examination and specification of the "what should be" might still be possible to achieve, if realistic, meaningful, standardized protocols for nursing education software can be described and proposed(5).

Careful attention to software evaluation and selection is extremely important for other reasons. Mace contends that "instead of asking which hardware to buy, schools are choosing software first, then finding the hardware to run it

on" (6). If this is indeed so, and it appears that it is, then the initial
software selection process is a primary determinant of the direction for
instructional computing in that educational setting's future. If early software
selections and evaluations are done poorly, the implications are evident and
far-reaching. It is apparent then, there is much to be gained from developing
protocols for the selection, development and evaluation of software for nursing
education. Although the base of nursing experience with computer software is
somewhat lean at this point, a broad general perspective for nursing software
expectations can emerge and provide a strong foundation upon which nursing
authors, developers and publishers can build(A13).

One additional point needs clarification before continuing. The basic
perspective from what protocols are constructed is extremely important to
consider. The perspective sets the basic parameters for the inclusion of the
criteria protocols. For example, Perry in an introductory article in a computer
trade magazine, outlined three distinct approaches for selecting computer
software(7). Each represents a different philosophical approach. The first, is
selection of a "canned program" which cannot be changed by its users. Its
general nature and wide applicability at reasonable cost, allows it to be quite
readily adopted. The second, costly in development time, exists when software
is designed and perhaps programmed and coded by its authors who are also
teachers. The end result consists of software with limited general usefulness,
but tailored specifically to local needs. The third approach known as an
authoring system, exists when a framework is provided for guiding a teacher-
author through creation of software. Although this third approach still
requires development time, the complexities of instructional design, computer
programming and coding have been reduced. The end result, a software program
tailored to the author's local needs, is adaptable, perhaps of general use and
probably quite easily revised, edited and updated. Selection and use of these
approaches either individually or in combination, constitute a top level
administrative decision, and affect what is subsequently included in protocols
designed for software selection and development. Thus, the basic philosophical
approach to software establishes an initial filter for subsequent decisions
about software selection and development. However, regardless of which approach
is chosen, protocols for software evaluation do remain fairly consistent.

In order to provide a context for examining computer software for nursing
education it is helpful to define what is included in the broad context known as
educational computing. Kniefel and Just propose that educational computing can
be categorized as administrative (60%) and academic (40%)(8). Academic can be
further subdivided into instruction (30%) and research (10%). Within the
category of instruction there are three components consisting of: 1) teaching
about computers i.e., computer science 2) teaching with computers i.e. computer
assisted instruction (CAI) and computer managed instruction (CMI) and 3)
teaching problem solving i.e. using computers to solve quantitative problems.
Table 1 illustrates these categories.

Although the percentages may differ slightly now in 1982, the paper focuses upon
the academic category and propose protocols for selecting, developing and
evaluating computer based software for instruction in nursing education. The
scope of the paper is further limited to include examination of the software
itself, and not the hardware systems. The paper does not compare nursing
education software for stand alone microcomputers with software for main frame
computer systems, confining itself to a discussion of the software properties
alone. Overlap among the arbitrary categories of computer software selection,
development and evaluation is inevitable. However, given the nature of the
different purposes of each of the actions, it is quite possible to minimize
duplication. First, for constructing software selection protocols, the world of
software will be examined from administrators' and educators' perspectives.
Finally software evaluation will be considered from instructional designers',
programmers' educational evaluators' and users' perspectives.

These pragmatic perspectives will assist in providing a common frame of reference for establishing a broad understanding about instructional software. This in turn can lead to the formulation of precise individualized protocols as well as an understanding of other associated criteria, useful in examining computer based software for nursing in general.

TABLE 1

EDUCATIONAL COMPUTING CATEGORIES (9)

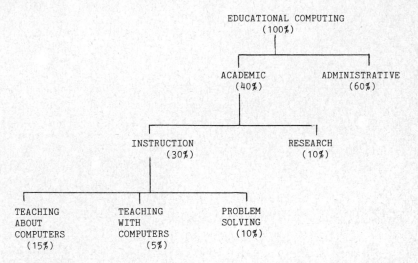

Selection

A brief introductory description of the various perspectives is useful for examining software. It precedes a more detailed description of each the publisher, purchaser, user and educator's perspectives. Each perspective contributes valuable information for understanding what might be included in the protocol for software selection.

First, the software publisher's perspective is related primarily to software development costs and sales volume projections. A purchaser's viewpoint also includes concerns related to cost, but includes additional factors such as adaptability, ease of adoption, compatibility, transferability and replaceability. The user's perspective generally includes concerns identified as "user friendliness", flexibility, clarity and ease of use. More experienced users may also be concerned with documentation, available vendor services, the software's actual marketing status and evaluation of the program from similar users. Finally, an educator is concerned about content accuracy and currency, instructional design, previous evaluations and revisions, and the software's suitability for curricular purposes.

Some software characteristics such as the type and kinds of feedback and cues provided for the user, could be considered from either an educator or user's perspective to those selected characteristics associated with an individual's actual use of the software. The user's perspective will not include instructional design features of the software. The specific software design

features which relate to the type of interaction required of the learner will be
considered from an educator's perspective.

a.   Publisher's Perspective

The software publishers (i.e. distributor's) perspective is tempered primarily
by costs and related budgetary concerns.   Specific factors affecting both
software development costs and sales volume projections are primary concerns of
publishers.   Decisions made regarding software production and distribution are
often determined on the basis of the traditional book publishing model.   This
reflects a unit cost equation which includes development expenditures balanced
by forecasted sales volumes.

CAI software, unlike books and print materials does not fit the somewhat
standard development and sales volume model.   However, with CAI software more
variables enter both sides of the cost equation.   For example, the edit and
review cycle prior to book publication is not truly equivalent to testing the
implementation of CAI programs.   CAI software with its programming differences
and potentialities, has so many variations in its execution that often "bugs" or
deficits are not all identified until the program has been marketed and is being
used by a variety of individuals.   Therefore, an updating process for software
is essential.   However, it must be accomplished without appreciably increasing
development costs or decreasing sales volume income potentials.   Software
development costs also include expenditures not present with book publication.
Often more than just one content expert is required for the development of
software.   Costs are associated with instructional design, development,
programming and coding, testing, updating, and servicing of the software
materials(9).

Software updating alone can be quite costly to publishers.   Depending on how
updating is designed and implemented it can also affect the sales-volume half of
the equation.   The provision of backup disks made necessary by the expendable
nature can also affect sales volume projections.   Publishers of CAI software
therefore have some difficult decisions to make.   Their choices include
decreasing development expenditures, heavily protecting disks to prevent
copying, closely monitoring and controlling updating, or increasing the unit
costs of the software.   Unfortunately, as noted previously, major educational
publishing houses and distributors are only begining to become involved in
computer software development and marketing for university education.   The
lateness of their direction in this area has allowed many smaller entrepreneurs
(often computer programmers without instructional design competence) to fill the
demand for software with almost any type of materials.   One result is addressed
in an Educational Products Information Exchange (EPIE) report on microcomputer
courseware.

> "Unhappily, the development and implementation of software packages has
> not been commensurate with the sales of the hardware.   The production of
> 'educational software' is a fractured cottage industry dominated by
> enterprising programmers, not educators.   Instructional design concerns
> are only occasionally addressed in the single concept tapes or disks.
> Even now that educational publishers, experienced in designing print
> instructional materials, are marketing large K8 courseware packages, there
> have been no accepted criteria as to what constitutes an effective
> instructional program"(10).

The publisher or distributor is, therefore, caught in the middle, half way
between choosing to market software and not quite knowing how to adjust to a
different model for producing it, and projecting sales volumes.   Additionally,
since computer software development is in its infancy, the producers and
distributors do not have much experience or a clear perspective about what

constitutes effective software programs which can be marketed on a development cost recovery and profit basis. Importantly, at this juncture, the market is being driven by purchasers' decisions.

b.   Purchaser's Perspective

The purchaser views software from a different vantage point than a distributor or publisher.   Many factors related to the actual software package being examined for purchase and adoption are important.   A purchaser's initial concerns are related to installation, compatibility and operation of the software with existing hardware.   For this, the component parts of a software package must be examined by the purchaser.   What is included in the package? Are there guides and adequate documentation for the installer and the user?

A second area of concern for a purchaser relates to how the software was developed or authored.   What information has the developer provided regarding the prototype testing, evaluation and revision of the software?   Have intended users been identified and included in the early testing of the software?   Did initial use of the materials require or prompt any revisions of the materials? If so, what changes and how many?   What version or revision is this?   Does the product compare favorably with other materials already on the market?   Does this distributor have other effective materials?   Is the software unique?   What are its limitations?   What type and level of preparation are required for its adoption and effective utilization?   Was it developed with sophisticated users in mind?   Are there any explicit or projected factors which may interfere with its effective adoption?

Other factors which need to be considered from a purchaser's perspective relate to the difficulty level required for a program's use.   Does the format of the software program require complex skills for its operation?   Does the program "boot up" easily, or does it require programming skills to manipulate files for specific instructional uses?   Is use of the software format appropriate for its intended purposes?   If the software program is intended for improving problem solving skills, does it in fact do so, or is it an elaborate page turner for knowledge and fact level tasks?   Next, if the package requires any preplanning on the part of the user does an explicit guide accompany the package?   Several available statistical simulation packages immediately come to mind.   Each requires that data be supplied by the purchaser for the learners to use in setting up and implementing statistical program runs.   In examining package materials are the directions and examples clear enough so that the required tasks can be accomplished readily?   If the software requires any other preplanning on the purchaser's part is it clearly specified?   Are necessary tasks able to be reasonably accomplished?   Finally, are there any learner or user guides required for the software's effective use?   Are there any other associated materials which must accompany the software?   How are these provided? Must they be purchased individually for distribution or can they be reproduced without any additional charges?

The purchaser's perspective overlaps somewhat with the user's, particularly if the purchaser and user are in fact the same individual.   However, regardless of the overlap it is possible to identify several user characteristics which can be examined closely before software is selected.

c.   User's Perspective

From a user's perspective, one of the first criteria usually mentioned is that the software be "user friendly", that is, the software should be interminably patient with its users without penalizing learners or ignoring naive user's input.   "Friendliness" is also interpreted to include several features which are now commonly included in most software programs and keep users informed of its operations, especially when slight pauses or delays are necessary for processing tasks. It should not require overly rigid entry formats, for example, if the software is concerned with mathematical calculations it should allow the user to enter the answers to problems from left to right instead of from right to left. Programs should accept reasonable input and provide comments which are not offensive to users. A good question to ask is "how does the software accept common abbreviations, typing errors, misspellings?" Are common terms and their synonyms acceptable? What happens if the input is still not recognizeable? Does the software stay operational?

Users should expect to be able to alter the pace of the presentation, and to answer with responses at their own rate. The software should contain some humor along with changes in pace. If there are attempts at personalization, are they realistic? Is any of the language used in the software either sterotypical, time or place bound? Are text and visuals clearly presented, formatted well, and readable? Video monitors used with computers often have poor resolution. Formatting and frame displays with this decreased resolution therefore should not add to user's visual difficulties. Screens should have a pleasing visual effect and printed text should be adequately spaced. Text should not entirely fill a screen and should not scroll unless it is under the user's control. One should be able to move easily and readily among the different portions of the material being presented, and be reasonably free to exit from a program as they wish. Importantly, the software should serve as more than just a page turner.

Are there online glossaries and help systems provided which offer reasonable and useful assistance to users? Are they flexible and constantly available? Can users access the help system at any time by exiting the activity in progress and then easily return to the original activity? How individualized are the materials? Is the user confined to a linear path in using the materials or is the design such that a choice is available? Can users follow different routes through the materials depending on their individualized responses?

An EPIE report on evaluating microcomputer software makes an excellent suggestion:

> "An important student option is to be able to exit an activity ... a book can be closed, a chapter skipped, a workbook page ignored. On the microcomputer, it is extremely frustrating to be forced through one activity after another with no choice but to continue"(11).

How are graphics, color and sound used in the software? Are they enhancements or integral parts of the program? Does their use serve to distract users from learning or contribute to user motivation and satisfaction with the program?

Are software programs easily loaded into the machine's memory, quick to respond to users, and structured to provide maximal learner involvement? What is the quality of feedback to users? When feedback is provided, are the correct responses provided with some remediation or explanation? Research findings do not provide specific suggestions about how feedback should be presented. However, the value of providing such feedback continues to be demonstrated.

Table 2 summarizing selected author's views on the major software characteristics from a user's perspective follows. Consistency among authors on user control, feedback and remediation, learner interaction and flexibility of input formats is evident. Full use of the technology is an expectation of each of the authors. Clarity of instructions as well as adequacy of documentation are also consistently mentioned as important features of software from a user's perspective.

It is evident that any protocol for the selection of software must include a user's review and trial of the package. Comparison of naive and experienced users' reactions to the software using the characteristics outlined in this section would provided a good initial, review protocol for selecting computer based software.

TABLE 2

AUTHORS' VIEWS REGARDING

SOFTWARE CHARACTERISTICS FOR USERS

	BORK (13)	CRAWFORD (14)	TEA (15)	KEHRBERG (16)	EPIE (17)
User Control	X	X	X	X	X
Interaction					
Variable sequenc	X	X		X	X
Variable exit(s)	X		X		X
Instructions					
Clear	X	X	X	X	X
On-line help			X		X
Variable Input	X	X	X	X	X
Perceptual Input					
Text	X	X	X	X	X
Format	X	X	X	X	X
Feedback					
Remediation	X	X	X	X	X
Difficulty Level		X			
Documentation					
Users			X	X	X
Debugging	X	X	X	X	X
Appropriate Technology	X	X	X	X	X
Record Keeping and Reporting					
Evidence					
User		X	X		
Attempted evaluation	X	X	X	X	X
Debugging and revision		X	X		

d. Educator's Perspective

An educator's concern about computer software selection includes considerations about the adequacy of the content, instructional design and the resulting interactive characteristics of the program. What is the primary instructional method of the software? Is it appropriate to the content and objectives? What is the level of student interaction associated with the selected instructional method? What is required of users? Where does control of the users sequence

exist?   Are   learners   forced   through   activities   with   no   options?   Are
individualized cues and prompts, provided through the system, instructionally
sound?   Are they designed and delivered in a positive and reinforcing manner?
Does the software reflect sound instructional design criteria?

The EPIE criteria for evaluating instructional materials from an educator's
perspective includes the following:

"Is there a description of:

a.   developer's rationale
b.   learning objectives
c.   both content and intended audience
d.   methods and activities included
e.   any evaluative methods or management system"(12)

Adequacy of content includes examination of its accuracy, currency and
suitability. Crawford was very explicit in outlining inaccuracies which detract
from content adequacy.   Included are: factual errors; ommissions; inappropriate
placement of topics; and, among others, incomplete indices, glossaries and
tables of contents(13).

A recommended method for assessing adequacy of content along with instructional
design adequacy includes seeking evidence of extensive review of the software by
educators and users.   Congruency between the stated instructional objectives and
achievement of those goals by users should be evident from such reviews.
Following initial peer and user review, an effective method includes subsequent
extensive validation and evaluation by users following a structured formative
evaluation process.   This review provides a means for revising the materials
using contributions from users, instructional designers, computer programmers
and content and evaluation experts.   Evidence of such revision is desirable for
any instructional design and software selection protocol.

Crawford describes other criteria which educators also need to consider in
reviewing available software for selection.   Included are:

a.   appropriateness of the software for its intended purpose
b.   scope of the program and its sequencing
c.   specific instructional methodologies used and their appropriateness for
      both content and users
d.   additional teacher preparation required for use of the program, and
e.   the specific type of evaluational methods which are included(14).

It is quite apparent by now that an educator's view of software needs to be
quite comprehensive.   It is the educator who makes an evaluative judgement about
whether the materials are suitable for purchase.   The decisions about whether
the software contents are accurate, current and designed well enough to maximize
the instructional potential for users is a difficult decision.   In essence, an
educator's decision is based upon sensitivity to, and an understanding of, the
intended uses, as well as a realistic and analytic purchaser and developers
perspective.

What criteria then should the educator use in examining the different kinds of
instructional software?   What characteristics are or should be associated with
each different instructional approach.   Table 3 provides initial information for
use in comparing and contrasting the different instructional types of computer
based software programs and some selected instructional software and hardware
characteristics.

TABLE 3

CHARACTERISTICS OF INSTRUCTIONAL SOFTWARE ASSOCIATED WITH DIFFERING TYPES
OF COMPUTER BASED PROGRAMS (21)

	Drill Practice	Tutorial	Simulation	Testing	Problem Solving	Research (Statistical Packages)	Information Retrieval	Programming
Cognitive Domain of Learning Objectives:								
Knowledge Level	X			X			X	
Understanding Level	X	X	X	X				
Comprehension		X	X	X	X	X		X
Application Level		X	X	X	X	X		X
User Sequence Determined:								
Random Generation	X	X	X	X	X	X		
User Responses	X	X		X	X			
User Choices	X	X			X			
Fixed (Sequence)	X				X	X	X	X
Branching Variable:								
Hi with User Response		X	X	X	X	X	X	X
Lo with User Response								
Records and Data:								
Stored	X			X				
Analyzed	X			X		X		
Retrievable	X			X		X	X	N/A
Interaction Level:								
Feedback	X	X	X	X	X	X		X
Referral	X	X		X	X	N/A		
Remediation	X	X	X				N/A	
Prompts	X	X						
Cues			X		X	X		
Error Messages								X
Machine Requirements:								
Usable Memory (RAM)	4-8K	16-32K	8-32K	16-32K	8K+	16-64K	16-64K	16-64K
Graphics		X	X	X	X			X
Hard Copy				X				X
Non-Integer Math		X	X	X	X			
Lower Case Characters		X	X	X	X			
Cassette and/or Disk	C	D	D	D	C/D	D	D	
Nursing Education Uses:								
Science Knowledge	X	X	X	X				
Psychosocial Behavior		X	X	X				
Clinical Decisions		X	X	X	X			

(21) Adapted from Thomas, p. 66.

The most common types of computer-based software are listed horizontally. Specific instructional and required machine characteristics comprise the remaining vertical scale. Notice that the types of software considered are consistent with the academic computing model presented earlier. Drill and practice, research, problem-solving with the computer as well as information retrieval are included. Concise definitions and examples of each instructional approach are included in Appendix A for use in interpreting Table 3.

Scrutinizing software using the distributor, purchaser, user, and educator's viewpoints provides a basis for understanding what should be included in protocols for selecting CAI software for nursing education. Though the paper has focused primarily on the software characteristics related to microcomputers, these same criteria can be applied to selecting software for use on large main-frame computers.

DEVELOPMENT

This brief section on the development of CAI software is organized with the knowledge that "software engineering" is in itself, a complex process. A definition of software engineering can be constructed by examining a brief list of recommended topics to be addressed by software engineers. Examination of the list is useful in providing a Gestalt for understanding all that is included in software development in order to determine what should be included in development protocols. Wasserman's software engineering topics are:-

"1. requirements analysis, definition, and specification (i.e., understanding the instructional problem precisely, developing an unambiguous statement of system functions, decomposing the problem into manageable subparts, and, specifying acceptable solutions);

2. software design (i.e., using well-defined methods for establishing the logical structure of a software system and, creating software "blueprints");

3. systematic programming methodology (i.e., using techniques for reliably producing programs that are correct, including stepwise refinement and structured programming);

4. program testing (i.e., programming verification, including constructing test cases to validate system performance and to assess that a program matches its specifications);

5. software certification (i.e., attesting that software meets stated qualities of reliability and performance); and,

6. documentation (i.e., user manuals, program descriptions, written specification, design representations, for program readability)" (16).

Regardless of what approach is chosen for software development, educators generally agree that the end result of the developmental activities should be programs which meet predetermined needs, are characterized by content adequacy, and show evidence of incorporating both learning theory and instructional design planning. Therefore development protocols should include each of these components in the established criteria.

Analysis prior to the decision to develop computer based programs should be quite explicit. Do needs justify development of the program? Are there other similar materials available which can be adapted? Will the anticipated use and program life expectancy justify the development time and investment? Does the necessity for updating the content relegate the program's useful life to a very initial time span? Why is it valuable to have this particular material presented in this format? Do the instructional methods chosen reflect the nature of the needs, goals and stated educational objectives? With development, other questions related to administrative cost and efficiency need to be asked. The process of software development can be a time consuming lengthy process. If individuals developing the materials do not have adequate expertise, then the preparation can extend the time line immeasureably, with development occurring on a trial and error basis. Resultant software outcomes may also be severe disappointments, since the complexity of the development process and the type and level of skills are quite specific. The idea that well intentioned effort results in good software outcomes is a common fallacy. It is well illustrated using a comment from an Air Force decision maker who had responsibility for overseeing computer software development activities. He said:

> "You software guys are too much like the weavers in the story about the Emperor and his new clothes. When I go out to check on software development the answers I get sound like, 'We're fantastically busy weaving this magic cloth. Just wait a while and it'll look terrific'. But there's nothing I can see or touch, no numbers I can relate to, no way to pick up signals that things aren't really all that great. And there are too many people I know who have come out at the end wearing a bunch of expensive rags or nothing at all"(17).

The unpredictability of software development efforts, combined with the number of failures has resulted in studies of software techniques. Wasserman proposes a deliberate approach to software development which requires early deliberate planning to develop a set of requirements, good specifications, a feasible design and a well qualified team of developers. "A well disciplined approach to software development places a greater percentage of effort up-front; on requirements definitions, specification and design, with correspondingly reduced time and effort on testing and debugging"(18). The implication then from this perspective of adequacy of preplanning establishes a common baseline for discussion of software development protocols.

Several different ways exist for approaching the development of CAI software and are presented in the following paragraphs. The author's personal and professional biases related to development from a team perspective are evident in explaining the last of the alternatives.

The first represents the novice approach to development. Avner, (19) an early pioneer in implementing the PLATO system provides interesting suggestions for beginners in CAI. These suggestion are loosely as follows:

> "Step 1. Art for the sake of art..Make full use of the medium...anything that can be done is worth doing.
>
> Step 2. Do your own thing...don't limit yourself to the needs, interests and abilities of your learner...don't think about where you are going until after you have finished.
>
> Step 3. The Procrustean bed...Adapt your existing media to the new medium, ignore the unique capabilities of the new medium.
>
> Step 4. Damn the torpedos...Don't try versions out on students or others...Forge ahead, finish the tasks.
>
> Step 5. Hitch a ride on a bandwagon...Don't worry about knowing how to accomplish the task, just keep up with the latest trends...".

The common denominator lacking for each of these suggestions is the absence of systematic design and planning.

In summing up what is to be included in a protocol for developing CAI software for nursing education, one would stress the necessity for a deliberate systematic approach, ideally accomplished by a team, with contributions from at least a nursing content specialist, an instructional designer and an educational evaluator. Computer coding of the designed materials should be carried out by skilled and experienced computer programmers. Each member of such a development team brings an essential component to the design. The nursing individual brings an understanding of the nursing discipline, as well as expertise in its teaching. The instructional designer brings an understanding of learning as well as knowledge of research findings regarding the design and structuring of material for effective learning. The educational evaluator assists with the analysis of the instructional tasks to be accomplished and has the responsibility for monitoring the fidelity of the design with originally stated objectives and intents. The computer programmer is responsible for establishing the instructional program's architectural structure and the actual coding of the materials for computer delivery and implementation.

Following this brief overview of the team, the next obvious question is can one person develop software for nursing? The author's answer would be in the affirmative, if one person could effectively do each of the above necessary tasks. However, the likelihood of this happening is indeed quite remote. How then does one proceed? First, it is necessary to define and operationalize the term "development". It can be considered as a series of decisions, beginning first with determination of the need for the materials followed by a specification of their purpose. Various authors suggest differing sequences for the process of development. Three will be cited for illustratives purposes.

Reed, Ertel and Collart suggest a preliminary state of CAI course development followed by an authorship sequence(20). This latter sequence includes a testing and revision cycle followed by course release and another evaluation cycle. Their charts, illustrates their approach to the overall development(21). Approximately one-third of their focus is on pre-planning activities and task designations related to planning, authoring and evaluation. The team members involved include author, instructional planner, and content consultants. Revisions are an integral part of the authorship sequence. Course release and external validation comprise their third sequence of actions.

A second instructional systems approach which can be used for developing CAI is know an the Interservice Procedures for Instructional Systems Development Model (IPISD). The model consists of five major phases: analyze, design, develop, implement and control(22). Each phase is then further subdivided into fairly detailed instructional design activities. Table 2.1 illustrating the phases and the blocks in each phase follows.

TABLE 4

IPISD MODEL

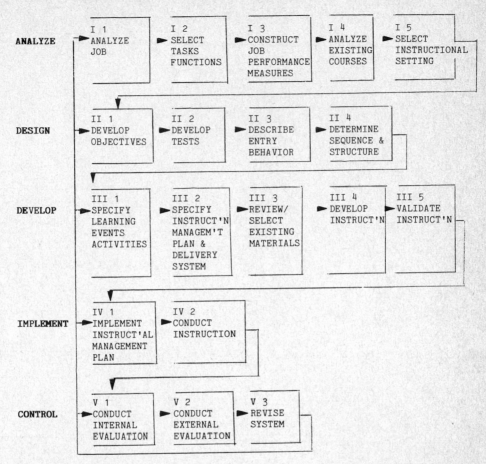

The reader should notice the similarity between the phases of the IPISD and the step of the nursing process model.

```
Analyze ..... Assess
Design ...... Diagnose
Develop ..... Plan
Implement ... Implement
Control ..... Evaluate
```

This design process can be easily understood and can be translated by individuals developing CAI on nursing. Its instructional task orientation within each of these steps however, makes it somewhat difficult for other than primarily instructional designers to understand and implement. It does, however, provide an effective guide for the flow of the actual design activities. The guide could be useful in establishing a common task orientation and communication among the members of any development team.

A last approach, which the author's team uses for developing nursing CAI materials is known as the structured decomposition model(23). Borich describes it as a systems methodology which can be used to perform a detailed analysis of a whole, for purposes of determining the nature, structure and sequence of its parts. Borich claims that it is "especially suited to helping understand the design of complex instructional and training programs in which it is often difficult to see the forest for the trees."(23). According to Borich:

> "Structured decomposition systematically breaks down a complex training program into its component parts. The process starts with a general or abstract description of the program. This serves as a working model from which successively more detailed portions of the program are conceived. Graphically, this process involves division of a cell representing the overall program into a number of more detailed cells, each symbolizing a major program activity within the parent cell. The extent of analysis within any step of the structured decomposition process is limited to a small number of program activities, each of which is further broken down in succeeding steps of the process.

> The approach ensures uniform systematic exposition of successive levels of detail. Structured decomposition utilizers a graphic language designed to expose detail gradually in a controlled manner, to encourage conciseness and precision, to focus attention on the relationships between program activities, and to provide an analysis and design vocabulary for use by program planners, developers and evaluators"(23)

A brief general illustration of how the model was applied to developing CAI on nursing process follows.

The first step of decomposition is to graphically break down the global concept (in this case, nursing process), into its individual parts, called activities or transactions. Thus nursing process, in this first step of decomposition are assessment, diagnosis, planning, intervention and evaluation.

Each block in the nursing process model represents an activity or a transaction. The flow of transactions from beginning to end is mapped. This reveals the interaction and relationships among activities. Thus the flow of instructional activities regarding nursing process would be mapped following the model (24).

Each transaction (or block) is further analyzed to identify constraints and to specify its inputs and behavioral outputs. Sources of influence which affect the implementation of the particular transaction or activity are identified as constraints(23, I10). Examples of transactions with inputs, outputs and constraints are illustrated in Table 5.

In its implementation by a team of developers, the decomposition process continues forcing a united activity of planners, designers, and evaluators while building both a common vocabulary and a concise graphic illustration of the program's training components. Decomposition also clarifies interrelationships among activities and allows for the gradual introduction of detail consistently across all areas of the planning. The top down design with the gradual accretion of details allows instructional development to proceed rationally without focusing on detailed differences at the outset of planning, thereby possibly interfering with the team's intent.

TABLE 5

TRANSACTION EXAMPLES

(CONSTRAINTS)

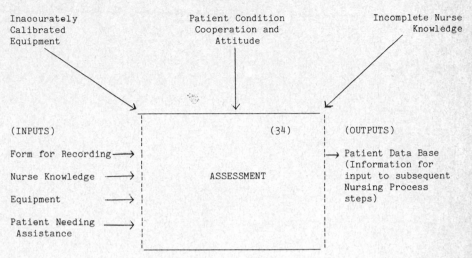

| Inaccurately Calibrated Equipment | Patient Condition Cooperation and Attitude | Incomplete Nurse Knowledge |

(INPUTS)   (34)   (OUTPUTS)

Form for Recording⟶   ⟶ Patient Data Base (Information for input to subsequent Nursing Process steps)

Nurse Knowledge ⟶   ASSESSMENT

Equipment   ⟶

Patient Needing ⟶ Assistance

In summary, a protocol for computer software development should include criteria which reflect a systematic deliberative approach to design and implementation. Adequacy of the specifications, feasible and rational instructional design characteristics, and implementation by a qualified team are essential. Formative evaluation processes using a sample of intended users are highly desirable. Finally, critical appraisal of the outcome product must be used as supplementary evidence.

EVALUATION

Protocols for software evaluation should be established based on goals and the intent of the evaluation. The distinction between formative and summative evaluation processes made by Scriven implies two different approaches and differing logical structures for performing the associated evaluative tasks (25). The formative evaluation process is considered to be a review of materials during the process of development for purposes of providing feedback to the developer. One of the goals of the formative process is improving the product under development. Summative evaluation involves collection of data about either the completed product or its outcomes. An example of the summative evaluation process is examining the software itself for its effects on a user.

Sanders and Cunningham suggest a framework for conducting formative evaluations (26). Their proposed structure is particularly helpful for identifying sources of information useful for the examining questions and establishing criteria for the formative part of an evaluative protocol. According to Sanders and Conningham, predevelopmental activities include both a needs assessment and a subsequent evaluation of the identified needs. Objectives established based on the identified needs are evaluated from both a logical and empirical perspective. This analysis of objectives is designed to answer questions such as: 1) logically, is there a rationale for the objectives and 2) empirically, do relevant others (i.e., peer groups and specialists) agree with the objectives as proposed?   Next interim evaluation consists of collecting information regarding 1) the expected pay-off value of the product's development and 2) the products contents. Information collected in response to these criteria is used primarily as feedback to the developer for consideration during development. The last stage consists of descriptive validation and cost analyses studies. Information collected from validation and cost analyses is again referred to the developer as feedback. The last step could also be called "field testing" which Sanders and Cunningham suggest be conducted at first informally, but followed by more realistic trials in the intended contexts.

Sanders and Cunningham's model is inclusive. Concrete suggestions for varied sources of information which can be accessed and used in each stage of the formative evaluation process are provided and categorized. Their sources could be incorporated as suggestions for sources for information in design of an evaluative protocol.

Two additional examples of established evaluative protocols for computer based software follow. The first is from CONDUIT, (an acronym for a consortium consisting of the following original members: Computers at Oregon State University, North Carolina Educational Computing Services, Dartmouth College, The University of Iowa, and the University of Texas at Austin) the second is from the International Council for Computers in Education. Although both are useful in refining any evaluative protocol for CAI software, the first could be categorized as formative evaluation protocol, while the second might be considered a summative one.

The first example developed by CONDUIT, whose original purpose was the facilitation of instructional computing at the university level. An outcome of the project was the design and testing of standards, guidelines, processes and procedures for the enhancement and exchange of computer based college level instructional materials. The published standards, although originally designed to be used for product evaluation purposes, require that many of the formative evaluation feedback processes have occured. In fact, a review of the computer materials for possible distribution by CONDUIT can be construed as a formative evaluation process using Sander's and Cunningham's external contextual sources of information.

CONDUIT standards and guidelines are presented in its Author's Guide(27). The guide is explicit in providing a "cook book" approach to both developing and reviewing computer based instructional materials. Concrete examples and excellent graphic examples are provided in each of the manual's sections. Suggestions included refer to design, development, style, packaging and review. In addition, each section of the guide contains very select annotated sources for further reference.

A second excellent source for establishing an evaluative protocol was developed by MicroSIFT (28), a project of the International Council for Computers in Education. These standards are primarily used in examining completed software, thereby implying summative evaluation. The Evaluator's Guide details several elements of a summative evaluation process. It provides definitions, descriptive formats and a sample guide with rating scales. The three major categories proposed for software evaluation include content, instructional, and technical quality. Samples of the type of criteria from the manual within each category follow:

Content:
    . . . is accurate
    . . . has educational value
    . . . is free of stereotyping

Instructional quality:
    . . . purpose is well defined
    . . . achieves its purpose
    . . . presentation is clear and logical
    . . . level of difficulty is appropriate
    . . . feedback is effectively employed
    . . . learning is generalizeable

Technical quality:
    . . . user oriented support materials
    . . . information display is effective
    . . . is reliable in normal use
    . . . intended users can easily operate.

Each category's major descriptors as listed are further delineated and include very specific descriptive criterion statements. Evaluator recommendations and descriptions of the strengths and weaknesses of programs are necessary as a part of this summative evaluative process.

One final but essential component of any protocol is user trial of the software. Very useful evaluative information about computer software is obtained from actual use and trial of the materials by intended users. Although this appears as very non-objective, this user trial mechanism provides a valid and most reliable source of information. If user trial before purchase or selection is not possible, then information from previous users should definitely be sought.

In summary, both formative and summative processes should be incorporated in any evaluation protocol. Information from a variety of sources should be used. Informally structured, early formative evaluational processes should gradually lead to more formalized protocols. Just as preplanning activities are an integral part of development, so too evaluation processes should be considered as both an early and integral part of development. A strong formative evaluative component actually reduces the necessity for extended periods of debugging, retrial and later revision. Time is well spent very early in planning activities and during development processes.

The evaluative protocol must also include a summative evaluation information. User trial is essential. Thus, the final criteria for the evaluative protocol can and probably should reflect a weighted listing based on individualised objectives, needs, and intended use. Good common sense tempered with intuitive judgements about the software from a broad knowledge of the publisher, developer, user and educator's perspective is absolutely essential.

REFERENCES

1.   Roblyer, M.D. Instructional design vs. authoring of courseware: some crucial differences, Association for Educational Data Systems Journal, 13. (1981) 243-7. p 243.
2.   Garraway, H. Its as easy as . . . 1, 2, 3. Instructional Innovator, 25 (No. 6, 1980) 20-21. p21.
3.   Crawford, S. A standard's guide for the authoring of instructional software: reference manual volume III. (Discovery Park, University of Victoria, P.O. Box 1700, Victoria, B.C. V8W2Y2 Canada, 1981) p2.

4.   Kleiman, G., Humphrey, M. and Van Buskirk, T. Evaluating educational software, Creative Computing 7 (October, 1981) 84-90. p84.

5.   Mace, S. Major book publishers are getting into the software business, Info World 4 (May 10, 1982) 13-19. (Info World, 375 Cochituate Road, Box 880, Framingham, MA 01701) p13.

6.   Ibid., p 16.

7.   Perry, T. and Zawalka, G. CAI: choosing hardware and software, Apple Orchard 3 (March-April, 1982) 22-24. p22.

8.   Kneifel, D.R., and Just, S.B.   Impact of microcomputers on educational computer networks, Association for Educational Data System Journal 13 (Fall, 1979) 41-52. p46.

9.   Steffin, S.A.   The educator and the software publisher: a critical relationship, T.H.E. Journal 9 (March, 1982) 63-64.   (Technological Horizons in Education, P.O. Box 992, Acton, Ma 01720) p63.

10.   E.P.I.E. Report, Microcomputer Courseware-Microprocessor Games, 98-99m. Educational Products Information Exchange, Box 620, Stony Brook, NY 11790, 1981. p4.

11.   Ibid., p 5.

12.   Ibid., p 7.

13.   Crawford, S.   A standard's guide for the authoring of instructional software: reference manual volume III.   (Discovery Park, University of Victoria, P.O. Box 1700, Victoria, B.C. V8W2Y2 Canada, 1981) p120.

14.   Ibid., p 101-2.

15.   Thomas, D. B. and McClain, D.H.   Selecting microcomputers for the classroom.   Association for Educational Data Systems Journal 13 (Fall, 1979) 55-68. p66.

16.   Wasserman, A.I. and Freeman, P.   Software engineering: status and prospects in Freeman, P. and Wasserman, A.I. (eds.), Tutorial on Software Design.   (Institute of Electrical and Electronics Engineers, Inc., N.Y., 1980) 445-452.   (IEEE Service Center, 445 Hoes Lane, Piscataway, N.J., 08854.) p445.

17.   Boehm, B.W.   Software and its impact: A quatitative assessment in Freeman, P. and Wasserman, A.I. (eds.), Tutorial on Software Design. (Institute of Electrical and Electronics Engineers, Inc., N.Y., 1980) 5-16.   (IEEE Service Center, 445 Hoes Lane, Piscataway, N.J., 08854.) p5.

18.   Wasserman, A.I. and Freeman, P.   Software engineering: status and prospects in Freeman, P. and Wasserman, A.I. (eds.), Tutorial on Software Design.   (Institute of Electrical and Electronics Engineers, Inc., N.Y., 1980) 445-452.   (IEEE Service Center, 445 Hoes Lane, Piscataway, N.J., 08854.) p443.

19.   Avner, R.A.   How to produce ineffective CAI materials, Educational Technology (August, 1974.) 26-27.   (140 Sylvan Ave., Englewood Cliffs, NJ 07632) p26 (Volume 14).

20.   Reed, F.C., Ertel, P.Y., and Collart, M.E.   A model for the development of computer assisted instruction programs, Educational Technology (March, 1974) 12-20. p13 (Volume 14)

21.   Ibid., p 13.

22.   Schultz, R.E. Computer aids for developing tests and instruction in O'Neil, H.F., Jr. (ed.) Procedures for Instructional System Development, (Academic Press, N.Y., 1979) 39-63. p42.

23.   Borich, G.D.   A systems approach to the evaluation of training, in O'Neil, H.F., Jr (ed.)   Procedures for Instructional Systems Development (Academic Press, N.Y., 1979).   205-231. p209, 210, 214,211.

24.   Grobe, S., Hudgings, C., Neusch, D., and Tarp, J.   Development of a Generic Nursing Process Model Using Cognitive Tasks: An Introduction, CAI Project, University of Texas at Austin, School of Nursing (1982). (Development funded by Division of Nursing HHS-D-10-NU 26044-01. p3.

25.   Scriven, M.   The methodology of evaluation, in Strake, R.E. (ed.) AERA Monograph Series on Curriculum Evaluation No I (Rand McNally, Chicago, IL, 1967).

26.   Sanders, J.R. and Cunningham, D.J.   A structure for formative evaluation
      in product development, Review of Educational Research 43 (No 2) 217-235.
27.   Peters, H.J. and Johnson, J.W. Author's Guide: design, development, style,
      packaging, review (CONDUIT Co., P.O. Box 388, Iowa City, Iowa 52244,
      1981).
28.   MicroSIFT: Evaluator's guide for microcomputer-based instructional
      materials, International Council for Computers in Education, Department of
      Computer and Information Science (University of Oregon, Eugene, OR 97403).

APPENDIX A

Instructional Methods:
Definitions* and Examples
from Nursing Education

DRILL AND PRACTICE: repetitive practice with feedback regarding correctness of
      responses (answers can be sensitive to users previous choices or randomly
      generated)

      EXAMPLE: A set of metric to apothecary conversions for computing drug
      dosages.   Users receiver positive feedback and are required to progress
      through increasingly complex calculations.

TUTORIAL: textual and graphic materials with response sensitive branching which
      is similar to a somewhat structure Socratic method on inquiry.

      EXAMPLE: An administrative decision-making sequence.

SIMULATION: model of complex phenomena for realism with interaction; compress
      time or model complexity of dangerous nature.

      EXAMPLE: A complex chemical reaction can be demonstrated without danger
      of explosion or injury to participants.

TESTING: provision of alternative testing; collapsed testing; item selection by
      reliability estimates and instantaneous scoring.

      EXAMPLE: Learners knowledge and understanding can be evaluated using
      randomly generated, individualized examinations.

PROBLEM SOLVING: the learning of rules and principles to apply to short
      algorithms to solve problems with a body of given data.

      EXAMPLE: An epidemiological investigation of neonatal diarrhea for
      community based nurses.   The nurse uses an available data base and
      proceeds through an inquiry process following specific protocols for
      investigation of the cause.

RESEARCH-DATA ANALYSIS: use of standardized statistical packages (i.e., SPSS,
      SAS, BMD, EXPERSIM.)

      EXAMPLE: Learners can collect data regarding the effects of specific
      nursing care on patients; can code the data and then analyze the data for
      either accepting or rejecting hypotheses regarding nursing care effects.

INFORMATION RETRIEVAL: search of large data bases using specific identifiers or
      flags to access a class or category of materials.

EXAMPLE: Users can access bibliographic data bases for citations related to a particular research area of interest.

PROGRAMMING: use of computer language used to control operations of the computer.

EXAMPLE: Nurse administrators can use programming algorithms to access different types of information from a stored data base.

*Source: Adapted from Thomas, 1979, p.58.

The Impact of Computers on Nursing
M. Scholes, Y. Bryant and B. Barber (eds.)
Elsevier Science Publishers B.V. (North-Holland)
© IFIP-IMIA, 1983

11.6.

COMPUTER ASSISTED INSTRUCTION IN NURSING EDUCATION – AN APPROACH

Susan E. Norman

> "If a patient is cold, if a patient is
> feverish, if a patient is faint, if he is
> sick after taking food, if he has a bed-sore,
> it is generally the fault not of the disease,
> but of the nursing".

Florence Nightingale
Notes on Nursing, 1859

Introduction

If one of the main aims in the nursing profession is to produce and maintain safe, well-informed practitioners then the profession has an obligation to explore and use new teaching and learning methods.

This paper is concerned with the use of computers in assisting instruction. Certain problems in pre and post-registration nurse education in the United Kingdom are identified and suggestions made as to how CAI (Computer Assisted Instruction) may minimise these. Considerations on software creation, programming, hardware and financial support are addressed.

CAI - Why Use It?

CAI has been in existence since the early 1960's, but has not developed into a major component of instructional method. The main reason for this has been the high cost of hardware. There are, however, several other factors identified by Porter which are as evident now as they were then and these will be discussed later(I25). What evidence is there to suggest that one should consider using CAI in nurse education? To what extent is student achievement enhanced? Almost all general education evaluation studies (1, 2) based on this factor conclude that CAI is more than equally effective as an alternative to traditional instruction. Similar studies in nurse education are few. However, two studies concerning nurse education in the United States came to the following conclusions:-

a) Although students using CAI did not learn more than the traditionally taught group, they took less time to learn the same material(I3).
b) Students were able to transfer their knowledge to clinical practice significantly better(I15).

If this last finding is substantiated in practice then CAI could have a significant beneficial effect on patient care. It could also help to bridge the gap between theory and practice, a problemm perhaps more significant in the United Kingdom due to the nature of nurse training. The lack of CAI evaluation studies in nurse education behoves one to collaborate with and learn from colleagues in secondary and further education who have knowledge and expertise in using CAI. It also demonstrates an area of much needed nursing research.

Problems in Nursing Education - CAI Advantages

As nurse education in the United Kingdom stands at present there are particular problems in both pre and post-registration learning that could be minimised with the use of CAI.

Pre-Registration

1   Mixed Ability Entry

CAI Advantage - Individualised Instruction.
An introductory course for State Registration may consist of students with educational attainments ranging from the minimum entry qualifications to an honours degree. This presents tutorial staff with a complicated mix of learning needs which, given the present tutor/student ratio, is almost impossible to meet let alone diagnose. Nor is this feature of nurse education likely to change for the better, since the suggestions of the United Kingdom Central Council working group on nurse education are for several varied routes to registration.

With sensitive and creative design and programming, CAI can provide a learning experience appropriate to the individual's needs(H3). There is opportunity for the repetition of part or whole of the program as often as desired without fear of peer or tutorial censure. CAI acts as a self-placed, one-to-one communication which can be at the students' rather than the teachers' convenience.

2   Application of Theory to Practice and its Evaluation

CAI Advantages   - Guided, Simulated Reality Practice
                                 - Recording of Results
                                 - Active Learning

The theory/practice gap is a common feature in nurse education and, as stated before, has particular significance in this country. For example, the length of training for state registration is approximately 146 weeks. Around twenty-eight of those weeks will be spent in the school or college of nursing, the remainder, by far the largest part, is spent gaining experience by giving paid service in the clinical area. This is largely unsupervised by those who teach the theory, therefore the practice gained clinically may bear little relation to that taught theoretically, and vice versa. When the practice is supervised, however well this might be, those doing so may have no idea of what has been taught. At best, some continuity is lost, at worst, conflict arises in the students due to two opposing areas of influence.

CAI programs written by nurse teachers in collaboration with clinical staff would help to promote continuity and reduce conflict. Not only could this provide guided, simulated practice in advance of an allocation but, better still, evaluate how well knowledge is being applied to clinical practice during and after that allocation - something which at present is difficult to do even with the advent of continuous assessment. A recent study by Olivieri and Sweeney(124) demonstrated how patient simulations in CAI can be used to evaluate the clinical expertise of the students the teachers plan to instruct.

One of the main features that differentiates CAI from other instructional methods is interactive learning. No response from a student will alter the material on a page, film or tape. With a CAI program however, progression is dependent on a student response. No opportunity for 'micro sleeps!' This sense of involvement is invaluable not only for learning but also for giving a feeling of reality to what is essentially a practice-based education. Two studies of medical students in Glasgow explored this active involvement. In the first(3) students who had used CAI made comments as follows:-

"Had to solve it ourselves - in the clinic the problem is already solved."
"Taught to think and think in terms of priorities."
"Could not side-step any of the decisions."

In the second(4), the interactive feature of CAI led to students using each other as a resource. A small group of three or four students seated around a microcomputer working on the same program promoted useful argument and discussion, an element of competition and not least of all, enjoyment.

3   Nursing Process and Decision Making

CAI Advantage - Guided, Simulated Practice

Much of the previous section applies to this one, but the nursing process requires particular mention. In providing a logical framework for teaching, learning and delivery of patient care it has revealed the need for students to learn and develop decision making skills. Practising this kind of skill on vulnerable individuals in unacceptable. Guided practice in a controlled environment is more desirable. Although students seem to have little difficulty in grasping the logic behind the nursing process they do have problems putting it into practice.

Again CAI programs written in collaboration with clinical staff could serve two purposes. Firstly, to provide guided, simulated practice and secondly help involve and educate trained staff who have not 'grown-up' with the nursing process. The latter point would hopefully help to promote continuity of supervision and reduce student conflict. The development of validated authoring systems at the School of Nursing, University of Texas at Austin,(Chapter 11.5) using the nursing process is regarded as a positive step forward.

4   Limited Supervised Practice

CAI Advantage - Optimisation of a Scarse Resource

As already stated there is a lack of continuity in supervision between theory and clinical practice. Added to this, tutor/student contact is limited due to the dual role of the learner necessitating long periods away from a conventional learning environment. The obvious answer is either to have more nurse teachers working as clinical practitioners in joint service/education appointments, or to make the students supernumery giving them more time to practice problem identification and management. This latter also requires increased supervision. The obvious is not always possible. Firstly there is a national shortage of nurse teachers running at 1,700 and improvement seems unlikely. Secondly, although there are moves afoot (UKCC suggestions from the working group on nurse education) to alter basic nurse education and reduce the service commitment, this will take considerable time. Meanwhile, students still have to be adequately prepared to provide the best possible care for their patients.

If one could have a series of CAI programs, graded in difficulty, simulating patient situations where students had to identify the patient's problems or needs and make decisions on nursing intervention required, correlation of theory and practice would take place in a manner that does not require the presence of a supervisor. It must be emphasised however, that CAI should be an adjunct to supervision not a replacement. CAI does not obviate the need for tutorial contact but rather it extends and makes better use of a scarce resourse - nurse teachers.

Post—Registration

1.   Maintenance of Competence and Updating

CAI Advantage - Challenge
             - Inform

Patients, trained nurses and employing authorities alike need to be assured of competent practice. Problem solving exercises that challenge the knowledge and decision making skills of trained staff can be developed on the computer as can the recording of those using the programs and their responses.   Similarly, policies and practices that change frequently, for example, intravenous drug administration can be put on a program and easily updated as and when required by new knowledge and developments.

2   Motivation and Time

CAI Advantage - Fun
             - Availability

No amount of microcomputers, terminals and CAI programs will motivate unwilling individuals to update or be challenged; but if they were to be 'frog-marched' to the terminal they might enjoy the experience, once there, more than attending a lecture. Most teachers who have dealt with computers have been struck by their strong motivational properties, something Levine and Wiener(I20) attribute to immediate feedback and the interactive 'pinball machine effect'.   Terminals or microcomputers can be available when teachers are not. One unit in a Glasgow hospital found nursing staff using programs developed for medical students. The nursing officer of the unit seized on the idea for in-service and continuing education.   Alas, there is no software available and little if any being developed for nurses by nurses.

3   Orientation

CAI Advantage - Labour Saving

This is probably the one area in which CAI would be rapidly cost-effective. With repetitive sessions on fire regulations, drug policies and general orientation, a CAI program that relieves the teacher of at least one of these and also records and evaluates responses could be a considerable saving.

4   Adult Learning, Mixed Ability and Experience.

CAI Advantage - Private
             - Individual

It is well known that adult learners are more reluctant than most to show their ignorance or lack of understanding. The privacy that CAI provides is therefore an advantage.   Many trained staff have greater difficulty than students in getting to grips with the nursing process for a number of reasons. CAI programs could help them practice application of the principles to patient care and help bring them in line with what the students are learning. Varied learning needs do not diminish with registration.   Rather, they are compounded by mixed experience, breaks in service or long service in one area. The same advantages of individualised instruction that CAI can provide apply to both pre-registration students and trained staff.

The Neglect Of CAI

By now CAI must appear as the panacea for all nurse education ills! Why, therefore, as mentioned earlier, has it not become a major instructional method? The five reasons that Porter (I25) identified are as follows:-

    Lack of: - stable financial support
             - experienced staff
             - standardisation of hardware and software
             - incentive to prepare programs
             - time.

The problems are no different today. The great danger is that now the major obstruction of hardware cost has been removed, nurse education establishments will be tempted to purchase systems without considering the above points. The manifold capabilities of microcomputers are widely advertised; the labour intensity of software production and evaluation is not.

Collaboration and Sharing

To date there is little nurse generated software in this country despite considerable widespread interest. A sizeable number of letters and telephone enquiries resulted from a paragraph the author wrote in a CAI newsheet (5). This surprisingly large response demonstrated an interest in CAI not only in schools of nursing, but also in educational establishments involved or hoping to be involved in nurse education.

There is much that can be learnt from colleagues in secondary and further education who are already engaged in software production. In certain subjects such as the biological sciences one could even share programs which in turn would help to cut costs and aid development. Valuable lessons could also be learned from the use of CAI in nurse education in other countries.

Most important of all, those interested in using CAI need to pool ideas and resources, to share development and to prevent wasteful and costly 're-inventions of the wheel'. The formation of local or regional CAI interest or user groups consisting of nurse teachers and teachers from further education would help to achieve this.

Considerations on Software, Programming, Hardware and Financial Support

Software

This must be considered **before** purchasing hardware. Who is going to write the programs? How much time will be allocated for this? To create one hour of educationally useful software takes between 200-400 hours (I17). What are the subject areas and teaching strategies to be used? Will this be an appropriate use of the computer? Collaboration with computer specialists is essential for classification of this last point. Most nurse educators do not have sufficient expertise to make this assessment.

Programming

Since the creation of educationally valuable software is time consuming and expensive, then ideally nurse authors should be programmers, but to achieve this would mean the authors spending so much time away from teaching that they would cease to be useful as nurse teachers and CAI authors. There are, however, several ways around this problem. One is to use authoring languages that require no programming expertise. Although limiting in teaching strategy, they are particularly useful for tutorial type programs. However, the sophistication

of the programs is probably limited by the degree of expertise the author does
or does not gain.

Another way round the programming is to buy professional help. This is useful
but expensive and potentially disruptive if author and programmer do not
collaborate well.   Ideally one needs to be lucky enough to have an in-house
programmer who is good at creating interactive programs, interested and clearly
understands the author's educational objectives.   There is a danger though in
authors becoming programmer dependent. If the programmer leaves, is unsuitable,
or ceases to be funded, then software production will cease.

Hardware

In the present state of ignorance, it is easy to be drawn into purchasing
unsuitable hardware.   It is vital that potential CAI authors clearly identify
their aims and objectives for CAI use **before** committing themselves to a
particular system.

Three points worth considering are:-

1.   What machines are other nurse education establishments using?
2.   Does the Regional Health Authority (or employing authority) have a policy
        regarding the type of computer hardware purchased?
3.   What computer systems are likely to have educational software developed
        for them?

Buying the same hardware as other CAI users in the same field aids development
of software enormously.   Each teacher knows what the other is talking about.
Programs can be exchanged, tried out, evaluated and eventually valuable
educational and programming standards set.   One area in which software has
developed well is secondary education where the type of hardware used is
virtually the same throughout due to Government policy. Following the employing
authority's policy on hardware, purchase can help standardisation, at least
locally, and also facilitate funding.

It stands to reason that if a system has been developed with mainly educational
use in mind, software will follow, some of which may well be suitable for nurse
education and if this is the case, then considerable savings on software
production can be made.

Financial Support

Most innovations involve add-on value for add-on cost and CAI is no
exception(1).   All the more reason then to collaborate with other nursing,
medical or technical colleges and universities, to share ideas, resources and
evaluation techniques.   In the present rush of enthusiasm 'one-off' funds for
hardware are not difficult to find. The financing of labour intensive software
production however, is quite a different matter. Hence the need to consider
software before hardware purchase, otherwise computers in nurse education could
suffer the same fate as some expensive but now redundant audio-visual aid
equipment.

In Conclusion

CAI is an interesting, exciting and valid use of the computer. If they are to
make the best use of its learning and teaching potential, then nurse teachers
must become involved in software creation and evaluation.   Ignorance of CAI's
potential could allow the profession to be swamped by a mass of inappropriate
software generated by commercially interested parties. Knowledge, on the other
hand, can give one the opportunity to use this potential to achieve one of the
profession's main aims - safe, well informed practitioners of nursing.

REFERENCES

1.   McDONALD, B., "The Educational Evaluation of NDPCAL"   British Journal of
      Educational Technology, 8.3. October 1977.
2   FRENZEL, L., "The Personal Computer - Last Chance for C.A.I.?"   Byte
      Publications, Inc., Peterborough, New Hampshire, U.S.A.   July 1980. 86-96.
3.   MURRAY,   T.S.,   BARBER,   J.H.,   DUNN,   W.R.,   "Attitudes   of   Medical
      Undergraduates   in   Glasgow   to   Computer-assisted   Learning".   Medical
      Education, 1978, 12. 6-9.
4.   KENNY,   G.N.C.,   SCHULMULIAN,   D.,   "Computer-assisted   Learning   in   the
      Teaching of Anaesthesia".   Anaesthesia, 34, 159-162. 1979.
5.   NORMAN, S.E., CALNEWS, 18. January 1982.

The Impact of Computers on Nursing
M. Scholes, Y. Bryant and B. Barber (eds.)
Elsevier Science Publishers B.V. (North-Holland)
© IFIP-IMIA, 1983

11.7.

THE SECOND COMING

Resurrection or Reservation?

Ian Townsend

> "Those who cannot remember the past are condemned to fulfil it".
> Santayana.

INTRODUCTION

The advent of a new strategy of teaching has always been regarded by some sectors of the educational community as an opportunity to hail the demise of the teacher, and welcome her replacement by sophisticated (albeit inanimate) technology. What even a cursory review of educational history shows is that if we are to succeed with computer assisted instruction,(CAI), this time round, then we have to remember the primacy of the teaching-learning relationship. Man, not technology, is the epicentre of this revolution, and man's continuing relationship with his students is not to be denied. If we fail to recognise this then CAI in nursing will suffer the same fate as the dinosaur, the dodo or (more appropriately perhaps) the leech - a footnote in the pages of history. Let us learn from the lessons of the past rather than repeat its mistakes. This paper will sound a cautionary note. Those willing to look back on the past 3 decades' history of educational development might be forgiven for saying "we've heard it all before - its been said time after time - and we're still waiting for the early promises to be met". So are we, in 1982, rediscovering the wheel? Can the past teach us anything at all? Or do we have to make the same mistakes all over again? An examination of some past innovations provide some points for computer based learning.

PROGRAMMED INSTRUCTION

The field of programmed instruction (PI) represents a considerable body of research spanning more than four decades. Within this research one finds significant pointers to present and future use of computer assisted learning,(CAL) and, indeed, many of the early workers in this field are currently commenting on the similarity between the present position and the early days of programmed instruction. Brian Lewis(35), Senior Professor at the Open University, writes:

> "I still enjoy recalling the heady razzle-dazzle excitement of those pioneering days. First, there were the travelling circuses - unlikely mixes of lecturers, salespersons, and technicians, moving all over the country to proclaim the Good News that PI had 'arrived'. And there was the equipment itself - machines of all shapes and sizes . . .
> The self-congratulatory conferences were no less memorable. Almost anything seemed to be possible".

Whilst enthusiasm is a laudable thing, we would do well to learn the lesson of the 1950's and 1960's - for what of programmed instruction now? Lewis points out that it contributed a "whole wealth of systems, guidelines, hints and 'simplification procedures' ... to help inform the practice of effective instruction" but he bewails the lack of effect this has had on education. "What stays with me, above all else, is the large number of valuable ideas that the PI movement either gave birth to or fostered - ideas which most present-day teachers seem hardly to know about".

This work provided guiding principles on the analysis, structuring, design and presentation of information through the printed page, the automatic teaching machine, the slide, filmstrip, or moving image. Correspondingly, Jurgemeyer (31) notes that "except for those involved in computer-assisted instruction, many of us have forgotten or discarded principles of programmed instruction as no longer being of value". Similar findings and sentiments had already been expressed some four years earlier, when Marson(36) reviewed her long involvement with PI in nurse education. Indeed, the only material thing from the PI movement to assume an important place in education was the emphasis on curricular objectives. While this is of course vital to the production of any sort of mediated instruction, the PI movement did generate so much more.

Many reasons have been given to explain why PI didn't maintain its early promises but Lewis gives two important ones. Insufficient academic recognition was given to the writers of first class material and hence leading proponents were not prepared to sponsor this educational development, also the situation was exacerbated by a general lack of good commercial software.

EDUCATIONAL MEDIA

The term is used here as a 'cover-all' for the use of simple audio-visual aids, the use of more complex equipment (such as CCTV), the more advanced use of learning packages and the sophisticated use of all of these in the context of individualised education in a resource centre. Each single item marks an educational development which whilst prominent over the past two decades only lingeringly continues in the present. The reasons for this failure have been discussed extensively (43,45,47, & 48) but there appear to be three main problems.

Firstly, much use of educational media has happened in the absence of clear-cut and publicly-debated research work. Indeed it is questionable whether we will ever be able to demonstrate the proven superiority of one method over another in terms of straightforward academic measurement of learning effectiveness.

Secondly, much of the failure of these early innovations can be traced to a failure of their originators and practitioners adequately to direct the underlying theory - the systematic use of educational technology - to address the vital areas of philosophy, curriculum and organisation. Furthermore, these early innovations failed to develop coherently.

Thirdly, any committment to a conceptually limited scheme "binds teacher, taught, and process into stereotypes which are pale reflections of what they could be"(43).

One of the most recent educational developments in this country has been that of the Learning Resource Centre. It has received much attention at all levels of general education as well as within nursing. In a two-year study of its evolution within nursing (42) it was noted for its limited dissemination. Shortly after this study Thornbury (40) demonstrated that as an innovation, the Resource Centre had failed to survive into the 1980s in its original form. What had happened was it changed from its concept as a source of self-directed learning to becoming a support system for the individual teacher. This view was also supported by a series of anonymous interviews conducted with individuals who had long been active in the resources movement (48). Even in universities where self-directed learning might have been thought to have had a better chance of survival, things proved to be grim.

In summary, it is necessary to think much more carefully about the financial implications of adopting a new strategy of instruction, making sure that it will deliver what it promises to. As recent experience shows

> "Schools across the country have hastened to adopt the new technology, often straining budgets . . problems resulting from this rapid transition include (1) Lack of standardisation of hardware, making software unusable in some cases; (2) Purchase of hardware before software is selected; (3) Inadequate preparation of faculty and (4) Repair and maintenance difficulties"(22).

Ackermann(1), quoting Ahl's (1977) survey (1,000 interviews), reports that

> "The quality of education is diminishing and at the same time the quantity of knowledge is increasing . . the technology that was generally in use in the classroom in the 70s was not very different from that which was generally in use in 1959 or 1940 or even 1930 . . teachers do not like technology, do not welcome it, and do not want anything that will change or usurp even part of their job".

It is by no means clear that things have changed significantly since the survey. It is most important to identify the objectives of any innovation, as Kaufman (32) suggests.

COMPUTER-BASED LEARNING: INTRODUCTION

This is no place for a full history of computer-based learning (CBL) but there is some merit in noting the early stages of today's developments. In the late 1950s and the 1960s many of the programmes generated by the young (and largely paper-based) PI movement became implemented on the computers of the day, with government funding assisting the process in the USA - but the size and cost of those early computers proved the method to be impractical. Even so, the early adoption by the computer of the theoretical approach of PI did mean that CBL was one of the few places were the pragmatic methodology of the early systems theorist survived.

The late 1960s and into the 1970s saw several extremely significant curriculum innovations. In the United States, Control Data Corporation introduced a powerful and sophisticated system - PLATO (based on the University of Illinois) which gave a hint of the power and versatility of CBL. Recently the system has produced in a microcomputer version, and CDC have just announced an ambitious project in association with the University of California to develop courses in high-technology subjects(19). Again in the States, MITRE Corporations TICCIT system (showing quite clearly the excellent influence of PI strategies mentioned in Jurgemeyer(31)) has shown what is possible(37).

In the United Kingdom, CBL has not attracted quite such a high level of funding and interest but despite this we have seen its use in the Open University (13), throughout the University system (in NDPCAL), and the Department of Education & Science-funded Microelectronics Education Programme(23) with its Scottish counterpart.

Another expansion of interest and use of CAI is becoming evident but before this is considered attention should be paid to the comments of those who have worked with it over the intervening years.

GENERAL ASSESSMENT

Looked at impassively there really is not a lot of evidence supportive of widespread and efficient use of this technology. Rushby(56) comments, "given that CBL is accepted as a powerful learning medium, it seems reasonable to ask why it has made so little impact in our teaching at all levels of education".

This is not an isolated criticism as can be seen from the many papers of CBL workers(50). Diem, noted(16), "Those schools which did try computer-assisted instruction, computer-managed instruction, or various methodological combinations that used computer technology as an integral part of daily classroom procedures were disappointed that technology could not solve all or even many of their instructional problems . . the residue of their disappointments helped create the reluctance toward using computers in classrooms which we are still experiencing to some degree today"(16).

Hiynka & Hurly(29) looking at the lack of impact that videotex and in particular at the Canadian Governments TELIDON system(12) suggest that three areas have contributed to its lack of impact. These they identify as the "gadget syndrome" where a preoccupation with shiny gadgetry overwhelms the potential user who is then seen by his colleagues as a "technician playing with toys" - a point of view also identified by the author(44). The second area deals with the general mythology that AV media can do wondrous things - followed closely by the third area which illustrates the inadequacy of media research indicating that research has been done on the wrong things and for the wrong reasons.

Neuhauser, comments that "the last twenty years have witnessed much effort devoted to increasing educational effectiveness and/or efficiency through a strong alliance with technology ... considering the makeshift nature of a good deal of the early CAI material courseware and the technology by which it had to be delivered ... it is surprising that performance wasn't worse"(38). In all fairness, however, he goes on to point out that more recent efforts (such as TICCIT and PLATO) "have also demonstrated that there is far more to teaching and, particularly learning, than we might have thought".

Frenzel(24), claims that CAI has not demonstrated any superiority over other teaching approaches. "Drill and practice" CAI was seen as unimaginative in use, the computer as an inefficient and expensive electronics page turner only able to deliver limited text and simple graphics. Furthermore Frenzel criticises the then-available author languages on the ground of time: quoting a ratio of from 100 to 200 to 1: even greater than that given for other forms of mediated instruction. It is worthwhile, in passing, to note that Neuhauser gave an estimate of 300-500 hours of preparation time for one hour of PLATO-delivered instruction, and Babb(6) inflates this even further to a figure of 100 to 1,000 hours preparation per terminal hour. Additionally, Kenyons(33) experience in the use of computer-generated multiple-choice question banks identifies a further time constraint:

> "it also requires a great deal of secretarial time to put in suitable banks of questions which must be quite large if frequent repetition of the same question is to be avoided".

However, Frenzel identifies two more areas which are even more important to pay attention to. The first is that of authorisation, the second is that of applicability.

AUTHORING

Frenzel points out that the preparation of a good computer based teaching package depends (like the preparation of any other sort of mediated instruction) on quite rare individuals. That is, individuals who not only possess expert subject knowledge (or who can effectively work with such experts), but who are capable of analysing and synthesising the teaching logic of the knowledge to be presented, arrange it with regard to good graphic presentation and learner interactivity, and then adapt all this for the computer by transcribing it into the most appropriate author language. As he says, "few good course programmes have become available ... what ... is available is only fair to poor and, most of it is too simple"(24).

Nievergelt supports this view, in his comment that "today it makes no sense to start a CAI project unless one is willing to write most of the necessary courseware"(39). From this we can see that the adoption of CAI in any form may well be a necessarily expensive project. Certainly the hardware is becoming cheaper, but the software costs are expensive and they are expected to rise.

APPLICABILITY

The body of CAI research has not looked into those areas where one suspects positive gains could be demonstrated - the areas of motivation and attitude. This is largely due to the fact that its early development based it on theories which paid little attention to these areas. PI theory did pay attention to motivation but this awareness has not survived into the 1980s. Nievergelt criticises the field as having no relevant theory to guide the designer, administrator, or user(39).

This failure of educational technology to address a wide base has been demonstrated elsewhere (29,45,54) and is summed up by Tom Stoniers' comment (60) "we can no longer afford a society where progress depends upon technologists who are humanistic illiterates". Indeed the simplistic use of CAI in its essentially programmed-learning based drill and practice mode has led Papert(62) to remark that this use of CBL does great violence to the potential of the computer.

ACCEPTANCE

Another group of problems lies with getting teacher-acceptance. Aiken & Braun (2) point out that this is probably the biggest challenge to be met by advocates of CAI, and Benington(8) in his study of the effectiveness of independent learning packages in a polytechnic reminds us that this has long been a problem in areas other than CAI. Rushby(56) gives a possible reason for this in saying that CAI is "perceived by many teachers as being beyond their ken, and only for a select few who are versed in computing or mathematics".

A further, compounding factor must be the change in role that is demanded of the teacher who accepts involvement with this medium. Well noted in the literature of educational media and individualised instruction, it involves switching from being a primary source of knowledge to that of a facilitator and consultant (7, 54,59,15). This change is a major watershed and it requires extensive preparation.

The relevance of this may be seen in a recent account of an attempt to introduce microcomputers into an American high school(25).

Hawkins carried out a major questionnaire-based survey of 61 centres of CBL in tertiary education. In his preparatory work he generated a 500-title bibliography, and, in assessing the first 100 titles from it, concluded that "whatever other things were reported, the problems and barriers encountered in computer-based learning and how they could best be overcome, were not among them(26).

He noted that much of the flowering of the movement depended not on establishment support but on individual effort (a finding also echoed in earlier research with educational media and learning resource centres). He was critical of the work done in CBL, noting that projects were developed without the benefit of the systems approach and without feasibility studies(27). He also noted that "the lack of curriculum building skills was a greater problem than lack of computer skills"(26).

LESSONS FROM CURRICULUM INNOVATION

The UK has a long history of curriculum innovation. The past 3 decades have seen all manner of schemes at primary, secondary and tertiary level come and go, alter and evolve - and die. What, if anything, can the evaluation studies of these innovations teach us, now we are faced with the possibility of CAL appearing on the nursing scene? Eraut(64) carried out an analysis of studies that had been made of seven major curriculum projects. He underlined the need for in-service support and he also identified the need rationally to consider all sides of the argument when faced with a potential innovation.

Steadman(67), in an investigation into the impact and takeup of a range of Schools Council-funded activities (drawing from a random sample of schools) found a confused picture, but a lack of awareness of published work was identified as a major problem. This lack of awareness of the published literature is one which recurrs in the history of innovation.

Ruddock & Kelly(66) in yet another massive survey of a range of educational innovations (this time occuring in 6 European countries) commented that

"Its main purpose must be to point to the need for more extensive, empirical studies of dissemination . . information about dissemination and diffusion . . appears to be negligable, or, at least, not very accessible".

The most stunning account of a curriculum innovation of most recent times is written up in Hebenstreit(65). In this account, Hebenstreit gives details of the introduction of CAI into the French educational system. He covers the first stages of the experiment (1970-1976) in which some 5,000 teachers were trained, a specific programming language developed (to ensure transferability of programs), 7000 copies of 500 programs distributed, and around 700 computer terminals activated. The experiment was evaluated, and a significant finding related to the amount of time spent at the terminal:

"the mean use of each (terminal) is about 20 hours per week . . . the evaluation of terminal use during NDPCAL (a 6-year British project aimed mainly at university-level use) showed a mean use of 500 hours per year: during France's experiment the terminals . . . also figured out to be about 500 hours per year".

The second stage of the experiment (1979-1985) aims to install 10,000 microcomputers within secondary schools:

"Even though 10,000 microcomputers will be in French schools by 1985, CAI will still be a scarce resource at that time. By 1985, there will be one microcomputer for every 73 students, allowing each student 15 minutes of use per week. For each student to have one hour of daily use, 200,000 computers would be needed. However, what is most likely to occur within the next five years is that some students will have a few hours of use each week and others will have none at all".

Finally, Stenhouse(68), in his masterly assessment of 16 major curriculum projects, claims that curriculum innovation has improved teacher development, revolutionised curriculum studies and teaching materials, changed the conduct of educational bodies (who have become more consciously self-explorative) and has led students to expect high-quality knowledge, attractively packaged.

WHAT OF COMPUTER USE IN NURSING?

Turning now to problem areas in the use of computers and the exciting possibilities these offer. Norman & Townsend (H5) identified 50 papers dealing with the use of computers in nurse education. Few of these are in any sense detailed. Nonetheless the following issues are addressed, or at least identified:-

1. The need to consider very deeply the impact of the computer on nursing-as-a-whole (B5,B4,I31,51,B34,9)
2. Educational (I18,H3,I25).
3. Technical (53)
4. Linguistic aspects(B12) limitations.

No nursing author accessed has pointed out the need for educationally sound design of computer programs and provided instances of this. Two recent papers (14,63) do provide the type of easily understandable design information that is needed. In terms of printed information, one of the best repositories of useful hints and tips is to be found in Rowntree(55).

BUT WHAT OF THE FUTURE?

It is interesting to reflect on how much of the work discussed above is appropriate to the rapidly changing scene - the advent of the microcomputer has much to answer for. The basic concepts relating to systems design are unaltered but of course the opportunities available to the designer are much wider with present day technology. These opportunities will expand as faster, greater capacity and more versatile computer hardware becomes available at a reasonable cost allowing more versatile software to be developed. Furthermore, simpler and more convenient ways of communicating with computers will become available.

Deeson(15) reported that in general education in the UK, 50% of British Schools had computer power available - with an increase, over the 5 year period 1975-1980 in the number of entries at examination level (for computer studies) rising by 28,000. Microcomputers will penetrate the educational scene even if no one does anything at all to help them. It is noteworthy that magazines on microcomputers now outsell other traditional leaders in the field.

As Bostock points out, regarding an earlier phase of the revolution

"Microtechnology actually first came knocking at the classroom door some six or seven years ago when children began to bring pocket calculators to school . . all has now settled to a point where the calculator lies unobserved in the pencil case, to be called up as a resource along with the biro and the compass"(10).

Ackerman, writing this year, was predicting "a new generation of computers every 5 years"(1), - too late, as it turned out. For two years previous to this, Aiken & Braun(2) had delineated the three generations of computers which have swept the market since 1975, and in the intervening period the market has remained far from static: with Commodore, Acorn and Sinclair launching new models. It used to be said that computers were becoming so cheap that their purchase could be financed for nursing through fund-raising activities such as raffles and bring-and-buy sales. Now it is more than likely that they will soon be cheap enough to buy out of petty cash. However, two words of warning are necessary:

1   "How does the cost of a fully computerised programme of nursing education compare with the cost of existing programmes? I don't know the answer, moreover it seems to be a premature question. It is based on an assumption that, given the money, we could buy a fully developed system and perhaps buy into an established computer network. However, converting to computerised systems of nursing education seems to be analagous to adding a child to the family: the money is over and above the inconvenience, waiting, and perhaps pain and nausea of it"(1).

2   "A 'citizens actions committee' has been formed in California aimed at halting what it calls the bandwaggon effect being promulgated by the microcomputer industry to put 'costly general purpose computers into virtually every American classroom' . . . 'There is definately a role for the computer in education but suddenly, only because its manufacturers have told us so, it is being proposed as an instructional aid for basic skills. I say this is overskill at its worst and someone has to begin questioning it before massive sums of money are spent prematurely'"(20).

The problem is that there is no one central location to which schools of nursing can go for nursing-specific information. Most microcomputers in nursing seem to have been purchased with a view to aiding allocations, time-tabling, and, perhaps, "being used in the classroom". There is no doubt that they do have the potential, if properly provided and organised, to deliver a sophisticated, accurate and highly motivating style of learning. However there are few commercially available computer programs on nursing subjects and schools wishing to experiment will have to develop their own. In a time of chronic understaffing, with class sizes in some cases approaching 70 - how many schools will be able to make use of the microcomputer? If schools are to explore curricular use they need advice, encouragement, support, and contact with kindred spirits eleswhere(Babb 6).

Table 1 provides a check list for the acceptance of information technology derived from the literature search.

THE SECOND COMING - POSSIBILITIES & POTENTIALS

That CAL has been used (albeit at random, and in isolation) in nursing cannot be denied as the following summary will show. What needs stressing is that each of the developments referenced here are in all too many cases simply isolated examples of good practice: an unfortunate feature of most innovatory procedures. Nevertheless, in looking to what has gone before, one can often gain insight on possible roads to take to the future.

COMPUTER LITERACY

Ronald's(H8) paper is a very important one, describing as it does the setting up of an experimental course on computer literacy for nurses. This is unique in the literature.

WIDE-RANGING EFFECTS

Timke & Janney (41) have reported that CAI seems useful in reducing problems of
student anxiety and embarassment. Buchholz(I5) notes its possible benefit to
enthusiastic motivation of learning.

Hofstetter(30) suggests that CAI can effect transfer of learning to actual
situations and that it is better adapted to yield self-pacing for mastery
learning and it enhances creativity on the part of both teacher and taught.
This is supported by Oliviera & Sweeney(I24) on computer simulation, and by
Donabedian(17), Lamy(34) and Taylor(61) in their papers describing aspects of
problem-solving with CAL.

SHARING INFORMATION

Some interesting work has been carried out in this area. Alvar(4) describes a
computerised resource network, banking and sharing data from nurse educators
related to course goals and objectives. Saba(57) shows how a three-year project
led to the establishment of an on-line, searchable database of information files
related to nursing orientated literature, abstracts, and 'fugitive' documents.

EMERGENT AREAS

Kamp & Burnside(I16) in an excellent paper (the only reported application)
describe the use of CAI in psychiatric nursing. Silva(59) also addresses the
important issue of how to support the development of trust and freedom in
learning with computer-assisted instruction.

There is a further point not considered so far - and aptly illustrated in a
recent issue of 'Educational Technology':

> "The computer could not have come at a more opportune time. Into a field
> beset with countless troubles, including, most importantly, demoralised
> teaching staffs at all levels, has come SOMETHING new.
> For the first time in years we see many educators interested in and
> excited about their jobs"(21).

How far this applies to the profession of nursing remains to be seen, but it is
indicative of the effect of CAL on the moral of staff in other areas.

What else can be gathered from the general literature? Leaving aside such
esoteric developments as computer-interactive videodisc, there are three
interesting developments reported:

1   Alty(3) remarks that users joined together in networks will become
     important - giving more computing ability at lower price.

2   Edmonds(18) observes that with CAL it is possible to present the
     appearance of student freedom in what seems to be an unstructured learning
     environment. It is not only seems important to motivate the student and
     give her responsibility for her own learning, it also makes use of the
     great power of the computer when coupled with modern authoring languages.
     Additionally it makes possible the identification - by the student - of
     her own unique learning processes. With the developments by Shaw (58) and
     Taylor(61) of computerised approaches to Kelly Repetory Grid Techniques,
     more insight is now available to the individual on how she communicates
     with herself and others.

3   Boyd(11) in a unique paper, elaborates on the societal impact of the differing styles of CAI and points to the possibility of using computers to provide specialised personal support systems.

It is in all these areas that CAI has much to offer - and about which there is so much to learn. Over and above the excellent uses of CAI - ranging from the simple 'drill-and-practice' excercises to the much more complex simulations, from its motivational effect on our students to its support of our-and-their-management of learning, we need to remember that, as Frank Herbert has it, human beings

>   " . . . evolved to confront infinity. Computers work within mechanical limits"(28).

In nursing, surely the most humanistic of all professions, it would not do to forget this in the wave of enthusiasm that computer-generated interest brings.

TABLE 1: GUIDELINES FOR GETTING INFORMATION TECHNOLOGY ACCEPTED.

1)   Realise that "hope" is not the same as reality.
2)   Not all change is good or useful.
3)   Means and ends are different - but are related (or they should be).
4)   Some people do object to everything new and different.
5)   At what level (anecdotal, personal, research) is your proposed use of CAL supported?
6)   Read the literature on similar work before starting.
7)   Read outside of your field.
8)   Evaluate your innovation.
9)   If you are going to 'research' - at least make sure you're not doing another dry 'comparison of CAI with . . .' be creative in asking the right questions.
10)   Don't believe people will read - persuade them personally.
11)   Avoid presenting yourself as a "technican playing with toys".
12)   Be aware of the total educational, technical and sociological implications of what you are proposing.
13)   Not all innovation contributes to useful organisational results.
14)   Make sure that the change you are suggesting links to individual effort, organisational effort, and professional impact. If it doesn't - revise it.
15)   Try to arrange for coherent support of your innovation by considering its possible effects on the philosophy, curriculum, and organisational setting of your establishment.
16)   Not every resistor to change is bloody-minded: it is sometimes useful to have active resistors to help you conceptualise and justify what otherwise might be enthusiasm gone astray.
17)   If you show people the reasons for change in terms of what might happen - they may well be more likely to listen to you.
18)   Listen to the people who are being asked to change.
19)   Pay attention to points against your innovation as well as points for.
20)   Carefully conceptualise your model of introduction.
21)   Carefully plan your rate of introduction.
22)   Once it's working well, how are you going to get continuing use out of it?
23)   Support your enthusiastic but isolated innovator.
24)   Plan to teach curriculum building skills rather than computing ones.
25)   Have a definate plan for in-service training.
26)   Arrange for specialised secretarial support.
27)   Identify the software you are going to use BEFORE you buy the hardware.
28)   Ensure that good quality software is available.
29)   If you take delivery of poor quality commerical software - send it back.

30) If there is no appropriate software available, ensure you have access to the appropriate skills.
31) Prepare the presentation of your content according to good theory: much useful information is being ignored.
32) Prepare your teaching material according to the precepts of PI: careful analysis, small steps, systematic approach to content.
33) Use an appropriate, but compatible, language.
34) Press for academic/professional recognition for program-writers.
35) Ensure that hardware and software are compatible before signing that cheque.

REFERENCES

1.   Ackerman W.B. (1982): "Technology & Nursing Education: A Scenario for 1990". J. Advanced Nursing. 7, 59-68.
2.   Aiken R. & Braun L. (1980): "Into the 80s with Microcomputer-Based Learning". Computer. July, 11-16.
3.   Alty J.L. (1982): "The Impact of Microtechnology: A Case For Reassessing the Roles of Computers in Learning". Computers & Education. Vol 6, 1-5.
4.   Alvar H. (1976): "A Simple CISNE Computerised Information Service for Nursing Educators Nursing Course". ERIC No: ED 121 388.
5.   Aston M. (1981): "Viewdata: Implications for Education". Computer Education. February, 43-44.
6.   Babb P.W. (1982): "The Accidental Revolution and Higher Education: Administration Fiddles while Computers Doze". Educational Technology. April, 11-14.
7.   Bavin C. (1973): "Clinical Teaching and the Use of AV Aids". Nursing Times. 12 July, 912-913.
8.   Benington M. (1982): "Lecturers Attitudes to Independent Learning Packages in H.E.". P.L.E.T. Vol 19, No 2, June, 148-157.
9.   Bennet L.R. (1970): "This I Believe . . . That Nurses May Become Extinct". Nursing Outlook. January, 28-32.
10. Bostock M. (1982): "Microtechnology: The Challenge to Education". Computer Education. June, 5-6.
11. Boyd G. (1982): "Four ways of Providing Computer-Assisted Learning and their Probable Impacts". Computers and Education. Vol 6, 305-310.
12. Brahan J.W. & Godfrey D. (1982): "A Marriage of Convenience: Videotex and Computer Assisted Learning". Computers and Education. Vol 6, 33-38.
13. Bramer M. (1980): "Using Computers in Distance Education: The First Ten Years of the British Open University". Computers and Education. Vol 4, 293-301.
14. Burkhardt H. et al (1982): "Teaching Style and Program Design". Computers and Education. Vol 6, 77-84.
15. Deeson E. (1981) "School Computers: Some Lessons to be learnt". Your Computer. December, 45-46.
16. Diem R.A. (1982): "Education and Computer Technology: Some Unresolved issues". Educational Technology. June, 19-21.
17. Donabedian D. (1976): "Computer-Taught Epidemiology". Nursing Outlook. December, Vol 24, No 12, 749-751.
18. Edmonds E. (1980): "Where Next in C.A.L.?". Brit. J. Educ. Technology. Vol 11, No 2, May, 97-104.
19. Educational Technology (1982): "Computer News". May, p6.
20. Educational Technology (1982): "News Notes". June, 7-9.
21. Educational Technology (1982): "Technically Speaking". April, 40-41.
22. Farrell J.J. (1981): "Media in the Nursing Curriculum". Nurse Educator. July/August, 15-19.
23. Fothergill R. & Anderson J.S.A. (1981): "Strategy for the Microelectronics Education Programme (M.E.P.)". P.L.E.T. Vol 13, No 3, August, 121-135.

24. Frenzel L. (1980): "The Personal Computer - Last Chance for C.A.I.?. Byte. July, 86-96.

25. Grossnickle D.R. et al (1982): "Profile of Change in Education: a High School Faculty adopts/rejects Microcomputers". Educational Technology. June, 17-19.

26. Hawkins C.A. (1978): "C.B.L. Why and Where is it Alive and Well?". Computers and Education. Vol 2, 187-196.

27. Hawkins C.A. (1978): "A Survey of the Development, Applications and Evaluation of C.B.L. in Tertiary Education in the U.K., the U.S.A., The Netherlands and Canada". in 'Aspects of Educational Technology' Vol X11, Kogan Page, 323-329.

28. Herbert F. & Barnard M. (1981): "The Home Computer Handbook". London: Victor Gollancz Ltd.

29. Hiynka D. & Hurly P. (1982): "Correspondence Education and Mass Media: Some Issues and Concerns". P.L.E.T. Vol 19, No 2, June 158-165.

30. Hoftsetter F.T. (1979): "Fourth Summative Report of the Delaware Plato Project". Eric Ed 202-472.

31. Jurgemeyer F.H. (1982): "Programmed Instruction: Lessons it can Teach Us" Educational Technology. May, 20-22.

32. Kaufman R. (1982): "Means and Ends: To Change or not to Change?. Educational Technology. February, 34-36.

33. Kenyon et al (1982): "Computer-Aided Self Assessment". Medical Teacher Vol 4, No 2, 67-70.

34. Lamy V. (1976): "Is Problem Solving Something That can be Taught?". Am. Lung Assn. Bulletin. Vol 62, No 10, 8-9.

35. Lewis B.N. (1982): "Its Seems to Me . . .". Educational Technology. February, 36-37.

36. Marson S.N. (1979): "P.I. Prohise, Predagation and Progress". in Page & Whitlock (eds) "Aspects of Educational Technology XIII" Kogan Page.

37. Merrill M.D. (1980): "Learner Control in Computer-Based Learning". Computers and Education. Vol 4, 77-95.

38. Neuhauser J.J. (1977): "A Necessary Redirection for Certain Educational Technologies". Computers and Education. Vol 1, 187-192.

39. Nievergelt (1980): "A Pragmatic Introduction to Courseware Design". Computer. September, 7-21.

40. Thornbury R., Gillespie J., Wilkinson G. (1979): "Resource Organisation in Secondary Schools: Report of an Investigation". Working Paper 16, C.E.T.

41. Timke J. & Janney P. (1981): "Teach Drug Dosages by Computer". Nursing Outlook. June, 376-377.

42. Townsend I.J. (1978): "Caring to Learn: The Evolution and Practice of Resource-Based Learning in Nurse Education". Unpub. MA Thesis. University of York, Dept. of Education.

43. Townsend I.J. (1979): "The AV Revolution: Do we Really Need It?". J. Adv. Nursing. 4, 181-192.

44. Townsend I.J. (1980): "Come into My Parlour, Said the Spider . . .". P.L.E.T. Vol 17, No 3, November, 271-274.

45. Townsend I.J. (1980): "The Learning Resources Movement: Its Relationships to Nurse Education". J. Adv. Nursing. 5, 513-529.

46. Townsend I.J. (1980): "Rediscovering the Wheel". Feedback No 3. May/June. NHS LRU.

47. Townsend I.J. (1981): "Microprocessors - state of the art". NHS LRU. Sheffield.

48. Townsend I.J. (1981): "The LRC: Historical perspective and current demand". Nurse Education Today.

49. Walker D. & Megarry J. (1981): "The Scottish Microelectronics Development Programme". P.L.E.T. Vol 18, No 3, August, 130-135.

50. Wiezenbaum J. (1976): 'Computer Power & Human Reason". W H Freeman.

51. Wheway I. (1979): "The Computer: Servant or Master?". Health Visitor. September, Vol 52, 364-365.

52.   N.R.I.G. (Edinburgh): Newsletter, December, '81. 2 pps.
53.   Piankian R. (1978): "Computer Hardware: Operation, Applications and Problems". J. Nursing Administration. February, 8-13.
54.   Roberts K. (1981): "'Futurizing' the Curriculum - Nursing Education for the year 2000". Aust. Nurses J. Vol 11, No 3, September, 49-52.
55.   Rowntree D. (1966): "Basically Branching". MacDonald: London.
56.   Rushby N. (1980): "Getting Started with Computer-Based Learning". Visual Education. p8.
57.   Saba V.K. & Skapik K.A. (1979): "Nursing Information Center". Am. J. Nursing. January 86-87.
58.   Shaw M. (1979): "Personal Learning Through the Computer". Computers and Education. Vol 3, 267-272.
59.   Silva M.C. (1973): "Nursing Education in the Computer Age". Nursing Outlook. 94-97.
60.   Stonier T. (1979) in Schuller & Megarry (Eds) (World Yearbook on Education Recurrent Education and Lifelong Learning) "Changes in Western Society: Educational Implications" Kogan Page. 31-44.
61.   Taylor A.P. (1980): "C.A.L. Clinical Simulations for Nursing". In Winterburn & Evans (Ed.) Aspects of Educational Technology Vol.XLV Kogan Page. ETIC '80.
62.   Paport S. (1980): "Mindstorms". Harvester Press Ltd.
63.   Kidd M. E. & Holmes G. (1982): "Courseware Design - Exploiting the Colour Micro". Computers and Education. Vol. 6, 299-303.
64.   Eraut M., (1976): "Some Recent Evaluation studies of Curriculum Projects - a Review" in Tawney, D., "Curriculum Evaluation Today - Trends & Implications, Macmillan Education, pp 102-124.
65.   Hebenstreit J., (1980): "10,000 Microcomputers for the French Secondary Schools", Computer, July.
66.   Ruddock J., & Kelly P., (1976): "The Dissemination of Curriculum Development", N.F.E.R.
67.   Steadman S.D., et al. (1978): "Impact and Take Up Project", S.C. Publications
68.   Stenhouse L., (1980): "Curriculum Research & Development in Action", Heinemann.

The Impact of Computers on Nursing
M. Scholes, Y. Bryant and B. Barber (eds.)
Elsevier Science Publishers B.V. (North-Holland)
© IFIP-IMIA, 1983

11.8.

COMPUTER ASSISTED LEARNING

Discussion

Software development

Three examples of current processes employed for software development were (1) development by manufacturers with input from consultants and educators; (2) acquisition and distribution by publishers; and, (3) development and distribution by individual educators, or groups of educators. It was noted that individuals may have difficulty distributing the software they develop, and could make use of The Harvard Directory of Software Products as well as other distribution resources cited in Susan Grobe's article. The need was emphasised for any developer of software to get input from potential users (i.e. nursing faculty) during the planning and formative evaluation stages.

Creative ways of approaching the goal of developing high quality software in a cost-effective manner were examined. Nurses based in university settings noted that they have valuable colleagues in other fields available as resources, as well as inexpensive staff in the form of graduate students in computer science, instructional technology, audio-visual technology, and other relevant areas.

Staying Abreast of Changing Technology

Peripheral equipment (such as video discs and video tape technology) that enhance educational effects are becoming increasingly available. In addition, authoring systems that enable people without great computer expertise to develop programs are proving useful.

Logistics of Funding/Management in Educational Computing Projects

Experienced managers of computing projects commented that it is important to establish a broad, flexible time-schedule for completion of a project. The time needed for software development can prove hard to predict; always allow more than initially projected. Additionally some management experience, or understanding of certain basic managerial concepts, helps ensure smooth running and successful completion of projects.

What if funding from usual sources is not available? Creativity in the search for funds is imperative. Suggestions include exploring foundation funding or liaison with industry or publishing companies.

Dissemination

Product usefulness is enhanced if the development and distribution of software products is aimed at a specific audience. One diskette cannot always serve the needs of persons from several education and experience levels. When creating materials aimed at health care consumers (such as patient education content), consider the users' general background and level of understanding.

There are many issues relating to copyright to be considered. Existing copyright law regarding electronic media is unclear and difficult to enforce. A similar, but less complex, situation arose following the appearance of photocopiers on the market. Legislation related to copyright of electronic media needs clarification at both national and international levels followed by dissemination of this information to those working in the electronic media field.

Resources

To what resources can education realistically turn for advice on hardware/software selection and the development, evaluation, distribution and implementation of software packages? Nurse educators will find a multidisciplinary approach valuable to increase knowledge and expertise by drawing upon resources in the general educational and computing sectors, formal and informal "networking" in meeting information needs and getting necessary support. There are lenders such as TERC (Technical Education Resource Centre) in Cambridge, Massachusetts, USA and similar facilities are understood to be available in other countries and in particular work is progressing on this subject on the UK, where visitors can try out hardware and software in computer laboratories and get information from unbiased, experienced and knowledgeable personnel.

Education

There is a need to define the scope of nursing and to establish a base line to evaluate the outcomes from using computer assisted learning.

Ethical issues are raised regarding education, and evaluation of student progress based on information resulting from students' interaction with educational programmes. Since students may understand their interaction with the computer to be private, educators who plan to use the information produced to assess learning programme lesson quality, or for other reasons, should be certain students are informed of this possibility.

CHAPTER 12

EDUCATION PROGRAMMES AND RECORDS

One essential feature of all education programmes is accurate and easily retrievable records.

The central training records are required in the UK and these together with the records required locally by nurse educators are described below.

The Impact of Computers on Nursing
M. Scholes, Y. Bryant and B. Barber (eds.)
Elsevier Science Publishers B.V. (North-Holland)
© IFIP-IMIA, 1983

12.1.

COMPUTER BASED SYSTEMS FOR PROFESSIONAL EDUCATION AND TRAINING

Sheila Collins O.B.E.

Introduction

All professionals need on-going education, updating and re-training in times of change and development. Changes in society, both national and international, research findings, scientific and technological advances, and the increasing awareness and expectancy of individuals, present challenges to us all. Not the least of these, is the need for speedier and more reliable information and communication. Although a pony and trap (or horse and buggy) may seem an attractive means of transportation, particularly during a rail strike, it is not particularly appropriate in this era of space travel. Professional education should anticipate future trends, as well as reflect current needs. Nursing education programmes, as we approach the year 2000 AD, will continue to focus on the central component of nursing, on the person as a potential or actual patient, needing compassion, caring and competence. The latter part of the 20th century has brought an explosion of discoveries in medical and allied sciences which demand skilful knowledge and understanding on the part of nurses in their care of patients. Technology can help to provide the nurse with systems within which plans can be formulated for basic and continuing education, and for updating by self-directed learning. Some of the different ways in which computer based systems are being used in nursing education and training include:-

a) information storage and retrieval for teaching and learning purposes, for example, drug interaction data; training aids for SI units.
b) recording health surveillance, or patient progress plans, for example, immunisation programmes in primary health care, patient care planning in general and psychiatric nursing.
c) assessing and recording students' progress, for example computer based marking of tests, validating item banks.
d) research and evaluation by analysing data, and providing comparative statistics, for example, by analysing test scores, and making comparisons between cohorts, or between differing tests for each cohort.
e) the management and use of resources, for example, by providing comparative data to enable choices to be made, and control to be exercised, in planning.

It is on this latter aspect that this paper will attempt to concentrate, since it forms the basis on which planning for reality in nursing education and training rests, and on which the nurse, the nurse educator and the nurse manager build for the future. The resources which the system needs to provide for professional nursing education are described in the following section.

The Basic Level

The nursing student should be provided with opportunities for learning about:-

a) health, health education and the prevention of illness;

b)   humanity - the nurse needs to be a 'people person', recognising individual differences, needs and responses, for example, to disability;

c)   the effects of illness on the individual and his life-style and family;

d)   measures of treatment or relief of pain and discomfort, and for rehabilitation or support.

European Community Directives for the Nurse for General Care

In Europe, nurses are seeking to harmonise their approaches to nursing education so that free movement of qualified nurses can occur within the countries in the Community. These directives require that a balance is achieved between the theoretical instruction provided in nursing schools and defined as "where students acquire the knowledge, understanding, and professional skills needed to plan, provide and assess total nursing care", and between the clinical instruction wherein the students, "as part of a team, in direct contact with a healthy or sick individual" learn to give that care "on the basis of their acquired knowledge and skills"(1).

Each of the countries within the Community seeks to achieve such a balanced programme to suit the needs of the country, and of the competent authority within the framework of the laws in force. In the UK, the modular system, or modifications of it, in England, Wales and Northern Ireland, the wider basic training programmes in Scotland, and in France the new training plans, with ten "stages", are examples of the ways in which the directives are being interpreted. To achieve a balanced programme, the planner needs a data base. The planning of a total training course, over three years, or 4,600 hours, for each student offering planned study sessions with the relevant clinical experiences, and choices of alternative holiday dates, is a time consuming exercise. With the combined skills of an operational research team, a nurse educator and an allocator can provide the knowledge required by a systems analyst or programmer to enable him to work out a system wherein a variety of choices are offered by a computer program. The choice of plan can then be made on the basis of knowledge, and the facts, that is the quantifiable data which does exist, the potential data that would emerge due to foreseeable circumstances which might develop and with possible modifications to the plan for such eventualities if they do occur. Professional judgement and choice can only be made effectively, however, if the basis of the original remit was clear, concise and understood. Communication between a nurse educator and a systems analyst or programmer is likely to be fairly slow process - no matter how willing and expert the pupil! Each has to learn the other's language for compatibility to occur.

Systems Support

How can such systems help to provide a balanced programme of study and relevant clinical nursing experience?

By forecasting the effects of:-

a)   change in the size of cohorts due to wastage,

b)   change in the type of clinical experience offered - due to closure or change of use of wards or hospitals,

c)   change in the requirements for training by the responsible statutory body,

d)   change caused by the introduction of new or experimental schemes of training in response to changing needs in the health-care system, which adds to the complexity of the planned alloction in some units.

By comparisons between forecast predictions and actual outcomes, for example:-

a) in the numbers available for particular experiences during training,
b) between the forecast and actual number qualifying on completion of training,
c) by the number of posts available on the staff, revealing staff turnover, fluctuations, with consequent budget alterations.

Budgetary Control

Planning the best use of resources by keeping a steady flow of nursing students through the agreed placements for clinical experience inevitably affects the nursing budget. Nursing students in the UK are not a cheap commodity! However, it is not only financially undesirable to have too many nursing students in one clinical unit, it is also an uneconomic use of their time for learning about particular patients and their needs. It is often as much of a trial to their supervisors to have too many searching for the limited material available as to have too few available for the material offered. Therefore, the nurse educator is vitally interested in having the optimum number of learners in any one place at one time. Bottlenecks causing a backlog and a build up of those waiting for the experience can ruin any nursing education programme. The well-documented dilemma of the university student who cannot get hold of the books he needs to read before his next essay is as nothing compared with the frustration of the nursing student facing an examination paper on which her professional future rests, without the confidence of the required clinical experience behind her to enable her to attempt one or more of the questions. During the past decade assistance from computer teams has developed in many nursing schools in the UK, and the level of interest is rising in the use of computer programs to try to overcome these problems.

Developments at The London Hospital in Tower Hamlets

In 1975, a 'Batch System' for creating a data base was developed and used by one school of nursing. The school had 1,000 learners, seven basic nursing courses, and seven hospital sites for clinical experience. Collaboration between the operational research and computer teams and the Director of Nursing Education led to the creation of a data base for all learners. From this base a system of stream-lining the study programmes, with planned clinical experience and annual leave was evolved. This reduced the pressure on the wards and departments by the swings from "peaks" to "troughs". The system also provided for the forecasting of "critical weeks" during a period when the health district was changing the use of hospitals, decreasing the amount of acute care and increasing the provision for long stay psychogeriatric care, and care of the elderly sick and frail.

The allocation office, and the communication network to the seven hospital sites had relied on manual systems of recording, and on personal, or telephone, communication to notify plans, or changes, or modifications to the plan. A complicated diagram (fig. 1) of the network produced by this activity was sufficient to spur the group on to further plans. By using the batch system, manual recording was still required, but was simplified and coded. The benefits of the system were:-

a) Fewer interruptions and telephone calls to the allocation office resulting in more time for planned work.
b) The data base provided an aid for allocation.
c) Short term and longer term forecasts were readily available of numbers, and of needs for students' experience.
d) Sickness absence and wastage statistics for learners were readily available.

Fig. 1

Outline of Manual System, showing contact between School,
Offices and Hospitals

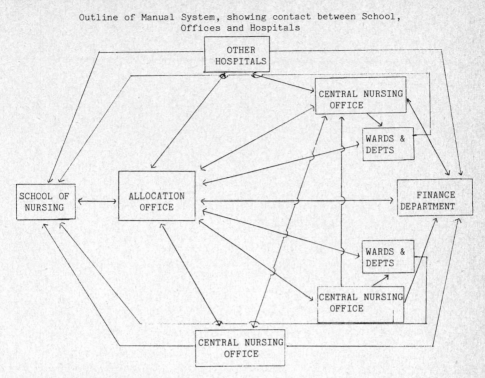

The main difficulty was that with the batch system running at weekly intervals, there was a time-lag between the in-put and the out-put of information, so that the outcome of changes was sometimes felt before it was documented for the recipient.   The data was consistent, legible and useful information, and accurate on the date of input, but not necessarily on the date of receipt.   It also involved large amounts of paper both as forms for entering data, and as computer print-outs.   The contribution of this batch system was in providing evidence of the advantages of computerising records, and from this, the health district supported the development of a real time system of computerising a data based system for all nursing staff within the District.   In setting up the system the defined objectives were:-

a)   Easy access to accurate information.
b)   Reduction in clerical work, and duplication of manual records.
c)   Aid to allocation.
d)   Sickness absence statistics for all nursing staff.
e)   Wastage statistics for nursing students.
f)   Data base for nursing manpower planning.

The benefits of immediate recording in the real-time system were obvious at once.   The visual display units on each major site provided the keyholder with access to that part of the system over which he or she was required to have control, for example, for entering sickness absence, but not for changing personal data. The choice of display frames included those details which any nurse manager would need to view at any time during the day or night, e.g. next of kin, or current address and telephone number, but a confidential key would be required for any change of data, to be held by a named person by the head of the department. No personal details, progress record or other sensitive information would be readily available on display.

A National Nursing Record

The General Nursing Council for England and Wales developed a computerised record system to maintain its register of nurses. This scheme was developed from a data base created when entrants to training were indexed at the beginning of the course. Data regarding each student for every type of course in every school of nursing in England and Wales was collected, and all subsequent changes updated on the computer records, as they were received from the nursing schools where these records were maintained manually. Some schools with access to computer systems in their own health districts were, however, able to send a computer printout of such records to the GNC. It was also the intention that, in due course, such systems would be able to communicate directly with the Council's computer, for example by magnetic tape. Currently many schools are showing a great interest in the development of on-line systems between the Council and themselves.

The Post-Basic Level

During the past twenty years there has been a growing awareness of the need for the nurse's clinical skills to be developed in response to new developments and advances in medicine, surgery, psychiatry and neonatal care. This has led to the establishment in the UK of the Joint Board of Clinical Nursing Studies in England and Wales and the Committee for Clinical Nursing Studies in Scotland, and the development of specialised clinical nursing courses for example in stoma therapy, the care of the elderly, special intensive care of the newborn, intensive care, community psychiatric nursing courses, to name but a few. The qualified nurses who gain such certificates on the completion of a course in England and Wales have this recorded on their professional computer record held by the General Nursing Council for England and Wales.

The New Statutory Framework

The Nurses, Midwives and Health Visitors Act 1979(2) established a new statutory framework for nursing, midwifery and health visiting, which will come into operation in 1983. The national boards in each country in the United Kingdom are charged under the act with the provision of courses for nurses, midwives and health visitors at institutions approved for the purpose. Currently the members appointed to the UK Central Council for Nursing, Midwifery and Health Visiting, and to the four national boards, are discussing the computerisation of current and future records. The Act places on the UKCC the obligation to:-

"prepare and maintain a register of nurses, midwives and health visitors".

It also spells out clearly the functions of the Council, including:-

"to establish and improve standards of training for nurses, midwives and health visitors"
"to ensure standards meet any community obligation of the UK"
"to determine the kind and standard of training with a view to registration"
"to make provision for the kind and standard of training available to persons already registered".

Therefore, to enable these functions to be carried out effectively and to facilitate accurate recording and the rapid and simultaneous communication of information between the Council and the four national boards, a computer based record system is clearly necessary for the storage and retrieval of information. The computers benefit the Boards and these institutions not only by providing information for the management of courses but also by assisting in the learning process for the students.

Conclusion

Nursing education needs support systems which enable the best use to be made of those resources currently available and which are sufficiently flexible to respond readily to future needs. Professional judgement, informed by facts and by research, a search for truth on the basis of sound knowledge, influences people - be they our patients, or our politicians. The nurse, now and in the future, needs to be alert, knowledgeable and capable of cogent argument, supported by facts, to take part in groups where he or she has an important part to play in shaping the future service offered to mankind.

References:

1. European Economic Community: Directives for the nurse for general care. 1979 European Commission, Brussels.
2. Nurses, Midwives and Health Visitor's Act 1979, H.M.S.O. London UK.

The Impact of Computers on Nursing
M. Scholes, Y. Bryant and B. Barber (eds.)
Elsevier Science Publishers B.V. (North-Holland)
© IFIP-IMIA, 1983

12.2.

A STEP TOWARDS COMPUTERISED LEARNER NURSE ALLOCATION

Colin J. Fildes

Introduction

In July 1980 the computer department at Trent Regional Health Authority was
asked by it's Regional Nurse Training Committee to investigate the possibility
of providing computer assistance in the schools of nursing, paying particular
attention to the area of learner nurse allocation. Initial enquiries at several
schools indicated that there existed such a need, not only in the area of nurse
allocation, but also in the area of record keeping for the learners. Some
months were then spent reviewing the computer systems that were already
available in this field to see whether these needs could be satisfied quickly by
obtaining an existing system. The only computer assistance then found to be
available came in the form of desk-top microcomputers which were limited to
record keeping and word processor functions. This is apparently still the case.
With the exception of a system at The London Hospital, Whitechapel, no evidence
of computer assistance in the area of learner nurse allocation was found.

It was quickly realised that the record keeping part of a computer system would
be relatively straight forward in design, but that in tackling learner nurse
allocation one was dealing with something infinitely more complicated.
Agreement to proceed with this development was made on the basis that if it were
possible to design a computer system which went a significant way towards
automatic learner allocation, the record keeping aspect would follow afterwards.
In other words, starting off by tackling the hardest bit first.

A need was also identified for more than one person at the school to obtain
information from the computer at any time, which meant that it was not possible
to recommend the purchase of a desk top microcomputer. As a result of an open
tender, a Digital Equipment Corporation's PDP 11/23 computer with 20M bytes of
disk storage was purchased. This computer had the capability to run up to eight
terminals and sufficient disk storage to cope with the anticipated demand for
word processing, the retention on-line, of learners who leave, statistical
analyses and so on. All the programs were written in the MUMPS programming
language.

An Overview of the Computerised Allocation System

The system is fundamentally based upon the assumption that there exist plans of
training which intakes of learners follow for the duration of their training.
Provided that these plans exist, it is a relatively straight forward process to
enter them into the computer. By stating the date that the intake starts in the
school, the system automatically calculates the key 'change' dates. This
process continues for each of the school's intakes.

Having entered this information, the allocation officer is then able to request
a print out of all the learners who are due to change from one area of their
training plan to another in any specified period. In conjunction with this a
report specifies how many learners have been allocated to the wards serviced by
the school for each week in a thirteen week period. Using these two documents

the allocation officer is then able to state to which ward each learner is to be allocated. This information is then re-entered to the computer and change lists for the period can then be automatically printed by the computer. This system enables the allocation officer to retain control over the actual ward to which the learner is sent whilst removing the drudgery of compiling lists.

The System in Detail

Training Plans

For the sake of clarity in what can easily become a complicated and confusing concept, Fig. 1 shows an example of an intake of SRN Students and the plan they would follow.

Fig 1.   **SRN TRAINING PLAN**

WEEK NO:

| 1 | 8 | 9 | 17 | 18 | 25 | 26 | 28 | 29 | 31 | 32 |

INTRODUCTORY COURSE	GENERAL MEDICINE	GENERAL SURGERY	ANNUAL LEAVE	BLOCK 1
	GENERAL SURGERY	GENERAL MEDICINE		

WEEK NO:

| 142 | 144 | 145 | 147 | 148 | 156 | 157 | 164 | 165 | 167 | 168 --> |

ANNUAL LEAVE	BLOCK 6	GENERAL MEDICINE	GENERAL SURGERY (INC 1 WEEK COMMUNITY)	ANNUAL LEAVE	FREE ALLOCATION
		GENERAL SURGERY (INC 1 WEEK COMMUNITY)	GENERAL MEDICINE		

This information is entered into the computer system in the following format:

for each 'element' in the training plan (an 'element' is defined as a discreet period of training, for example, weeks 9-17 in Fig. 1 is one element, weeks 29-31 is another), the computer requires:

- the duration of the allocation in weeks;
- a group number in the range 1 to 4 which relates to the number of 'splits' within the element (for example there is a two way split in the 9-17 week element);
- a character to identify whether the allocation is to a speciality, a period of annual leave, or to a study block;
- the speciality or study block code.

For weeks 1-8 in our example, the entry to the computer would be as shown in Fig 2.

Fig 2.   DATA FOR COMPUTER

Number of Weeks	Group Number	Speciality/holiday or Block	Code
8	1	B	IB (introductory block)

Weeks 9-17 would be entered as

9	1	S	GM (general medicine)
	2	S	GS (general surgery)

and weeks 148-156 would be entered as

9	1	S	GM (general medicine)
	2	S	GS (general surgery)
	2	S	CØ (community)

In Fig 2, the computer is being informed that when the intake reaches week 148 in their training, one group of learners will be going for a period of nine weeks to general medicine, the other group will be going for nine weeks to general surgery, plus, at some time during this spell, they will be going to work in the community. The implications of this grouping procedure are explained later.

'Starting' an intake of learners

Once a training plan has been entered, it then becomes possible to 'start' an intake of learners. Most schools have some form of shorthand coding system to identify the different intakes on their various courses. In this respect, the computer system is no exception. The coding structure settled on was YY/MM/CC where YY is the year that the intake started, MM the month within that year, and CC the code for the type of course being followed. Using this format, an intake of SRN students who started in May 1981 might be given the code of 81/05/SR.

Having entered this code, the computer needs to be told which training plan the intake is following. This information enables the same training plan to be used for a number of intakes. The allocation officer is then asked to enter the start-date for the intake. At this point, a check is carried out to ensure that the date entered is a Monday because it is assumed that all changes occurring throughout the course of training take place over a Sunday night, Monday morning. Once a Monday's date has been entered, the computer 'copies' the training plan and calculates the start date and end date of each element of training. It is then possible to print out the intake's training plan as shown in Fig 3.

It is possible to build up, within the computer, all the start and end dates of every period of allocation for every intake in the school.

Fig 3

INTAKE TRAINING PLAN

INTAKE: 81/05/SR

COURSE: STATE REGISTERED
VERSION NUMBER: 1

FROM	TO	WEEKS	GROUP	SPECIALITY CODE/NAME
04/05/81	28/06/81	8	1	IB INTRO. BLOCK
29/06/81	30/08/81	9	1	GM GEN. MED.
			2	GS GEN. SURG.
31/08/81	25/10/81	8	1	GS GEN. SURG.
			2	GM GEN. MED.
26/10/81	15/11/81	3	1	AL ANNUAL LEAVE
16/11/81	06/12/81	3	1	B1 BLOCK 1
07/12/81	07/02/82	9	1	GE GERIATRICS
			2	GM GEN. MED.
			2	GS GEN. SURG.

Identifying learners due to change

Suppose that an allocation officer wishes to allocate learner nurses to wards and then produce change lists for the month of November. The first task that is to be performed is to ask the computer to print out all learners on all intakes who, according to their training plan, are due to change from one training plan element to another in the four week period starting on 1st November, 1982 (again, this date must be a Monday). This in fact, is all that the allocation officer is required to do, namely to state the start date and the number of weeks. The computer will then print out the data as shown in Fig 4. This shows the nurses due to change each week, by intake, starting with 1st November. It gives details of:-

- where they are changing 'from'
- where, according to their training plan they should be going 'to'
- for how many weeks
- the names of all the wards that the learner has previously been allocated to for this speciality (where applicable)
- any comments that the allocation officer has put into the system relevant to the learner.

It would be possible to produce this information as a display on the VDU screen, but the allocation officers wished it to be in printed form so that they could consider the allocation of an intake as a whole. A display would have only given them one, or possibly two learners' changes at once. The print-out is used by the allocation officer as a working document to write on the name(s) of the ward(s) to which the learner is to be allocated and for which weeks. Naturally it is possible to allocate a learner to more than one ward during, say, an eight week allocation. It is also permissible to allocate a learner to a completely different speciality if desired. In this way, the power of decision about the final destination of a learner rests with the allocation officer and not the computer.

It is appreciated that a significant proportion of all allocations involves transferring learners into periods of study block or annual leave. The system incorporates a short cut method which may be used to allocate learners to study block or annual leave.

Fig 4

CHANGE LIST

NOTTINGHAM SCHOOL OF NURSING   R22 PRINTED ON 12-Aug-82

PLAN PROGRAMME FOR 01/11/82 TO 28/11/82 (4 WEEKS)

CHANGES DUE 01/11/82

	FROM	TO	WKS.	PREVIOUS WARD(S)	TO WARD	FROM/TO	TO WARD	FROM/TO
INTAKE 80/01/SR								
1/2 ALEXANDER Lesley Jane	BLOCK 5	GEN. MED	8	(WARD 1 INFIRMARY) (WARD 5C INFIRMARY)	NIGHTINGALE	1/8	MUST TAKE TEST	
1/2 BARNES Alan Trevor (M)	BLOCK 5	GEN. MED	8	(WARD 21 GEN HOSP) (NIGHTINGALE GEN.)	5C (INF)	1/8		
1/2 EVANS Gillian Margaret	BLOCK 5	GEN. MED	8	(WARD 1 INFIRMARY) (NIGHTINGALE GEN.)	21 (GEN)	1/4	5C (INF)	5/8
2/2 BAKER Denise Allison	BLOCK 5	GEN. SURG.	8	(WARD WEST 4 GEN.) (WARD EAST 1 INF.)	7A (GEN)	1/8	ALL NIGHT DUTY	
2/2 WATSON Ann Linda	BLOCK 5	GEN. SURG.	8	(WARD EAST 1 INF.) (WARD 7A GEN.)	1 (INF)	1/4	21 (GEN)	5/8
INTAKE 81/09/SE								
1/1 COTTON Susan Elizabeth	LEAVE	BLOCK 3	2					
1/1 DAVISON Martin Bryan (M)	LEAVE	BLOCK 3	2					
1/1 FANSHAWE Tracy Amanda	LEAVE	BLOCK 3	2					

There are two further facilities available for the use of the allocation
officer. The first of these is concerned with night duty on the ward. It has
been found that on some occasions allocation officers know that within say an
eight week period of allocation, a learner may be due to work two of those weeks
on night duty. The allocation officer may also know which two weeks in
particular these are. In either event, a note to that effect on the print-out
will suffice. The way the system handles this information is described later.
The second facility available allows the allocation officer to pass on to the
ward sister a comment concerning a particular learner. Again, by writing this
comment onto the print-out, the system can handle the information so that it
appears subsequently on the change list, as shown in Fig 4.

You recall that when the training plan for this intake was entered, it stated
that group 1 would be going to, say, general medicine while group 2 went to
general surgery. When an intake of learners starts training, and their personal
information; for example, name, date of birth, country of birth, address and so
on has been entered, the allocation officer must decide which line of the
training plan each learner is to follow; in other words, which group they are to
go into. Unless the allocation officer alters the groupings of a learner, the
computer will assume that each learner will follow that line of their training
plan continuously.

Putting the allocations back into the computer

Once the allocation officer has completed the allocations for the period, it
then becomes necessary to tell the computer the outcome of these decisions. To
do this, an interactive updating program is used. The VDU screen displays the
name of the next learner, in the sequence that appears on the print-out,
together with the learner's anticipated area of allocation (for example, general
medicine). The information written onto the print-out for the learner is then
entered in the appropriate places on the display. A checking procedure is then
carried out to ensure that no week number is included in more than one place
(that is, no overlapping). An example showing how the system can handle a
rather complicated allocation is shown in Fig. 5. Notice the two types of night
duty entries and the input of comments to the ward.

Fig 5

UPDATE PLAN PROGRAMME

```
INTAKE 81/05/SR    CHANGES DUE 1/11/82
NAME    THOMPSON Geraldine Caroline    ALLOCATION FOR 9 WEEKS

SPEC/HOL/BLOCK          WARD(S)/DEPT(S)         FROM TO    COMMENTS FOR SERVICE
                                                           STAFF
[S] [GEN MED  ]         [WARD 1 (ROYAL INF)]    [ 1][ 2]   [                    ]
                        [WARD 2 (ROYAL INF)]    [ 6][ 6]   [MUST TAKE WARD TEST

INCLUDES [  1] WEEKS NIGHTS STARTING AT WK.[  2] AND [   ] WEEKS STARTING AT WK


[S][GEN.SURG.]          [WARD 8 (GEN HOSP) ]    [ 3][ 5]   [                   ]
        INCLUDING [  1] WEEKS ON NIGHTS STARTING AT WK. NO. [   ]

[H][ANNUAL LEAVE]       [                  ]    [ 7][ 7]   [                   ]
                        [                  ]    [ ][ ]     [                   ]

[S][GEN.MED.]  ]        [WARD 1 (ROYAL INF)]    [ 8][ 9]   [                   ]
        INCLUDING [   ] WEEKS ON NIGHTS STARTING AT WK. NO. [       ]
```

Where the computer recognises that an intake is due to transfer into study block or annual leave, a display will be brought up to allow the user to allocate all the learners on the intake at one go.

Producing change lists

Having told the computer the destination of all the learners due to change, the system is now capable of producing change lists. At most of the schools visited, it was found that once a complete set of change lists had been drawn up and typed, it was then photocopied, distributed to ward sisters, unit nursing officers, senior tutors, pinned up on the noticeboards and a copy kept in the allocation office. It was apparent that a number of people were receiving irrelevant or superfluous information. For example, ward sisters had to flick through several pages of changes to pick out those which affected their ward directly. Using this system it is possible to produce a change list for each ward detailing the names of the learners leaving on the Sunday (if any) and those starting the following day - as shown in Fig 6.

Fig 6   **INDIVIDUAL WARD CHANGE LIST**

NOTTINGHAM SCHOOL OF NURSING   R30   PRINTED ON 12-Sep-82

    WARD/DEPT. CHANGE LIST FOR WEEK COMMENCING 1-Nov-82

WARD/DEPT: NIGHTINGALE WARD   TO: SISTER JOHNSTONE

LEAVING ON 31-Oct-82

80/04/SR   WARD/HOL/BLOCK TO   WEEKS

BAKER Susan Joan   BLOCK 5   3

JACOBS Andrew David (M)   BLOCK 5   3

COMMENCING ON 1-Nov-82

80/09/SR   WEEKS   TESTS LEFT   COMMENTS

MASTERSON Denise Joy   8   1   TEST TO BE TAKEN
                                                    IN THIS ALLOC
WOODHOUSE Sarah Elizabeth   8   1   TEST TO BE TAKEN
                                                    IN THIS ALLOC
                                                    (NIGHT DUTY FOR
                                                    2 WEEKS)

The system is also capable of producing a change list for a particular intake; for a unit nursing officer who may cover several wards; for a senior tutor who may be responsible for a number of intakes, or in the traditional form for the noticeboard. It may of course prove necessary to alter the allocations for some learners after the publication of these change lists. This may be done very simply and a new change list need only be produced for those wards affected by such alterations.

A problem encountered

Wards need to be told of changes which affect them some weeks in advance. It is not unrealistic that allocation officers produce a nine week change list for publication four weeks in advance. It may take two weeks to produce the change list prior to publication, so at an extreme, changes could be made for a period up to fifteen weeks ahead. The problem we encountered was how to allocate those learners who were not due to start training until after the change lists had been published, yet had a change onto a ward due in the period of that change list. Naturally this problem exists irrespective of whether one uses a computer system or a manual one. The problem has been overcome as follows; at the time the allocation officer starts the new intake, one usually knows approximately how many learners will be starting. At this stage the system asks the allocation officer to state how many learners are expected to start and generates that number of notional, or 'dummy', records. Provided this is done for intakes due to start within, say the next three months, when the allocation officer prints out the learners due to change, the print will include these 'dummy' records which may be allocated in the normal way. When the actual names of the learners are known, a matching process is performed to connect the real learners to their 'dummy' allocated records.

Functions Available other than Allocation

1. There is a full GNC record keeping system for each learner including the production of a GNC acceptable print of the learners record of training. Sickness and absence recording is also incorporated.
2. Various immediate statistical displays, for example the whereabouts of any learner, the whereabouts of all learners on an intake.
3. Automatic calculation of the number of hours worked by any learner in each speciality, the number of hours spent on sick leave, annual leave, and study block.

Anticipated Future Developments

1. The incorporation of word processing facilities into the system.
2. Based on the concept of training plans, the development of a modelling facility to allow the user to state
    i)   when intakes are due to start over an 'n' year period.
    ii) how many learners are anticipated in each, and
    iii) which training plan they will be following.

With this information it is possible to calculate how many learners one expects to be allocated to the various specialties each week over the 'n' year period. This could then be used to adjust the structure of the training plan, change the numbers on each intake, change the frequency of the intakes and so on, in order to produce a more even flow of learners to the service side. These figures could also be adjusted to take account of an estimated wastage rate.

Conclusion

This system has been in live operation at the schools of nursing in Nottingham, Leicester and Derby for some months. Development of new parts of the system continues alongside amendments requested by the schools in the light of their experience of working with the system. It's development so far has been achieved thanks to close co-operation with, and the enthusiastic involvement of, allocation staff in each of these schools. Allocating learner nurses to wards can be a time consuming, repetitive chore. It is hoped that this computer system goes some way to removing this burden from nursing officers in schools of nursing and provides them with more time for planning and liaison with learners and the service side.

The Impact of Computers on Nursing
M. Scholes, Y. Bryant and B. Barber (eds.)
Elsevier Science Publishers B.V. (North-Holland)
© IFIP-IMIA, 1983

12.3.

COMPUTERIZED NURSE ALLOCATION AND THE IDENTIFICATION OF RELATED SERVICE TOOLS

Jean Roberts

Introduction

The Lancaster Health Authority (the District) serves a catchment population of approximately 220,000. It does not contain a teaching hospital and has therefore not the specializations or limitations accruing from that. The District contains eleven hospital locations and supports a large number of general practitioners. In the current UK situation there are limited resources of a financial, manpower and clinical nature.

The management team has defined the local computing policy to state that computer projects implemented in the District must not require specialist computer operations support staff. [This is feasible as large data processing functions such as payroll and stock control are carried out on other hardware which is not the responsibility of the District].

This paper discusses a resource management tool available to nurse managers, highlights the projected development and sets this in the perspective of the centrally coordinated and integrated computer support to health care in the District(2).

Requirement for the Facility

There are two hundred nurses in training in the District at any one time. The assessment of the implications of integrated ongoing and projected learner nursing training plans is a very time consuming manual task. The specification and manual drawing up of a schematic representation of the effects of projected new course plans and the ongoing training schemes may take three man-weeks. To develop a total manpower planner, the availability of trained staff must be considered. A possible extension of this would be to allocate staff of whatever grade to ward locations on the basis of degree of nursing care required by the patients daily.

A computer program has already been implemented to map training schemes (both actual and projected) onto each other to arrive at an indication of peaks and troughs of load on facilities(J6). This program incorporates options to facilitate the alteration of start dates, course contents and duration. It is written in Coral-66 on the District development machine, a Ferranti Argus 700E with 64K of core. The program does not take up all the space and could be transferred if the nurses were to gain better accessibility on another machine.

Development

The initial phase of computerized nurse allocation is that of determining the implications of potential training schemes,

     (a) on nurse availability to the wards, and
     (b) on the load to be placed on the education facility.

This procedure overlays the current status of training groups and the projected training schemes onto a theoretical plan of the expected course contents for future intakes. At best this mapping produces a good estimate of the possible situation in the future.

Fig 1. Training Courses to be considered.

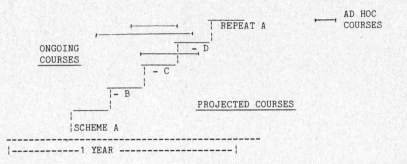

The procedure could be applied to any identified locations available for training. Because of the limited and specific nature of our teaching resources, the program considers 'location' to the level of ward and day or night duty. The resultant chart shows areas of shortfall or overload in learner nurse allocation. Data on nurses of all grades could be considered under the same scheme. It is intended that this facility be added. As a result of the small numbers (approx. 16) per intake of learners it is not possible to introduce any wastage modelling criteria.

The information can be acted upon, to ensure the most practical cover both for patient nursing care and the availability of staff to assist in the ward-based training of the learners. This operational function may well include the redeployment of trained and auxiliary nurses both on staff and in the pool to cope with the projected situation. Efforts must be made to reduce the time between having to base considerations on theoretical information and the real current information being available. To this end visual display units at the volatile locations - nurse allocations office, training school and divisional nursing offices, will make data input more efficient. Current manual systems generate numerous memos which get transmitted relatively slowly, so decisions are made on non-current and perhaps incomplete information.

Report Requirements

The identified output from learner nurse allocation systems are various:-

For the learner: personal training scheme details

For the nurse manager   change lists of those transferring in and out of the
and the learner: 'area' in the next period

For the allocations   details of the ongoing schemes showing projected
and nursing officers: numbers by specialty and area

Ad-hoc updates: changes necessary between the formal change list
                                          production times.

An unexpected priority arose from putting the above list to the nursing managers at Lancaster. An area was identified where information was not always readily available under the current manual system. In order to produce the above reports the training scheme lines must be identified with a particular named individual. The nurse information required is less than that required for registration but is not just name and number.

The information requested is:

a)   Intake group identifier (year, intake within year, learner number).
b)   Learner name and home address.
c)   Marital status.
d)   Whether resident or non-resident in hospital accommodation.
e)   Emergency control details.
f)   Payroll number - as nurse managers have to provide details to the finance
        department.
g)   Previous qualifications (whether of nursing relevance or not).

Rather than make all this information available on every report which would generate inordinately large quantities of paper, the nursing service officers asked for a register of all nurses in training by intake group containing all the above information to be a priority output from any computer system. This information is to be held by each nurse manager for use if required when that group comes into her area for training. In a manual system, this information is only available by reference to a central (not permanently manned) location.

Discussion

Initial work went into a scheme for developing computer assistance in projecting numbers and throughputs (with or without wastage and other inbuilt modelling factors(J11). The emphasis at Lancaster, a provincial mid-size district general hospital, seems to have been altered to a personalized information bank to assist nurse managers in the identification and deployment of their staff. This change of direction in no way contradicts the long term aim of balancing nursing skills available with the patient care requirement of those currently having hospital treatment(L18).

The system development suggested will be of localized use. In no way is it intended to duplicate the information or procedures being designed for the SNIPPET (Standard Nursing Information Planning, Evaluating and Training) system or those required by the UK Central Council for Nursing, Midwifery and Health Visiting. The aim is to use available resources to satisfy a locally identified need.

Comments

Nurses in the Lancaster District, as elsewhere, are increasingly being faced by interaction with computer facilities for example:-

a)   printouts of reports:-
        - cross infection monitoring
        - intravenous feeding regime calculations.

b)   Visual display terminals:-
        - currently in use for the acquisition of pathology results
        - potentially available for CAI using simulations of in-service
          systems.

It is necessary to introduce all staff to computer technology in general and to systems they will personally have to interact with. In the area of health care provision the size of Lancaster, it is suggested that computer specialist support solely for the nursing group is not feasible(2). Support and information dissemination must be shared with all other disciplines to make cost-effective use of facilities, both hardware and software, and computer specialist time.

From the viewpoint of computer specialists and health care professionals alike, it is necessary

a)   to understand the usage, and inter-relationships of information generated by different disciplines.
b)   to have complete, consistent, correct data on both patients and staff.

Within the framework of limited resources, it is necessary that all who interact, either

a)   directly by operating terminals, or
b)   indirectly by providing/receiving data/information,

must be made aware of the power and limitations of the facilities available to them.

Conclusion

A greater amount of available information on both manpower and user requirements can result in more efficient use of available resources. Education of users to their required level of competance results in better understanding and tolerance of computer power and may result in user-initiated development suggestions.

The introduction of computer facilities as an information 'tool' of direct benefit to the people using them makes those people more receptive to other computer-aided developments which they may previously have felt reticent about.

REFERENCES

1.   "Standard Nurse Information Package for Planning, Evaluating and Training" A/D.N.O. Working Party on Manpower Planning/Information Systems NWRHA July 1982.
2.   "District Computer Services in Practice" Broadey K., Brook S., and Roberts J. Hospital and Health Services Review. March 82 73-75

CHAPTER 13

PLANNING THE NURSING SERVICE

Manpower planning has been defined as a strategy for the acquisition, utilisation, improvement and retention of the human resources of an enterprise.

Nurse managers need to analyse and take stock of their present situation, then set objectives and call upon other relevant professional skills to assist them, for example, operational research and mathematical modelling - these aspects will be expanded in Chapter 15. The following papers describe some alternative ways in which nurse managers have considered the use of computers to assist them when planning the nursing service.

The Impact of Computers on Nursing
M. Scholes, Y. Bryant and B. Barber (eds.)
Elsevier Science Publishers B.V. (North-Holland)

13.1.

THE USE OF COMPUTERS FOR PLANNING NURSING SERVICES

Barbara Rivett

Summary

The purpose of this paper is to focus on the problems of taking a long-term view
of nursing services. It outlines planning processes, attempts to identify
information requirements, and suggests that computer-based nursing systems have
a valuable part to play in health care planning.

Introduction

Dame Catherine Hall's keynote address emphasised the importance of looking ahead
and of satisfying ourselves that existing systems of professional education are
relevant to today's and tomorrow's needs. If changes seem to be necessary, they
should be initiated now so that the nursing profession moves towards the 21st
Century equipped to respond to the demands made upon it.(see Chapter 2) What is
true of education is also true of our systems of nursing practice and nursing
management. Identifying the changes necessary to achieve longer term goals are
steps in the planning process. Although enthusiasm for planning has a tendency
to wax and wane(1), planning processes offer a logical way of deciding how the
future should change and how the necessary changes are to be achieved.

A definition of planning

Planning may be defined as "deciding how the future pattern of activities should
differ from the present, identifying the changes necessary to accomplish this
and specifying how the changes should be brought about"(3). Planning is
therefore not only about deciding how the future should be better than the
present, but it is also about the management of change which is itself a complex
task. There is good reason to hope that well constructed long term plans based
on good and up-to-date information, could be helpful in breaking down the
initial resistance to change which we all sometimes demonstrate and which can be
a significant bar to progress.

While planning is not new to the health services, a comprehensive health care
planning system was introduced for the first time in the National Health Service
(NHS) in 1976(3). The planning system was introduced at a time of substantial
real growth in financial resources and in spite of the evidence of the oil
crisis, the NHS felt growth would continue, if only at a slightly lower level.
Planners had become accustomed to incremental thinking and planning; they
addressed themselves to questions about where the extra money should be spent.
But times have changed and those nurses who have experience of planning for
services ten years hence know that the attempt is surrounded by difficulty and
uncertainty because life does not stand still. Changes in demography, advances
in medical science and technology, changes in the availability of manpower and
alterations in the money we believe will be available all add to uncertainty in
planning. Today, planners are more concerned with questions about the balance
of resources between the different services, how existing financial and manpower
resources might be redistributed to meet tomorrow's needs and efficiency in the
use of the funds available. Demand when measured by public expectation

consistently outstrips the availability of resources and failure to demonstrate the best use of money is inevitably criticised. This, together with the problem of changing resource assumptions makes a flexible approach to planning essential.

Planners now appreciate more clearly than they did that a decision to spend more money on one service means that there will be less available for another. The aim therefore must be to produce long term plans which make priorities clear and are feasible enough to cope with uncertainties about future resources(4).

The planning process

The planning process attempts to answer four basic questions(5):-

1. Where are we now?
   Taking stock of the present situation
2. Where do we want to be?
   Setting objectives and mapping out a course of action within a framework of national(6) and local guidelines.
3. How do we get there?
   Constructing a plan setting out the means of achieving objectives.
4. How are we doing? Making an assessment to check that objectives are being achieved.

These were the questions which health authorities attempted to answer during the first round of strategic planning in 1977. Not surprisingly the plans were tentative and incomplete because of the scale of the exercise and because most people were in the learning phase(7). Too great a depth of information was requested by those who designed the planning system, and there were significant gaps in the availability of data not least the manpower information which is of particular concern to nurses. Information about different aspects of health service management could not be linked. Service, capital and manpower plans were seldom adequately related to the money available. Because of these difficulties the idea of a 'minimum core' of information was introduced into the second round of strategic planning in 1978. The aim was to enable planning objectives to be linked to manpower, activity and financial information.

The problem and difficulties experienced in the introduction of the planning system, through lack of appropriate and timely information, have a number of lessons for nurse managers and nurse educationalists who have developed discrete computer systems for nursing. Nurses may wish to expand their systems, but there may be problems in linking individual systems which use data-sets unrelated to each other. The development of nursing systems which provide information for planning purposes are likely to be increasingly important. New computer systems which are being planned should include an analysis of existing information and a specification of likely information requirements for policy making, planning, management and operational control of the nursing services. The ability to link data-sets is an important principle in the development of nursing information systems.

The nursing role in planning health services

Nurses are not unfamiliar with planning procedures. For example, many are engaged in constructing patient care plans as part of the nursing process. Others are involved in the preparation of plans for nurse education and in nurse manpower planning. The challenge now is for nurses at all levels and in all branches of the profession to become actively involved in the wider aspects of health care planning. In so doing, they will develop greater insight into the demands that are likely to be made on nursing services in the longer term.

The nurses' role in planning is still evolving. It was through the introduction of a national health care planning system that nurses in England were required to participate in the full range of planning activities. Role specifications for nurse planners included specific duties such as participants in the setting of objectives for service planning and evaluating performance against agreed objectives(8).

One of the first tasks tackled by nurse planners was forecasting ten years ahead the number of nurses required in each of the nursing specialisms, for the acute and long stay sectors, the hospital services and the community. Ideally, manpower forecasts should be based upon an assessment of the services needed, but in many cases the projections represented a best guess for the data available did not allow anything more accurate. The tendency is still for nurse manpower planning to be carried out in isolation but the aim should be to **integrate** manpower, service and financial planning. For example, the use of hospital and community activity analyses allows us to observe trends and to see which services are expanding and which are contracting.

Nurse educationalists have an important contribution to make in planning. Developing long term plans for nursing services requires joint planning between nurse managers and nurse educationalists for how can a service be provided without trained manpower? Strategies for nursing services should be in harmony with the strategic objectives for the development of health services. Inevitably these objectives have implications for nursing manpower. Nurse educationalists have the crucial task of planning nurse education programmes to meet future demands for qualified nurses, midwives and health visitors.

Nursing information as a component in planning

Where do we go from here and how do we define the nursing information that planners, not just nurse-planners, will need?

Ten years ago nursing experience in the use of computers in hospital and community services was virtually non-existent. Nursing computer systems were therefore developed as individual applications, a nursing orders system here, a nurse allocation system there. Indeed, projects centrally funded through the Department of Health experimental programme, were encouraged to develop different systems. As a result nurses had an opportunity to gain practical experience of the use of computers in hospital and community settings. The ultimate aim, a somewhat ambitious one, was to combine a number of nursing, administrative and medical systems into a composite hospital or health service computer system. The systems, developed out of particular tasks or functions, sometimes provided nurse managers with information for day-to-day management of nursing services. Little was done to assess the use of stored data for other purposes such as planning. A lot went to waste, but there is now a wealth of data waiting to be tapped and presented in a form for use in long term planning of services. For example, a nursing orders system could give the workload indicators over time and by specialty. Information derived from nurse allocation systems could provide input into manpower planning systems. Patient administration systems could give trends in length of stay, bed utilisation and so forth.

Whatever nursing computer systems are being planned, it is imperative to look beyond immediate objectives. A definition of information required from a system for day-to-day management of nursing services must be followed by an examination of the potential of the system to provide information required for short and long term planning and for policy making. Information for planning may require additional items of data, but very often it does not; it requires different presentation in summary or tabular form, showing trends over time. Using information for planning requires the correlation of a number of variables and nurses would find operational research scientists, statisticians and health economists valuable allies with much helpful advice to offer(9). But, if nurses are to be accepted as useful colleagues in planning, and planning not only nursing services but the wider health services as well, it is up to them to demonstrate that the information available to them is vital to all. Health care is a team undertaking and not an individual event. Data knows no disciplinary boundaries, neither do computers and nor should nurses.

CONCLUSION

Over the past decade, considerable progress has been made in the introduction of computer-based nursing systems. In the main, systems were developed as single applications designed to assist particular nursing tasks or functions. They gave nurses an opportunity to gain practical experience of using computers in a variety of hospital and community settings. This experience has enabled nurses to explore the wider uses of computers for managing and planning services. New issues are beginning to emerge. It is now being recognised that further benefits would accrue from individual nursing systems if the data from each could be co-ordinated and presented in a form suitable for policy making, long term planning and management purposes. Thus plans for expanding the use of nursing and other computer systems will require careful study of information requirements related to decision-making processes at all levels of the nursing services.

Nurses, through their knowledge of the needs of patients at the point at which care is delivered, have a unique contribution to make to the wider aspects of health care planning. The effectiveness of this contribution will largely depend upon the availability to their colleagues of relevant, accurate and timely information about nursing services.

In ten years time we may be largely concerned with the analysis and use of computer-derived information and its place in decision making processes in nursing.

REFERENCES

1. Barnard, K., Lee, K., Mills, A., Reynolds, J., N.H.S. Planning: an assessment. Hospital and Health Service Review. August and September 1980.
2. The N.H.S. Planning System. Department of Health and Social Security. London June 1976. Her Majesty's Stationery Office. (HMSO)
3. Ibid.
4. Health Services Development: The N.H.S. Planning System. Health Circular (82)6. Department of Health and Social Security, London. 1982.
5. The N.H.S. Planning System. Department of Health and Social Security. London. June 1976. HMSO
6. Priorities for Health and Personal Social Services in England. A Consultative Document. Department of Health and Social Security. 1976. London. HMSO
7. Priorities in the Health and Social Services. The Way Forward. Department of Health and Social Security. September 1977. HMSO
8. Management Arrangements: Nursing and Midwifery Management Structures. N.H.S. Reorganisation Circular HRC (74)31.
9. Pendreigh, D.M. The Health Economist and N.H.S. Planning. Hospital and Health Services Review. June 1980.

The Impact of Computers on Nursing
M. Scholes, Y. Bryant and B. Barber (eds.)
Elsevier Science Publishers B.V. (North-Holland)
© IFIP-IMIA, 1983

13.2.

COMPUTERS IN HEALTH SERVICE MANAGEMENT FROM A NURSING PERSPECTIVE

Patricia Hardcastle

1. SUMMARY

This paper attempts to put into perspective the position of the nurse when Hospital Information Systems are being planned and particularly where nurses are not aware of what computers can do. The present experience at Groote Schuur Hospital is illuminating factors in the planning and implementation of information systems which have been documented by others who have already travelled this road.

2. IN THE BEGINNING
COMPUTERS - WHERE DO NURSES BEGIN TO ACHIEVE UNDERSTANDING?

The very word computer conjures up a feeling of anxiety in most nurses. The square box of tricks which flashes words and figures on a screen at the touch of a few keys seems immediately to set up a barrier and the nurse closes her mind to and hopes it will go away. Many questions are triggered off:

-   Isn't it cheaper to use people rather than machines especially in a country which has a large pool of unskilled labour?
-   Do the potential benefits justify the cost of computerised information systems?
-   Who is responsible for designing and implementing systems - the computer experts or the end users?
-   Where do nurses fit into the scheme of things?
-   If nursing systems are introduced for direct patient care will nurses be more concerned with the machine than with the patient?
-   What happens when the computer is "down", do we have to write the information up, and would it not have been better to write it in the first place?

Being a novice at this stage, my investigations in writing this paper have afforded me the opportunity to read some of the literature. I do not expect that my feelings are any different from the rest of the nurses who have little knowledge of computers and their uses. It is in looking for the answers that I am in England to attend the Conference and to visit various centres where applications of computers to nursing are in operation. One reads about them but do they really work? Do the staff who operate them feel that they are beneficial in the giving of better care and better communication?

3. COMPUTERISATION AT GROOTE SCHUUR HOSPITAL IN 1982

Groote Schuur Hospital is a large Teaching Hospital attached to the University of Cape Town for the training of undergraduate and post graduate medical students. It is a training school for nurses, both basic and post basic nursing students. It also provides facilities for the training of students in Medical technology and the paramedical professions. The hospital was first opened in 1938 and from that date has almost doubled the number of beds it contains. It is the centre of a region and is linked with five smaller hospitals. Groote

Schuur itself has 1400 beds with a further 200 in the smaller hospitals making a total of 1600 beds. Groote Schuur is one of three large hospitals in the Cape Town area which share a central computer in the Computer Centre of the Cape Provincial Administration. The other hospitals are the Tygerberg Hospital and the Red Cross War Memorial Children's Hospital. In 1972 a group of outside consultants undertook the first Hospital Information Systems Study but in the nine years that followed only four real-time systems have been implemented, these were for:

(i)   Patient registration and
(ii)   Folder Control
(iii)   Outpatient Administration (Tygerberg Hospital only)
(iv)   Inpatient Records (Red Cross Hospital only)

Why was this? In his book "Hospital Information Systems" Homer H Schmitz has identified two possible reasons. The first was an assumption that people with knowledge of computerisation in industry could step in and set up hospital systems. The second reason was that "only rarely did hospital personnel know enough about the new computer technology to be any real help in developing new systems"(1). Both these factors affected development of the Cape Hospital System and during 1980 the need for review of the original proposals and current development was clearly perceived. In March 1981, the Chief Medical Superintendent, Dr. H Reeve Sanders selected a team of "Senior hospital managers, clinical user representatives, Senior University representatives and some members with special knowledge of and expertise in information systems concepts and technology"(5). This team was to review the needs and priorities for hospital information system development. The reasons for setting up the study were that:

1. Outside consultants had done an initial study in 1972.
2. The hospital environment had changed, increasing costs, heavier workloads, changes in technology and many other developments, were putting additional pressures on management.
3. Data processing philosophies were changing "Until comparatively recently data processing was regarded as a service function, with little recognition of the potential benefits to be gained by sharing information between systems, or providing information for management control"(5).
4. At Groote Schuur the development of real-time systems had been very slow.

The Hospital Information Planning Study (HIPS) began in June 1981. The objectives which were set are as follows:-

(i)   Review the hospital, it's environment, goals and objectives, it's managers and their information needs, and from the input establishment requirements and priorities for information systems (I/S).
(ii) Identify systems that are capable of producing substantial benefits for the hospital, and are both feasible and manageable.
(iii) Ensure that information system resources available to the hospital will be managed for the most efficient and effective support of hospital goals.
(iv) Provide the hospital with a relevant and up-to-date information systems plan which will indicate priorities and procedures for system development and give general direction to I/S activities.
(v)   Improve relationships between the Department of Computer Services and hospital users by providing systems responsive to requirements and priorities of users"(5).

By the end of 1981 a report had been published and a direction had been set for the development of other sub-systems. The mission of Groote Schuur Hospital had also been determined. "This hospital seeks, as a referral centre, to provide comprehensive health care of the highest quality and to offer teaching, training, research and specialised diagnostic and therapeutic services. It also aims to meet the less specialised health care needs as far as facilities allow and training of health care personnel requires, and to support and develop other health services in the community(6).

The hospital's goals are:

"To ensure effective management of all resources specifically money, manpower, materials, facilities and information.

To determine the needs for all categories of health professionals and to provide training opportunities to meet the need in collaboration with other training institutions.

To maintain good relationships with external organisations and the community to ensure that maximum support - political, financial and social is obtained.

To promote the reputation and standing of the hospital by producing trained health care professionals and research and patient care of high quality, thereby attracting outstanding academic and other staff, and students"(6).

I have purposely quoted the mission and goals in full because they "provided the framework within which information systems were identified and prioritised"(6). The basic concept adopted during the HIPS study was that information must be regarded as a resource, and is as important as any other resource used in the provision of health care. The information must be accurate and readily available. With the planning and commissioning of the new Groote Schuur Hospital the need for such information is increasing daily. I asked myself what an information system is and returned to Schmitz' book. He uses a definition given by Birch and Strater. "The primary function of information, hence of an information system, is to increase the knowledge of the user and reduce the uncertainty of the user"(2).

If the system does not perform this function then it is not a good system.

4.   IMPLICATIONS FOR NURSING

From the Nursing point of view, HIPS was a significant step forward.

1.   The Matron-in-Chief Miss L J du Preez was a member of the team. She kept Senior and Middle Nursing Management informed of the progress of the study.
2.   Interest in systems already in use in other hospitals was aroused and visits were arranged to local hospitals with computerised HIS for nursing.
3.   The Department of Computer Services began a series of regular lunch time lectures to which nursing staff were invited.
4.   The development of a matrix showing where nurses would have a minor involvement, major involvement or be directly involved in major decisions was important.

This information was gathered through a series of interviews with key personnel. These developments commenced bridging the gap in knowledge and understanding which the nursing staff had, and are a necessary adjunct to introducing new systems. The attitudinal change which is required is not an overnight phenomenon, but a continuous seeding of the minds of the staff with knowledge, and the provision of an environment which will be conducive to the growth of that knowledge.

Virts in his paper "Introducing the Hospital wide Information System to Hospital and Medical Staffs" says that there are "two major implementation considerations:

1. Creating an Environment of Acceptance, Principles of Participation, Direction and Control, Co-ordination, Communication, Realistic Expectations and Hospital/Vendor Relations.
2. Training Principles of Responsibilities, Relevance, Reinforcement and Reality Stock"(9).

5. THE INTRODUCTION OF COMPUTER TERMINALS INTO THE WARDS

This had only occurred as recently as 1980. The creation of suitable space was a problem, but with redeployment of storage space in the wards the problem was solved. The computer terminals are used for the two modules already mentioned with a third application which has since been developed. This is for the receipt of laboratory results from the Chemical Pathology Laboratories. The main user of this terminal is the ward secretary who records the patient admissions and deals with the patient folders. The doctor, who requires laboratory results may also use the terminal. Nurses use the terminal when the ward secretary is off duty. A question which we need to answer for our new hospital, is, where is the best place for a terminal when more systems will be operating? Will each category of staff, doctor, nurse, secretary have to use the same terminal?

6. PRESENT APPLICATIONS TO NURSING AT GROOTE SCHUUR HOSPITAL

1. Student Nurse Record System

During 1981 a team from the Computer Science Department at the University of Cape Town investigated the development of a real-time record system for Student Nurses. The paper work involved in the employment, registration, training programmes and completions of students in training is immense. Matrons and clerical staff are involved in all the phases of documentation. The retrieval of information is laborious and time consuming. The development of a student nurse record system is essential and was recognised by such as HIPS. The investigation into the development of this system forced the Matron's involved with the personnel work and training schedules to look very closely at what the different tasks were in performing this function. The module will supply the following records:-

Group 1: The Nursing Record

| 1. | The kardex | 2. | Sick leave list |
| 3. | Experience list | 4. | Completed nurse record |

Group 2: Information for allocations

5. College and leave allocation list
6. Availability for night duty
7. Accumulative Vacation due report
8. Rotation list

Group 3: Statistical Reports

9.	Absence List	10.	Summary of allocations per ward
11.	Monthly statistics	12.	List of exits
13.	Location list		

This system is not yet in operation but is expected to be operational shortly in real-time mode but separate from the real-time Cape Hospital System.

2.   Inpatient Administration Systems

The nursing staff will have to be directly involved with the module for inpatient movements, and the Department of Computer Services has consulted with the nursing staff users as to the type of information required for this module, as regards bed occupancy. This is of importance for statistical purposes and to enable Medical and Nursing staff to call up information on the bed state at any time so that the Matron and Medical Superintendents can ascertain where there are empty beds. This system will also give information on patient workloads for the allocation of staff which will also be extremely useful. Liaison between the Department of Computer Services and the Nursing staff is effected by a registered nurse who is part of their team. This is in line with the principles developed empirically by Virts in implementing HIS in 6 hospitals in the U.S.A.

"1.   of Participation - minimise the number of decisions but maximise participation in those which must be made.
2.   Principle of direction and control - Implementation success is directly related to the organisational position, leadership strength and interest level of the individual who directs and controls the effort.
3.   Principle of co-ordination - Co-ordination should be carried out by the staff project group whose responsibilities derive from, remain with, the established hospital and medical staff organisation.
4.   Principle of communication - The environment of acceptance increases in proportion to the quality, consistency and honesty of communication about the system.
5.   Principle of realistic expectation - The shortest route to acceptance and positive attitudes is for the results to equal or exceed expectation"(7).

7.   ESTABLISHMENT OF PRIORITIES FOR FUTURE DEVELOPMENT

The HIPS also established priorities for development keeping in mind the objectives that were set.

"The sub-systems to be developed in order of priority are:

1.   Laboratory results communication.
2.   Computer based pathology handbook.
3.   Radiology report communication and storage.
4.   Hospital pharmaceutical index.
5.   Cumulative reporting of laboratory results.
6.   Real-time patient summaries.
7.   Inpatient administration.
8.   Preformatted clerking booklets.
9.   O.P.D. patient description.
10.   Dispensing and control of pharmaceuticals.
11.   Real-time O.P.D. Clinic notes.
12.   Real-time clerking booklets"(7).

In this list of priorities there are no systems exclusively for nursing. The priorities had been derived by the study team from the Information Architecture which was determined from the interviews with key personnel, and an objective cost/benefit ranking method.

A second priority list for follow on studies was also established.

"1.   Nursing care plans and records.   *
2.   Patient medical record review.
3.   Demographic, economic and epidemiological data base.
4.   Equipment management.
5.   Outpatient appointment.   *
6.   Trained nursing staff scheduling.   *
7.   Inpatient catering.   *
8.   Transport scheduling.   *
9.   Inventory control.   *
10.   Manpower data.   *"(7)

Many of the above systems (indicated with an asterisk) will have a direct
bearing upon the nursing team both in the field of patient care and also in the
management field. The ability of nurses to provide the necessary information to
the Department of Computer Services in order for them to develop these systems
is an important factor.

4.   Other possibilities with potential benefits' for nursing are:

1.   Direct linkage with the South African Nursing Council, the body with whom
      all nurses are registered and the South African Nursing Association, of
      which all practising nurses are members, would save hours of clerical
      work. Both these organisations are situated 1000 miles away from Cape
      Town, and are fully computerised.
2.   Storage of information required for Policy Manuals comprising Hospital
      Notices, Memoranda, Procedures, and the South African Nursing Council
      regulations all of which require amending periodically.
3.   Community services in the Cape Town area are not yet linked to the Central
      Computer at the Head Office of the Cape Provincial Administration but
      liaison with these services with the aid of a computer facility would aid
      discharge planning and follow up care for our patients.
4.   Nurses Education.
      Nurses in South Africa have not yet ventured into the educational computer
      field but in a local primary school for boys "Apple" computers have been
      installed and eight and nine year old children are using them by booking
      time and doing various educational programmes.

      The University of the Western Cape has installed the "Plato System". Some
      sixty-five terminals are used by students for a wide variety of
      programmes. The system also stores student records and permits
      conversations between student and teacher in different venues. This
      system will eventually be linked to similar systems in other centres in
      South Africa.

8.   SYSTEM IMPLEMENTATION

If systems with nursing applications are introduced, who teaches the staff how
to use the system and will the staff accept the system?

Schmitz says "One of the key requirements for successful system implementation
is to provide and enforce a thorough training program for personnel"(3).

Teaching the staff is not the problem, because there is no doubt that they can
be taught. Who does the teaching is important. Schmitz speaks from two
viewpoints which came out of research. Thoren, who came to the conclusion that
"a carefully planned, formal, classroom education programme is more likely to
effect a smooth introduction of a highly technical innovation than is an
informal, on the job training project"(3).

Thies, another researcher had concluded that "Hospital personnel ......perceived a greater overall contribution from working demonstrations and self-instruction through operational experience than from formal training sessions.   Training conducted by hospital personnel was generally better received than that conducted by an independent systems vendor"(3).

These are two conflicting but not incompatible points of view and the approach at Groote Schuur Hospital is to use both methods at different stages. Determining the attitudes of staff toward a system before implementation is an important factor.   If the staff view the introduction of a system negatively the implementors must employ an intensive education campaign to sell the system to those who will be using it.   This means that the reasons for introducing a system must be very clearly expressed, and show definite advantages over present methods.

The clinical area may well be one of the areas where personnel will be least inclined to accept computerisation.   Schmitz using data from research done by Thoren indicates that personnel directly involved in patient care may see computerisation as a threat to individuality, and increased automation, further diminishing the human factor in relationships.   They also may feel that computerisation will decrease their decision making.   Schmitz concludes that "behavioural factors must be given serious consideration when selecting systems for implementation.   In order to sell a system the user must clearly perceive the benefit to themselves(4).

9.   CONCLUSION

Having to do some research in developing this paper I have come to the following conclusions:

1.   That a nurse at top management level should be leading any computer training and implementation where nurses are involved.
2.   That the nurse should have knowledge of computers and their application before she can make a significant contribution to the development of any system.   As a start there should be a handbook for nurses with a glossary of terms because the subject of computerised information systems has a language of it's own.
3.   That the nurse must be able to articulate the reason for requesting a system with implications for nursing.
4.   That the nurse must be represented on any committee formed to investigate Hospital Information Systems.
5.   That the nurses in training must be introduced to the computer technology which is being used in the hospital setting.
6.   That the nurse must be able to describe her own function in detail before it can be programmed.
7.   That the nurse must be prepared for changes in attitude and approach.
8.   Confidentiality - is it possible? Do passwords keep information secure? In the Cape Times of April 26 1982 there is a paragraph about the cracking of computers(10).   It is claimed that "students of the University of California, Berkeley, have discovered how to read confidential material filed in the University computer, including such information as proposed exam papers, study ratings, and personal files. This method of cracking the computer is untraceable, even by the experts on the computer maintenance staff - leading to the position where nothing stored in the memory banks can be regarded as secure".

Finally, some of the questions I posed at the beginning of this paper have been answered for me.   I am much clearer on the position of the nurse in H.I.S. implementation and application and judging by the increasing amount of the advertising of hardware in the South African media this year, computers are

really here to stay, and data typists, word processor operators, systems
analysts and programmers are in great demand. There has also been a mushrooming
of educational facilities in the private sector to train people to do these
jobs.

REFERENCES

1. Schmitz Homer H, Hospital Information Systems, Aspen Publication p.25
2. ibid p.1.   3.   ibid p.88.   4.   ibid p.96
5. Groote Schuur Hospital Information Planning Study, July-August 1981 p.2-4
6. ibid p.64-65   7.   ibid p.76-82
8. Virts Samuel S., Introducing the Hospital-wide Information Systems to
    Hospital and Medical staffs. MEDINFO 77 Shires/Wolf editors
    North-Holland Publishing Company (1977)
9. Palma-Figueria, A., Weight, J., Groote Schuur Hospital
    Student Nurse Record System. September 1981. University of Cape Town
    Computer Science Department.
10. Molloy Bob. Science Focus. Cape Times April 26 1982 p.5

The Impact of Computers on Nursing
M. Scholes, Y. Bryant and B. Barber (eds.)
Elsevier Science Publishers B.V. (North-Holland)
© IFIP-IMIA, 1983

13.3.

THE NURSE MANAGER AND THE COMPUTER

Peter Squire

Introduction

Recognition of the need for the efficient use of the considerable resources which the community makes available to us is moving to a new level of urgency. The system of audit within the service is being strengthened, and we are rightly being required to account for the ways in which we use the money allocated to our service. The computer promises to be a most important aid to increased efficiency, an aid that we cannot afford to ignore or misuse. We are at a crossroad, which way should we turn? What should we be doing?

A multitude of salesmen claim to provide the definitive answer to all our needs for computer systems which will aid us in our efforts towards increased efficiency, but do we as nursing managers know the right questions to ask? In the majority of situations, the honest answer is no. This paper aims to discuss:-

1.   Why we should be using computers to aid the nurse manager.

2.   To outline some of the pitfalls and problems that face us and some of the decisions we will need to make if we are to exploit this most useful development in technology, the computer, as it can be applied to the problems of administering a nursing workforce.

3.   To describe how in Rugby we approached the task using a computer to support the nursing management, and how we have developed both our program and administrative systems.

4.   To outline how the immediate and intermediate future is seen in the context of the general availability of the technology rather than its application within centres of excellence only.

What to do with Computers

In considering what to do with computers, we should recognise what computers are particularly good at, and how this fits our needs as nurse managers. What computers are good at depends, to a large extent on the type of computer you use and the amount of memory store that is available. Even the small computers can be very good at manipulating information relating to staff and reproducing it in a variety of ways, they do this very quickly, far more quickly than is possible by using common office techniques.

The majority of uses to which computers have been put within the Health Service have required large mini or mainframe computers. The revolution which is now taking place in the technology of computers has made available at relatively low cost a capacity and facility which until a few years ago required hundreds of thousands, if not millions of pounds.

What type of computer system should we be introducing to aid the nursing manager?

Some people would seem to be moving towards systems which act as repositories for all the information that is available within the nursing administrative service relating to staff. It is suggested that this is probably inappropriate. Such systems require at the least mini computers with substantial memory storage facilities. These types of computers are expensive and when such systems are introduced into nurse management, their cost effectiveness can be lost or substantially reduced. No nursing organisation is going to dispense with its files or permanent information, correspondence, application forms, reference forms etc., which are held on all the staff within the Nursing Service. If the address of a particular member of staff is required, it is usually quicker to open a file cabinet than to use a computer. Very rarely do we write letters to all our staff at one time. This theme is developed later in the paper.

One cannot underestimate the necessity of ensuring that in introducing computers into a working situation, we do not create more work than we alleviate. When considering the use of a computer, serious thought should be given as to how it will fit into the organisation, rather than fitting the organisation to the computer. A nursing administrative system which existed at Rugby, and which is currently being developed within South Warwickshire, was based on the centralisation of contracts of employment. Employers have a statutory responsibility to provide staff with a contract of employment, and variations of the contract are also required when significant changes take place in working conditions. When a member of staff is employed, or changes hours/grade/address etc., a staff commencement form or a staff change form is completed and copies go to Finance and to the Nursing Office. It is from this source that the majority of information is collected. The system existed some time before the computer was introduced and so as far as the Nursing Officers are concerned, there has been very little change. The West Midlands Regional Health Authority also requires information as to the number of staff working in various wards/departments and so we arrange that any permanent change of location of staff is notified using the same return to keep the system simple.

The Rugby Development

The author, whilst District Nursing Officer in Rugby, purchased an inexpensive microcomputer, a 'Video Genie' and with a 16K of Random Access Memory then had to determine whether or not it was possible to produce a useful program which could be used in the better management of the nursing service. It was, he believed, a tribute to computing technology that he was able to produce a program which met his requirements. The program which was produced is planned to have the capacity of being modified and developed to meet changing needs.

The program published (L43) provides a visual display. It is very simple to modify this to provide a paper print-out. It utilises codes in order to save space and has its data stored within the program. This is a very inefficient mode of data storage and ways to overcome this weakness are discussed later in the paper.

The primary feature of this original program was that the personal/payroll number of each member of staff was used as a line number in the data part of the program. This is an advantage when it becomes necessary to change the information relating to a particular member of the staff. Each member of staff listed within the computer can be 'called' by their personal payroll number. The first 9999 lines of the program are reserved for data, that is information about the staff. The working section of the program listed within the articles takes up about 4,000 bytes of information leaving approximately 12,000 bytes for data. The various modifications to the program have increased its size thus within a small computer limiting the number of staff who can be listed within the program.

A similar theme is used throughout the program, a read, sort and print statement frequently repeated and asking for different pieces of information according to the requirements of the operator. The data recorded about each individual member of staff includes in addition to their personal number, their grade and the program displays codings which are used for grades. It is useful to make minor alterations to the codings in order to list nursing staff working in various parts of the hospitals and community. For example, nursing auxiliaries working within the maternity service could be classified as maternity nursing auxiliaries (MN/A) whereas auxiliaries working within the community could be community auxiliaries (CN/A). This facility is useful when there is a mix of units stored within a single data file. The program asks by which grade it is to analyse the data, the grade is entered and the computer then lists all the staff within the data of the grade to be examined. It provides the following information:-

Grade   Name   Unit   Location   Qualification   Age   WTE

and the sum of the whole time equivalent of that particular group of staff. Similarly, staff can be listed by unit. The unit program shows the code letters for the unit when this is inserted. Forty qualification codes are used.

'Location' is a particularly useful listing as it enables the manager to identify staff working within a particular ward by day or by night, or within a particular primary health care team. There are currently seventy location codes. A verification of the data within the computer is undertaken by checking the staff within individual wards against manual 'off duty' rotas.

Within the Rugby District the ward or departmental 'off duty' lists have space for the contracted hours or whole-time equivalent to be listed alongside each individual's name. This figure is added up to give the whole time equivalent allocated to each ward/department. A print-out of all the staff is made monthly by ward/department. These are sent to the Nursing Officers who check them against the ward 'off duty' lists, and it is a relatively simple matter to spot differences, which when they occur are rectified or explained. After the initial months of the new system, the alterations became less frequent, the work undertaken in relation to the maintenance and establishment by the nurse managers within the units has reduced, and the accuracy of the system much improved.

Monitoring Sick Leave Amongst Nursing Staff

'Monitoring the Sick Pattern' in the Nursing Mirror (L42) outlines a second development of the program which provides information relating to sickness and absence. It is in no way as comprehensive as the work which has been done by Telford(1,2). The program displays frequency/days lost and estimates percentage sick leave by District, Unit, Hospital, Area, Ward/Department, grade, qualification and age group. It also lists staff with more than or less than an identified number of periods of sick leave. One factor which came to light was the computer report concerning the frequency of periods of sickness which identified some members of staff who had a substantial number of periods of sick leave and yet had not been previously identified as having an attendance problem. It appeared that some of the staff known to their peers and managers as being poor attenders had displayed some other problem within their work.

This would seem to indicate that it is at times possible that a double standard may exist whereby the "popular" nurse or "troublefree" nurse may to an extent get away with a greater amount of periods of sickness than the nurse who had been less popular/trouble free with her peers and/or managers. By reviewing all staff the computer identifies all staff who equal or exceed the parameters set. This is an area of Personnel Management which warrants more research.

A further development of the program as yet unpublished provides an estimate of the cost of groups of nursing staff. It is an estimate which takes into account the basic salary, the night duty allowances, geriatric and psychiatric leads. It makes an estimate of extra duty payments based on a study of extra duty payments within the unit. It takes into account incremental point and is a far more accurate method of assessing the true cost of the salaries and wages element of the nursing service than the mid point of the scale approach which is used by so many Finance Officers to the detriment of the Nursing Service. The Rugby District has for two years now been using the SAS (Standard Accountancy System) accounts system. SAS is adequate on the expenditure side, but the preparation for the use of SAS, often neglected, is an accurate estimate of the actual costs of a particular nursing service, distributed by grade and unit.

The same simple basic pattern which forms the foundation of all three of the programs outlined can also be developed to monitor in-service training, management training, and the recording of individual nurses qualified to undertake additional nursing duties.

Nurstat, Nursick and Autoprint

The programs have now been considerably modified with the assistance of the Small Computer Group of the West Midlands R.H.A. to function on the CP/M operating system.

A large microcomputer with a rapid printer and a twin 8 inch disc unit is now used. The development of the original programs has continued, and the author is particularly indebted to Robin Toohill for his help.

The program within the Random Access Memory of the computer has been developed to operate from a separate data disc and this allows more information to be stored and makes updating of information far more efficient. The establishment control program NURSTAT, the sick leave program NURSICK and the cost estimating program is now working, although considerable verification is required on the latter before it is ready for publication. Both programs use the same data store. Instead of using the personal number as the file number, an input number is now used. This sorts the data produced and provides information in a more logical sequence than was possible in the original program.

Additionally, there is an autoprint program which provides the end of the month printout. This is particularly useful although far more complicated than originally imagined. Autoprint produces staffing lists by ward and area and produces summaries by area and District with a breakdown of staff by management, registered, enrolled, trained, learners and untrained for the District summary. A CP/M version of the Finance Program and a new program which will collate community nursing returns is currently being developed.

It is hoped to introduce the programs developed in Rugby to the authors' present District in order to continue developments of the program to aid him in the task of managing the District.

Programming and the Nurse

Learning the intricacies of "basic" programming is, a fascinating and most enjoyable hobby. Computers, contrary to the common belief, are invariably right, it is the people who deal with them who are wrong. They will only produce what they are asked to produce, and they will only produce that when they are "asked" properly. Programming is, in many ways, similar to chess, it is similar to writing off duties. It does require a lot of patience, and the ability to recognise ones own deficiencies.

The author recently received a telephone call asking advice about computer programs from a Nursing Officer, who was interested in using a computer, but not in any way interested in the technicalities of programming. It is not advocated that it should be part of a knapsack of every nurse manager that they should be able to program computers. However, within the nursing profession there is room for a number of nurse managers to learn the basic skills of programming in order that they can provide support and service to their colleagues. Ideally, this support should come from regional or sub-regional specialists. Every region in the country has a computer department employing systems analysts and computer programmers. They are however in such small numbers that it would be impossible for them to cope with the increasing number of small computers which are appearing within the Health Service. Because the "programmers" are over-committed, it is difficult for the ordinary manager to get access to them, and so consequently when a system or program has been developed, changes to the system and consequently to the program can only be achieved with great difficulty. Furthermore, professional computer programmers generally program in languages which are far more sophisticated than the amateur usually employs. It is likely that this will result in the amateur not having sufficient skill to make even the most minor modifications within the program to meet changing needs.

Because we are in the early days of computers in nurse management, it is important that the programs we use allow us to be flexible. To this end the author advocates the use of microsoft basic as the language of choice. Commercial programs may claim to offer flexibility but each program has its limits, particularly in their ability to handle the mathematics required to estimate costs in the nursing service.

If we could define exactly what we wish the program to do, no doubt a commercial program could be written but we do not know at this time what we want. Our needs will change as our knowledge of just what the technology is capable of develops. Microsoft basic enables local modification.

The Future

It is probable that in the future computer terminals will be available in most hospitals throughout the country. Some of these terminals could be intelligent terminals capable of independent activity. It is likely that the terminals will be linked to mini or mainframe computers situated either in large hospitals or in the District Headquarters with links to the Regional Health Authority. We have the technology, but it is likely to be some years before such a system becomes generally available.

We are at a difficult stage, the priority which individual health authorities will give to the introduction of the technology will differ between the Districts and the Regions. It is suggested that the best option available at this time is the use of micro computers as a first and interim step. In order to do this, there needs to be a degree of standardisation in the types of system used, so that there can be co-ordination and co-operation between Districts.

The Department of Health have offered a lead in this direction. In circular WKO(81)3, an obscure document for the eyes of District Works Officers entitled 'The Use of Small Computers in Health Service Works Organisations', they discuss the introduction of a collection of programs. These programms go under the names of WIMS (Works Information Management Systems), which were developed within the Department of Health to assist Works Officers in the management of their responsibilities. These programs have been designed to work on a particular type of microcomputer which operate on "microsoft" MBASIC language (Version 5.1) for a CP/M 2.2 computer operating system. The computer requires a 64K processor and twin 8 inch floppy disc units as stores for programs and data. Additionally, a line printer is required.

Such microcomputers would provide the type of computer support which would fulfil the immediate needs within nursing management for a number of years. The cost of such equipment is such that over a five year period it could be considered expendable, and could hopefully bridge the gap between now and when the large, more complex linked systems become available. A major advantage is that it is a microsoft basic language computer which is programmable by the amateur, and as such lends itself to the development of local programs. It is inappropriate for us to expend public money to develop systems that are only for our own use. If we develop something which is good and useful, we should, pass it on for use elsewhere within the service. Copyright law, of course, may apply to commercial systems. Relatively inexpensive programs are also available to convert such machines for use as word processors. This would be particularly useful in the production of the contracts of employment in a District Headquarters, nursing policies and procedures, and standard letters and documents required within the nursing service.

Although many advocate the use of the new technology we must be extremely careful, for computers can be a bandwagon on which it is popular to jump. Some salesmen are more than willing to sell computers which have either no immediately available and relevant programs or which require expensive additions if useful work is to be achieved.

To quote from a well known medical guideline "never do harm".

- we should not harm the service we provide by introducing untested systems which destroy the confidence of managers in the use of the technology.
- we should avoid the introduction of expensive systems until we can be sure that they can meet the needs of the service not only locally but in a way that allows inter-changeability and computer to computer communication.
- we must ensure that our systems are secure and that the information stored within them are only used for legitimate purposes controlled by an agreed Ethical policy.
- We should not destroy the credibility of the technology by introducing systems which create additional work or produce irrelevant information through it being either inaccurate or time-expired.

The use of computers within the Health Service is just about to take off in a big way. The decisions we take now will enhance or mar the use of this new technology. Money is not so readily available that we can afford to make costly mistakes. The only justification for introducing computers into nurse management is that they can, and if given the opportunity will, enable us as nurse managers to make far better use of the considerable resources that are made available to us. They will enable us to ensure that our nursing officers can spend more time in the management of nursing care than the administration of nurses.

Acknowledgement

I would like to acknowledge the major part that Mr. R.J. Toohill at the District Nursing Office, Rugby Health District has made in the development of the programs discussed within this paper.

REFERENCES

1.   Telford, W. A.,   Time Out a Matter for Management, East Birmingham
      Hospital (1980)
2.   Telford, W. A.,   Future Consideration of Time Out, East Birmingham
      Hospital (1981)

The Impact of Computers on Nursing
M. Scholes, Y. Bryant and B. Barber (eds.)
Elsevier Science Publishers B.V. (North-Holland)
© IFIP-IMIA, 1983

13.4.

NURSING DEMANDS ON DISTRIBUTED COMPUTER SERVICES

Ulla Gerdin-Jelger

Nursing Demands on Distributed Computer Systems

Centralized or distributed computer systems? Is there any difference to the
health care staff? If you ask a technician, the answer will be no, but if you
put the question to the trade unions they will say yes. In this paper I will
discuss the difference between the centralised and the distributed computer
solution, and especially the duty of the nurse in influencing the development of
health care computer systems.

15 Years of Health Care Computing

Sweden has, as many other countries, developed the main part of the health care
computer systems on a centralized base, with many different systems using the
same computer and database. Within Stockholm county, we have 400 terminals
distributed to hospitals, primary care units and long term hospitals. They are
all using the same programs for patient identity, control routines and patient
administrative routines. The terminals are handled by medical record officers
and in certain clinics by nurses and nursing aids.

The benefit of these systems is that you always can find out where and when the
patients have been treated before and for what.

The laboratories and the intensive care units have bought or developed their own
local computer systems for use only by each department for its own requirements.
They have seldom any connection with the central computer and are handled by all
members of the staff.

There is a great demand for computer support for various medical and
administrative problems today but the technique for development and the computer
technique itself is not yet ready to meet the essential demands from medical
operation and the health care workers.

The health care worker's essential demands on a computer system are the same as
ten years ago.

* The staff must be able to get information in and out of the system 24 hours a
  day. There is not very much activity going on in a hospital during night
  hours, but it is certainly not the time for extra routines.
* The system must be easy to develop and to make changes to. The daily unit
  operation is alive and the system must be able to follow all changes.
* The computer system must be a part of the daily routines, not something extra
  without connections.
* The professional knowledge must not be decreased due to the computer system.
* The development resources must include time for the health care workers
  involved to take part.
* The involved staff must, within the project, get the education they need.

* The health care workers must have the right to say no to a solution or a
  system that does not fit in.

From the nurses point of view, the big centralized computer system that we use
today is, as I have said before, mainly an administrative tool without any
special interest to nursing work. For over ten years we have had computer
systems and there have been many requests for clinical applications but for
several reasons, some of them listed below, it has not been possible.

* The centralized computer system demands a uniformity, which means that within
  a reasonable price you can not get a particular application which is suitable
  to your own requirements.
* The system should serve many different interests and there are always limited
  resources where the administrative applications have priority.
* The complexity of the system makes it expensive to develop, expand and even to
  make small changes to.
* The vulnerability of the system makes it unreliable in a nursing situation.
* The accessibility is not enough.
* There is no one within the clinical departments that has the responsibility
  for the design of work routines in and around the computer system.
* There are too many hands and communication between the nurse on the floor and
  the computer technicians takes too long.

It is worth remembering that within Stockholm county, every patient is
registered in the system with all the administrative data, including X-rays,
during the last thirteen years. But that is on an administrative level. With
the same computer philosphy you can not work out the problems on the clinical
level.

Distribution - just a philosophy and some new technique

The control of the computer system must be given to those who will use it. This
sounds very natural and simple; but when it comes to computer systems, it is
not, and probably will not be for many years. The light I can see is what the
technicians call the distributed system. This requires the same effort and cost
as the centralized system and the same possibilities to communicate with other
systems. It will physically be placed close to the operation level and each
clinical department will have a suitable version of a system where the unit
operation as well as the work conditions and the work environment can be taken
into consideration.

With the progress that the computer technique has and will have, distribution of
the systems will give the health care workers a chance to influence their own
work condition. My own starting point is that we need a computer support in
health care, but the outcome now and in the future will depend on the health
care workers own engagement and possiblities to influence them.

Resourses for experimental development

We still miss a good technique for development of computer systems in health
care. So far, the health care worker's knowledge of her own operational tasks
as well as the complexity of the operational tasks have been underestimated.
The knowledge of the effects of the computer system are also not very efficient.
We must find a practical and useful way and a model for examination of the
effects.

We can not any longer afford to develop expensive computer tools that only will
be used as subroutines. In Sweden we have got a national project called DASIS.
it is supported by the Swedish government and has two purposes. One is to
develop a health care system which can be a product to the Swedish manufactures.

The second is to develop a system that will function in the health care environment. Most people with earlier experience of development in health care are gathered together on the DASIS project. The most important part of this project is that it has got resources to experiment with different techniques for system development and examination of effects.

The timetable of the project says that the specification of demands will be finished by the end of March 1983 and that an operational test will be carried out a year later. The DASIS project started in 1978 and will be concluded in 1985. All interested parties have got a place within the project. They have a duty to influence and to put the demands that will give the project a chance to succeed. The health care workers are represented through the whole project organization on the operational level by the staff working there and in each of the other levels by their trade unions. The trade unions have got their own consultants, paid by the project. These consultants shall co-ordinate with the unions and help them to find the necessary demands on the outcome of the project.

The most interesting part of the project is the review of the effects. This part has got its own resourses to develop methods to control and steer during the specification stage. Finally to report the effects in qualitative and quantitative terms as well as which are and are not possible to realize.

The system also gives potential for new technical development. We know that the technique we have today is not sufficient to the requirement of health care. Within the project we will need to experiment both with the system design and the in and output tools.

Stockholm county is one out of three counties within the DASIS project that will do local operational tests. We will test computer support in medical record handling, including routines for order entry to laboratories and medical consultants. The DASIS system will be a distributed computer system. The nurses participate in the project and have an obligation to put realistic demands on the result.

Nursing demands on distributed computer systems!

The new technique not only gives the computer system more power. It also makes it possible to develop systems that can take over a lot more of the complex routines. New facilities are for example,

* Composing
* Control routines
* Voice input

* Automatic mail
* Chips on a card
* Communication between different systems

This means that we will have to get used to the idea that nothing will be as before and that we have to say how we would want the health care sector to be as a place of work.

What are our possibilities to influence the development in Sweden?

* Since 1977 we have had a co-determination act that forces the employer to inform and to negotiate with the trade unions about changes in the work conditions including workroutines, organisations and employment.

* Since 1979 we have had a work environment act which gives each employee possibilities to influence her own work conditions.

These two acts do not really help us since we know too little (we have no experience) about the possibilities and consequences of the computer. Only operational tests can give us experience. We, the nurses, can not alone put the demands on the project result. We have to co-ordinate ourselves with the other interested parties. In Sweden we have four different categories working in the clinical department, including doctors, nurses R.N., nursing aids and medical record officers.

In this uncertain development situation everyone is as anxious about her or his,

* Professional role   * Professional knowledge
* Tasks and amount of work   * Work environment
* Education   * Contact with the patient
* Employment and the effects on the work organization

The different parties have conflicting interests in the outcome of development work. It is therefore very important that each party has prepared questions and are ready to negotiate. The parties will, in this case, be the trade unions.(1)

* What is our role today and how do we want it to be developed?
* Which tasks we are doing today and which do we want to be relieved from?
* What is important in the work today?
  - The contact with the patient?
  - The contact with other fellow workers?
  - The contents of the work?
  - The professional progress?
  - The team work?
* What is urgent to change?
  - The organizing?
  - The amount of administrative work?

The answers will be the found in the examination of the effects.

The Swedish nurses association and SHSTF, (the trade union), are working with a description of the future role of the nurse and her professional skills. Within two years, before the DASIS project has come into its final stage, the trade unions must have presented their demands on distributed computer systems (2), in the terms of:

* Unit operation   * Work conditions
* Service to the patient   * Economy and resources
* Security for both the patient
  and the health care staff   * Future development

Summary

The difference between centralized and distributed computer systems, to the health care staff, is the closeness to the users. The new facilities that the latest technical development have brought will, together with the distributed system philosophy, carry a whole new outlook on the health care work. There are already today projects going on that have started this change of procedures in different parts of the health care sector.

It is urgent that we, the nurses, together with the rest of the health care workers express our demands and requirements on what we want the health care sector to be as a place of work in the future. We have an obligation to use all possibilities to influence the development and to make and active role in the project work. To do this we need to be prepared for the discussion with the other trade unions on the several questions that have conflicting interests to ours, for the setting of demands on the project results and finally for examination and evaluation of effects.

REFERENCES:

1. A Trade Union EDP Policy, U. Gerdin-Jelger, U-B Johansson, A-C Boden, I Holmback, Proc. MEDINFO 80.
2. Dasis, A Warranty for a User Accepted Computer Application, U. Gerdin-Jelger. IMIA Working Conference, Stockholm 1982.

The Impact of Computers on Nursing
M. Scholes, Y. Bryant and B. Barber (eds.)
Elsevier Science Publishers B.V. (North-Holland)
© IFIP-IMIA, 1983

13.5.

THE DESIGN AND IMPLEMENTATION OF COMPUTER PROGRAMS FOR ORDER ENTRY AND REVIEW

Dickey Johnson

Introduction

Growing numbers of hospitals are installing computer systems to make procedures and record-keeping more efficient and accurate. Hospitals may purchase a pre-designed system that is marketed in a package which allows the purchasing hospital limited flexibility in program design. Other systems available to hospitals may be developed on-site which allows the hospital much design flexibility. These systems, however, require a great deal of analysis, design, and testing before hospital-wide implementation is successful.

LDS Hospital in Salt Lake City, Utah is a tertiary care facility of 570 beds. In conjunction with the University of Utah Department of Biophysics, a computer system is being developed and implemented on-site. An outdated computer was replaced with a completely flexible system that would accommodate previously designed medical decision making programs. This system will be marketed to other hospitals in the near future. Currently, the major emphasis in development is on design and implementation in order entry and order review programs. This is one of many phases in establishing an extensive computerized data base on patients.

Prior to order entry there was already an extensive data base on all patients in the hospital. Laboratory results, medications prescribed, and admit data are a few of the contributions to the data base. Most data entry was performed by the departments. Terminals and printers on each nursing division were used primarily for data retrieval.

The most unique aspect of this system is the HELP (Health Evaluation through Logical Processing) medical decision making system. Data from all areas can interact to produce sophisticated decisions that may assist doctors and nurses in caring for their patients. Algorithms have been designed to provide numerous laboratory and pharmacy alerts, the five most probable x-ray diagnoses on a patient, acid-base interpretations, various other pulmonary interpretations and ECG interpretations.

The main purposes for addition of order entry to the data base were to automated billing, expedite service to patients, and improve order record-keeping. Order review programs were to be developed so that orders could be reviewed, cancelled, and billed on-line by each department. Although the ideal situation would be to have physicians enter their own orders, it was felt that all attending physicians were not yet willing and that it would be difficult to train the large numbers of house staff that rotated in and out of the hospital. Programs were therefore designed for use by ward clerks and nurses.

The design and implementation of these programs has occurred in several phases, each phase being a learning experience adding to improve the methods for design and implementation of the next phase. The steps in design of the programs were in the order of system analysis, program design, and user review. The steps in implementation were program piloting, training, and hospital-wide implementation.

1.   Phase One

The first phase of the design and implementation of the order entry and review programs was carried out by one programmer and an assistant.   The system analysis was done by reviewing paper requisitions with the various hospital service departments.   This, along with feedback from department heads, established the data needed by the department when an order was made.   All chargeable procedures or items were given codes.   Two nurses and three ward clerks were contacted for input on ordering procedures on the nursing division.

After this analysis, three programs were written to allow for flexibility in design of ordering questionnaires, print capabilities, and review programs.   The flexibility was necessary to accommodate different needs of the departments. The "questionnaire" program for order entry allows for a series of questions and answers that appear in a menu selection format.   Brief instructions can be displayed with each question and menu choices are made by typing in the number of the desired option.   Choice of a certain option may automatically branch to another question specific to that option such as a size selection.   A "free text" (any combination of letters or words) question is also available for answers that must be typed in. (see Fig.1)

The second program to be developed provides the capability to print a hardcopy or "printout" of the order.   A program was designed to allow data from an order to be arranged in any manner on a hardcopy.   The hardcopy is sent to a printers at any specified location.

The basic review programs allow for review of orders according to department or patient.   Users of programs on the nursing division may change the time the order is to be done and review or cancel orders.   In addition, users in the departments have the ability to change the billing status of the order.   All orders have a status of "pending" as soon as they are stored by the order entry program.   When an order has been completed, the status is manually or automatically changed to complete (ready to bill) in the department.   Options such as crediting and adding a cost are also available to the departments.

With the completion of these programs, order entry questionnaires were designed for each hospital department.   In most cases, information from the paper requisitions comprised the questionnaire.   Hardcopies of the order were to print in the departments and each department designed their printout.   The review programs allowed for a general format that would apply to all departments.

User approval and implementation were the next steps.   The same nurses and ward clerks were shown these programs and the director of nursing was given hardcopies for each questionnaire.   Their approval was given.   Implementation was to cover all fifteen order entry questionnaires to be brought up hospital-wide over about two months.   Training was to be done by the Director of Education, an R.N. with experience in the computer department, and the ward clerk orientation instructor.

Problems with the designs and plans became apparent when the trainers began preparation for classes.   After drawing on their own experience and communicating with a few hospital departments, it was obvious that many changes or additions were necessary.   The programmers failed to fully comprehend user capabilities, user job responsibilities, different ordering needs in specific nursing areas, and details of billing in different departments.   The users approving the programs also were not fully aware of the implications and significance of the change to computer ordering.   Fundamental needs had been fulfilled, but there were more specific ones to be met.   The R.N. was assigned to be the Computer Co-ordinator and act as the liaison between the programmers and the hospital.   She began working with the questionaires and review programs

in depth.   She recognized that changes were necessary in several areas.   To
begin with, program prompts and instructions needed alteration for three
reasons:

Figure 1

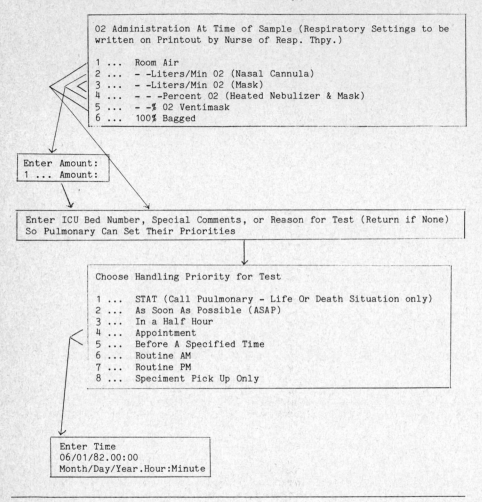

Screens from Blood Gas Order Entry Questionnaire

(i)   Hospital users have varied levels of expertise and rates of comprehension.

(ii)   Knowledge of typing terminology and basic typing skills varies, and

(iii) Many users had not used the terminals enough in the past to be familiar
       with basic computer functions and terminology.

A second issue was that the questionnaire would have required ward clerks to enter information not always provided in physician's orders. The clerks could not be held legally responsible for providing this information by making decisions on patients medical data. Other changes were found to be necessary because computer order entry replaced paper requisitions in duplicate and triplicate. The copies were used for a variety of purposes and their absence would require many changes in keeping records. Another problem was that the billing programs did not satisfy individual departmental requirements. In both ordering and billing there were many situations occurring only occasionally or even rarely that were not covered by the programs. In addition, many ordering situations were specific to one nursing area such as intensive care, nursery, surgery, or emergency room. Training and implementation was delayed until changes could be made. It was decided that order entry would be implemented for several departments at a time.

Phase Two

The second phase of order entry and review was the re-design of programs for the blood gas and cardiology departments. This phase took five months from analysis to implementation. The previously designed questionnaires and reviews were used as the basic framework to which additions and changes were made. The programs were originally designed to be flexible enough to allow for many changes.

1. System Analysis

The objective of the system analysis was to detail departmental and nursing procedures in greater depth so that the computer ordering would work similar to the current paper system. With the new design, some problems in the current system could even be alleviated. The Co-ordinator spent time in each department to learn how an order was handled upon receipt, what types of errors were made in ordering and billing, how patients were billed and credited, what records were kept, how copies of the requisition were used, and what information the department needed on their requisition. The next step was to talk with clerks on a variety of nursing divisions to find out what they wrote on requisitions, how the orders were communicated to the department, and what records were kept of orders made. Charts were reviewed to see how physicians wrote their orders.

The flow of events for the computer ordering and billing process was outlined. When the order was entered into the computer by the nurse or clerk, a hardcopy would print in the appropriate department. This hardcopy would be the notification and paper record. For blood gases, a hardcopy would also print on the nursing division so temperature and respirator settings could be filled in by the nurse. Upon completing the ordered procedure, department technicians would be responsible for changing the billing status of the order from "pending" to "complete-ready to bill".

2. Program Design

The pre-existing questionnaires were reviewed by the Co-ordinator and changes were discussed with the programmer. In addition, a method was agreed upon whereby a beginner could go step by step through each screen or the experienced user could enter a string of commands without viewing each screen.

Review programs were re-designed by a second programmer and allowed for review according to patient or department, order time or execute time (time procedure is to be done), and billing status. (See Fig. 2) Twelve review programs were designed with slight variations on format and function depending on who the users would be.

Figure 2 Printout of Orders from all Departments: Johnson, Evan

DESCRIPTION	ORDERED	EXECUTE	STATUS	TECH
1 2D/M-Mode Echo(Combo)	06/14 09:18	06/14 09:18 ASAP	BILL	DIA
2 EKG (12 Lead)	06/13 01:19	06/13 01:19 STAT	BILL	YWE
3 Partial Blood Gas	06/13 02:28	06/14 00:00 ROUTINE A.M.	COMP	YWE

The Co-ordinator and programmers also planned general considerations for all programs. Numerous methods for correcting entry errors were decided upon. Prompts or instructions for each screen were written using non-technical language. The ability to type in a " ? " to bring up a screen with additional detailed instructions was to be included in a number of places.

3.   User Review

The next step was to have a representative group of clerks and nurses review and critique programs. Two separate groups were formed with representatives from Medicine, Surgery, Intensive Care, Orthopedics, Obstetrics/Gynecology, and Management. The seven nurse representatives were comprised of head nurses and two assistant administrators. Staff nurses were asked to participate but there were no volunteers. Clerks asked to be representatives were chosen on the basis of expertise. Two meetings for each group were held approximately four weeks apart and requested changes were made in between meetings. At each meeting, questionnaires and programs were demonstrated by the Co-ordinator and then the users each had hands-on terminal practice. They entered orders collected from patient charts all over the hospital. They were then asked to apply hypothetical or real ordering situation from their own experiences.

The user reviews were extremely useful and informative. A number of ordering situations had not yet been considered in the program designs. The ICU representatives pointed out problems caused by their need for more data input for blood gas orders, their unusual ordering situations, and their need for speed in ordering due to large numbers of orders. Feedback from all users on steps in the data entry included the need for further changes in prompts or instructions on screens. They indicated that some steps were too complicated or confusing. At the first user meeting only the Co-ordinator was present and she was unable to answer a number of qestions about programming capabilities. When she relayed user requests to the programmers, they had difficulty in understanding or believing the importance of some requests. Therefore, the second meeting included the programmers so they could better understand user needs and provide feedback on what changes were possible. At the second meeting the users gave their approval. Only minor changes were made after that.

4.   Program Piloting

The implementation phase began with piloting of the two programs on a nursing division. The purpose of this was to enable users to discover further unforeseen problems while using the programs in a real-time situation. Before hospital-wide implementation took place, all necessary changes were to be made in order to minimize the difficulties caused by a need for re-training or notification of all users if post-implementation changes were made. The pilot would also give the departments time to practice and enable them to uncover problems.

The plan for the pilot was to have one medical nursing division use the program for at least two weeks. The clerks and nurses would be trained on site. Paper requisitions would accompany computer orders for the first week as a back-up. A comment sheet would be taped to each terminal for communication of ideas, questions, and problems. The Co-ordinator would make at least two rounds per day (morning and afternoon) to the division and departments.

Once the pilot began, many alterations were made in the plan. One nursing division did not generate enough orders so a second one was added. The time period expanded to four weeks because of numerous problems in billing patients. Also, one department supervisor was very resistant to the change and had been relatively uninterested when reviewing programs and procedures prior to the pilot. The pilot, however, aroused the supervisor's interest and raised many questions. Numerous changes had to be made for that particular department. Use of paper requisitions as a backup made the users begin to ignore the computer and rely on the old method. This was abandoned after two days and a phone call was instituted as a backup for three days only. This backup reassured users of the reliability of the computer and alerted departments to watch their printers for orders.

The comment sheet was very helpful and was used heavily mostly by the night and weekend shifts. The Co-ordinator checked the comments on her twice daily rounds and wrote replies to each one. Many of the comments gave rise to changes. The sheet also had dates and times of the occurance of specific problems which made it easier for follow-up by the Co-ordinator. For the pilot, the Co-ordinator was assisted by the ward clerk supervisor. At least two rounds, one in the morning and one in the afternoon, were made each day. On weekends, users were given the home phone numbers of the two trainers. There were few night and weekend calls. While doing the on-site training and answering questions, it became apparent what areas were to be concentrated on in training for the hospital-wide implementation. Certain changes in procedure and some terminal entries were more confusing than others.

Before beginning the classroom training, instructions were written for the two new questionnaires and the review programs. The purpose of this written documentation of procedures and computer entries was to provide users with a reference for problems or questions, and to enable users to learn more complicated entries after learning the basics. Designing the format of the instructions was difficult as there were no other manuals available for reference nor were there any published articles on the subject. A five column format was designed that would enable the user to quickly find the screen in question. Because questions branched in various directions, consecutive step by step instructions were not possible. Each step was numbered, however, and the number of the next step was given for each question. (See Fig. 3) Branch diagrams were attempted but the majority were too complicated and large. Instructions were referred to during classroom training and manuals were placed on each nursing division. The manuals also contained other program instructions for transfer, discharge, and lab review along with a glossary of terms, terminal instructions, and printer instructions.

Figure 3: Manual Instructions for ECG Order Entry

LDS HOSPITAL

ORDER ENTRY - EKG/CARDIOLOGY

STEP	COMPUTER MESSAGE	EXPLANATION	ENTRY EXAMPLES
		-->= refer to entry column	
1	2. EKG/CARDIOLOGY		
2	1. EKG (12 LEAD) 2. RHYTHM STRIP 3. HOLTER MONITOR	These 3 orders go to the EKG lab. Go to step 4	
	4. ECHOCARDIOGRAM 5. 2DIM-ECHOCARDIOGRAM (only) 6. M-MODE ECHO 7. 2D/M-MODE ECHO (COMBINED) 8. CONTRAST ECHO 9. EXERCISE THALLIUM 10.PHONOCARDIOGRAM	These orders (4-10) go to cardiology Go to step 3	
	11.MISCELLANEOUS>>	This is free text for any order that does not fit in any of the above categories. There should **rarely** be a need to use this. Go to step 4.	
3	ENTER RETURN IF PATIENT TO BE TRANSPORTED OR CHOOSE 1: 1...PORTABLE EQUIPMENT REQUIRED	This option appears only with cardiology orders. If the patient is seriously ill and cannot be moved enter-->. Go to step 4.	1

5.   Training

Classroom training and hospital-wide implementation took place simultaneously over a period of six weeks. A total of approximately 250 clerks, night nurses, head nurses, and nursing supervisors were trained. The head nurses were responsible for seeing that all their staff received instruction. There was not adequate in-service funding to allow for classroom training of all nurses. Nursing supervisors were to be responsible for answering questions and referring problems to the trainee during the afternoon, night, and weekend shifts. The training room had six terminals for hands-on practice and a large screen video monitor for demonstrations. The classes were to be an hour long with a maximum of 8 trainees per class. Past experience in training proved that two hour classes were too long and that material was forgotten if training took place more than four or five days prior to implementation. Seven A.M. classes were scheduled for those working the 11pm-7am shift. When classes were scheduled before the shift at 10 pm, most staff did not show up. On the other hand, it was difficult for the night shift to stay awake during the Seven A.M. classes. The trainers were the Co-ordinator and the ward clerk supervisor. One trainer would teach a class while the other made rounds on all the floors that had been started on computer ordering within the previous two weeks.

The method of instruction was to discuss changes in procedures, demonstrate the data entry on the overhead monitor, and then have users have hands-on practice entering orders. During each class, these steps were carried out separately for blood gas ordering, ECG ordering, and order review. The hands-on practice was very helpful but the bulk of actual learning seemed to take place when the users were computer ordering on a real-time basis. The users that used their terminals during the demonstration (they were instructed to just listen) tended to have more problems during the hands-on practice because they had tried to listen and practice at the same time. The trainers also discovered that one trainer was not enough to supervise the hands-on practice because there were usually one or two people who were slower to learn. After this became apparent, the other trainer would try to be present during the hands-on practice.

6   Implementation

The implementation schedule had three to four of the nursing divisions begin computer ordering on Mondays and Tuesdays. A majority of the classes were held at the end of the week on Thursdays and Fridays. Frequent rounds were made to "new" divisions the first week and at least one morning and afternoon round the second and third weeks. Both trainers were also available by beeper during weekdays. Comment sheets were placed on all divisions, but were used rarely -- probably because most problems had already been worked out.

Frequent rounds were also made to the departments. Department supervisors were considered the computer "resource" person within the department so they handled most problems and contacted a trainer when necessary. The comment sheets were most helpful as the department technicians could specify which clerks were making mistakes when ordering. The comments also pointed out procedures that were not working well. In this case, an alternative was decided upon and divisions were notified during the trainer's rounds and through messages on the terminal screens. It was somewhat difficult for the departments to operate using both the old and new ordering procedures for the implementation period. At the end of the six weeks, things were running smoothly and only a few minor changes were yet to be made.

The reactions from clerks, and nurses were interesting. The clerks, as a whole, felt the computer ordering was faster for them and resulted in a much faster response from the departments. They particularly liked the fact that there was no question as to whether an order was sent because it was stored in the computer and available for review. The ICU nurses frequently order their own blood gases and the ones that had not been trained were very angry at the change. They felt it was unnecessary and time consuming. The majority of these nurses, however, liked the ordering once they learned the reasons behind it and the quick method for using the questionnaires.

Phase Three

The third phase of order entry was the design and implementation of programs for X-ray and Central Service. Steps were taken similar to those in Phase Two. Changes were made, however, to avoid some of the problems previously encountered. The third phase took six months from system analysis to hospital-wide implementation.

1   Analysis and Design - X-ray

The analysis and design of the X-ray program was the sole responsibility of a programmer assigned to X-ray. The department had a large number of programming requirements specific to their needs. Because these needs were so specific, ordering from the nursing divisions would be in the form of "electronic mail." Physicians would be required to fill out a requisition, which was the current practice, and this information would be entered into the computer verbatim by the clerk or nurse.   Upon receipt of the electronic mail order, the X-ray department would enter the order into the computer with their specifications. This entry generated appropriate labels and forms to print in the department. The divisions would have the same review and cancel functions after the order was entered by the department.

A few problems became apparent when the X-ray programmer demonstrated the finished electronic mail questionnaire to the Co-ordinator.   The ordering questionnaire was written from the point of view of the programmer and the X-ray department supervisor. The questionnaire was time consuming and asked for some data not available on the requisition. Revisions were made so that the format of the questionnaire was in the same order and worded the same as the requisition. Free text entry was provided for any portion of the requisition where the physician could write in his request (e.g., exam, reason, time to be done).   Other parts of the requisition were menu selection and this was easily copied into the questionnaire.

2   Analysis and Design - Central Services

Analysis and design of Central Service (C.S.) was carried out by the Co-ordinator.   It was difficult, as in the Second Phase, to get both the C.S. department head and supervisor involved in the specifics of the design of ordering and review programs.   They were very busy with their management and billing responsibilities and as with the other users who helped plan and review programs, it was difficult for them to realize the actual degree of change that computer ordering and billing would induce. Discovery of billing needs not yet encountered in other departments required introduction of several new billing statuses and three new variations of the review programs.   These billing needs occurred for situations such as items ordered in quantity, items temporarily out of stock, and machines or equipment rented by patients on a daily, weekly, or monthly basis.

The most time consuming job was to obtain and organize an accurate inventory of all C.S. items. The C.S. management could not give this their complete attention so the Co-ordinator updated the information obtained when the first phase was carried out two years before. In addition, the description of each items had to be understandable for all users - clerks, nurses, and C.S. technicians. The old method of ordering consisted of writing a description of the item on a requisition. This, however, allowed for a diverse range of descriptions for any item. Also, to assure the user of finding a specific item when ordering in the computer, the 525 items were alphabetized and sorted into various groups. There were twenty groups including, for example: Most Common Items, Dressings & Gauze, Orthopedics, Patient Personal & Comfort Items, and Trays & Sets.   The C.S. requisition was in duplicate so users for each copy had to be traced. Billing was done from one slip and the second was used for keeping track of rental machines and for Infectious Disease records. Review programs had to be written to accommodate uses of the second copy.

3   User Review

The same group of users met to review the programs. One additional ICU head
nurse was invited to join the user group because she was very dissatisfied with
the previously implemented programs. The Co-ordinator thought it would be
helpful for her to understand why the programs were designed the way they were
and it would also encourage her to give constructive criticism instead of just
complaints. The users met twice and gave helpful suggestions. Some volunteered
to review the list of C.S. items to comment on descriptions and help group
items. The two ICU head nurses voiced great concern over how to handle the
large amounts of items ordered to restock the "mini-C.S." closets in the ICU's.
Various methods were discussed and it was decided that one method would be
implemented on a trial basis. Anticipated reactions from the users were
discussed because both order questionnaires would take slightly longer than the
current system. The users agreed that the overall benefits of the change would
minimize this concern.

The C.S. department head and supervisor reviewed the ordering and review
programs. They decided that all C.S. technicians would be trained to review and
change the billing status of orders. They voiced concern over the fact that the
C.S. staff had no prior experience with the computer so approximately six weeks
before training for the program pilot, all C.S. employees were given a forty-
five minute class with basic typing and computer entry instruction and hands-on
practice. The C.S. terminal was installed in the department so they could
practice using simple patient location programs.

4   Program Pilot

Two nursing divisions were chosen to pilot both ordering programs for a minimum
of two weeks. Since piloting programs was often frustrating for clerks and
nurses, different divisions than those used in the second phase were chosen.
Clerks and nurses were taught on the divisions.

All C.S. personnel attended a 90 minute class with hands-on practice. The
ordering questionnaires and all aspects of changing the billing status of orders
were presented. The technicians had had no previous experience with patient
billing so they had difficulty understanding credits and debits. They had also
had little time to practice on their department terminal and were, therefore,
very unskilled and anxious. Despite this, they all were very willing to learn.

Due to a very tight hospital budget, the Co-ordinator conducted the pilot
without assistance. The nursing divisions had few problems with ordering.
Their biggest problem was finding a specific C.S. item in the various menus.
The X-ray department encountered problems in their collection and organization
of exam requests. While the X-ray programmer spent long hours changing his
programs, the Co-ordinator spent a majority of her time in the C.S. department.
The C.S. staff still needed a great deal of help and were very apprehensive
about the change.

It was felt, after two weeks, that addition of another division was necessary to
really test the impact of the ordering on both departments. A nursing division
was chosen that was large and very busy. The increase in orders received helped
the departments be better prepared for the implementation. The pilot was
extended for one week.

5   Implementation

The Director of Education and the Co-ordinator decided that no classes would be
held for third phase implementation. Most nursing division users were
experienced as they had been ordering ECGs, echocardiograms, and blood gases for

six months. They had also been using the review programs to review and cancel orders. Since it had been difficult to take clerks and especially nurses away from their divisions to come to class, it was decided that training would take place on the nursing divisions. All clerks would be trained on a one-to-one basis and an attempt would be made to train as many nurses as possible.

It was also decided that implementation would take four instead of six weeks. The Co-ordinator wanted to avoid prolonging the confusion in the departments caused by use of both the old and new methods. The hospital administration was also very concerned with the fact that the project was falling behind schedule.

Previous trainers were not available to assist in the implementation so two new ones were temporarily hired to assist the Co-ordinator. One ward clerk and one R.N. were involved because of their expressed interest in the computer. Both had been involved in the user groups and both were on a division piloting the C.S. and X-ray programs. Several meetings were held during the piloting to discuss departmental procedures and plans for implementation. A schedule was made out so that trainers were available 8 a.m. to 5 p.m. seven days a week. The nursing supervisors would again be trained and would answer calls on evenings, and nights. They could call the trainers at home if necessary. The X-ray programmer would be responsible for any problems within that department.

The implementation went as planned although some problems occurred. After the second week, X-ray order entry had to be stopped because of the department's inability to handle the large number of incoming orders. Many changes had to be made in the X-ray programs. Management and personnel problems in the C.S. Department along with major changes in their procedures caused much disruption. The coordinator spent the majority of her time assisting the C.S. employees in their use of the computer. Also, during the implementation, few nurses were trained as they were rarely at the nurse's station with time to spare and, as before, they assumed they could just learn from the clerks. The trainers were not available during night shift hours so morning clerks were encouraged to demonstrate the programs to the night nurses. Few learned from this approach.

The X-ray Department was not ready for implementation for another 5 weeks. The training assistants had since gone back to their regular duties. Therefore, only the coordinator and X-ray supervisor attempted to assist the users in learning the programs. A message on all terminals announced the commencing of computer ordering for X-ray. X-ray employees would phone nursing divisions still using the old method to remind them of the change. These employees were also instructed in the use of the ordering program so questions phoned to them could be answered. This was probably the most helpful aspect of this implementation. The order entry program on the whole was very simple and self-explanatory and there was only one procedure change.

In an effort to evaluate the phase three implementation, a questionnaire was distributed. Respondents (136 total) consisted of nurses (61%) and clerks (39%). A majority of the clerks felt the training had been adequate for both C.S. and X-ray. The nurses however, felt the training had not been adequate. Of those clerks and nurses who felt the training was not adequate, most would have been willing to come to a class. A large majority of both groups felt programs to be self-explanatory. An interesting response was that 74% rarely or never referred to the instruction manual.

Conclusion

As a result of the various methods used here in design and implementation, I have a number of suggestions for those about to embark on such an effort.

Initially, before design and implementation, it is most important to establish strong administrative support from both hospital and nursing administrators. If these administrators are directly involved in the initial planning of the system they will understand, from the beginning, the intended goals. As development progresses, the administrative group must be kept informed of strengths and weaknesses. They must also be involved in making decisions about such topics as priority of needs, changes in job responsibilities, and changes in procedures.

When designing programs for clinical use it is essential that a nurse be directly involved because nursing as a whole will ultimately be affected. When functioning as a liaison/coordinator between the hospital and computer department, it is most helpful if the nurse has had considerable experience in the institution. Since most nurses have no experience with systems analysis, at this stage a consultant could be hired to assist the nurse coordinator.

It is also very important that departments be actively involved in the design of any program that will affect them. A department representative should review and test programs on a regular basis during the design phase. The coordinator should discuss all possible implications of the change with the department manager so both parties will know what to expect.

User groups are, of course, invaluable and at LDS Hospital they have final say as to whether or not a program is ready for use. Frequency of meetings depends on the speed at which program changes are being made. The meetings should be frequent enough so that the users can become very familiar with the programs and can apply a wide variety of situations to them. It may be wise to continue these user meetings during and after implementation to assure a steady flow of feedback.

For the phase of program piloting, at least 3 weeks on two nursing divisions should be planned. This may vary due to the complexity of the programs being tested. Nursing divisions that will use the programs the most should be selected, although the same division should not be used repeatedly for piloting. Piloting programs can be very frustrating at times. Departments should be fully trained before the pilot and a resource person within the department should be appointed - preferably the same person who worked on designing the programs. Comment sheets for nursing divisions and departments are very useful.

Training assistants should be involved in the user groups and available to assist the coordinator during the pilot. This will give them sufficient experience with the programs so that they can handle most questions and problems arising during hospital-wide implementation. At least a full-time and a part-time assistant should be available for the hospital-wide implementation.

Training classes should be considered rather than on-site training for the hospital-wide implementation. Too many distractions and interruptions occur during on-site training. Terminals for every 1-2 persons should be available for hands-on practice. In order to train a greater number of nurses, a slide presentation of screens could be held on the nursing division at a regularly scheduled inservice time. Night and weekend staff nurses must be trained as there is less clerical and computer assistance during those shifts. Training should be given as close to the time of implementation as possible.

The coordinator should be available on a permanent basis to follow up on problems, keep programs up to date, and to train new nursing personnel. This is particularly important in a development setting such as that at LDS Hospital. The coordinator keeps up to date on all developments and makes sure that input from nursing is given when needed.

The Impact of Computers on Nursing
M. Scholes, Y. Bryant and B. Barber (eds.)
Elsevier Science Publishers B.V. (North-Holland)
© IFIP-IMIA, 1983

13.6.

AMENDING AND EXTENDING AN EXISTING PATIENT ADMINISTRATION SYSTEM

Deirdre M. Gossington

Introduction

The North Staffordshire Health Authority, one of the largest in the country, with a population of 469,000 was chosen by the D.H.S.S in the late 1960s as an experimental site for the development of a real-time patient administration system to serve two acute hospitals, the City General Hospital with 597 beds, the North Staffordshire Royal Infirmary with 475 beds and the Central Out-Patients Department all of which are managed as one unit and form part of the Hospital Centre.

The system consists of a Master Patient Index which provides common routine details like name, age, sex, address, G.P. for every patient making an in-patient or out-patient contact. Data related to each admission or out-patient attendance is added to the record to build up a patient history. Information from the in-patient element provides bed occupancy figures, H.A.A. statistics, real-time bed states and lists of patients currently in hospital. The out-patient element is used to book clinics within consultant rules, reschedule clinics, print patients calling letters and prepare statistics. The waiting list system schedules patients from their addition to the list to their admission to hospital. The systems operate in real-time and are available all day every day.

Original System

The original mainframe machine was installed in a building in the grounds of the North Staffordshire Royal Infirmary. VDU's and teleprinters were supplied to all out-patient clinics and admission offices and the in-patient system was driven by a network of datapens on all the 50 wards and teleprinters in locked cabinets in hospital corridors for the shared use of several wards. From 1974 to 1982 these facilities provided a successful real time patient administration system for the 35,000 in-patient admissions and 190,000 plus out-patient attendances per year.

By 1980 the mainframe machine, datapens and teleprinters were due for replacement, providing an opportunity to reassess the existing system in the light of future priorities for development already identified by the District. A decision was made to replace the mainframe machine and, at the same time, to replace the ward datapens and teleprinters with VDU's. A hospital information system could then be introduced, followed by manpower availability, resource usage and patient dependency modules leading in time to a comprehensive management information system. The datapens were easy to use requiring only the passage of a fibre-optic pen across an appropriate bar-coded label in a manual (as used in supermarkets) but they were limited in their application in comparison to a V.D.U. which is capable of both receiving and transmitting information.

Conversion

The Computer Department's remit was to convert the existing system to the new machine for implementation in 1982. There was some opportunity for limited modification to increase effectiveness and the system was to be 'packaged' in modules to ease transferability.

The task was enormous and would only be successful if the users were fully involved in working closely with the in-patient, out-patient and waiting list teams set up within the computer department to design the new systems.

Consultation

Nurses are not directly involved in operating the out-patient or waiting list systems but they are responsible for ensuring that information related to a patient's stay in hospital is recorded on the computer. The majority of the input from nurses to the conversion came therefore in the in-patient system so a working group of nursing officers, sisters, ward clerks and computer staff met regularly to view the proposals for the contents of screens and suggest alternative formats for each conversion, using a manufacturer's simulation package on a VDU. Many innovative suggestions were made by sisters and ward clerks which often changed the thinking of the systems designers. A menu-type format was adopted which gives users the option of choosing the information or action they wish to take from a list or menu (Figure 1) displayed on the screen and typing in the appropriate number to begin the transaction. Thereafter instructions are displayed on the screen along with relevant information so that the user is led from one stage to another without reference to a guidance manual. Experienced operators are able to bypass the menu by typing in a transaction identifier and qualifying details immediately so the program design meets the needs of staff with varying levels of expertise.

Figure 1

Transactions available to this terminal

```
1     IN          - To accept a patient on your ward
2     OUT         - To transfer or discharge a patient
3     INF         - To input and view general information
4     RAP         - Referral appointment for an inpatient
5     FAP         - Follow up appointment for an inpatient
6     QU          - Shows/Amends/Cancels O/P appointments
7     QL          - Shows a list of patients on your ward
8     QW          - Shows patient's present hospital/ward
9     QC          - Shows patient's consultant and specialty
10    QD          - Shows patient's registration details
11    QDIS        - Shows summary of discharges/transfers
12    CANCEL      - Cancels last action on an inpatient
13    CHCONS      - To change a patient's consultant
14    BEDS        - Shows count of beds available on ward
15    FREEBED     - To view current hospital bedstate
16    ADDCONS     - Additional consultant for a patient
17    WDLEAVE     - To record a patient's ward leave
18    CHCAT       - To change a patient's category
19    COL         - To view messages sent to your terminal

              Enter required number / e(X)it / (N)ext page
```

At the same time a similar user group of medical records staff was meeting to assist in the development of the out-patient system. At senior management level a liaison committee met regularly to ratify the user group decisions and to monitor the progress of the conversion.

Once the broad outline of the system was settled a method of training nurses to use the VDU's was required. A training committee was set up with a nucleus of members drawn from the original user group supplemented by In-Service Training and general tutors, nurse managers and computer staff which defined its objectives as:

1. To train approximately 1,200 trained staff and learners in the use of V.D.U.s in the 9 months before 'live' date on January 1st, 1982.

2. To encourage a positive attitude towards the VDU's rather than a passive acceptance of the change.

3. To reinforce the sisters responsibility for the prompt and accurate input of patient information into the system.

4. To make arrangements for on-going training for new recruits to the District after January 1st, 1982.

Nursing management was responsible for providing training for all its staff from within its existing manpower and finance levels, aided by the part-time assistance of one member of the Computer Department's in-patient team.

Cascade Method of Training

It was agreed that a 'cascade' method of training could overcome the manpower and finance constraints by spreading the teaching load over a gradually increasing number of people. First, two in-service training tutors would teach a group of 22 core trainers, mainly nursing officers, who would then pass on those skills to ward sisters in their respective units, who in turn would teach the trained staff in their charge. A working party of committee members produced a training package:

1. suitable for use by core trainers and sisters

2. easily understood by nurses with different levels of expertise

3. divisible into modules for teaching over a period of time

4. easily and inexpensively reproducible so that all core trainers and sisters could have a copy

5. suitable for some element of self-instruction and practice.

A series of overhead projector sheets introduced the philosophy and mechanics of the system and a set of work cards allowed staff to work through structured examples at their own pace. A pilot study suggested that three 1 hour sessions were necessary to gain competence and that no more than four people could be trained at once. The only facility for practical training at this time was the 4 VDU's in the Computer Department's training room available for approximately 3 hours each weekday. No limits were set on the amount of instruction trainers could receive and they were actively encouraged to attend as often as they felt necessary.

The bulk of the training of the 22 core trainers was carried out in the summer and autumn of 1981. By this time it had become obvious that there were insufficent core trainers and the number was increased to 49 (24 on night duty). When the implementation data of the new system was deferred to June 1st, some momentum was lost but thankfully the pressure on the in-service training tutors was reduced. In retrospect, it would have been difficult to meet the January 1st deadline. Core trainers were offered refresher sessions in December and the training of sisters began in January. By this time experience had shown that the overhead projector sheets were unnecessary and demonstration on the VDU was a more effective alternative. By February VDU's were installed on the wards for training purposes only which greatly increased the available training locations and more training time was made available at weekends and during evenings and nights. Each ward had an individual training programme on its VDU, which mirrored the patients and consultants found there and set of worksheets to suit. Core trainers had the choice of teaching their sisters in the training room or on the wards. In practice they tended to teach in modules as time became available and nurses practised on the ward VDU, with or without supervision, in their free moments. As more people became familiar with the system, modifications were identified and incorporated into the program design.

The ward clerk supervisor had attended core trainers meetings regularly and was familiar with the training package used by nurses. The ward clerks were trained using the same work cards as the nurses and this led to them practising together and helping each other. Each nurse and ward clerk was given a booklet which reinforced their teaching and gave helpful hints in the event of problems. All the day staff and the ward clerks were trained within their normal hours of duty but night staff had some sessions arranged the hour before their spell of duty began because of the difficulty of removing them from the ward situation.

The training worked well. Staff were surprised to find how easy the system was to use and enthusiastic about the added advantages of the VDU's and the information system. It had been anticipated that difficulties would arise on night duty because of a large number of nurses requiring tuition in a situation of staff shortages. In the event, this area was the most successful.

A policy statement from the senior nurse manager underlined the ward sister's responsibility for the maintenance of patients' records on the computer and the ward clerk supervisor emphasised to her staff that whilst the ward clerk might have those duties delegated to her she was acting on behalf of the sister.

Anxiety temporarily replaced confidence amongst the staff in the run up to the changeover on June 1st, but the transition went very smoothly. The Computer Department provided a 24 hour a day trouble-shooting service for the first two weeks to sort out technical problems and core trainers were present on each ward as the VDU was phased in to help the staff check the patient information, get transactions up-to-date and offer assistance as required in the ensuing days. It was a great help that all nursing officers were also core trainers and could monitor the situation on the wards as part of their normal duties.

A core trainers' meeting at the end of the first week reported that data was being input promptly and accurately and the few problems encounted on the wards were generally attributable to teething troubles with the database rather than ignorance of the working of the system. In some cases, core trainers had not fully realised their teaching responsibilities in time and fifty nurses were not fully trained. Two ward clerks were possessive of their VDU's and reluctant to allow nurses to use them. A common mistake was an insistence on turning off the VDU when not in use which prevented communication between computer and ward. The reason given was a wish to save electricity!

The continuing effectiveness of the computer system depends on maintaining the level of training and grasping the opportunities offered by the new system. Learners will continue to be taught computer competence on the VDU's in the Nurse Training School and all trained staff joining the organisation from other Districts have the subject included in their induction course. Nurse managers are now planning to exploit the information element of the system by involving users in deciding what is to be developed. Early suggestions include - nursing policies and procedures, drug information, patients' menus, hazard warnings and a 'What's On' diary. Each sister also has the opportunity to develop a computer information system specific to her own ward and arrangements will be made for experiences and advice to be shared. The longer term strategy for developing the patient administration system to produce integrated management information is being pursued through the appropriate Regional channels.

Evaluation

The District is sufficiently happy with its experience of the 'cascade' method of teaching to use it again in preparation for the extension of computerisation to three more hospitals in the District in October of this year. The original training package is being modified to cater for staff with no previous experience of automated systems and the user group is looking at the extent to which manual record keeping can be reduced.

An early evaluation of the changeover from one mainframe machine to another and the replacement of datapens by VDU's in North Staffordshire suggests that success from the nursing viewpoint depends on:

1.   an awareness of the complexity and time consuming nature of the change

2.   the early and continuing involvement of the users in every aspect of the system design

3.   the creation of a simple, comprehensive standardised training package for all nurses and adequate time to teach it

4.   careful choice of core trainers who must be committed to the system and able and willing to fulfil the teaching role

5.   the earliest possible installation of VDU's on the wards so that staff can practise their skills and become familiar with the system

6.   close co-operation with ward clerk supervisors to ensure uniformity of teaching and advice

7.   the provision of adequate and continuous support for the first few weeks after implementation

Conclusion

There are now many nurses in North Staffordshire to whom computer maintenance of patient's records is the norm. They have never worked with manual systems because their whole work experience has been within the same Authority. It is only long-serving members of staff and those who have been recruited from outside who remember the multiplicity of ward record books in the old days and who are now able to appreciate the value of the computer system.

CHAPTER 14

RESOURCE MANAGEMENT

Within the health care systems in use globally it can be stated that the nursing services are users of and deployers of resources on a large scale.

It would seem appropriate, therefore, to work towards the construction of data systems to process information on all facets of resource utilisation; thus providing nurse managers with accurate, timely information to assist them in deploying nursing resources in the best possible way.

The papers in this chapter highlight the need for nurse managers to become involved in the provision of the system that they will be using.

Some of the systems in this chapter are related to matters discussed in Chapter 3.

The Impact of Computers on Nursing
M. Scholes, Y. Bryant and B. Barber (eds.)
Elsevier Science Publishers B.V. (North-Holland)
© IFIP-IMIA, 1983

14.1.

THE USE OF COMPUTER SYSTEMS IN NURSING ADMINISTRATION

Joy L. Brown

Introduction

We live in an era where technological change is endemic, leadership styles are changing and the nurses' role is expanding to accommodate these changes. The computer is no longer a tool for research and education or purely business. It has for some time played a small part within the health care field as 'fiscal management' of the hospital business office. With further introduction, this health care distributed system has become an integrated network of applications, functions and procedures, serving almost every hospital department. It's biggest impact in recent years has been on the nursing department, with order entry as its prime function. With this interface organisational changes occurred and the ability for nurse managers to work with historical data has become very important.

In planning for further applications for the nursing department, it is important that these applications be CRT-orientated, must be on-line with full communications capability and integrated with patient care information, patient demographic information and financial system. Benefit studies should be done to eliminate the 'nice to have' and promote the 'need to have' with long-term benefits in the lead. This then will leave management with the challenge of creating organizational structures and management techniques which will place information systems at the center of the organization plans.

Historically, each organization has a 'MEMORY' in which data is placed (INPUT) for storage. Examples of such storage areas are books, files, pieces of paper, ledgers and in the minds of persons comprising that organization. Access time is high, retrieval of information is useless by the time lag and the nature of storage (PROCESS) resulted in incomplete or misleading information (OUTPUT). Computer and computer storage systems have been shown to offer particular advantages for the storage and processing of organization information and for the manipulation of such information for decision-making purposes.

The information needs of a health care manager vary by levels of managerial activity. Since the level of the management activity influences the characteristics of the information used, information system must be designed to provide different types of information at different levels.

Four General Managerial Levels

1.   STRATEGIC PLANNING:
     long-range planning
     setting of organizational goals
     identifying general range of appropriate organizational activities.

2.   TACTICAL OR MANAGERIAL CONTROL:
     short-range activities for acquiring and allocating resources
     analysis of budgets and variances from budget

3. OPERATIONAL CONTROL:
    ensuring specific tasks are implemented effectively and efficiently.
    ensuring quality of service at point of delivery
    allocating personnel to predetermined programmatic plans
    determining reasons for variation of expenditures from budgeted amounts.

4. CLERICAL INPUTS:
    completing data capture forms according to prescribed procedures
    performing assigned functional tasks.

Clerical systems feed information into the decision-oriented information systems
at higher levels of the organization. As management activity moves from the
lower levels of the organization to higher levels, the decision emphasis turns
from operations to control - to planning and policy-making - while planning and
control operate throughout the entire organization. The emphasis is decidedly
different at the varying activity levels. Data is condensed and filtered until
it becomes information for decision-making.

Transactions refer to interactions with the system in connection with its
operation (patient using services, purchases from outside vendors, salaries,
etc.)

Scheduled Reports refer to outputs from the processing system in a fixed format
at a fixed time (census reports, drug inventory status, payroll summaries,
budget variances, etc.)
Demand Reports refer to outputs based on special requests (explanation of
admission, cost of a certain service, etc.)

Having reviewed therefore computers, its impact on the health care institution,
information and its importance to managers, we will look to the future as we
review some applications which are the critical segment for effective management
control. The goal of the nursing department is to achieve a high quality of
nursing care; therefore, it is important that the information be available in a
form carefully structured for decision-making.

Nursing workload measurement, quality assessment, nurse scheduling and material
requirement planning in the surgical suite, are the major component of a
management information system, for nursing administration. However, these
quality control tools must be manually sound, before they are computerized. A
good manual system will be a good computerized system. These subsystems are
already operational across North America, and are adaptable. There are three
types of automated data processing in operation:

        computers
        programmable calculators
        time-share reporting services

Therefore, the entire subsystem could be computerized or the reporting segment.

Workload Measurement is a tool that will determine predictable demands of care
generated by patient needs per shift and an integrated system which supports the
function of measurement of frequency of task performance, the identification of
participating levels of mix, the computation of workload values based on minutes
of nursing care per patient day and the setting of weekly and monthly cumulative
reports.(2) Automation is a way to increase the speed and accuracy of routine
calculations, thereby enabling timely feedback on operations.

Computer Systems: Adapt the manual workable system to the terminal, making
changes if needed, and leaving the system in an 'add mode'. Each element of
care is assigned a 4-digit code which identifies the unit, category of care and
specific activity.

Figure 1 Demonstrates the conceptualization of data to information
          process through varying levels of Managerial activity(1).

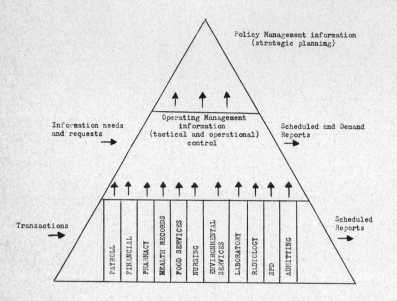

Example: Cleanliness (Category) = 3000 (Code)

Code	Specific Activity	Unit
3101	Bathes self	Med/Surg

Having established codes for the elements and activities, each activity is appointed a numerical value which represents points as per the manual system.

The nurse, assessing the patient, accesses the patient from the census screen and then selects the care plan from the function screen, as it appears. Items reflecting the patient's specific care are selected and according to the command listed in the programme, once entered, calculation begins. Unless a new admission is being processed, only updates are necessary as the previous entries are automatically entered if not changed. To access or update a line item the appropriate 4-digit code is entered on the keyboard. The CPU will automatically record and total the minutes of care required by that patient for the next 24 hours. The CPU also computes the number of staff by shift based on predetermined percentage distributions, stored in memory. Staff results are accessible only through the central staffing coordinator's terminal which can produce hard copy documentation(3).

Programmable Calculators: Texas Instruments advertisement for these calculators reads "You will be amazed at the convenience". At present there are 2 models – TI 58C and TI 59, which sells for approximately $200. These calculators could be programmed to allow input of total points, patient days and the number of days reported in the period. The formula for converting points to hours of care and factors for converting hours to FTE, could be permanently stored in the calculator, to permit automatic calculation of required FTE's and other information needed for the report. The keyboard is also programmable. Constant memory feature retains data and program information even when shut off, provides power in solving mathematical, statistical, financial and other problems. The programme can be written by a consultant, or one can programme the calculator after studying the Texas Instrument manual and some trial and error. However, once the programme is written, along with detailed instructions for preparing the reports, as well as reprogramming the calculator in case the programmes were accidentally erased, anyone with minimal orientation to the calculator could assume responsibility for the reports. Users, however, view computers as being superior to programmable calculators. It relieves them of the necessity of knowing or referring to a precise sequence of data entry.

Time-Share Reporting Services: Team up with a shared computer service, have them develop the program and sell the reports to you on a shared basis. I have seen reports from a service who used a 'dual disc drive intetech data microcomputer' with integral data printer for its data processing and printing.

The computer cannot ensure the correct classification of patients. This remains with the nursing staff, however, the reports generated from the system, alert managers of apparent potential problem areas, allowing for effective management control and decision-making.

Reports: Having decided on the report formats and information needed along with manipulated data from the nurse scheduling system, the following reports will generate.

Daily Unit Report:

- Actual Patient care units
- Actual Nursing care units
- Budgeted Nursing care units
- Staff Variance
- Utilization Index

- The average hours of care per patient day required
- The average hours of care per patient day given.

Daily Admitting Reports:

A daily report is available to the Admitting Department clerks to provide them
with guidelines for admitting patients to various units in order to balance the
workload among units.

Weekly Administration Report will print per nursing unit, listing

- Total weekly census
- Occupancy rate, based on the Unit's bed capacity
- Summary of weekly shift utilization
- Summary of weekly shift P.C.U's
- Summary of weekly shift N.C.U's
- Summary of weekly shift Variance
- Total P.C.U's
- Total N.C.U's
- Total Staff Utilization Index
- Weekly hours of care per patient day required
- Weekly hours of care per patient day given
- Budgeted N.C.U's versus Actual N.C.U's
- Variance + or -

Monthly Cumulative

- will display previous months' information
- number of days in month
- average daily census
- occupancy rate
- staff utilization percentage
- average hours of care per patient day required and given
- actual N.C.U's available
- actual P.C.U's
- variance whether over or under-staffed
- current period FTE's
- could accommodate the Quality Assessment percentage

Controls

Staffing guidelines.   Personnel policies and procedures, operating budget
allocated to each unit.

Workload measurement will accomplish two objectives:

1.   Prospective allocation of nursing resources.
2.   Monitoring of staff productivity and workload trends retrospectively:
      -    the prospective system will forecast staff requirement prior to the
           start of each shift
      -    the retrospective staff utilization reports will monitor past nurse
           utilization performance as input to future staffing decisions.

Guidelines for Staff Utilization Index

Objective: To review for extremely high - 120% or low - 80% utilization indices
            and its relationship to census and quality of care.

The baseline is 100%, but quality of care is optimized between 90% - 110% and compromised when utilization is less than 80% or greater than 120%.

Below 80% = excess staff - therefore productivity and quality are compromised
Between 80% - 90% = excess staff
Between 90% - 110% = adequate and sufficient staff. All patients needs should be met
Between 110% - 120% = insufficient staff, but workload manageable
Above 120% = insufficient staff, quality of care compromised and staff unable to meet minimal patient care needs for all patients

Quality Assessment

Quality assessment programs within a hospital is evidence that there is an organized program designed to enhance patient care through the ongoing objective assessment of important aspects of patient care and the correction of identified problems.

Once the quality assessment program has been debugged and implemented manually, and is properly coordinated, proving that duplication is minimised, information gathered is assimilated, communication is enhanced, there should then be a search for potential cost savings.

Most quality assessment programs consist of criterias and subcriterias, and the assessment is done concurrently and/or retrospectively. The entire program or the reporting segment could be computerized.

Benefits: Administration
-    a means to evaluate quality of care
-    measure improvements in quality
-    identify managerial effectiveness

Benefits: Nursing Staff
-    assists in providing a basis for documenting staff needs
-    documents what is not being done and provides for action plans to improve the situation

Reports

All information processing handled through the system provides data for analysis and compilation as required. Reports are generated for different managerial levels and vary from detailed reports to summary reports. Results of the assessment could be in quantitative or numerical manner, reporting the percentage of positive responses and identifying problem areas.

Managerial Level Reports:

Head Nurse:
-    Current criteria action report
-    YTD criteria action report
-    Summary report
    These reports will list recommended levels, % satisfactory levels, number of satisfactory levels, current % and YTD %, displaying the type of plan specific to her/his unit.

Assistant Director Report:
-    Will list all units, and the details as listed per head nurses' report.

Director Report:
- Will list subdivision and units
  Example - Obstetrics: Post partum
                         Labour and delivery
                         Nursery
  These reports will highlight units with below-recommended levels and
  satisfactory % of current and YTD levels.

Executive Report:
- Will list satisfactory % of current and YTD levels and those units with
  below-recommended levels(4).

Action Expected

Eliminate or reduce identified problems by educational/training programs, new or
revised policies or procedures, staffing changes, equipment or facility change
or adjustments in clinical privileges.

Computerised Scheduling

This tool could be centralized (staffing office) or decentralized (on-line at
the unit level), depending largely on the organizational structure. The data
base should be easily manipulated for payroll and workload index abstracting.
The system is flexible, allowing for requests, changes in rotation pattern -
full or partial rotation (job sharing) permits scheduling of staff between and
among units.

- allows for cancellation of part-time staff based on workload index
- allows for available days to be changed to work days
- schedules are available in advance and printed
- changes are made on-line(5).

On the following day of the last pay period, updates to the schedules are done
and entered into the system for computation and payroll run begins. The systems
being so well integrated, data capturing is easily facilitated. Following the
bi-weekly payroll run, the nurse administrator receives a bi-weekly hours
summary sheet of each nursing unit. This report reflects:-

- point census at midnight
- direct nursing hours per shift per employee status
- total direct nursing hours
- sick time hours per employee status
- vacation hours per employee status
- statutory holidays hours per employee status
- overtime hours per employee status
- orientation per employee status
- paid education days per employee status
- total paid hours
- average paid hours
- average direct nursing hours
- budgeted paid hours available
- budgeted position to date - over/under hour

Hospital administrators have begun to recognise the need to borrow proven
management techniques from business to survive in the health care market(6).
Since the computer is commonly used in the business environment, material
management is an effective management information system.

Surgical Suite

The operating room - an entity unto itself - is an area which is well suited for the development of a computerised information system, not only for scheduling but also for material requirement planning. The cost effective, maximum use of operating rooms requires much detailed statistical information which, up to now, has either not been collected or is collected periodically requiring secretarial time(7).

Surgical Scheduling:
- includes the date, operating room number, scheduled time, patient room number, patient's name, procedure, surgeon and anaesthesia.
- should include a calendar file (one-month cycle) to assist with checking on the particular day a surgeon has a block allocated.

Material Requirements File:
- This is also known as instrument and case card files. This file contains the materials and supplies needed for various procedures. It identifies quantities of each item needed for a procedure as well as the specific size or brand of the item.
- The file also contains the materials used by all surgeons when performing a procedure along with preference items reflecting surgeons differences in material requirements.

Inventory Status File:
- Is a record of each item available for use in the surgical suite, displaying the description of the item, quantity in hand, vendor information, lead times, and per unit cost.

Surgical Suite Reports:

Utilization: Number and types of cases, % of time used in each room and % of allocated times used for all surgeons

Planning Reports: Forecasting inventory and specific material requirement

Performance Reports: Material Usage reports

Exception Reports: Identifying excessive inventory, late or overdue orders, etc.

Frequency of Reports: Weekly, monthly, or annually

Objectives for these Reports:
1. To monitor operating room utilization.
2. To monitor cutting in and out by surgeons prior to scheduling by computer.
3. To assist in the study on surgeons' time requirements for specific cases.
4. To determine staffing pattern.
5. To monitor to what extent each surgeon is utilizing his blocks.

Who gets these Reports:
1. O.R. Supervisor
2. Patient Scheduling
3. Chief of Surgery
4. Nurse Administrator
5. Chief Anaesthetist - who reviews patterns of anaesthesia, methods and types.

Other Reports

Labour Distribution system distributes hours and dollars to nursing for budget purposes. Prints the budget file report and a monthly actual and projected staffing level report, enabling nursing to maintain an accurate record of employment hours and dollars by position code, i.e., RN, RNA, U.S., etc.

Employee Health Record

The personnel system is updated from the payroll system, thereby all new employees or terminated employees or change of status employees will be recorded in the personnel system. A monthly medical report is printed, showing employees who are due for X-rays, T.B. tests and physicals.

How reports are generated –

Depending on the type of system, reports are created by one or two methods.

1   Collect the data as the transactions occur – insert the information in sequence in the report data base – extract the information for any indicated period.
2. Generate the data as a snapshot of the current situation or for a specific previous time period – delete any information remaining from a previous time period – replace or update the new time period in sequence into the report data base.

The reports are intended to provide hard copy records for reference purposes as well as control listings to reflect the current situation. Full edit capabilities are provided to ensure entry of accurate data during the application encounter. Full correctional capabilities are provided. All relevant data is automatically stored in the report data base to enable the on-line generation of reports whenever required. Purging of data is at the hospitals' option.

Information Accessibility

The degree of accuracy and timeliness with which Nursing Administration reports status is maintained is dependent on the manual information flow. The system remains as up to date as the people who have update access are advised of new information. The levels of retrieval and update access are at the same plateau as that level established for information entry. The degree of control is established by each hospital. The system controls access based upon terminal identification and operator sign-on and password.

It is my hope that as you explore the different types of tools that the computer will be seen as one tool which will assist you in attaining your goal of improved patient care and good management practice.

REFERENCES

1. Head, R., Datamation, May 1967.
2. Meyer, D., Grasp: A Patient Information and Workload Management System, 1978.
3. Meyer, D., Grasp Too: A Patient Information and Workload Management System, 1981.
4. Sullivan, D.J., and Associates Inc., Quality Assessment Series. 1978.
5. I.B.M. Canada: Nurse Scheduling, 1977
6. Goldsmith, J.C.: The Health Care Market: Can Hospitals Survive? Harvard Business Review, September-October, 1980
7. Meijers, A., Operating Room Management Systems, 1981.

The Impact of Computers on Nursing
M. Scholes, Y. Bryant and B. Barber (eds.)
Elsevier Science Publishers B.V. (North-Holland)
© IFIP-IMIA, 1983

14.2.

A COMPUTERISED OPERATING THEATRE MANAGEMENT SYSTEM

Elizabeth Butler

Description of the Operating Theatres at St. Thomas's Hospital

The operating theatres consist of twelve main theatres, two outpatient theatres, and one ophthalmic theatre. The main theatres are situated on the second floor of the North Wing treatment block and on the second floor of the East Wing block. These two areas are connected by a link corridor. The outpatient theatres are on the ground floor of the treatment block they provide a comprehensive service for day cases dealing with minor surgery and endoscopies. The ophthalmic theatre is a self contained unit on the 8th Floor of the North Wing ward block. It is adjacent to the ophthalmic ward. There is a twenty four hour, seven day a week Recovery Room service in the North and East Wing theatres; patients stay in these areas for any length of time up to twenty four hours, after which they are transferred to their ward or to the intensive care unit. All aspects of general surgery are performed in the main theatres, and all specialities excluding Neurosurgery.

The specialties include:
        Cardiothoracic Surgery
        Paediatric Surgery
        Plastic/Micro Surgery
        Orthopaedic Surgery
        Genito-urinary Surgery
        Gynaecological Surgery
        ENT Surgery
        Vascular Surgery
        Oral/Fascio-Maxillary Surgery.

The theatres provide basic experience for student and pupil nurses and there is an Operating Department Assistant training school.

Introduction

Since 1974 a computerised theatre statistics system has been in operation throughout the theatres producing quarterly tables of workload by theatre and surgical firm. The data was collected on a specially designed form. Various fields were coded and the information was then keyed into the computer where the respective tabulations were derived and printed out. In 1979 in order to improve the data collection aspects of this system (as suggested by Mather [L31]) and in particular to reduce duplication of effort, a change of procedure was proposed by the then Senior Nursing Officer for the Theatres. Until this time, the practice had been to hold the Theatre Register book centrally which presented difficulties in completing the entries. This required doctors and nurses to enter details of each patient on an operation list, at the end of each session in each theatre.

The Proposed New System

The new system was designed to streamline theatre information procedures and avoid duplication in the provision of information within the theatre complex. Its principal feature was a data collection document (the theatre register form) which would double as a theatre register. This would enable the entries for each patient to be made in each theatre after each individual operation, thus avoiding the task of entering, at a central point, all the patient's details from a complete operation list at the end of a theatre session.

Development of the Project

A statement of need was considered by the Theatre Statistics Working Group. The membership of this group was the senior nursing officer (Theatres and Specialist Units) in the chair, the senior nursing officer (Computing), the chief systems analyst, the systems analyst for the theatre system, and the administrator (Treatment and Amenity Services). With the formation of a District Computer Steering Committee, a Theatre User Group was set up with similar membership under the chairmanship of a consultant to monitor and report back on the progress of the system.

The objectives of the proposed system were seen as:
1.   Management control of the theatres
  a)   evaluation of theatre usage
  b)   establishment of data for forecasting
  c)   clinical information for Joint Board of Clinical Nursing Studies courses

2.   Information for control of infection
  a)   microbiological evaluation and tracing

3.   Theatre Information and Statistical evaluation
  a)   for statutory purposes
  b)   departmental workload
  c)   clinical patterns
  d)   research facilities

It was agreed that a pilot trial of the theatre register form should be undertaken.

Pilot Trial

A representative set of sessions including inpatient and outpatient and ophthalmic theatres were chosen in which to test the proposed input form. The operating list for each session was used to set up a file which would provide lists of patients and expected operations in the computer from which the initial version of the theatre register could be printed. The theatre register form was then completed manually in the selected theatres. Thirty five sessions were covered in two weeks. Normal coding was carried out to ensure that the details met the system requirements.

The trial indicated that:
i)   minor revision should be made to the theatre register form for the main and Ophthalmic Theatres
ii)   major changes should be made to the theatre register form for the Outpatients Theatre and a further trial would be needed
iii) the timing of the arrival of the operating theatre lists should be examined.

Following the pilot trial it was agreed to implement the system in July 1980, in the Main and the Ophthalmic Theatres.

Preparation for Implementation May/June 1980

A theatre sister was released one day a week to assist the SNO (Computing) in implementing the system and to provide on-going support for the system. She was trained by the Systems Analyst who designed the theatre system in the full use of the System. She planned a series of educational sessions for 99 members of the theatre staff – these included:

SNO (Theatres and Specialist Units)	1
Nursing officers	5
Sisters	20
Clinical tutors	3
State Registered Nurses	47
Enrolled Nurses	
Surgery ODAs	5
Anaesthetic ODAs	11
Receptionists	6
ODA course co-ordinator	1

They were taught in groups of four for a period of up to one hour. The demonstrations included a full explanation of the system, and allowed each person to enter an operation list, and generate a theatre register form. Since the implementation phase the theatre sister designated to monitor the theatre system has planned an on-going educational programme for all new theatre nursing staff. This has been extended to include doctors and medical students. Some Housemen now enter the operations lists, printout the number of copies required, and sign the top copy to authenticate it. This has alleviated the problems associated with the interpretation of hand written operation lists.

Implementation

On 1st July 1980 the theatre register forms were introduced, and the theatre register and previously used form discontinued. The new forms were completed in each Theatre, and collected at the end of the day and checked for completeness. They were then numbered, and the top copy was filed in the Senior Nursing Officer's office and the bottom copy was sent to the computing department where the details were coded and entered onto the computer file. On 11th July the computer print program was put into operation and approximately eight copies of each operation list was printed out for use in the theatres. On 21st August the program for printing the theatre forms, from the input from the operation lists, was put into operation.

The Data Collection Document

The theatre register form was printed on two part NCR stationery. (Fig 1.) The heading is 'St. Thomas' Hospital Theatre Register'. Beneath is shown:

    Theatre by number
    date
    name of the list surgeon
    page number and selection of morning, afternoon and all day.

Each form has four sections, each section providing a profile on one patient. The information for each patient is divided into four units. Section one includes:

PATIENT INFORMATION
     Name
     Central Bureau number
     Sex
     Date of Birth
     Ward
     Listed Operation
     Consultant Surgeon   Box for coded initials
     Operating Surgeon   Box for coded initials

Section two includes:

OPERATION DETAILS
     Theatre book number
     Start time (24 hour clock)
     3 lines marked 1, 2, 3
     These lines are used in the following ways:
     -     a tick(s) is entered to indicate that the listed operation(s) has
           been performed
     -     unlisted operation(s) is written out in full
     -     a combination of listed and unlisted operations are entered

     There are 3 boxes for operation codes as defined in the Classification of
     Surgical Operations published by the Office of Population Censuses and
     Surveys for use in Hospital Activity Analysis and in the Hospital
     Inpatient Enquiry.
     Anaesthetist   Box for coding initials

Section three includes:
     Swab Count/Type of Anaesthetic/Instrument Nurse Section
     Instruments   counted correct YES/NO
     Needles and Swabs
     Signed
     Name of Instrument Nurse
     Anaesthetic (Box to enter)   General
                            Spinal
                            Local (L.A.)

     Finish time (24 hr clock)
     Emergency: Yes/No

Section four includes:

RUNNER NURSE INFORMATION
     Signed: Name for First Runner
     Signed: Name for Second Runner

The Outpatient Theatre
The system for this area was implemented on 1st March 1982. The printout is
compiled under the following headings: (Fig 2)

     Order number   Operation and Comments
     Surname, First Name CB Number
     Age   Ward code
     Locker   Surgeon
     Escort arranged   Appointment time

The lists can be compiled well ahead of time and as the information becomes
available. The order in which the operations will be carried out can be entered

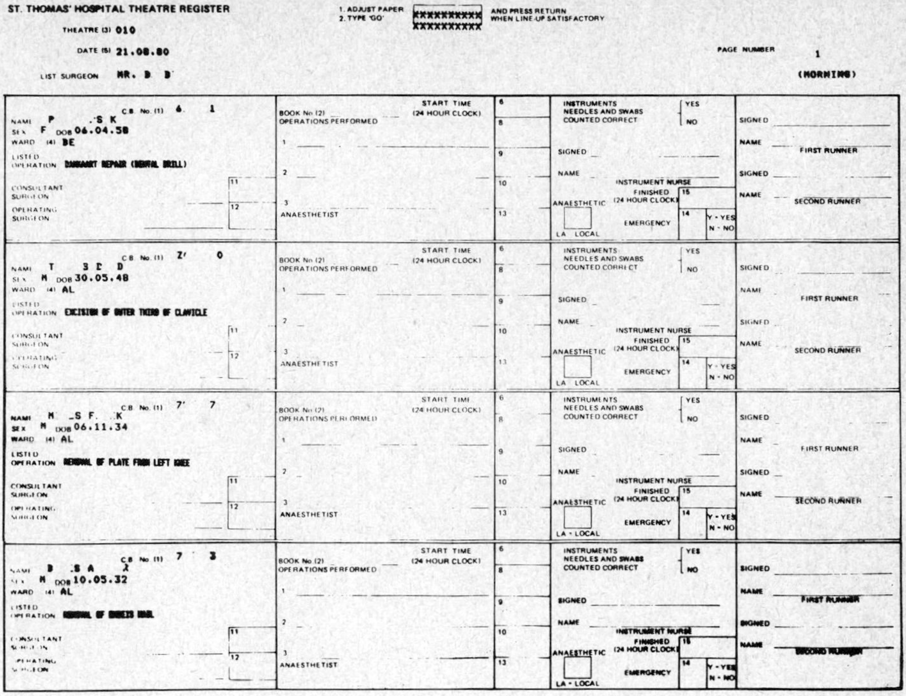

ST. THOMAS' HOSPITAL THEATRE REGISTER

1. ADJUST PAPER XXXXXXXXXX AND PRESS RETURN
2. TYPE 'GO' XXXXXXXXXX WHEN LINE-UP SATISFACTORY

THEATRE (3) 010

DATE (5) 21.08.80

PAGE NUMBER 1

LIST SURGEON MR. B D

(MORNING)

C.B. No. (1) 6 1
NAME P .S K
SEX F DOB 06.04.58
WARD (4) BE
LISTED OPERATION [illegible] REPAIR ([illegible] DRILL)
CONSULTANT SURGEON 11
OPERATING SURGEON 12
BOOK No (2)
OPERATIONS PERFORMED
1
2
3
ANAESTHETIST
START TIME (24 HOUR CLOCK) 6
8
9
10
13
INSTRUMENTS NEEDLES AND SWABS COUNTED CORRECT YES / NO
SIGNED
NAME
INSTRUMENT NURSE
FINISHED (24 HOUR CLOCK) 15
ANAESTHETIC
LA - LOCAL
EMERGENCY 14 Y - YES N - NO
SIGNED
NAME FIRST RUNNER
SIGNED
NAME SECOND RUNNER

C.B. No. (1) Z 0
NAME T 3 C D
SEX M DOB 30.05.48
WARD (4) AL
LISTED OPERATION EXCISION OF OUTER THIRD OF CLAVICLE
CONSULTANT SURGEON 11
OPERATING SURGEON 12
BOOK No (2)
OPERATIONS PERFORMED
1
2
3
ANAESTHETIST
START TIME (24 HOUR CLOCK) 6
8
9
10
13
INSTRUMENTS NEEDLES AND SWABS COUNTED CORRECT YES / NO
SIGNED
NAME
INSTRUMENT NURSE
FINISHED (24 HOUR CLOCK) 15
ANAESTHETIC
LA - LOCAL
EMERGENCY 14 Y - YES N - NO
SIGNED
NAME FIRST RUNNER
SIGNED
NAME SECOND RUNNER

C.B. No. (1) 7 7
NAME M .S F. K
SEX M DOB 06.11.34
WARD (4) AL
LISTED OPERATION REMOVAL OF PLATE FROM LEFT KNEE
CONSULTANT SURGEON 11
OPERATING SURGEON 12
BOOK No (2)
OPERATIONS PERFORMED
1
2
3
ANAESTHETIST
START TIME (24 HOUR CLOCK) 6
8
9
10
13
INSTRUMENTS NEEDLES AND SWABS COUNTED CORRECT YES / NO
SIGNED
NAME
INSTRUMENT NURSE
FINISHED (24 HOUR CLOCK) 15
ANAESTHETIC
LA - LOCAL
EMERGENCY 14 Y - YES N - NO
SIGNED
NAME FIRST RUNNER
SIGNED
NAME SECOND RUNNER

C.B. No. (1) 7 3
NAME B .S A X
SEX M DOB 10.05.32
WARD (4) AL
LISTED OPERATION REMOVAL OF [illegible]
CONSULTANT SURGEON 11
OPERATING SURGEON 12
BOOK No (2)
OPERATIONS PERFORMED
1
2
3
ANAESTHETIST
START TIME (24 HOUR CLOCK) 6
8
9
10
13
INSTRUMENTS NEEDLES AND SWABS COUNTED CORRECT YES / NO
SIGNED
NAME
INSTRUMENT NURSE
FINISHED (24 HOUR CLOCK) 15
ANAESTHETIC
LA - LOCAL
EMERGENCY 14 Y - YES N - NO
SIGNED
NAME FIRST RUNNER
SIGNED
NAME SECOND RUNNER

Fig. 1. Theatre Register Form.

E. Butler

```
                              ST.THOMAS' HOSPITAL
                                OPERATION LIST
        DATE 21.06.82             OUTPATIENTS THEATRE
ORDER  I                      I   I    IESCORTI                                          I         IWARDI    IAPPT.
NO. I   ISURNAME & FIRST NAME IAGEILCKRIARR.  I OPERATION & COMMENTS                    IC.B.NO. ICODEISURGEONITIME
                                                   09:30    PAIN CLINIC

   I   IS   I V   T          I 36I    I     I COELIAC AXIS BLOCK                        IZ     5 I     I      I09:30
   I   I                     I     I  I     I                                          I       I     I      I
   I   IB    T G   A J.      I 36I    I     I RENAL DENERVATION                        I1     5  I     I      I09:30
   I   I                     I     I  I     I * ? WARD PATIENT                         I       I     I      I
   I   IW    M J. E          I 40I    I     I FACET JOINT INJECTION                    IZ     9 I     I      I09:30
   I   I                     I     I  I     I                                          I       I     I      I
   I   IR'  .S J  N          I 41I    I     I MARCAIN RIGHT LUMBAR SYMPATHECTOMY       IZ'    7 I     I      I09:30
   I   I                     I     I  I     I                                          I       I     I      I
   I   IB'   'S   A          I 34I    I     I REPEAT CRYO INTERCOSTAL BLOCK            IZ     5 I     I      I09:30
   I   I                     I     I  I     I                                          I       I     I      I
   I   IH'  'I H' Y          I     I  I     I MARCAIN SYMPATHECTOMY                    I       I     I      I09:30
   I   I                     I     I  I     I * ? INPATIENT                            I       I     I      I
   I   IS.  'S R  .D         I 56I    I     I CRYO TO C3                               I6    '8 I     I      I09:30
   I   I                     I     I  I     I Y                                        I       I     I      I
   I   IW'  E M              I 62I    I     I TRANSACRAL INJECTION S 2                 IZ    '2 I     I      I09:30
   I   I                     I     I  I     I                                          I       I     I      I
   I   IS   .N S. .A         I     I  I     I FACET JOINT INJECTION                    I&Z.   5I     I      I11:30
   I   I                     I     I  I     I                                          I       I     I      I
   I   IT.   .L D  'D        I     I  I     I FACET JOINMT INJECTION                   I&O'   1 I     I      I11:30
   I   I                     I     I  I     I                                          I       I     I      I
```

Fig. 2. Operation List – Outpatient Theatre.

on the day the operation is to be performed. The program allows operations to be entered initially without a name. It is also possible to enter DNA (did not attend) against the name of any patient who defaults, and the system is therefore suitable to be used as an appointment register.

The Computer System

The programs for the theatre system are written in both COBOL and FORTRAN programming languages and consist of list entry, Register Printing, Statistics entry and Statistics print-out.

The list entry program accepts and checks formatted input for the theatre session and patients, which is then output as the required number of copies of the theatre list.

Additionally the list data is re-formatted and all registers for the next session output on demand ready for distribution to the individual theatre where details of the surgical procedures, firm and other details are captured.

The second copy of the completed register is manually coded to become the input document for the Statistics file, which holds details of each patient and procedure as codes.

The statistics print-out programs are in two parts; one consists of the file audit and statistics printout programs which inspect the records and indicate anomalies, such as numbers missing from the sequence for each of the theatre groups, and mismatches in the consultant firm and surgeon firm. Once an audit shows acceptable results the second program prints the several statistics tables for distribution to the management of the Theatres. Circulation of the information is controlled by the Surgeon's Committee.

The second part of the statistics printout programs is a facility to select individual records according to a defined criterion (or several combined) e.g. records for one specific operation, or firm, or surgeon and print selected parts of the record either as codes or expanded to the full description.

Equipment: There are four visual display units (CIFER 2605s) - one in each of the North Wing Theatre, the East Wing Theatre, the Royal Eye Ward and the Outpatient Theatre

In addition there are five DECWRITER III printer terminals - two in the North Wing Theatre - one dedicated to pre-printed stationery (Theatre Registers) and one each in the East Wing Theatre, the Royal Eye Ward and Outpatient Theatre.

These are linked to the hospital's mainframe computer, a Xerox Sigma 6 on which the programs are run. Various other terminals are also linked to the Sigma 6 thus providing the capability of assessing the theatre system from other locations if required.

Output/Analysis: The system provides up to 20 each of operating lists at one time and the pre-printed theatre register forms from the lists file.

Analyses: Quarterly theatre statistics include;
1.   Usage of individual theatres/or groups of theatres
2.   Analysis of emergency operations
3.   The number of cases performed by individual surgeons within firms in the main theatres, outpatient theatres, and ophthalmic theatres.
4.   The total time in theatre by individual surgeons within firms.

5.   Listings of patients undergoing specialist surgery by patient name, date,
      CB number, operation, consultant surgeon, and length of operation.

Ad hoc requests include specific operations by length of time by surgeon and
lists of all operations for JBCNS purposes.

Laboratory/Theatres Output

This listing details patient name in alphabetical order, CB number, sex, age,
ward from/to, emergency operation Yes/No, theatre number, consultant initials,
surgeons initials, firm, anaesthetists initials, firm, date details of
operation.

This information is provided through the microbiology computer system from the
theatre system, and this output is provided on a weekly and monthly basis for
the Control of Infection Nursing Officer.

Future Plans

1.   The computer data files are being extended to accommodate a code for each
      of the nurse signatories and programs will be amended or written to
      convert these codes to the nurses' name using an identity dictionary to
      enable computer reports to match the written register records. In time it
      is hoped to combine this information with the identification of the
      initials of doctors and anaesthetists in order to assist in the work of
      the Control of Infection Nursing Officer.
2.   A new transaction is in the process of design and construction to enable
      fewer key depressions to be used in the compilation of the lists, viz.
      entering the ward and bed number (4 key depressions) will transfer patient
      details from the bedstate file to the operation list file. Similarly the
      use of an operation code will provide the written description of the
      operation from the operation code dictionary (eight key depressions).
3.   To meet a possible requirement from the Anaesthetic Department, all of the
      next days list may be produced at the end of the day after normal
      computing services have ceased.
4.   There is a tentative proposal to prepare the Hospital Activity Analysis
      report relating to surgical procedures for the Regional Authority form the
      data collected.

Conclusions

The system described above was built upon a simple statistical system.   The
users had become aware of the limitations of the statistical system but sensed
that it could be a basis on which to build a more extensive and meaningful
system.   So the new system came into being and operated in two parts:

i)   the operation list module   ii) the register data collection module

and the statistical data recording and analysis module was continued.

This combination of modules has streamlined the collection of theatre
information, avoided duplication of entries, and overcome the dangers of
illegible handwriting. Details of each patient and his operation are collected
in the individual theatre at the time of operating or immediately afterwards.
Thus the information is timely and has achieved a high level of accuracy. This,
in turn led to the provision of accurate statistics and analyses of workload and
theatre usage for medical and nursing management.

The expansion of the system has resulted from the positive attitude of the Theatre User Group, backed up by a close liaison within the theatre nursing structure and the Computing Department, which has supported the on-going education of all staff. The introduction of greater simplicity in the method of accessing the system will lead to its wider use. The knowledge gained by the user will hopefully deepen his understanding of computing and thus strengthen links with computing professionals which will result in future systems that are tailored to provide specific information with the overall objective of assisting in the many aspects of patient/client care.

The Impact of Computers on Nursing
M. Scholes, Y. Bryant and B. Barber (eds.)
Elsevier Science Publishers B.V. (North-Holland)
© IFIP-IMIA, 1983

14.3.

COMPUTER-ASSISTED TRAINING AND MANPOWER PLANNING FOR STUDENT NURSES IN LEIDEN HOSPITAL

Elly Pluyter-Wenting

1.   Summary

This paper describes the development and use of a computerized training and manpower planning for student nurses. It is designed to help nursing management assign student nurses equally to the hospital departments. It has to keep in balance the personnel needs to the wards and the practical training requirements for student nurses. The system has been developed during the period 1974 to 1977 and has been operational in the University Hospital Leiden since 1977. It has proved to be a useful and flexible management tool with which most users are very satisfied.

2.   Introduction

A brief outline of the Dutch educational program for student nurses and some background information about the University Hospital Leiden.

The education program for student nurses in the Netherlands is as follows(1):-
During the last ten years, the Dutch Government has changed the training program for student nurses several times. At the moment the length of the course is 3.5 years. The theoretical part of the course comprises 1060 terms of 50 minutes. The practical training comprises at least:

medical ward	- 24 weeks
surgical ward	- 24 weeks
maternity ward	- 16 weeks
childrens ward	- 12 weeks

If the practical results are adequate the student gets a written examination at the end of the first and second year. At the end of the third year, after the prescribed practical periods in the wards have been completed, the student obtains permission to take the national-multiple-choice tests. At the end of the 3.5 years, an oral examination takes place. This is based on a case-study or nursing report. This type of nursing education is called an "in-service" program. Student nurses are employees of the hospital and are paid for their duties (a type of apprenticeship). This way of training nurses is gradually being faded out in Holland and in its place is a form of training where the student nurse is not attached to a hospital but to a school. Nursing schools are found all over the country now, but nevertheless training periods in hospitals will always be part of the program, so computerized planning programs for trainees will always be useful.

General outline of the University Hospital Leiden

The University Hospital Leiden has existed for more than 200 years. For the moment the hospital is situated in several pavilions built during the years 1910-1930, which makes hospital communications difficult. The hospital has 933 beds distributed among all kinds of specializations. The 933 beds are divided among 37 wards. Most of the wards contain about 30 beds, but some less than 15 and a few about 60 beds. (see fig.1).

Fig. 1.

List of in-patient nursing departments of the University Hospital Leiden where student nurses have training periods

Wards	Number of beds	Number of student nurses	
		Minimum	Maximum
S U R G I C A L			
General surgical A	26	7	11
General surgical B	36	7	11
General surgical K1	24	6	10
Urology ward	26	5	8
Thorax-surgical ward	29	5	9
Orthopaedics	40	8	13
Surgical childrens ward	20	5	9
Ear/Nose/Throat	57	9	15
Gynaecology	29	4	8
Neuro-surgical ward	37	8	13
Eye-surgical ward	50	6	10
Traumatology	24	5	8
M E D I C A L			
Endocrinology	29	6	9
Cardiology	11	3	6
Infectious disease	20	5	9
Rheumatology	18	3	5
Oncology	14	1	2
Nephrology/Haematology	34	7	11
Pulmonology	31	7	11
General medioal ward K1	27	7	10
Gasto-enterology	13	3	5
Neurology I	29	6	9
Neurology-childrens ward	21	6	9
Dermatology	22	3	5
Obstetric department	38	15	20
Paediatric department			
General paediatric 1	30	15	20
General paediatric 2	17	15	20

A school for nursing educaton is related to the hospital. This school has about 300 students in training. Training programs start three times a year, in September and December with 40 students and in March with 20 students. Every week about 60 students get theoretical education in the school and are not available for work. During the summer months, every week about 60 students are on holiday. However, every week of the year about 240 student nurses are divided among 30 nursing wards.

At the end of the sixties a manual planning system was used for this purpose. Although the system worked satisfactorily it was complicated and took a lot of time. Providing the wards with a constant even flow of students, taking into account the type of patient care, number of beds of each ward and honouring the training regulations of the government was very complex.

Some problems of those days:

- "training bottlenecks", short supply of a special type of clinical experience (maternity and paediatric departments (2).
- short time crisis if a ward was short of staff they asked for more students. Interruption of a students training on her original ward had to be avoided. How to fill those gaps?
  If the allocation officer did not move students, the ward sister "borrowed" students from other wards (2).
- communication problems, allocation of student nurses has to be sufficiently flexible. It was a great problem to inform in time all the person and departments who needed this information (about 60 addresses).

The nursing allocation officer was under great pressure, constantly facing crisis.

3.   General Question

The management question in 1974 was, is it possible to divide 240 student nurses equally among 30 wards using a computer program while taking into account all the different individual training categories of the students and the personnel needs of all the different wards?

In 1974 we started with the development of a computer design for manpower allocation of student nurses. The knowledge of the manual planning system was a great help as there was little knowledge of this subject at that time.

4.   Main Considerations

During the years 1974/1977 a complex computer program was created by a computer science specialist. Together with the nursing allocation officer some main considerations were specified:

- an annual computerized system of manpower planning had to be made one year in advance.
- an annual schedule had to be divided in week schedules; every ward had to get its own schedule one year in advance, divided into 52 weeks.
- a week schedule for a ward had to give the following information:
  . number of students
  . names of students
  . training level of each student
  . date of leaving the ward
  . reason of leaving the ward
- all students had to get their own schedule

- every department had to get a stable number of students. The training
  levels of the student nurses placed on the same department had to be well
  mixed; some first year, some second year and some third/fourth year
  students.
- the system had to be very flexible for each individual student theoretical
  periods and holiday weeks had to be specified in the schedule as well
- training regulations of the Government had to be respected strictly
  theoretical education concerning maternity wards or paediatric departments
  had to be given before a student can be allocated to this type of ward
- every training period must be more than twelve and less than twenty weeks
- for management reasons a small reserve pool had to be made.

5.   Development of Design

At first a scheme of all existing and expected groups of students was made for
one year in advance. For each group - identified by the date of starting
education - we planned the theoretical and holiday periods for one year in
advance.

A well designed block and holiday plan is of great importance to get a well
balanced student manpower planning (2).

As was mentioned before our hospital has no standard numbers of beds so besides
the type of patients also the number of beds of one ward play an important part
in the student-manpower planning. For this reason we introduced a list with the
necessary minimum number of students and possible maximum number for each ward.

The next step was to divide the wards in three levels.

As a university hospital we have different types of wards:

level I   :   general medical/surgical wards
level II   :   specialized wards (paediatric, maternity, neuro-surgery ward
                 etc.)
level III   :   super-specialized wards (intensive care units and recovery
                 rooms etc.)

The level II and III wards are of less importance for the general training of
student nurses than the level I wards. However two types (level I and II) had
to be provided with students for the nursing care of the patients. So we
decided that for the level I wards every student had to pass at least two
different general surgical wards and two different general medical wards.
Concerning level II, wards we decided that every student gets as much as
possible. For information reason you are told that on level III wards no
students are allocated.

The third step was to transfer all individual training history data of each
student nurse into the computer data base. The computer program is connected
with the personnel records of the hospital and is written in the language
Fortran. It is operational on the PDP 11/70 equipment located in our hospital.
Until now the program has been run by computer personnel of the hospital under
supervision of the same computer science specialist who built and supervised the
construction of the original design.

To construct the system we needed the following information:

- history and present state of training periods of every individual student
  nurse
- date of theoretical periods and holidays

- personnel needs of each ward, how many student nurses are necessary for a ward.   What is the minimum number of students for each ward and what is the maximum number of students a ward can train (see fig. 1).
- what type of training level is required for students for each department
- does the student need an additional theoretical period before starting a special training period (maternity or paediatric ward).

After one year of study and experience a reasonable well balanced and flexible system was constructed. The program correctly links student nurses to wards. This results in annual schedules.

6.   Results

- The program divides available students equally among the nursing departments.   The training regulations of the Government are strictly respected.
- It is possible to change annual schedules of students on-line. Necessary updates and printouts are done automatically.
- If necessary, after six months, a new schedule can easily be made for the rest of the year.
- Communication between nursing school, nursing management, wards and many other hospital departments has improved.

7.   Illustration of the Planning Process

To give more details and to describe how the system works, some layouts are presented. The first list given by the program is a weekly review of the number of student nurses for each ward (fig. 2). In this way the nursing allocation officer can see if the students are equally allocated to the wards throughout the year. Usually the parameters are adjusted and we need some re-runs to see if better results are possible.

Fig. 2 WEEKLY REVIEW (Extract from weekly review).

```
-------------------------------------------------------------------------------
|                                                                             |
|         AFDELINGSOVERZICHT DER STAGEPLANNING   ROOSTERJAAR: 1981-1982        |
|                                                                             |
|            **** HEELKUNDE KINDEREN   HKIN   153 ****   D.D. 17.05.82         |
|                                                                             |
|                    HET AANTAL LEERLINGEN PER WEEK:                           |
|                                                                             |
| WEEKNUMMER : 1 VAN  29.11.81  T/M  06.12.81   AANTAL : 6   *                 |
|                                                                             |
| WEEKNUMMER : 2 VAN  06.12.81  T/M  13.12.81   AANTAL : 6   *                 |
|                                                                             |
| WEEKNUMMER : 3 VAN  13.12.81  T/M  20.12.81   AANTAL : 6   *                 |
|                                                                             |
| WEEKNUMMER : 4 VAN  20.12.81  T/M  27.12.81   AANTAL : 7   *                 |
|                                                                             |
| WEEKNUMMER : 5 VAN  27.12.81  T/M  03.01.82   AANTAL : 6   *                 |
|                                                                             |
| WEEKNUMMER : 6 VAN  03.01.82  T/M  10.01.82   AANTAL : 9   *                 |
|                                                                             |
-------------------------------------------------------------------------------
```

As soon as the basic review is accepted we give the order to print out the individual student nurse annual schedules (fig. 3).

Fig. 3 INDIVIDUAL STUDENT NURSE ANNUAL SCHEDULE

```
-----------------------------------------------------------------------
|                    Stageplanning 1981 - 1982                        |
|                                                                     |
| 1E JAARS SEP'81  GROEP A                        MICRO-S. NR?: 470635 |
|                                                                     |
| *** DE VOLGENDE AFDELINGEN, BLOKKEN EN VAKANTIES ZIJN GEPLAND***     |
|                                                                     |
| VAN 29.11.81. T/M  30.01.82:  HEELKUNDE KINDEREN                    |
| VAN 31.01.82. T/M  20.02.82:  BLOK 1                                |
| VAN 21.02.82. T/M  27-02-82:  VAKANTIE                              |
| VAN 28.02.82. T/M  27.03.82:  HEELKUNDE KINDEREN                    |
| VAN 28.03.82. T/M  20.04.82:  BLOK 2                                |
| VAN 21.04.82. T/M  01.05.82:  HEELKUNDE KINDEREN          TOT 15    |
| VAN 02.05.82. T/M  07.06.82:  ALG.HEELK.VERPLEEGAFD. A (M)          |
| VAN 08.06.82. T/M  26.06.82:  VAKANTIE                              |
| VAN 27.06.82. T/M  23.09.82:  ALG.HEELK.VERPLEEGAFD. A (M)  TOT 18  |
| VAN 24.07.82. T/M  06.11.82:  LONGZIEKTEN VERPLEEGAFDELING  TOT  6  |
| VAN 07.11.82. T/M  27.11.82:  BLOK 3                                |
|                                                                     |
|                            D.D. 28.05.1982                          |
-----------------------------------------------------------------------
```

On each annual schedule the name and address of the student nurse are printed. Besides the training periods the theoretical and holiday periods are planned. For reasons of management control the total number of weeks is given when a training period is finished.

The next print we get is the annual schedule for each ward (see fig. 4) divided in week lists.

The three figures together make it possible for the allocation nursing officer to see if the planning is correct. Usually some checks are necessary to be able to accept the planning. After accepting, copies of the individual schedules are printed and sent to the student nurses and the nursing school. Copies of the ward schedules are sent to the ward, the nursing officer and to the personnel department who needs the information for financial and other reasons. In this way management information is now available for many departments. Getting the same information at the same time makes hospital communication more efficient and saves time.

8. Conclusions

- The program is implemented and accepted all over the hospital. As said before the communication concerning training periods of student nurses is much easier now.
- Student nurses are allocated equally over the wards. During the last five years the program has become more complicated as training regulations got more rigid.
- The reserve pool (about 3 persons a week) is needed to help wards with manpower problems.
- The allocation nursing officer can always change the individual annual schedule of the student nurse on-line. There is a possibility for a student nurse to change a holiday period we planned. Of course, the allocation nursing officer has to agree with this request and has to change the schedule using the computer.
- Every ward sister can see on the display terminal if the information of the individual annual schedule (fig. 3) of the student is the same as the information of the weeklist of her ward.

Figure 4: Annual Schedule for each Ward

D.D. 28.05.82.   BLZ: 1

```
        *** STAGEPLANNING 1981 - 1982 ***
        *** ALG.HEELK.VERPLEEGAFD. A (M) **

IN WEEK:  1  VAN  29.11.1981 T/M  05.12.1981  ZYN DE VOLGENDE LEERLINGEN AANWEZIG:

                                    VERTREK     NAAR            (EVT.VERVOLGENS NAAR)

J.       ???     19??????????????   28.02.82
A.       4E JAARS MRT'79  GROEP A   24.01.82    INFECTIE-ZIEKTEN VERPLEEGAFD.
E.P.     4E JAARS DEC'80  GROEP A   03-01.82    BLOK 3        VERLOSKUNDE-VERPLEEGAFD
A.A.M.   2E JAARS DEC'80  GROEP B   03-01.82    NEUROLOGIE DAMES:VERPL.AFD. II
P.M.     2E JAARS DEC'80  GROEP B   03.01.82    K.N.O.-VERPLEEGAFD.
A.W.     2E JAARS SEP'80  GROEP A   07.02.82    VAKANTIE      BLOK 4
J.P.     1E JAARS SEP'81  GROEP A   31.01.82    BLOK 1        VAKANTIE
Y.A.M.   1E JAARS SEP'81  GROEP B   28.02.82    VAKANTIE      BLOK 1
F.D.J.   2E JAARS MRT'81  GROEP A   03.01.82    BLOK 2        ALG.HEELK.VERPLEEGAFD. A (M)


IN WEEK:  2  VAN  06.12.1981 T/M  12.12.1981  ZYN DE VOLGENDE LEERLINGEN AANWEZIG:

                                    VERTREK     NAAR            (EVT.VERVOLGENS NAAR)

J.       ???     19??????????????   28.02.82
A.       4E JAARS MRT'79  GROEP A   24.01.82    INEFECTIE-ZIEKTEN VERPLEEGAFD
E.P.     2E JAARS DEC'80  GROEP A   03.01.82    BLOK 3        VERLOSKUNDE-VER/:EEGAFD.
A.A.M.   2E JAARS DEC'80  GROEP B   03.01.82    NEUROLOGIE DAMES:VERPL.AFD. II
P.M.     2E JAARS DEC'80  GROEP B   03.01.82    K.N.O.-VERPLEEGAFD.
A.W.     2E JAARS SEP'80  GROEP A   07.02.82    VAKANTIE      BLOK 4
J.P.     1E JAARS SEP'81  GROEP A   31.01.82    BLOK 1        VAKANTIE
Y.A.M.   1E JAARS SEP'81  GROEP B   28.02.82    VAKANTIE      BLOK 1
F.D.J.   2E JAARS MRT'81  GROEP A   03.01.82    BLOK 2        ALG.HEELK-VERPLEEGAFD. A (M)
```

- The program does need the attention of the nursing officer, but it has proved to be a great help in planning nursing manpower.
- The nursing management, the student nurses and the head nurses of the wards are all reasonably satisfied with the system.

Acknowledgement

The author would like to acknowledge the computer science specialist who constructed the system: Martin Mulder, B.A.Z.I.S., University Hospital Leiden, Holland.

References

1.   Ministerie van Volksgezondheid en Milieuhygiêe
      Training regulations:
      Regeling opleiding diploma A-verpleegkundige d.d. 28.12.73 nr. 41006 afd.
      DGVgz/MBO Ministerie van Volksgezondheid en Milieuhygiêe (Staatscourant
      nr. 12 d.d. 12.01.74), zoals laatstelijk gewijzigd bij Besluit van
      18.02.81, Stcrt. 1981 nr. 44
2.   Ian Banks MA: Nurse allocation, first published 1972
3.   Concluding report on the NOBIN-ZIS-project 1972 - 1976
4.   Nationaal Ziekenhuisinstituut: Handboek Roosterplanning.

The Impact of Computers on Nursing
M. Scholes, Y. Bryant and B. Barber (eds.)
Elsevier Science Publishers B.V. (North-Holland)
© IFIP-IMIA, 1983

14.4.

COMPUTERS AND NURSING ADMINISTRATION

Sally Mizrahi

1.   Computers and Nursing Administration

If Florence Nightingale and her nursing colleagues of the last century, could
see what nurses are achieving with sophisticated information handling techniques
and computers in the 1980's, what do you suppose their reaction might be?

> One of disbelief
> One of surprise
> Or one of complete approval!

Miss Nightingale herself, was a skilful administrator. With the help
of Sydney Herbert, she persuaded the British Government of the day to closely
examine the Army Medical system and was therefore instrumental in initiating
much needed reform. Today, more than ever, we must look closely at the various
practices which exist within hospitals and be prepared to institute improvement
and beneficial change. Nursing Administration today is involved in managing a
myriad of activities within the hospital. A major part of this management is
the co-ordinating responsibility which nursing administration undertakes as the
organizer of the largest hospital department. However in carrying out this
responsibility, it must never be forgotten that the patient is not just one of
the many concerns of a nursing service department. The patient is CENTRAL to
the total function of nursing administration.

In developing systems and computer programs for Nursing Administration, there
may be a tendency to lose sight of the fundamental importance of the patient.
However indirectly related to the patient the various programs may be, it is
essential to achieve a balance between systems for nursing management and those
concerned with the clinical sphere. As the task of administering a nursing
department in a hospital becomes increasingly complex, it becomes decidedly more
difficult for a Director of Nursing to maintain control of every aspect of
nursing department management. The nursing director, as head of the nursing
service and as one who wishes to be effective, must endeavour to get the right
things done, through the right people and at the correct time.

Elaine Orr, the former Director of Nursing at the Royal Children's Hospital, and
a nurse with over twenty five years of experience in the nursing administrative
'hot seat', refers to administration which is expected to have happened
'yesterday' as Nescafe Administration. The instant variety! Whilst
acknowledging that computers are not the complete answer to what ails hospital
administrators, Miss Orr does believe that computers have a constructive use in
modern day hospital management. We are endeavouring to prove that this is
indeed so, in the nursing services of the Royal Children's Hospital. The basis
of what we have developed is an integrated payroll/personnel, allocation system,
consisting of over 50 programs.

Figure 1

NURSE ALLOCATION PROGRAMS

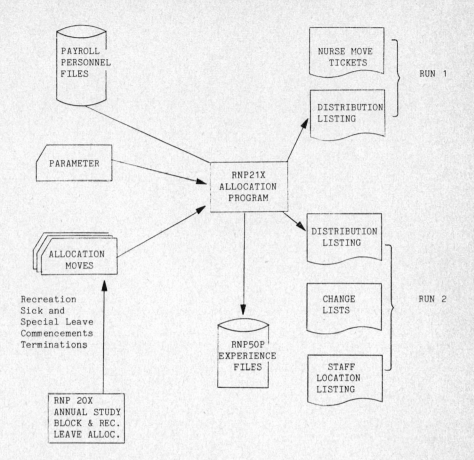

The allocation component is naturally of great value to the nursing office. Nurse allocation as a component of staffing control is one of the most persistent and critical concerns facing nursing administrative staff. The process of allocation is a constant cycle which must take place, week after week, and is an essential component of both service and educational programs. The cycle undertaken at the Royal Children's hospital is as follows. Friday morning, the Rostering Assistant Director of Nursing receives a nursing staff distribution listing and a set of nurse move tickets. The listing shows all nurses in every hospital location including recreation leave and study block. The system provides for 40 locations, 25 of these being wards and departments. This listing serves as a work sheet and is known as Run 1 of the system. The set of nurse move tickets, act as a reminder to the rostering assistant director, indicating that Nurse Thompson is due for a move of location in two weeks. The student nurses past clinical experience in numbers of weeks is set out on each ticket. Asterisks * printed on the distribution listing, correlate with each move ticket.

Figure 2

```
------------------------------------------------------------------------------
|ROYAL CHILDRENS HOSPITAL |Type|Serial No.|Name|Transfer To|Date From|Date To |
|                         |N20 |151920    |THOM| 5E  |  1  |  090882 | 031082 |
|-----------------------------------------------------------------------------|
| ST. NURSE    J R. THOMPSON        (6)            CLINICAL EXPER.    17.4 |
| SENIORITY    1/82                                INCLUDES N/D        0.0 |
| LAST LOC - MOUNT ROYAL HOSPITAL  26/07/82  8/08/82   STUDY BLOCK    10.0 |
|                                                  RECREATION LVE      0.0 |
|NURSE MOVE SELECTION                              LVE OF ABSENCE      0.0 |
|                                                  SICK LEAVE          0.6 |
|           EXPERIENCE: AS AT 9/08/82              EXPER. IN WEEEKS   27.4 |
|                                                                          |
| MED/SURG       0.0  TOTAL                                                 |
|                                                                          |
| MEDICAL        4.0  TOTAL  9E  .. 4.0,                                    |
|                                                                          |
| SURGICAL       9.4  TOTAL  7W  .. 4.8, 8W .. 4.6,                         |
|                                                                          |
| SPECIAL        2.0  TOTAL  MTR .. 2.0,                                    |
|                                                                          |
| DEPARTMENTS    2.0  TOTAL CSD  .. GLC .. 1.0,                             |
------------------------------------------------------------------------------
```

The system is entirely flexible and is left to the rostering assistant director to decide whether a nurse is to move keeping in mind the requirements of the clinical rotation program. The assistant director prepares the moves over the next two work days. On the Wednesday morning of the following week, a one to two hour data input session is performed. This session also serves as a checking system to ensure that all data is transcribed correctly, thus eliminating errors from the input. The nurse move select programs are part of a batch mode system and the data is processed at weekly intervals. The input data, consists of new moves, commencements, amendments, cancellations, moves to and from recreation leave and records of sick and special leave.

Run 11, known as the Complete run of the system, is performed on the Thursday morning and distributed that afternoon to all wards and departments. (see figure 1) We are able to communicate messages on the distribution listing and the computer automatically prints the dates and venue of forthcoming Charge and Supervisory Nurse meetings.

The previous manual system took 4-5 days to prepare, and produced from 5-6 foolscap pages of typewritten change list, which was at times inaccurate. The charge nurse preparing a roster had to sift through pages, looking for the names of those nurses moving either in or out of the area. The allocation work now takes from 2-3 days, is very much simplified, does not involve the duplication that existed with the manual system and has freed the rostering assistant director for other duties.

The charge nurse at ward or department level, now receives one to two pages of concise printout, with the actual ward staff and their seniority set out, along with the number of weeks in the location at a date two weeks in advance. Also included on the printout is the day a student nurse is to attend study day, which is essential information for the person who is to prepare the roster. The printout is a saving of 2-3 hours typing, and collating per week, to the nursing administration clerical staff, which frees these personnel for other tasks.

A great advantage of the automated system, as against the previous method, is the accuracy of the information and its availability to wards and departments, one complete day earlier, than was the case with the manual system. This is excellent from the charge nurses point of view, as it means the roster can be prepared prior to the forthcoming weekend instead of Sunday evening or even the Monday or Tuesday of the following week. The computer system enables the projected roster to be prepared 12-13 days in advance, which improves morale, as a nurse can plan for his/her days off much earlier.

Some people may consider that nurse allocation is a reasonably simple cyclical process which can be handled by an input/output device such as this, used by us before 1974.

Figure 3   Mixmaster

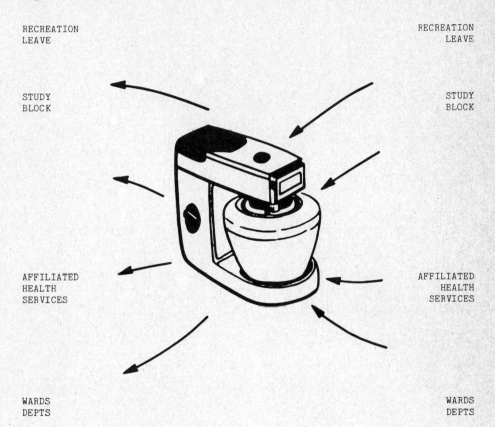

RECREATION
LEAVE

RECREATION
LEAVE

STUDY
BLOCK

STUDY
BLOCK

AFFILIATED
HEALTH
SERVICES

AFFILIATED
HEALTH
SERVICES

WARDS
DEPTS

WARDS
DEPTS

Today, however, nurse allocation is a very much more exacting and complex task, and should, whenever possible, be undertaken with the aid of more sophisticated hardware.

Figure 4   Computer Hardware

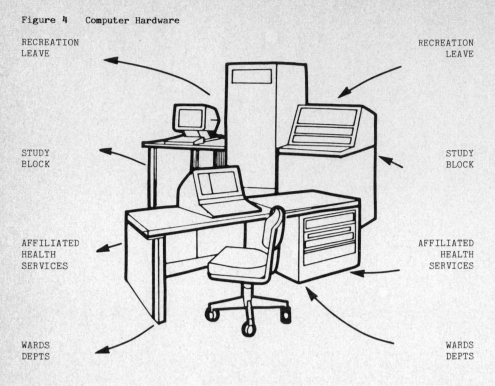

RECREATION   RECREATION
LEAVE   LEAVE

STUDY   STUDY
BLOCK   BLOCK

AFFILIATED   AFFILIATED
HEALTH   HEALTH
SERVICES   SERVICES

WARDS   WARDS
DEPTS   DEPTS

Nurse allocation is a major undertaking particularly when the nursing department
is responsible for a basic school of nursing and clinical and theoretical
programs of rotation.   The diploma type of nursing education, i.e. the
apprenticeship scheme is still the norm in Australian hospitals, and is based on
the British model.   There are only a few institutions which are independent
schools of nursing and provide a college type nursing education.   The central
focus of all nursing service activities is the provision of patient care.   This
nursing care must be maintained throughout the 24 hour period, 7 days a week, to
implement this coverage.   Allocation is a vital component.   The Nurse Allocation
system which has been developed at the Royal Children's Hospital, is a nurse
management tool that allocates nursing manpower to hospital locations, and
records individual accumulated experience.

Information provided by the Nurse Allocation system is derived from two basic
sources.   The hospital payroll system supplies the personnel details, and the
allocation system itself supplies locations, manning requirements, and summary
of experience for individuals due to move.   The system provides the following
sort of information:

        NURSE MASTER FILE LISTING
        ALLOCATION, WORK RUN 1, AND COMPLETE RUN 11
        PERSONNEL LISTING
        PERSONNEL DETAILS ON GUMMED LABELS
        EXPERIENCE REPORTS
        JOURNAL LISTING
        STUDENT NURSE DATE LIST
        NURSING STAFF RETURN

There are three other programs, which although not creating any output of direct benefit to the Nursing Department, are nevertheless vital parts of the overall system.

EVALUATION REPORTS UPDATE
ANNUAL INPUT OF THEORETICAL CURRICULUM AND RECREATION LEAVE
CREATION OF MAG. TAPE FOR ARCHIVED RECORDS

The function of this suite of programs is two-fold: One, to record the movement of individuals as they are transferred from location (be it a ward/unit or department) to location; and two, to accumulate the above information so as to provide a history of time spent in the various locations (experience). To accomplish one, the system accepts a number of records to maintain and update a location record for each individual. The location record for an individual contains an accumulating table showing the various locations in which the individual has worked. This portion of an individual record will account for every day that the individual is employed by the hospital and includes clinical experience, recreation leave, sick leave and special leave.

It may be useful to think of the individual records in terms of a 'body' and its 'tail'. In the former, details relating to the individual are kept (for example, employee number, given names, surname, date of birth, etc.). The 'tail' portion consists of a maximum number of 200 location entries, each consisting of the location (in abbreviated form), the date of the first day in the location (cease date), the type of experience, be it day duty of night duty and the number of hours the individual may, for whatever reason, be absent from a location, i.e. sickness or study days. This tail (sometimes referred to as the history table), will form a continuous block of time, that is the end date of location A is back-to-back with the start date of location B, the end date of location B is back-to-back with the start date of location C and so on. It follows that weekends (or any 2 days off per week) will be included in the start end dates of a location and, therefore, all calculations consider that for every 7 day's 5 will be work days.

The program revolves around the concepts of location entries forming continuous lengths of time and the seven day week. We have endeavoured to look closely at the data already captured in the payroll/personnel allocation files and design programmes and reports which will provide up to date documentation to the nursing administration office. The use of a report generator program has greatly enhanced this capability.

Gradually we have dispensed with the duplication which existed. This process takes time, as does any worthwhile changes for the better. Those of you who have experienced implementation of automated programs are aware that a manual system must be run parallel to the 'new' automated system for a varying period of time. This length of time depends on the commitment of the user's working with the system and the degree of time it takes for these users to become completely confident in the automated system. However, after a defined period of time, a cut off date should be decided upon.

In describing the nursing system, it is interesting to note the definite similarities which the computer system has to the human organism. A tremendous amount of energy goes into error avoidance and error repair, just to keep systems viable. Error catastrophe occurs in the human mechanism when the amount of error is such that the system is unable to function effectively. Error catastrophe may also occur and does occur in computer systems. System catastrophe! An occasion on which the program generates reports sending all the nurses to study block and leaves none for nursing service in the wards and departments! Another catastrophe when the reports printed all the students names twice! It is comforting to know that in this particular instance, the computer was sympathetic to the staffing shortages. Unfortunately, the extra students only appeared on paper! Obviously the computer is well aware that we have enough chiefs and not enough indians. However, just as we continue to strive for excellence in patient care, we should continue this development of nursing management programs, which will help in the delivery of that patient care.

A modern day nurse, involved in computers and nursing, Rita Zeilstorff states that 'the crucial determinant is active participation by qualified nurses at every stage of planning and developing computer based systems'. Whether these systems be for Nursing Administration or for the clinical sphere, we as a professional body have a wealth of knowledge in hospital information handling. It is up to us to have those resources tapped, to come forward and speak up, to have our ideas heard, so that nurses play an active role in health care computing and nursing management, both now and in the future.

The Impact of Computers on Nursing
M. Scholes, Y. Bryant and B. Barber (eds.)
Elsevier Science Publishers B.V. (North-Holland)
© IFIP-IMIA, 1983

14.5.

THE COMPUTER – A TOOL FOR NURSE MANAGERS TO IMPROVE STANDARDS OF CARE

Jean G. Jarvis

This paper describes how nurse managers can use the data collected from care plans as a means to monitor and improve standards of care. It is the duty of all nurse managers to use resources efficiently and performance is assessed using this criterion. The advantages of receiving information about ward workloads immediately raises the question "are the staffing levels right, and are the right skills available?". It is obvious that a manpower system is also necessary.

1. Background to the Exeter Computer Systems

In the early 1970's fully integrated computer systems were developed at Exeter on the ICL 1904 A main frame computer. Application areas include:

(1) Primary Care Record Keeping
(2) Hospital Administration
(3) Ward based systems:-   i)   Nursing orders record
                           ii) Urgent Pathology Laboratory results
                           iii) Nursing Procedures
                           iv) Enquiry systems, e.g. General Practitioner
                                Lists, Drug Information, "What's On".

During the last two years further developments have taken place including Learner allocation and a nurse personnel record system. The systems are available seven days a week 21 hours per day real time.

2. The Nursing Record System

The design of the nursing system was based on the maintenance of a nursing record planned according to individual patients requirements. It can be evaluated and updated as conditions change. In addition the data collected provides information on workload that indicates the style of nursing, the standard of care, and the skills required to execute the plan of care. The system has previously been described(C.5) (C.12). Similar installations of computerised systems of nursing have taken place at Ninewells Teaching Hospital Dundee(D4) and Queen Elizabeth Hospital, Birmingham.

The design has provision for the following:

i)   Admission, Transfer into a ward and change of admission details
ii) Change of record position of patients beds within a ward
iii) Set up and amend patient care plans
iv) Print care plans, name lists, etc. in several different ways.
v)   Report on prescribed care
vi) Automatic printing of summary of care on patients discharge or transfer.

FIGURE I: NURSING CARE ORDERS

```
-----------------------------------------------------------------------
|                           INTAKE - DIET                             |
|                                                                     |
|DIET : 1 NORMAL                    DIET :15 HIGH PROTEIN             |
|     : 2 LIGHT                          :16 HIGH RESIDUE             |
|     : 3 SOFT                           :17 LOW CALCIUM              |
|     : 4 PUREE                          :18 LOW CHOLESTEROL          |
|     : 5 LIQUIDISED                     :19 LOW FAT                  |
|     : 6 FLUID (?)-CALORIES             :20 LOW LACTOSE              |
|     : 7 GASTRIC                        :21 LOW PHENYLALANINE        |
|     : 8 TODDLER                        :22 LOW POTASSIUM            |
|     : 9 VEGETARIAN                     :23 LOW PROTEIN (?)-GRAMS    |
|     :10 FAT FREE                       :24 LOW RESIDUE              |
|     :11 GLUTEN FREE                    :25 LOW SODIUM               |
|     :12 REDUCING (?)-CALORIES          :26 NO ADDED SALT            |
|     :13 DIABETIC (?)-GRAMS CARBOHYDRATE :27 VIVONEX                 |
|14 DIET: NO MEAT/YEAST EXTRACTS,TINNED FISH, :28 SMALL PORTION       |
|CHEESE,YOGHOURT,BROAD BEANS,BANANAS,PINEAPPLE, :29 HELP FEED PATIENT |
|ALCOHOL                                                              |
|     :30 LIGHT BREAKFAST      :36 NOTHING BY MOUTH                   |
|     :31 LIGHT LUNCH          :37 NOTHING BY MOUTH FROM (?)-HOURS    |
|     :32 LIGHT SUPPER         :38 LAST DRINK AT (?)- HOURS           |
|     :33 DRY BREAKFAST        :39 TEACH PATIENT TO GIVE OWN FEEDS    |
|     :34 DRY LUNCH            :40 FEED ORALLY,OTHERWISE BY NASO-GASTRIC |
|     :35 SOUP & SWEET             TUBE                               |
|                                                                     |
|                                                                     |
|                          INTAKE - FLUIDS                            |
|                                                                     |
| 1 INTRAVENOUS FLUIDS AS PRESCRIPTION SHEET    :                     |
| 2 ICE TO SUCK                                 :                     |
| 3 WATER ONLY                                  :                     |
| 4 WATER ONLY,(?)ml (?)-HOURLY                 :20 ICED              |
| 5 CLEAR FLUIDS ONLY                           :21 THROUGH FEED TUBE |
| 6 CLEAR FLUIDS ONLY,(?)ml (?)-HOURLY          :22 AT LEAST          |
| 7 MIXED FLUIDS                                :23 AT MOST           |
| 8 MIXED FLUIDS,(?)ml (?)-HOURLY               :24 AT (?,?,?,?,)-HOURS |
| 9 SKIMMED MILK SUPPLEMENTS                    :25 (?)-HOURLY        |
|10 MILK (?)-HOURLY                             :26 (?)ml IN (?)-HOURS |
|11 CONTINUOUS MILK FEED,(?)-LITRES IN 24 HOURS :27 COPIOUS          |
|12 COMPLAN                                     :28 RESTRICTED        |
|13 NOURISHING DRINKS AT (?,?,?,?,?,?,?)-HOURS  :                     |
|14 TUBE FED (?)ml (?)-HOURLY                   :                     |
|15 INFANT FEEDS AS DIRECTED                    :                     |
|16 (named feed)                                :                     |
|   30 ALCOHOLIC BEVERAGE AS PRESCRIPTION SHEET :35 NOTHING BY MOUTH  |
|   31 FEED ORALLY,OTHERWISE BY NASO-GASTRIC TUBE :36 HYCAL           |
|   32 TEACH PATIENT TO GIVE OWN FEEDS          :37 FIZZY DRINKS      |
|   33 LAST DRINK AT (?)-HOURS                  :38 HELP FEED PATIENT |
|   34 NOTHING BY MOUTH FROM (?)-HOURS                                |
|                                                                     |
-----------------------------------------------------------------------
```

The Committee on Nursing in 1972 (2) emphasised the need for patient orientated approach "The important thing is to keep the focus on the patient at all times as the centre and origin of all the activities undertaken". The activities generated by the nurse to provide nursing care can be identified. Quantative measures can take place and have been achieved by the use of patient dependency studies and work measurement. The Aberdeen Formula(3) and other dependency systems, such as Barr's, classify patients into dependency categories and a workload is associated with each category of patient. From this information the nursing hours required are calculated. There are distinct disadvantages in using these systems because they are dependant on the manual completion of forms. Nurse managers are well aware of skewed figures resulting from a tired sister or staff nurse who resents the time spent away from direct patient care. However, a computer system, that can produce automatically a workload indicator from care ordered for the patients, must have advantages.

To obtain a care plan the nurse makes an initial assessment of individual patients nursing needs on admission and then select from pages of orders the appropriate care (Fig. I). It is also possible for her to identify specific problems that may need special consideration, and if the correct phrase is not found free text may be used.

At the Visual Display Unit the nurse admits her patient (Fig. II).

FIGURE II: ADMISSION SHEET

```
-------------------------------------------------------------------------------
¦)MR  WILLIAM JAMES JONES           M  39 YEARS   WHO  333333                  ¦
¦10.11.81.------Today--                                                        ¦
¦(  )WEARS CONTACT LENS(ES), BOTH,NOT TO WEAR LENSES WHILE DROWSY,REPLACE AS   ¦
¦SOON AS SAFE.                                                                 ¦
¦(  )MOBILITY,INFECTED FOOT ULCER:CONTROL INFECTION.                           ¦
¦(  )THIN,RELIEVE PRESSURE.                                                    ¦
¦(  )DIABETIC.                                                                 ¦
¦(  )APPLY SHEEPSKIN BOOT(S), LEFT.                                            ¦
¦(  )NURSE PATIENT ON SHEEPSKIN                                          **  ¦
¦Mark deletions,terminations; accept orders,from Today,Tomorrow, or date  WRONG
¦BED BATH---------------------------------------(/)    (  )   ( 11.81)  (  )¦
¦MOUTHWASH, AS REQUIRED-------------------------(/)    (  )   ( 11.81)  (  )¦
¦CHANGE POSITION OF PATIENT 2-HOURLY------------(/)    (  )   ( 11.81)  (  )¦
¦BED REST---------------------------------------(/)    (  )   ( 11.81)  (  )¦
¦INTRAVENOUS FLUIDS AS PRESCRIPTION SHEET---------(/)    (  )   ( 11.81)  (  )¦
¦RECORD TEMPERATURE,PULSE, BLOOD PRESSURE 6xDAILY (/)    (  )   ( 11.81)  (  )¦
¦RECORD WEIGHT WEEKLY ON MON.----------------------(/)    (  )   ( 11.81)  (  )¦
¦ROUTINE URINE TES-------------------------------(/)    (  )   ( 11.81)  (  )¦
¦MIDSTREAM SPECIMEN OF URINE----------------------(  )    (  )   ( 11.81)  (  )¦
¦PASS NASO-GASTRIC TUBE---------------------------(  )    (  )   ( 11.81)  (  )¦
¦NOTHING BY MOUTH, TILL SEEN BY DR.----------------(/)    (  )   ( 11.81)  (  )¦
¦CHECK CONSENT FORM-------------------------------(/)    (  )   ( 11.81)  (  )¦
¦PREMEDICATION-----------------------------------(/)    (  )   ( 11.81)  (  )¦
¦INFORM RELATIVES OF PRECEDURE--------------------(/)    (  )   ( 11.81)  (  )¦
-------------------------------------------------------------------------------
```

The ward screen indicates the position of the patients in the ward. The screen can be raised at any VDU and is useful for nurse managers to ascertain where there are empty beds. Nurse then sets up initial necessary care by selecting from pages of orders. Following acceptance of order including the identification of certain special problems, the nurse obtains a print of the Care Plan (Fig. III).

FIGURE III: NURSING CARE PLAN

```
-------------------------------------------------------------------------------
|-1557-HOURS-   BAY G            WARD AVON                                     |
|                                                                             |
|BILL J JONES       333333    WHO------1557-HOURS-10.11.81----Tuesday         |
|_____|
|                                                                             |
|      Special Needs & Precautions                                            |
|WEARS CONTACT LENS(ES), BOTH, NOT TO WEAR LENSES WHILE                       |
|  DROWSY, REPLACE AS SOON AS SAFE.                                           |
|MOBILITY, INFECTED FOOT ULCER: CONTROL INFECTION.                            |
|THIN, RELIEVE PRESSSURE.                                                      |
|DIABETIC.                                                                     |
|                                                                             |
|      Basic Care                                                             |
|BED BATH      (AEH)                                                          |
|MOUTHWASH, AS REQUIRED    (AEH)                                              |
|CHANGE POSITION OF PATIENT 2-HOURLY                    (chart)               |
|APPLY SHEEPSKIN BOOT(S), LEFT                          (AEH)                 |
|NURSE PATIENT ON SHEEPSKIN                             (AEH)                 |
|KEEP RIGHT HEEL OFF BED   (AEH)                                              |
|                                                                             |
|      Mobility                                                               |
|BED REST      (AEH)                                                          |
|                                                                             |
|      Diet & Fluids                                                          |
|INTRAVENOUS FLUIDS AS PRESCRIPTION SHEET               (TTT)                 |
|                                                                             |
|      Observations & Recordings                                              |
|RECORD TEMPERATURE,PULSE,BLOOD PRESSURE 6 DAILY        (TTT,TTT,AEH,AEH,      |
|      18,22)                                                                 |
|RECORD WEIGHT WEEKLY ON MON.                           (--)                  |
|                                                                             |
|      Tests & Investigations                                                 |
|ROUTINE URINE TEST          (TTT)                                           |
|TEST URINE FOR SUGAR & KETONE BODIES, EVERY                                  |
|SPECIMEN      (TTT)                                                          |
|BLOOD GLUCOSE ESTIMATIONS (B.M.STIX)                   (AEH)                 |
|                                                                             |
|      Technical Care                                                         |
|NOTHING BY MOUTH, TILL SEEN BY DR.                                          |
|CHECK CONSENT FORM        (AEH)                                             |
|PREMEDICATION             (chart)                                           |
|INFORM RELATIVES OF PROCEDURE                          (AEH)                 |
|                                                                             |
-------------------------------------------------------------------------------
```

Traditionally patient classification systems have focussed on hygiene, nutrition, mobility, monitoring of vital signs and prescribed treatment. The plan has placed these orders under traditional headings but "special needs and precautions" can focus on physiological and psychological needs as well as handicapping conditions that will influence patient classification and are vital for an accurate workload. Computer classification occurs by the use of markers against certain orders. There are 24 markers in total including:-

Special	Unconscious/totally dependent	
Needs	Emotionally disturbed	Confused

Mobility	Up more than 6 hours	Up less than 3 hours
	Up more than 3 less than 6 hours	
	Chairfast	Bedfast

Toilet	Help with washing, etc.	Washed by nurse
	Bedpan/Commode	Incontinent

Feeding	Assistance	Fed by nurse

Treatment	Tube Fed	I.V.
	Suction/Aspiration	Oxygen
	Drainage	

Observations	Pulse/BP 4 hourly	Peritoneal dialysis
	Monitoring (machine)	

Age Code:	0	Under 12
	1	75
	2	70 - 75
	3	12 - 59
	4	No age
	5	60 - 69

The accumulation of these markers together with the patients age automatically places the patient into one of five dependency levels. The Barr System (4) was used as it was considered a more accurate means of classification than a three grouping. The dependency levels are categorised as follows:-

Care Group 1	Self Care
Care Group 2	Intermediate Care - Ambulatory
Care Group 3	Intermediate Care - Others
Care Group 4	Intermediate Care - Bedfast
Care Group 5	Intensive Care

3.   The Reporting System

The design of the system includes a reporting facility. Fig. III also illustrates the space on the screen provided for the nurse to indicate the order has been completed. The nurse signs on with her individual password and marks by the side of the order carried out. The reporting system supplies her initials and her unique identity is retained for professional accountability and legal purposes. In the future it is anticipated this facility may also be used as a record for learners ward experience. The record is eventually microfiched for long term storage.

It was recognised by nurse managers that workload information automatically produced from care plans required validation. Random audit checks were introduced and sisters were asked to place selected patients into dependency categories using manually the Barr Dependency System. These classifications were compared with the computer category and matching occurred in approximately 85% of cases. The errors tended to be over estimation of dependency by the computer rather than under estimation.

4.   The Exeter Workload Indicator

From the patients nursing record daily workload figures are produced for all patients and for all wards. A print out is produced on a monthly basis (Fig.IV) for nurse managers.

FIGURE IV: WORKLOAD INDICATOR FORM

```
---------------------------------------------------------------------------------
|                                                                               |
|                  MONTHLY TOTALS OF WORKLOAD (EXTRACT)                          |
|                                                                               |
|                          WARD:- YEO/YARTY                                      |
|                          MONTH:-                                               |
|                                                                               |
| WARD    DATE            GROUP              TOTAL        WORKLOAD               |
| NO            1    2    3    4    5       PATS      TOTAL    AVGE              |
|                                                                               |
| 15     01/12/81   3    0    4   21    0    28         99     3.54             |
| 15     02/12/81   0    0    3   22    0    25         97     3.88             |
| 15     03/12/81   2    0    4   23    0    29        106     3.66             |
| 15     04/12/81   4    0    4   19    1    28         97     3.46             |
| 15     05/12/81   1    0    4   19    0    24         89     3.71             |
| 15     06/12/81   1    0    2   20    0    23         87     3.78             |
|                                                                               |
|                              THROUGH TO                                        |
|                                                                               |
| 15     28/12/81   1    0    3    9    0    13         46     3.54             |
| 15     29/12/81   1    0    3   11    0    17         56     3.28             |
| 15...30/12/81     8    0    3   14    0    25         73     2.92             |
|                                                                               |
| 15              53    2  108  473    4   640       2293   107.50             |
|                                                                               |
|                             GRAND TOTALS                                       |
|                                                                               |
|                 53    2  108  473    4   640       2293   107.50             |
|                                                                               |
---------------------------------------------------------------------------------
```

Each patient is classified and the workload is calculated by multiplying the number of patients by their dependency category. The totals provide the ward workload and an average is also indicated. This information can also be produced in histogram form (Fig. V).

The information generated by the computerised nursing record system may be used by nurse managers in various ways but the following are typical examples:-

i)   Establishing a distribution of staff to match the actual workload pattern, for example the weekend ward use, and if pool nurses are available they can be allocated to wards with the highest workload.

ii)   Equalising the workload between wards.

iii)   Establishing standards of care by evaluation of care plans.

iv)   Prediction of workload by knowledge of dependency levels associated with individual cases. Standard Care Profiles are being developed for specific cases.

v)   Balancing workload between wards through correct distribution of admissions.

vi)   Carrying out comparative studies of care plans associated with identical cases but following differing patterns of prescribed care to evaluate the efficiency of nursing practice.

vii)   Identification of changes required in nurse training and professional skills to meet technical advances.

viii) Assessing the implications on nursing workload of technical advances.
ix)　The maintenance of continuity of care by the provision of the patients
　　　discharge summary of care to nurse managers in the Community.

The Exeter Nursing Record system demonstrates how nursing input can be
quantified thus providing managers with a valuable tool in determining staffing
levels and the skills required to maintain and improve standards of care. One
facet of the qualitative measure of patient care is the ability of nurses to
carry out the care according to the individual plan. In the future, nurse
managers can monitor this aspect of care by using the reporting system.

FIGURE V: WORKLOAD INDICATOR HISTOGRAM

```
-------------------------------------------------------------------------
|                                                                         |
|RETURN OF DAILY TOTAL WORKLOAD (EXTRACT)                                  |
|                                                                         |
|  DATE    TOTAL                                                          |
|          WLD   0  10  20  30  40  50  60  70  80  90  100 110 120 130 140|
|                .   .   .   .   .   .   .   .   .   .   .   .   .   .   . |
|                                                                         |
|                                                                         |
|01/12/81   99   **************************************                    |
|02/12/81   97   *************************************                     |
|03/12/81  106   ********************************************              |
|04/12/81   97   *************************************                     |
|05/12/81   89   ********************************                          |
|06/12/81   87   *******************************                          |
|07/12/81   97   *************************************                     |
|08/12/81   89   ********************************                          |
|09/12/81   87   *******************************                          |
|10/12/81   97   *************************************                     |
|                                                                         |
-------------------------------------------------------------------------
```

5.　The Personnel Record System

The need to have the right nurse in the right place at the right time is a
service commitment essential for meeting the needs of patients. A system which
identifies the extent to which current staffing levels meet the present need and
ultimately forecasts how the size and mix of staff must change to meet future
needs must be the aim of all nurse managers. M.G. Auld in 1978(5) stated that
one of the difficulties in manpower forecasting has been the lack of positive
information about "expected standards, about stated objectives and about
criteria for evaluation of nursing input".

In Exeter there was clearly a need to develop a manpower planning system which
would complement the nursing workload information. Nurse managers would then be
in a position to plan for a cost effective use of resources and prepare
recommendations for budgets which would truly reflect the needs of the service
rather than being subjective judgements related to historical establishments.
Discussions took place with the Computer Project Team to examine the
possibilities of providing a computerised manpower planning system. It was
understood from the outset that any development would have to be maintained
within the capacity of the main frame computer and without any further revenue
consequences.

The resulting Computerised Personnel Record which has been adapted from the Primary Care Record system demonstrates the benefits gained from the larger computer which supports a network of linking terminals. Real Time access and data analysis as well as batch information can be provided. The aim was to produce a personnel file containing a record for each nurse and auxiliary working in the General Division. The records would provide a variety of data agreed necessary for managers to optimize patient care:-

i)   Identification data (e.g. name, status, address)
ii)   Grade, place of work, contracted hours
iii) Qualifications, record of training (e.g. Joint Board of Clinical Nursing
      Studies, extended role)
iv)   Employment History
v)   Special Attributes e.g. Languages spoken, car driver
vi)   Sickness and absence record
vii) Annual Leave Record.

Four types of screen are used:-

i)   Registration details (Fig. VI)
ii)   Employment History and Training Record (Fig.VII)
iii) Absence Record (Fig. VIII))
iv)   Personnel details (Fig. IX)

FIGURE VI: REGISTRATION DETIALS

```
------------------------------------------------------------------
|                                                                |
|DRAFT SCREENS:   1)  Registration                               |
|                 2)  Employment - Training                      |
|                 3)  Personal History                           |
|                 4)  Sickness/Absence                           |
|                                                                |
|                                  * * * * * * * * * *           |
|1) REGISTRATION                                                 |
|                                                                |
|   NAME          Prefix.......(e.g. MR. MRS. MISS).....         |
|                 Surname..................................      |
|                 Forename(s)............................        |
|                 Registration/Enrolment Number.........         |
|                 Grade : Day/Night Duty...............          |
|                 Ward/Department.......................         |
|                 Registered Disabled...................         |
|ADDRESS          Thoroughfare (house No. Road).........         |
|                 Locality Code.........................         |
|                 District..............................         |
|                 Post Town.............................         |
|                 County................................         |
|                 Postcode..............................         |
|                 Telephone.............................         |
|DETAILS          Date of Birth.........................         |
|                 Sex...................................         |
|                 Status................................         |
|                 Contract Hours........................         |
|                 Unit Code.............................         |
|                 Management Code.......................         |
------------------------------------------------------------------
```

FIGURE VII: EMPLOYMENT HISTORY AND TRAINING RECORD

```
--------------------------------------------------------------------------------
|                                                                              |
|Display Consultant                                       Hospital No 903706|
|                                                                              |
|        ZZ-JONES, Mrs ANGELS MARY "DAY", 1 SIDMOUTH ROAD, EXM                 |
|                                                                              |
|Document-Consultant No.2  Ref -                             Date 16.12.80|
|                                                                              |
|Hosp  EMPLOYMENT                                                              |
|Dept.  -                                                                      |
|From   -                                                                      |
|Posn.  -                                                                      |
|To     -                                                                      |
|                                                                              |
|post                       site             :number    : dates               |
|ENROLLED NURSE TRAINING    :PAIGNTON HOSPITAL     :123456   :04/66-09/68|
|B.T.A. CERTIFICATE         :HAWKMOOR CHEST HOSPITAL:3323    :09/68-03/69|
|THEATRE NURSE              :NEWTON ABBOTT HOSPITAL :        :04/69-09/70|
|NIGHT DUTY (MEDICAL)       :R.D.E.H.(WONFORD)      :        :07/74-01/76|
|S.E.N. GERIATRICS          :R.D.E.H. (HEAVITREE)   :        :02/76-03/77|
|S.E.N.                     :SAUDI ARABIA           :        :04/77-04/79|
|S.E.N.                     :ABU DHABI              :        :06/79-12/79|
|S.E.N. GERIATRICS          :R.D.E.H. (HEAVITREE)   :        :02/80-    |
|                                                                              |
|                                                                              |
|         Read Document-Consultant? No.=                                       |
|                                                                              |
--------------------------------------------------------------------------------
```

FIGURE VIII: ABSENCE RECORD

```
--------------------------------------------------------------------------------
|                                                                              |
|Display Consultant                                       Hospital No 903706|
|                                                                              |
|        ZZ-JONES, Miss ANGELA MARY "DAY", 1 SIDMOUTH RO-,FRE                  |
|Document-Consultant No. 1  Ref ENTITLEMENT 35 DAYS         Date 16.12.80|
|Hosp   SICKNESS/LEAVE                                                         |
|Dept  -                                                                       |
|From  -                                                                       |
|Posn  -                                                                       |
|To    -                                                                       |
|                                                                              |
|leave type  : start   :stop      :days    :details                           |
|ANNUAL      :01.08.80 :14.08.80 : 10    :                                     |
|STUDY       :01.07.80 :01.07.80 :  1    :APPRAISAL                            |
|STUDY       :19.09.80 :21.09.80 :  3    :STOMA COURSE                         |
|CERT        :02.04.80 :10.04.80 :  6    :                                     |
|SICK        :16.07.80 :18.07.80 :  3    :                                     |
|SICK        :03.06.80 :05.06.80 :  3    :                                     |
|            :        :        :       :                                       |
|            :        :        :       :                                       |
|                                                                              |
|                                                                              |
|              Read Document-Consultant? No.=                                  |
--------------------------------------------------------------------------------
```

FIGURE IX: PERSONNEL DETAILS

```
--------------------------------------------------------------------------------
|                                                                              |
|Display Consultant                                     Hospital No 903706|
|                                                                              |
|        ZZ-JONES, Mrs ANGELA MARY "DAY" 1, SIDMOUTH ROAD, EXM               |
|Document-Consultant No.3   Ref -                        Date 16.12.80|
|Hosp  N.O.K., FAMILY & O.P.                                                   |
|Dept  -                                                                       |
|From  -                                                                       |
|Posn  -                                                                       |
|To    -                                                                       |
|                                                                              |
|relation: DoB       :names,  address and notes                                |
|FATHER  :            :JACK (N.O.K.) 27, WARREN VIEW HEIGHTS, DAWLISH, DEVON  |
|        :            :                 TEL 913 6854                           |
|SON     :12.01.71   :JOHN BERNARD      AS MOTHER                             |
|DAUGHTER:09.06.73   :SARAH MILLICENT   AS MOTHER                             |
|G.P.    :            :DR MERRICK  MT. PLEASANT HO                             |
|                                                                              |
|                    Read Document-Consultant? No.=                            |
|                                                                              |
--------------------------------------------------------------------------------
```

6.   Input

It is possible to input on any ward terminal. Nursing Officers have been
trained to use the system and this provides immediacy of update information by
unit and avoids errors.   At present the input on sickness and absence is
obtained from a manual return completed by ward sisters or Nursing Officers.
This form is required for the Treasurer's department. However, it is hoped in
the future the computer system will collate this information and provide it in
an acceptable printed form for finance purposes. The real time system provides
scope for record inspection at any Terminal. Access is obtained by the use of
passwords. Each nurse record is identified by either a record number or name.
The mechanism makes use of the patients index system but there is strict control
to ensure nurse records are kept distinct.

7.   Output

Although data entered to the system is in real time, the majority of identified
output needs are produced by batch processes.

The data captured provides operational output including:-

i)   Return of staff in post by grade/sex/full or part time, by ward, unit and
       hospital site. (Fig. X)
ii)   Summaries of joiners and leavers by grade and unit.
iii)   Absence levels and reasons, individual and by ward, unit and site.
iv)   Turn-over rate in grades by age structure, etc.
v)   Experience and skill levels.
vi)   Retirement schedules.

FIGURE X: STAFF IN POST

```
--------------------------------------------------------------------------------
|                                                                              |
|15.12.81.                                                                     |
|                                                                    AGE NO|
|                          A L L   S T A F F                                   |
|                                                                              |
|           M A L E S              F E M A L E S             T O T A L          |
|                                                                              |
|        FULL TIME   PART TIME    FULL TIME   PART TIME                         |
|          NO        NO    WTE      NO       NO    WTE     NO      WTE          |
|                                                                              |
|13F  SRI    0        0   0.0       0        0   0.0      0       0.0           |
|13F  CHNI   0        0   0.0       0        0   0.0      0       0.0           |
|13F  SRII   0        0   0.0       5        2   1.0      7       6.0           |
|13F  CHII   0        0   0.0       0        0   0.0      0       0.0           |
|13F  SN     1        0   0.0       7        2   1.3     10       9.3           |
|13F  SSEN   0        1   0.4       0        1   0.9      2       1.3           |
|13F  SEN    0        0   0.0       7        0   0.0      7       7.0           |
|13F  NNEB   0        0   0.0       0        0   0.0      0       0.0           |
|13F  NA     0        0   0.0       1        6   4.2      7       5.2           |
|                                                                              |
|13F         1        1   0.4      20       11   7.4     33      28 8           |
|                                                                              |
--------------------------------------------------------------------------------
```

Before the computer facility was obtained collection of data and analysis necessitated time consuming surveys and routine manual returns. In the future it will be possible to keep an on-going record of sickness and absence. This will enable nurse managers to place realistic allowances for time spent out of the service. Close monitoring of sickness levels could obtain improvements in certain areas. This has been achieved in a system developed in East Birmingham by W.A. Telford[6].

8.   The Future

In the future it is planned to continue the development of the nursing systems towards closer integration with the patient administration systems. Admission, transfer and discharge activity input at ward level already produces automatically a bed state and valuable information on throughput for nurse managers and hospital administrators. It is hoped in the future the computerised patients nursing care plan will reflect more clearly the continuous pattern of assessment, planning, implementation and evaluation in line with the concept of the Nursing Process. Technically this is possible and has the support of nursing staff.

We believe the introduction of the computer system on all wards at the Royal Devon and Exeter Hospital, has helped nurse managers to establish an environment for the nurse to develop the skills she needs for carrying out planned nursing care based on individual patients needs. The reporting system has helped to establish the professional accountability of the clinical nurse. I hope financial resources will be available to enable future research and development to take place. The true value to nurse managers of computerised nursing systems will be realized when the workload data produced from patient care plans is analysed in relation to the information produced by a Manpower Planning System. Together these applications should ensure a cost effective use of the nursing resource based on the needs of individualised patient care.

9.   Conclusion

It is important that nurses take part in the formation of computer policies for
the future. Few Authorities/Hospitals can contemplate either the capital outlay
or the revenue consequences of a mini-computer, but computer technology is
advancing rapidly and maybe we can look forward to networks of linking micros.
In this way it might be possible to phase in computerised information systems.
It is vital that nurses do not lose sight of the advantages of ward based
systems. We need to know much more about the activities of the nurse at the
bedside to ensure our patients are receiving the best value from our limited
resources.

REFERENCES

(1)   Orlando I.J. (1961). The dynamic nurse - patient relationship. New York:
       Putnam's Sons.
(2)   Report of the Committee on Nursing. Paragraph 123.
(3)   The Aberdeen Formula: evaluation on the large scale. Nursing Times,
       London 1979.
(4)   Measurement of Nursing Care. Barr A. O.R. Research Unit Publication No.
       9. Oxford Regional Hospital Board 1967.
(5)   Perfecting the System. Auld M.G. Nursing Mirror 6.4.78.
(6)   Time Out - A Matter for Management. Telford W.A., D.N.O. East Birmingham
       Health District. July 1981.

The Impact of Computers on Nursing
M. Scholes, Y. Bryant and B. Barber (eds.)
Elsevier Science Publishers B.V. (North-Holland)
© IFIP-IMIA, 1983

14.6.

PRESENT PRACTICE AND POTENTIAL OF COMPUTER SYSTEMS IN NURSING – THE STATE OF THE ART IN ONE HEALTH BOARD AREA IN SCOTLAND

Catherine V. Cunningham

1. Introduction

It is said that the introduction of the computer and information management techniques can be a solution to some of the major health management problems. However, they should not be expected to resolve health care delivery problems. More reasonably, they can be expected to relieve the congestion in the medical/hospital/health care communication network and to assist the user in carrying out duties involving documentation and clerical functions. Much of the inherent paperwork involved in arranging, describing, monitoring and evaluating the service to patients and clients could conceivably be re-directed into automated systems. Where consistent standards are established for the storage and transmission of information, computerization reduces human error and legibility can be a certain positive benefit.

AUTOMATION in a health care setting provides an information processing capacity for ENTRY, STORAGE and RETRIEVAL of data - patient and personnel from admission or entry through to discharge or exit. A 'system' can decrease the responsibility for health care personnel in SORTING, MERGING and COMMUNICATING INFORMATION. Separate departments can be linked and tasks which are repetitive and clerical in nature will be automated, allowing personnel to increase their productivity and decrease communication errors. A totally comprehensive medical information system requires to be superimposed upon a fully computerised management information system. The logical and sequential organisation of medical functions and patient information is dependent on there being an accessible data bank in a manual system. An improved hospital information system can effect overall improvement in organisational procedures. Automation brings improvement in efficiency and effectiveness by accelerating transmission. Control is obtained by supplying staff with concise information concerning events as they are occurring - the data being distributed throughout the system for appropriate uses. The data base itself is constantly updated during operation from input data.

Ball(1) reports that a comprehensive total system does not presently exist but the beginning of an ultimate system is being explored. Acceptance of such a system is revolutionary and the entire approach to communication and information handling should be co-ordinated in a controlled collaborative exercise. Many disciplines are involved and this collaboration is probably the most difficult thing to arrange. In order to produce this type of system, an integrated flow of data processing needs to cover:

1. the collection of service data;
2. the transmission of information via terminals and other communication links to a central computer;
3. the establishment of a large, immediate-access data bank;
4. the development of computerised management information to be used for decision-making;
5. the unification of the physician and his staff with an on-line, real time computer complex.

There will have to be a number of computer assisted applications making up a potential health care information system and current developments in Britain might be considered in some perspective when related to the taxonomy for a total system provided by Ball and included here in Figure 1.

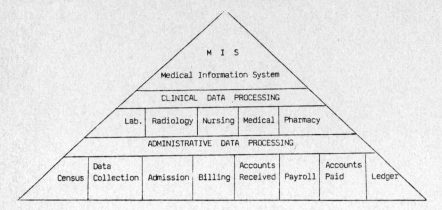

Fig. 1

In a MEDICAL INFORMATION SYSTEM some of the computer assisted applications contributing to the total system include:

1. Admissions and Bed Control
2. Billing and Accounts Receivable
3. Payroll/Personnel
4. Accounts Payable
5. Purchasing
6. Inventory Control
7. Maintenance/Engineering Department
8. Laboratory Medicine
9. Scheduling
10. Administrative Management
11. Pharmacy
12. Radiologic Diagnosis and Therapy
13. Multitesting and Health Screening
14. Nursing Services
15. Patient Support
16. Patient Monitoring
17. Medical Records
18. Electrocardiology
19. Electroencephalography
20. Respiratory Therapy
21. Physiological Monitoring
22. Food Service
23. Diagnostic Support
24. Medical Library

Hospital communication systems have already been devised to tie many of these functions together. The most popular approaches are:

1. Medical Records
2. Nursing
3. Fiscal
4. Multiphasic Screening
5. Research-oriented
6. Modular
7. Distributive Systems

and several computer companies have entered into the field of computer based health care systems.

A number of systems have been designed to organise and view many separate facts and problems into a united picture. One such system (Spectra - MIS, Medical Information System - Chicago) was designed by medical people - doctors, nurses, medical technologists and pharmacists. When using this particular system the practitioner maintains a precise scientific approach to diagnostic procedures and therapeutic management of patients. The primary goals and objectives are:

(i)   to improve patient care delivery and to assist those who practise medicine;
(ii)   to replace most of the manual record-keeping systems and clerical tasks involved in hospital operations, and to maximise the operational efficiency of the hospital;
(iii) to help alleviate problems of escalating costs and manpower shortages;
(iv)   to provide a hospital-wide communication network;
(v)   to help expedite patient services by improving accuracy and timeliness of information;
(vi)   to provide relevant, timely information for CONTROL and DECISION-MAKING by medical and hospital management;
(vii) to be cost effective.

2.   Contemporary Thinking

World Health Organisation, Copenhagen in 1980 published 'Information Systems for Health Services - Public Health in Europe 13' in order to reflect its policy of establishing common principles and providing basic information to help member states towards the settlement and implementation of their own national policies. In this document an overall picture of the present position, together with a selection of technical problems, are presented in the form of essays from technical experts with practical experience. The intention was that they should provide criteria for national systems against which shortcomings in policy and performance could be measured. Special attention is focussed on the role of WHO and on the experience related to information systems which has accumulated in the Federal Republic of Germany, in Scotland, and in the USSR.

WHO also report on the scale and complexity of arranging total systems. Because so many disciplines are involved in bringing together health information - epidemiologists, administrators, statisticians and physicians - the failures in internal communication constitute a fundamental weakness. The problem is compounded when shortcomings in the data themselves are recognised by the specialists and when the expectations of computing science in information handling is tantalisingly within reach. It may be that the more sophisticated aims such as outcome measures and health indicators, may be well beyond present competence or cost. To gather elements, to collate, assess and relate them in a quantifiable way may come to be seen as idealistic and a compromise in a less than total system may more readily be achieved.

The two mainstreams of information flow are for clinical purposes and managerial effectiveness. Both streams converge at certain points. Because total data capture would involve extensive and exhaustive expensive investment there is a need to develop sensible strategies in each system so that the kind of information which is selected will be of maximum operational use both in a clinical and managerial sense.

Data are not information. The main need in a health care service is to translate data into information which is simple and easy to understand. Much effort may be required to transform raw data into comprehensible information and similar effort may be required to program the sophisticated calculations applied to the data in order to produce a final finished report. Managers and management are more likely to benefit when they have understood the implications of the information. The production of information from data is a relatively young activity concerned with issues and techniques of great complexity. Total information seems an impossible goal. Selection is therefore necessary - despite the attendant limitations. Many disciplines are involved and some disciplines are still developing and emerging as separate entities with a specific contribution to make in the delivery of health care. An improved information system includes up-to-date methods of data collection and processing, the use of information for the health care management, for clinical research, for improved practice and for health care planning.

3.   In Scotland

The National Health Service in Scotland comprises 15 health boards covering geographic areas whose population varies from 17,000 in Shetland to 1 million in Greater Glasgow. Heasman(2) reports that the present health information system in Scotland has slowly evolved from a situation where vital statistics and limited data were mainly required for central government purposes and as a matter of historical record, towards a system now by which information for monitoring, evaluating planning and management of health services is more readily available in proper form. In Scotland the general policy is for statistical and computing services to come under the joint control of Information Services which are a health service responsibility. The information Services Division has five statistical branches employing 3 community medicine specialists and 2 statisticians and a small research group of social scientists who undertake **ad hoc** studies and assist in the utilization of statistical data. There is also a computer advisory group and a small computer unit.

The routine collection of health statistical data in Scotland can be divided into:

a)   National vital statistics collected and processed by the Registrar General for Scotland, which is an independent government department and is therefore not part of ISD but there are close formal and informal links between the two.
b)   Hospital inpatient statistics are collected via statistical case abstracts completed on discharge of a patient and processed centrally.
c)   Manpower data are collected for all grades of manpower in the Scottish Health Service. As far as possible, these data are related to that collected for payroll purposes.
d)   Other statistics are collected mainly in summary at health board level and transmitted centrally for collation. These include immunisation and vaccination status outpatient data, notification of infectious diseases, ophthalmology detail and work of public health nurses.

Developments include:

a)   Some pioneer work on the tabulation of existing data for the use of physicians in the hospital service, enabling them to review their work. Alternative systems of providing this kind of information are being pursued.
b)   A system enabling record linkage from individual case abstracts is used for **ad hoc** research studies. With further amendment of the methodology it is hoped that longitudinal morbidity statistics might be produced as routine.
c)   Personnel records have been designed to form the basis for more detailed manpower statistical information.
d)   A master patient index carrying detail of a large number of different health service contacts introduced in one health board.
e)   The design of a system able to collect and process data on hospital outpatients and in general practice is indicated but the scale of such an enterprise is almost inhibiting. There are difficulties more than the potential costs of setting up such a system.

The development of computers has opened up a new world for data processing but the cost of a 'total' system is still prohibitive and all disciplines are not working together. The selection of a restricted data base has tended to be favoured. This is the position within the Nursing Section and also with other disciplines in the Greater Glasgow Health Board and, of itself, is legitimate argument for independent, user-controlled micro systems.

4.   Where to Start: The Preliminaries

In order to employ advanced communication's concepts in the provision of health care, the scope and nature of each task must be carefully defined. Choice and implementation of a computer system must be preceded by a thorough analysis of the present manual operation. The initiator must be familiar with basic data processing principles. Without sufficient knowledge of how a computer system works, he is poorly equipped to compare available alternatives - other important considerations include realistic cost assessments and the quality of the in-service training available for staff. The support/dedication of medical staff and co-operation of administrative staff is essential.

A review of the existing procedures for collecting, handling, storing and retrieving information is also required. An approach described originally by F. W. Taylor as scientific management is most useful. Pritchard(B23), described systems analysis as a method by which careful scrutiny is applied to a procedure with a view to increasing efficiency and increasing economy. This may be achieved by redesigning the existing system or by replacing it by a new system. The exercise is neither simple nor superficial but should be carefully carried out before any modification is arranged, particularly if the use of computers is contemplated. Systems analysis is concerned with refining the operation of organisational components in relationship one with the other. The aims are to increase efficiency by reducing overlapping functions, producing more accurate information in up to date reports and to improve economy by eliminating unnecessary tasks, reducing the number of clerical operations and thereby increasing productivity.

The preparatory work involves an examination of the management objectives relating to the existing system; of the manuals and policies and of the people currently using the existing system. When the analysis is made the design or plan of the improved system can be presented in the form of flow charts showing the logical progression of data through the proposed system and highlighting the points at which decisions may be made; points at which additional data are added and points at which data may be sent elsewhere. Hardware requirements can then be made specific - if computers are to be used.

Computer scientists are able to advise on programming and will help define the form which the input data will take, the processing to be performed and the form of the output. Their collaboration, should not in terms of the best use of their time - be invited until the existing manual operation has been made as effective and efficient as possible. Computerisation will accelerate the process. The old system should be run in parallel for a limited period of time with the computerised system so that errors or problems in the automated system can be traced in the manual system. If they are run in tandem for a period, and only current data introduced in the new system gradually, over time the new system will include all the data input on an incremental basis. During this introductory period staff learn to become familiar with the new system.

5.   User Controlled Micro Systems

Microbased products are compact and relatively easy to accommodate within an office because developments in electronic technology have produced a dramatic fall in the size of components. A concomitant reduction in cost has also contributed to the current popularity and to the installaiton of micro systems in a range of settings within the National Health Service. It is claimed now that microbased products are more reliable. A single electronic component can do the job of many electrical and mechanical components. Electronics devices are very fast - several million operations each second can be arranged or programmed in a single micro processor. This programming function is the vital and most attractive feature of micro systems for although, increasingly, commercially available program packages are available for specific functions, the programming function permits individualised user-control and selectivity.

Standard hardware models purchased from commercial suppliers are increasingly being introduced into the Health Service into clinical areas, into laboratories, into nursing administration offices and staff are developing programming skills on their own initiative. Tentative 'computer awareness' sessions have been arranged on an **ad hoc** basis and attendance is arranged as study leave. Those who enlist for classes at Technical Colleges and Universities are encouraged and secondments have been arranged. Similarly, microcomputing experience for college students has been arranged during summer vacations in Industrial Placement schemes.

Overtures from institutions and from individuals are welcomed, for at this time nurses' knowledge and experience in harnessing computer science is limited. Exposure to some knowledge, to someones ideas about automation, about systems analysis, about alternative applications - is progress. When a link is established and it seems that the association is likely to be mutually beneficial, a nurse is assigned to the particular project for the expected duration. These appointments can be made in Glasgow partly because provision has been made since 1974 for 5 research nurses. This is a small number in a cohort of approximately 18000 but it is an encouraging beginning, and nurses are alert to this opportunity for further study and continuing education. Some use this for computer-related projects. Other nurses are identified by nurse managers, and secondments to Area Health Board officers are given priority. The day release, part-time appointments are resisted as counter productive and full-time concentrated periods of study are preferred. Clinical responsibilities have to be shed for the specified time and discretion about hours of work have to be relaxed. With these appointments there is the freedom to work and protection from distraction.

In early discussions it is clearly established for all parties that there are potential benefits for individuals, for the particular discipline and for the nursing division of the health board and that the onus is with the participants to derive full effect. Notes in diary form of progress and short-term objectives are made, shared and reviewed regularly. Each person is expected to produce a report at the end of the experience and these reports are the basis for academic papers, and the 'seed corn' for future investments of nurse time or health board resources. The reports describe the development of expertise and trace the progress of studies. These are tentative beginnings and are not yet fully evolved as training schemes or apprenticeships but they have proved useful and have already justified the investment of nurse time. Programs have been developed, tested and are now operational. For some nursing administrative and nurse manpower planning exercises there are computer assisted data processing packages and other are in stages of research and development.

A microcomputer with disk storage and printer was purchased in 1980. This hardware system is desk top, user driven and portable and operates from a power point:
- CBM Commodore Computer (Model 3032)
- CBM Floppy Disk Drive (Model 3040)
- CBM Tractor Printer (Model 3022) printing unit of 78 columns across page.
- DYSAN Floppy Disks
The total cost was £3,500 and maintenance costs are approximately £350 per annum. The purchase was made for the development of automated information systems related to nurse manpower planning and nursing research. A case has

since been made for the purchase of a data management software package for handling inventory detail, statistical analyses and personnel records for specialist subgroups within nursing. There are currently three separate projects in different stages of development:

a) Learner records/allocation to clinical areas.
b) Leaver records/stability indices.
c) Patient data processing: Aberdeen formula calculations and in-post nurse staffing comparisons.

The learner records and allocation to clinical areas system was developed from a mathematical model of the disposition of learners simulated on a mainframe. The General Nursing Council for Scotland recommended new Trainings and the effects of the proposed changes were simulated to show the learner contribution to service during the transition period and the long-term effect on the workforce in clinical areas when the old trainings run down. The learner flows through colleges and the increased teacher contact weeks were also highlighted. Close working relationships with the scientists at the Health Services Operational Research Unit, Strathclyde University, were established and a program is available which simulates the College programming/allocation function and produces output documents in a form that permits meaningful discussion between nurse educationists and service managers when arrangements for clinical experience are to be finalised. These documents have been useful in planning new college facilities and invaluable in manpower planning discussions related to workforce requirements.

The system has been transferred to a micro system and the Advisory Panel for Information Processing Scottish Home and Health Department has agreed to fund the exercise in its first operational stage in a College of Nursing and Midwifery. The Nursing Officer has been appointed for a further three years to allow gradual incremental data input, to instruct potential users on the College staff and to be consultant and catalyst in other settings. It is hoped that each of the five colleges in Glasgow will adopt this model of record keeping and that additionally, users will recognise other potential applications on site.

6. Automated Systems in Nurse Manpower Planning Developed on Micros

(i) Learners

In nurse manpower planning the first and most obvious tactic to increase numbers of trained staff has been to increase the learner cohort. In Glasgow increases have been planned and incremented over a five year period. The target ceiling of 4,000 in training has been achieved by centralising control and finance at Area and by setting up a monitoring and forecasting information system. A study of leaving rates and sickness/absence characteristics by college and by special trainings has brought some precision to the planning and to the predicted uptake of monies set aside for learner nurse salaries. Progress reports in the form of statistical compilations have been produced in a manual system each month in the monitoring function and forecast levels and authorised intake levels are derived and updated from current information continuously. These dynamic manual systems worked well in a laborious and clerical way and further refinement was related to reducing the possibility of human error and accelerating the interrelated processes.

The conversion of learner monitoring and forecasting to a computerised system was judged to be timely and the concomitant objectives - to provide microcomputing experience for a student from the Information Systems course at the College of Technology during a period of secondment to industry - to introduce a nurse(s) to computer science technology - to provide programming skills and user interest in micro computers in nurses, seemed feasible. A concentrated period of time was set aside for the two people to work together and a Learner Forecast program has been developed using the principles of modular programming. Individual processes have been coded and tested separately. Individual subroutines are assessed using a combination of computer instructions. The basic outline of the program is that there is a main program from which all subroutines can be assessed. The main program consists of displaying the options of inserting a new course, amending or reviewing an existing course and running the program complete. Appropriate questions are asked periodically to take the user through the processor. The programming language known as BASIC has been used. The Learner Monitoring and Forecasting problem requiring repetitive simple arithmetic is well suited to BASIC.

The advantages of converting this manual system of statistical compilation to a computerised system are related to the person doing the work, the nature of the work and the resulting image it projects. The co-worker on this project claims that it saves time. Once the program was written the pattern for compilation was established and now the in-put data are typed in. Boredom and human error are reduced and consequently job satisfaction has increased, largely because of the mental stimulation arising from converting a series of simple arithmetical exercises into an intellectually sophisticated method of calculation based on logical system analysis.

There are less direct but immediate advantages to the organisation. The basic work has not changed but the effect is produced more quickly and accuracy and currency have been improved. What was formerly many simple arithmetical exercises has become apparently more sophisticated and we are alert to the indictment that, in computerising this system, we may have over-technicalised this problem and introduced an aura of scientific respectability which is both unfounded and unnecessary. It is so very easy, once aware of the potential of computers for statistical analysis, to keep adding dimensions to the original problem, thereby getting distracted from the primary aims and objectives of the exercise. It is however, almost impossible to perceive what the next step could be until the plateau of achievement has been reached. Computers, because of their infinite capacity to work with numbers are well suited to statistical data collection and processing. They have a place therefore in all aspects of manpower planning.

(ii) Leavers
Recruitment of additional learners is one strategy for increasing the number of trained staff and this was arranged in Glasgow. Monitoring the leaving rate in trained staff in order to define more precisely the replacement numbers required is part of the overall manpower planning function. Information about numbers leaving, length of service, age, qualifications, contracted hours, location, is included in termination forms compiled by nurse managers and relayed to finance department. Data captured from personnel records at time of leaving could accumulate to describe vital statistics and grade profiles in trained staff careers. Interventionist policies might more effectively be defined when evidence about the numbers and characteristics of leavers is available for scrutiny, i.e. when data is made meaningful as information for nurse managers. The scale of such an undertaking in a manual system involves many hours of nurse time and findings are insulated and fragmented by location. Computer assisted processing was considered as a medium for standardising definitions which would allow comparisons between location and as a service to nurse managers.

A Nursing officer was assigned to set up a file of 80 records and to devise a program which would, in the first instance, analyse the data, identify those records which were incomplete or inaccurate. Eventually, the software included major and ad hoc programs.

The major programs are:

(a) a creator program to input individual records;
(b) a reader program to read records and print
(c) the data file;
(d) analysis programs which consider:
     entries and leavers by age
     entries and leavers by grade
     stability by age
     stability by grade
     stability by percentage grade in post
     reasons for leaving by age
     reasons for leaving by grade
     destinations of leavers by age
     destinations of leavers by grade.

Ad hoc programs includes listings (a - c)

(a) by individual name - will print out the record
(b) entry year - will print out individual entry year
(c) by current grade - will print out grade as at particular month or grade at
     date of leaving on exit, and
(d) a writer program which enables the production of reports.

This software was developed to analyse data held retrospectively over a five
year period. It is designed to accommodate current requirements in a monitoring
function. The Nursing officer had the advantage of working very closely with
two WHO Fellows from Burma who spent many long hours guiding, instructing,
experimenting and collaborating in the development of this personnel management
information system designed on micros.

The completion of the project gives information about previous patterns of nurse
behaviour and provides a basis for comparison with future patterns. The model
has been tested. Application in field trials is not yet arranged. Standardised
data collection is taking place in more than one location. The Nursing Officer
is still associated with the project but is currently undertaking full-time
study in computer science as an undergraduate. It is anticipated that the
project will run from year to year. Data will be submitted to a central
point(s) annually or as disruption occurs. Data forms have been reviewed and
provide clear and concise data. This project is relatively simple in an
automated system. Further progress rests upon access to hardware and user
instruction.

(iii) Patient Classification data processing for nurse manpower planning

Information on nurse manpower is incomplete without detail of nursing workload
derived from patients' and clients nursing time requirements. Formulae have
been devised for calculating nurse staffing requirements. In Scotland the
Aberdeen Formula is the recommended method for hospital staffing excluding
Psychiatry and Mental Deficiency and this uses, as a basis calculation, a
patient classification system. The classification is made by registered nurses
in patient areas over a 28 day period. Bed numbers and occupancy rates are
recognised as contributing quantitative factors but the overriding qualitative
factor is the patient dependency factor derived as a professional nursing
judgement made daily by the nurse in charge on site. Historically, bed numbers
and previous staffing levels have determined future staffing provision and
little cognisance has been given to the variations in requirements between
similar wards or departments particularly within the same hospital. The
Aberdeen Formula takes account of current practices and changing functions and
data should be collected annually. Because of the calculations involved, nurses

at all levels have shown some resistance to these numerical exercises and are understandably suspicious of all things 'scientific'. It was difficult to convince all nurse managers of the necessity to define a nurse staffing requirement when there was reluctance to give time to data collection and constraints of time applied also to data processing. Previous exercises had been arranged in Glasgow and many months had elapsed between data collection and the presentation of findings.   To be used in budget negotiations, the information has to be current.   Administrators and finance officers have historically defined nursing budgets on bed numbers and existing staffing levels and staff mix.   In order to change the focus of control nurses have to assume professional responsibility for defining nurse staffing requirement i.e. the demand side of the demand and supply equation in nurse manpower planning. Nurses have to be seen to do this in a systematic way and to produce evidence in support of claims. Nurse managers like administrators and finance officers have responded in the past to emotive appeals in a subjective way.   Now, with resources strained there is less optimism about a real response and conflicting claims are judged and measured in objective terms to identify priorities.

Professional judgement of patients' nursing care requirements is a part of the unique function of the nurse but the data handling was amenable to automation. This was arranged and an Aberdeen Calculation program is operational. Nursing Officers attend at the health board with the raw data and input ward detail. Allowances for additional duties, layout factor, sickness/absence, night duty and nursing administration are selected from tables where relevant and the solution of the formula is the nurse staffing requirement. Printouts show the results of the calculation and one copy is filed at health board and the other is held locally.   Nurse managers are gradually availing themselves of this facility and other health board officers are showing interest.   Copies of the programs have been made on floppy disk for those with compatible hardware.

Additionally, data are collected in one purpose-built 30-bed geriatric unit for a period of one year. It is hoped to describe staffing requirements over this time and to examine the data for pattern and consistency because staffing levels were defined arbitarily as an estimate of requirement.

When the staffing requirements were defined, the next step was to relate in-post levels to requirement and to describe the level as a percentage of requirement. This can now be done automatically and monthly comparisons are produced as output documents.

iv)   Software for micros

With the experience derived over two years and insight into the labour intensive procedure of systems design, program development and testing, 'bespoke tailoring' for every project has to be impractical.   Until now, it has been difficult to know and define precisely the particular requirements and to compare the commercially available software.   Neither have we been able to discriminate between what is claimed for a particular program and to decide whether it could be universal in its application. There was a feeling formerly, that neither scientist nor salesman should have the responsibility totally for computer developments in nursing. This being so, time in which to acquire the knowledge for parity in decision-making was necessary. A case for the purchase of a data management software package was made only recently and is shown in Figure 2. The users will be nurses, clerical officers and researchers.

Figure 2

DATA MANAGEMENT SYSTEM: A Case for Purchasing Software

1.   The software is commercially available at a cost of approximately £270

2.   It has been tried and tested in a number of settings for different data handling projects.

3.   Computer scientists advise that it is sufficiently flexible in use to accommodate to the data handling, for example,
(i)   for service requirements in monitoring exercises of staff in post in Colleges of Nursing and Midwifery by grade, location, appointment dates, dates of birth, professional skill/experience.
On Bank Nurse Register update and statistical analysis.
On equipment lists in Colleges where detail of location, officer responsible, equipment description, equipment make, serial number, suppliers name, address, purchase date, maintenance contract, warranty, performance in use.
(ii) For research exercises where the STORE, SELECT and SORT functions would assist in the data processing. The collection of data related to the centralisation of learner applications could be analysed by this program and the prospective information about actual applicants could be held for interrogation and updating as events related to the progress of individual applicants are reported.
iii) For office organisation within the nursing section ie. for the production of standard reports and statistical forms. Updating and modification of existing formats held on file can be arranged on the video display unit and copies produced on the printer when final adjustments are made.

4.   The potential applications are almost limitless.

5.   A computer scientist student is available to work now and is interested to assist in the setting up of particular files during his secondment. A nurse can be assigned to work with him. This would be a shared experience and the nurse would thereafter become the operator.

6.   The initial cost should be seen as cost-saving in terms of improved efficiency and increased output.

7.   This does not encroach on planned developments in personnel or manpower information systems on a local or national level.

8.   It is logical development in the introduction of microcomputing to nurse management and nursing research.

9.   The acquisition and use of commercially prepared software will allow nurses to enter a dialogue on current developments and specific applications for the health service.

10.   It seems important to take advantage of these opportunities and invest now.

(v)   Microdevelopments in Clinical areas

In an intensive care unit in Glasgow Royal Infirmary the input to a computer-controlled patient-monitoring device are measures of cardiovascular and respiratory functioning. The system provides staff with up-to-date, accurate information in the form of trend graphs and detail on lung resistance and complicance.   Complicated calculations related to cardiac output are

automatically produced for medical staff.   The Nursing Officer in this unit
secured a Florence Nightingale Memorial Committee Scholarship in 1981 sponsored
by the Joint Committee, Order of St. John and the British Red Cross Society to
visit and study computer assisted patient monitoring systems in use so that she
could assess the attitudes of nurses who were working with computer hardware and
so that she could have then identify and discuss the specific problems which
occurred locally before and during the technological implementation. She sought
eventually to acquire a better understanding of the implications of computer
technology on nursing practice and to begin to plan teaching programs for nurses
in clinical settings.   The primary purpose of the study tour was to examine
systems in critical care areas but it proved difficult to separate, to isolate
specific systems when these were contained and structured within large hospital-
based systems on mainframes.   In none of the centres in the USA were
microcomputers operational although there was a stated intention to develop in
this medium.   The mainframe systems which were examined in San Francisco,
Mountain View California, Salt Lake City, Utah, and in Birmingham, Alabama were
at least six years old and some of the hardware was becoming obsolete.   The
programs were well developed and validated and might be translated into a format
for use with modern machines including micros. In addition to the equipment in
critical care areas the nursing officer reported on nurses involvement with
total hospital systems, patient data management systems, computer-controlled
intervention systems and computer-assisted care plans.

Systems operational at The Royal Devon and Exeter Hospital, Devon - The London
Hospital - Ninewells Hospital, Dundee and Dijksigh University Hospital,
Rotterdam were also examined. In the report for the sponsors Mrs Shirley Watt
states that she was aware of several decisive factors which influenced the
successful implementation of new technology in clinical areas.

It was important that nurses arranged introductory training sessions as part of
a continuing in-service programme for nurses and that each nurse is gradually
introduced to the hardware before the system is operational at the patient's
bedside.   She felt too that there was a need for support during and after
implementation from someone with a computer science background. The technology
is often perceived as awe-inspiring and intimidating when the implementation is
proposed and a gradual, planned introduction helps dispel the aura of science
fiction associated with 'thinking machines'.

7.   Conclusion

A micro-computer with disk storage and printer was purchased in 1980 for the
development of automated information systems related to nurse manpower planning.
The hardware is desk top, user driven and portable. It is independent on
mainframe and operates from a power point. It may become standard nursing
office equipment. The Commodore PET in the Nursing Section at the health board
offices has been the concentrated focus for nurse activity. Three nurses have
'clocked' up terminal time and are well able to interact with the computer and
to construct simple programs. The learner record scheme has been brought to the
attention of the General Nursing Council for Scotland and has attracted funding
form SHHD. It is planned to replicate this in the five Glasgow Colleges of
Nursing and Midwifery. The learner monitoring and forecasting scheme provides
printout for management, education and finance departments and simulation
exercises have reduced the speculative component in recruitment and manpower
planning policies.

The nurse staffing requirement is calculated and information made available at
source so that current requirements can be defined. The inpost levels are
related to requirement and priority areas can be defined in 'league tables'.
Stability indices could be measured. The model needs testing in an operation
setting.

It is timely now to consider the selection and purchase of hardware for nursing sections at district and unit level and to guide the introduction and training of personnel. Hardware costs and scepticism are only two of the obstacles to be overcome. The author is cast in the role of the White Queen(3).

> 'One can't believe impossible things'
> said Alice to the White Queen.
> 'I dare say you haven't had much practice'
> said the Queen. 'When I was your age,
> I always did it for half an hour each day.
> Why, sometimes I've believed as many as
> six impossible things before breakfast.'

REFERENCES

1. BALL M (1974)   Medical   data   processing   in   the   United   States   -   Hospital Financial Management January 1974 Vol. 28. No.1 pp 10-30
2. HEASMAN M A 1980   The Strategy for Scotland in Information Systems for Health Services - Public Health in Europe 13 - Copenhagen
3. Carroll L. (1920) Alice Through the Looking Glass. p.101.

The Impact of Computers on Nursing
M. Scholes, Y. Bryant and B. Barber (eds.)
Elsevier Science Publishers B.V. (North-Holland)
© IFIP-IMIA, 1983

14.7.

COMPUTERS: A RESOURCE IN A NURSING DEPARTMENT REORGANIZATION

Fotine D. O'Connor

The shortage of hospital-employed nurses is a critical problem in the United States. The Los Angeles County-University of Southern California Medical Center has not been an exception and much time and effort has been directed toward finding and implementing solutions to the problems.

This is no small matter at the large University-affiliated Medical Center which has 2,105 licensed beds within four fully accredited acute hospitals. The nursing department is budgeted for 3,544 positions; of these positions, 1,724 are for registered nurses. The department provides and maintains all nursing services.

Two years ago, as one response to the nurse shortage problem a decision was made to reorganize the nursing department so that the management role of the ward head nurse would be considerably enlarged. The intent was to establish the head nurse as the manager of the ward on a 24-hour day, 7-day week basis with responsibility and authority for maximum decision-making at that level. The role of the supervisor in the new organizational structure was to be that of a consultant/teacher providing support and assistance to the head nurse. Basic goals of the reorganization were to improve decision making and facilitate participation management reflecting a belief that the satisfaction and thus the retention of nurses would be positively affected.

At that time the nursing department was organized in the traditional multi-level hierarchical structure of authority and responsibility. Within the clinical nursing areas the staff nurses reported to the head nurses, the head nurses reported to a unit supervisor who reported to a second supervisor who reported to the area nursing director. The area nursing director reported to the Associate Director who reported to the Director of Nursing Services and Education the top administrator of the nursing department. A role activity study revealed a maze of overlapping duties and responsbilities.

The reorganization of the department which has been implemented through a rather complex participation process is just now nearing completion. Though effective, the process was slow and it was not easy. Briefly, the process involved the participation of the head nurses and supervisors in small group activities and workshops designed to assist them to learn and to implement their new roles. The reorganization did not occur simultaneously in all areas; rather, it was initiated consecutively in each area at approximately six-month intervals.

In the current organizational structure, the head nurse is firmly established as the ward manager. In the smaller clinical areas the head nurse reports directly to the area nursing director who reports to the Director, Nursing Services and Education. In the larger clinical areas, the head nurse reports to a unit supervisor who reports to the area nursing director. All supervisors function in the consultant/teacher role although the unit supervisor and the evening and night supervisors provide administrative support to the area nursing director. In a recent evaluation there was clear evidence that the head nurses, the supervisors, and the area nursing directors perceive the reorganization to be a functional positive management process.

Early in the reorganization process there was a recognition of the need to provide management information support to the head nurse who was now expected to make effective management decisions. Management information was available to some extent at the area nursing office level and to a large extent at the Medical Center administration nursing office level.

At the head nurse level the primary management information needs were identified as 1) the need for a personnel data file, 2) the need for length of service and turnover data, 3) the need for nursing hour ratio and personnel utilization data.

Timely and accurate information about the nursing hour ratio and personnel utilization were especially important for the head nurse now charged with managing personnel resources in a time of extreme budgetary constraints. In addition to the realized nursing hour ratio, it was important for the head nurse to have information about the variance between the number of employee hours budgeted, the number of hours scheduled, the number of hours worked and the reason for the variance, i.e., sick, overtime, registry help, etc. Information about special training and special pay bonus programs were important also.

An information system that would meet the identified needs was developed through a pilot program with the collaboration of appropriate nursing personnel. Automating the system through the county-wide data processing department (the only computer access available to the nursing department) proved to be not feasible. A minicomputer was then purchased. Part-time programming service was obtained and the intent was to develop a program which they could then market, but the proposal contracts were too expensive. At present, the in-house project is continuing.

Experience with the management information and computer project to date suggests that in such a project the following areas need careful attention:

Information   What information is needed?
                  Why is the information needed?
                  In what form is the information needed?
                  When is the information needed?
                  Where is the information needed?
                  Who needs the information?

For example, the nursing hour ratio is needed to ensure that the mandated quantity of care is provided. A monthly report of daily nursing hour ratios (perhaps graphically displayed) is needed by the ward head nurse who makes the staffing decisions which affect the nursing hour ratio.

Data   Will raw data or summarized data be entered into the computer?
           Will data be entered directly into the computer (perhaps a computer on each ward) or onto a form to be delivered to a central computer area?
           How, when, where, and who will collect the data?

For example, one way to enter nursing hour ratio data into a central computer would involve the ward clerk completing a form each day for each ward showing the patient census and the employee hours worked. The form would then be delivered to the computer area.

Personnel   Who will collect the data?
                     Who will deliver data sheets, if this is necessary?
                     Who will enter data into the computer?
                     Who will have access to the output?
                     Who will manage an output system, generate reports, deliver
                     reports?

For example, if a central computer is used, arrangement must be made for possibly hiring and certainly training operators to enter data. Time intervals for generating and delivering reports must be established, such as a monthly hour ratio report to all head nurses.

In summary, reorganization of the nursing department established the ward head nurse as the person who is expected to make the decisions necessary to manage the ward effectively. Efficient management information systems and computerized data processing can provide timely and accurate information needed to support decision-making. At the Los Angeles County-University of Southern California Medical Center the computer is seen as a valuable resource in a reorganization intended to increase decision-making at the ward head nurse level.

LOS ANGELES COUNTY - UNIVERSITY OF SOUTHERN CALIFORNIA MEDICAL CENTER

DEPARTMENT OF NURSING SERVICES AND EDUCATION

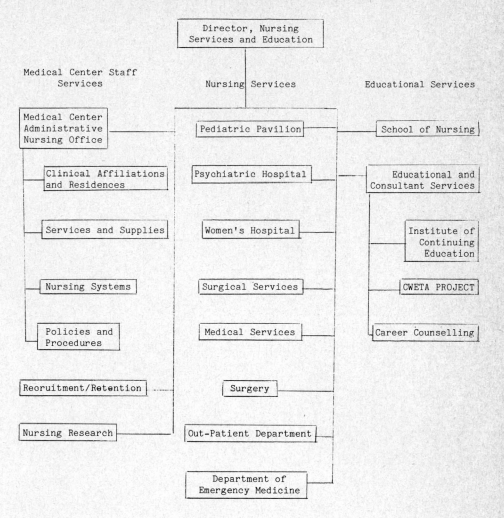

INTERNAL MEDICINE NURSING SERVICES

DIRECTOR OF NURSING SERVICES AND EDUCATION

UNIT NURSING DIRECTOR

STAFF ASSISTANTS   EXECUTIVE SECRETARY

AND II   AND II   AND I DAY

AND I EVENING

MED. ADM.	82/8300	4700	11-621	
D & E	8600	6000	14-600	
6200	8700	66/6640	18-400	AND I NIGHT
6700	8800	7000		
6800	TRIAGE	7200		
7800		11-4/11-600		

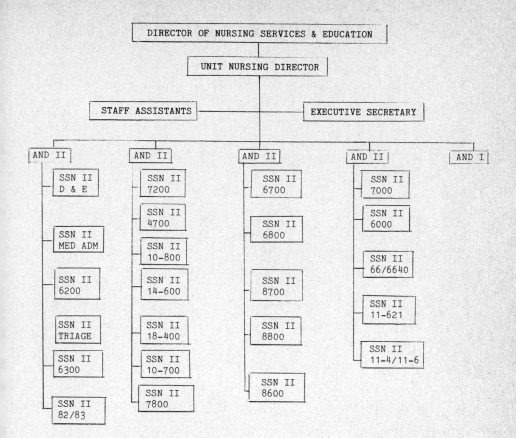

The Impact of Computers on Nursing
M. Scholes, Y. Bryant and B. Barber (eds.)
Elsevier Science Publishers B.V. (North-Holland)
© IFIP-IMIA, 1983

14.8.

BUDGETARY CONTROL SYSTEM AND THE DEVELOPMENT OF FINANCIAL MANAGEMENT SYSTEMS

Bernard Groves

Introduction

Nearly half a million pounds a year would have been spent in the North East Thames region if the bureau service used by several districts in 1978 to produce monthly statements to budget managers had been adopted by all authorities. Although each of the districts involved could justify the £10,000 to £25,000 per annum it was not economic to expand the system to provide all the additional financial information required. The Finance discipline examined proposals from computer manufacturers who were offering hardware and software packages which would provide Management Accountants with a Budgetary Control System. The Regional Computer Centre produced a specification for a demonstration system which included the following essential characteristics:

* The data must be on-line at all times
* The Management Accountant must be able to print Budget Statements in his own office.
* The Management Accountant must have facilities to correct and re-print statements.

The specification was accepted by 3 major computer companies who each programmed the required system and, in September 1978 they gave a demonstration of their hardware and of each of the technical requirements of the system. The decision was made to purchase from Digitial Equipment Company a PDP 11/70 which would run under the MUMPS data base management system. The Computer would be used to provide Financial Management Systems of which Budgetary Control would be the first development. The Management Accounts departments of 17 Districts, 6 Areas and the Region would each be supplied with a visual display unit and printing terminal, and data would be transmitted to and from the computer over telephone lines. It was agreed that for the first year, only 10 authorities would use the system and a representative from each Authority would meet under the chairmanship of a District Finance Officer, as a User Group, to monitor the developments of the system.

Budgetory Control System

In April 1979 the System went live. By comparison with what is available today, it was somewhat simple, but nevertheless the result of 5 months development was an interactive, on-line system, which provided:

* Budget Statements and Summaries of Budget Statements.
* Estimate 22 report for Region. (Aggregated Function Analysis).
* Unique report for each District Management Team.
* Full explosion facility of all totals for audit control.
* Journal and Commitment entry with on-line validation.
* Automatic capture of journal entries for input to the Ledger systems.

Most importantly, the system provided accurate and timely information which gave the Management Accountant more credibility when talking to his budget holder.

The first Authorities using the system were provided with a telephone connection to the computer. It was known that this dial-up facility would be subject to interference known as line noise, so private circuits were ordered at the same time to ultimately replace the dial-up lines. Today, the problem of line noise is solved by more sophisticated modems which carry out error-checking and retransmit data which has become garbled. Today's modems are much smaller and cheaper than the 1979 models. However, the transfer to private circuits eliminated the problem completely.

The development of the system through the first year was particularly interesting. The User Group met each month but initially each request for a small change or enhancement was voiced reluctantly, in case the request would involve great expense or delay more important items. Then it became apparent that with a system running under MUMPS it is relatively easy to make changes to report formats, totals, security passwords, on-line validation etc. The User Group gained confidence in the system and in their ability to plan out improvements and additional requirements. This was not to be a system thrust upon them that they were obliged to accept; instead it was their system, with each stage of development being discussed and achieved in timescales that kept motivation running high. During the early months quite a large percentage of the data processed from the Regional Accounting System into the Budgetary Control System had to be rejected because budget statements had not yet been designed for those ranges of expenditure codes. However there was a constant process of creating these statements and of updating the look-up tables that directed an expenditure item to the appropriate statement. Month by month Authorities' error reports became smaller and more statements were automatically printed. Today, with the entire Region using the system, the look-up table for expenditure codes contains over 200000 items for the current year and a similar number for the previous financial year. This table is accessed not only when processing monthly expenditure from the Regional Accounting System but also for on-line validation of all journals and commitments.

Towards the end of the first year the Authorities had the system producing all the reports they required for total basic control. There was a continual process of setting up still more reports for cross-checking purposes, and of creating further analyses of existing data.

The Management Accountants' Role

At this stage the question was being asked as to what effect this computerised system had made on the job of the Management Accountant? Before the system was introduced a time consuming part of the Management Accountants office routine was the manual maintenance of budgets and the extraction of expenditure from the ledger. Only the Regional returns, DMT reports, and some of the more important budget statements were typed. Most budget holders enjoyed a friendly relationship with the Management Accountant who would visit regularly and discuss the state of the budget. This was essentially a verbal reporting system. However, some Finance Officers noted that now everyone could have a smart, computer printed budget statement, some budget holders were receiving theirs through the post and were not being visited with the same regularity. Indeed, there was a suggestion that too much time was being spent with the new technology working at the Visual Display Unit instead of getting out into the field. This phenomena was of course due to the novelty of a changed working environment, and as the 'bleeps' from the visual display unit and the chattering of the printing terminal became an accepted feature of the office routine, the Management Accountants resumed their personal contacts.

The visits from the Management Accountant most certainly could not be replaced by a Budget Statement received through the post for although the format of the statements made allowance for showing both Manpower and Workload statistics,

none of these items was included automatically in the system. If they were to
be shown, they had to be input by the Management Accountant. A Budget statement
based entirely upon financial information, must be studied with regard to the
manpower and workload activity before a proper understanding of the performance
can be reached. In the Health Service, budgets are subject to hundreds of
different profiles (spending patterns) and are influenced by variable external
factors. It is the understanding of this very complex mixture of variables that
is the skill of the Management Accountant and it is precisely this complication
that makes it so difficult to computerise a statement which brings together all
the facts in a single meaningful document.

A nursing manager may hold a budget for service or educational purposes. It may
include salaries, agency staff equipment study leave and travelling expenses.
The salaries and wages budget is subject to quite complicated differing rates of
pay. For example, overtime is time plus one half, night duty is time plus one
third and bank holidays are paid at double time plus a day off in lieu. The
establishment of nurses is prone to change particularly in acute hospitals thus
making it difficult to fix a budget on an average grade. The cost, and
allocation of learner nurses is another complication to the budget and learners
who fail their examination and return to training for a further four months
effectively cause an over-staffing burden. The agency staff budget may exist to
cover holidays and sickness, and whereas the holiday leave is measureable and
scheduled in advance, sickness has to be estimated from past experience.
Similarly, the travelling expenses are estimated each year from the best
available records.

An energy budget for a hospital Engineer is an excellent example of a budget
that can go massively overspent, despite all the best efforts. The success of
energy conservation campaigns has led to a reduced thermal consumption each year
for the last four years. The Management Accountant studies historical data on
fuel consumption. Through the continued installation of thermostats and time-
switches, he may reasonably expect that consumption will continue to fall. The
cost of the fuel is bound to go up so he will make an allowance for that in
calculating the total financial budget for fuel oils. The profile for an energy
budget would obviously show consumption of more fuel in winter than in summer.
But what sort of winter will it be? How much will the fuel really cost? The
workload statistic is controlled by climatic conditions.

A final example of a department with different factors which affect a budget,
that the Management Accountant must bear in mind when considering performance,
is the X-Ray department. The cost of the machinery, its maintenance and the
cost of the staff are straight-forward items. But how many X-Ray films will be
used each day? In fact, as some X-Ray investigations take much longer to
perform than others, a scale of weighting factors has been produced for the
calculation of work statistics.

Extension of the System

As we entered the second year the computer centre began a training programme for
the remaining 14 Authorities who were to come onto the system. The User Group
swelled in number from 10 to 24 (plus computer staff, Regional Audit and
Chairman) and the meetings took on a new atmosphere. Most Authorities stayed
absolutely silent, feeling they were 12 months behind everyone else and that
they had a lot of catching up to do whereas the pioneer Authorities were anxious
to forge ahead and were concerned that the system's development had lost its
momentum. The computer staff were overwhelmed. The training requirement,
telephone support to user queries, issue of amendments to user manuals and a
constantly growing list of enhancements became cause for concern. A short
freeze was put on the system, to give new Users a chance to catch up and become
familiar with all the problems already overcome by the original users.

One day, when the computer was taken by the engineers for maintenance, the switchboard at the computer centre jammed as 13 Authorities each wanted to know if the machine had broken down. A system known as 'The News' was developed whereby each authority could leave messages or questions for any other authority. The messages are stored in the computer to be read by all. Today the system is used not only to give warning of maintenance periods, production run times, security backup times etc, but also to give notice of meetings and to include the Agenda. The news sheet is read at every Visual Display Unit and can be printed on the printing terminal. This has saved endless telephone calls, and a great deal of typing and postage. It has also been an excellent way of advising everyone exactly when each new development has become available.

The frequency of the User Group meetings changed to alternate months and it was agreed that a budget ledger system and adjustment ledger system should be built in as the next priority. The Budget Ledger is an historical record of every change to a budget since the start of the financial year. Whereas the adjustment ledger is a record of every budget that is changed, say for a wage award, thus providing the total cost of that wage award. The volume of data now being created and stored on-line, as users made variations through their visual display units, had grown enormously, and this in the same year that we had more than doubled the number of users. Computer staff were becoming concerned that there were no proper monitoring tools to measure the utilisation of the computer and thus decide if there was capacity for much more development. They were soon to learn! (Today, the latest version of DIGITAL'S MUMPS has excellent monitoring tools). The User Group was unanimous that with so much data being held on-line accessible from the comfort of their own offices they wanted an enquiry package so that they could make ad hoc interrogations.

User Programs

The Computer Centre felt that the easiest way for Authorities to access their data was to learn the MUMPS programming language and write their own programs. The problems would be in preserving systems integrity, audit controls and the privacy of one authority's data from another. The solution was developed in what is called the 'Mumps Filter Package' (MFP). The MFP allows most of the MUMPS language to be used and provides total security of data. An Authority cannot interrogate another Authority's data, neither can it corrupt or change its own data. The MFP provided very much more than an interrogation package as it allowed for the storage of new data so that authorities could create their own files in the computer data base. Interrogation programs, pilot studies and minor suites of programs were now the tool of the Management Accountant. Machine capacity was about to become a problem. MUMPS programming manuals were purchased and sent to every Authority. The QUEST package (developed by Joan Zimmerman & Bob Stimac of Washington University) was installed in the computer to provide tuition in MUMPS programming, and when students were ready they attended an intensive 3 day workshop at the Computer Centre to learn how to use the MFP and access their data.

Today more than 60 accountants have attended the training workshops which are still run every 4 months, and more than 300 MFP programs written by these accountants are in production. Some of the more interesting systems the users have written themselves are:

* Ward Costing - Southend Health District
* Capital Planning - City & London Area Health Authority
* Budget Preparation - Havering Health Authority
* Drug costing at St. Barholomews' - Pilot study for CIPFA examinations - City & London Area Health Authority.

480

The System Overloaded

The computer, which schedules itself, was finding that certain jobs were having to be held up for some seconds in order to cope with the processing demands. Users at the terminals became irritated at the jerky response at their screens and printing times were doubling.

Although the User Group had agreed not to run MFP programs during normal working hours and the computer centre examined many different design techniques and programming methods in a search for greater efficiency, there was little effect. Throughout this second year each Authority had dramatically increased its volume of data and reports. League tables were drawn up showing totals of expenditure codes, Budget Statements, Summary Statements, DMT report lines and number of MFP programs used by each authority and these were presented at each User Group. Veiled accusations were made by those authorities at the bottom of the lists that others must be mis-using the system, whilst those at the top of the lists quite correctly defended their position by pointing out that no limits had ever been specified for computer use.

In the third year we were an older and wiser User Group. Everyone had a good knowledge of the system, and of the effect it had made on the office routine. Many had a working understanding of the programming language, and there was a general awareness that computer power was seriously stretched and not to be abused between 9 am and 5 pm. There was, of course, plenty of capacity after 5 pm. Nevertheless, authorities stated that data volumes must increase still further as they had a real need for more information. At the same time the Region identified an urgent need for a system to manage Patients's Money in long stay hospitals. Management Accounts declared that they needed statements based on pay figures only and must have these much quicker than by extraction from the accounting ledgers on a monthly cycle, and it was not to be forgotten that the budget system still needed an automatic inclusion of manpower statistics and ultimately workload statistics. Therefore Planning began for the purchase of a second Digital PDP 11/70 to be installed at the Regional Computer Centre and linked to the first machine 20 miles away in London.

The Patients' Money system was developed in MUMPS for both on-line use from the office of the Patient Affairs Officer and for batch processing for those hospitals who were already sending Patients' Money data to some central point for control. The system is being used by 22 hospitals throughout the region and there are no plans to develop it further.

The production of early payroll statements was undertaken as a pilot study involving just 3 authorities. As 70% of all expenditure is for salaries and wages it clearly is important to be able to identify overspendings at the earliest possible moment. It was found that by taking expenditure data directly from the Payroll system and feeding it through a sub-system of budgetary control, the Management Accountant was able to produce pay-statements 2 weeks earlier than by waiting for the ledger data to go through the full Budgetary system. This not only gave him the opportunity to take earlier action on a problem but it also allowed him to examine, and if necessary correct pay data before the ledgers were run. In other words when the main Budgetary system was run he only had to check the non-pay items. This spreading-out of his workload was a major factor in the systems approval for full Regional Development.

Following the re-organisation of the Health Service in April 1982, we entered our fourth Financial year with just 16 District Authorities and the Region. The new computer has been installed as indeed have all the private circuits and, the two computers are inter-linked. Now this link is operational the additional computing power is available to provide the next priority systems which are Payroll budgets, Manpower statistics and Final Accounts.

CHAPTER 15

MANAGEMENT SCIENCES IN THE NURSING SERVICE

This section deals with the techniques that can be employed by or on behalf of nurse managers to assist them in tackling problems related to the provision of nursing services. The papers emphasise the need for a multidisciplinary approach in terms of the involvement of nurses, computer scientists, management scientists and financial experts. The outcome of such collaboration, when successful, will allow nurse managers to set objectives, monitor progress and regularly review the viability of those objectives in the light of current situations, financial constraints and changing needs. Some of the points covered here were introduced in Chapter 13.

The Impact of Computers on Nursing
M. Scholes, Y. Bryant and B. Barber (eds.)
Elsevier Science Publishers B.V. (North-Holland)
© IFIP-IMIA, 1983

15.1.

WHY NURSE AN ANALYST?

Barry Barber

Operations Analysis and Systems Analysis

Operations Analysis, or operational research (O.R.), as it is called in the U.K., is the study of complex systems, with a view to building models of the system in order to provide a better understanding of its operation and to improve its effectiveness or efficiency. Systems analysis is the study of a complex system with a view to utilising some computer system to improve its performance.

The improvement of the capability of a major organisation is a long, slow, development of staff attitudes and competence with new techniques. Logically, operations analysis should precede systems analysis but in practice it sometime turns out that the introduction of a low level data processing system may be much the most satisfactory initial approach as it can provide a mass of detailed information for analysis, it can help to encourage the spirit of enquiry and generally build up the confidence of the staff concerned - as well as providing some basic initial benefits. However, staff are often ready to believe that a computer system might be helpful without thinking that they could handle the technical work themselves. In contrast, most staff believe that they organise their own work and staff efficiently and regard it as insulting to suggest that anyone else could have worthwhile suggestions to make.

A computer system can be put into a somewhat lukewarm environment but successful operations analysis requires extensive collaboration. The medical, nursing and administrative staff have to be willing to become involved in quite detailed and technical aspects of the work of building models and utilising them to study the systems. Operations analysis itself cannot rectify a problem, it can only offer help to those who have the problem and wish to rectify it.

Operational research has, as yet, no clearly defined boundaries and its activities are published in a wide variety of places. It borders on mathematics, statistics, computing, economics, finance, management and social science and in the medical field it links with community medicine, medicine and nursing. Most text books describe relatively clear cut situations whereas, in practice, the obvious technical solutions may not be helpful because there is no data for the models, no acceptance of that formulation of the problem and often no interest in the problem at all (as is clearly the case in many of our Outpatient Clinics in this country). This doesn't mean that the model is faulty but rather that the analyst is an adviser who doesn't have the problem while the manager with the problem doesn't regard it as significant or worthy of his attention. Furthermore, in many situations analysts contribute to the discussion of organisational problems making practical suggestions arising from the logical structure of the problems encountered. Often this activity is of profound educational and conceptual importance without ever resulting in complex models or original papers. The advice is contributed to a working group or committee which then builds it into their thinking. Implementation frequently arises, but the operations analysis is 'obvious' and the basic material is unpublishable except as an action report and the analysts contribution cannot be clearly identified subsequently. Indeed, the best implementation strategy is to encourage the working group to take the concepts over as their own because the degree of implementation of a study is frequently directly related to the degree to which the study is seen as an organisational response to its own problems rather than as an identifiable outside academic exercise.

The word **INFORMATICS** embraces both these aspects of information technology and systems thinking and it has the merit of deflecting interest into the information and the wider systems aspects of the problem rather than the mechanics of computing. It is also noticeable that an exploration of a situation mathematically can be very cheap by comparison with the implementation of inappropriate information systems or worse still the building of inappropriate health care facilities. The mathematical techniques currently available are far in advance of current understanding of health care and it is rare that some standard technical approach cannot be adapted to the needs of a particular investigation - at least as a starting point.

Operations Analysts' Perspectives

One of the most extraordinary features of hospitals to an operations analyst is the fact that they work at all. They open their doors and accept whoever comes through as an emergency patient and they make appointments for outpatient visits and inpatient stay with relatively little consideration of the details of what has to be done for the patients on arrival. Regularly, hospital staff and departments are surprised at peaks of activity that happen regularly during the day, week or year. Staff rarely have the time or inclination to analyse their work and organise it more appropriately and even where computer systems have been installed there are few management scientists available to study hospital problems and provide solutions. Certainly, the course of an individual's disease and response to treatment is difficult or even impossible to predict but statistical analysis can reveal patterns of activity, disease and response which can be used to assist in the provision of care. However, the likely course of activity for inpatients can be studied and planned tentatively in advance so that instead of simply booking a bed, the likely critical facilities required during the inpatient stay can be booked provisionally prior to admission. This approach to the scheduling of patient care requires careful development but it should enable the service departments to plan their activities more smoothly, to staff their departments more appropriately and save wasted days in hospital while the patient waits for the next part of his care to be organised.

The effectiveness of this patient scheduling will depend on a careful analysis of patterns of patient care and it will inevitably involve nursing staff as the doctors outline proposals are converted into a practical sequence of health care activity. Mathematical techniques already exist for scheduling a variety of activities competing for the same resources and interactive programs can be designed to enable staff to explore the best way of scheduling planned admissions to enable the best use to be got out of the available resources. Such systems will not be automatic so much as semi-automatic where the mathematical analysis will come forward with suggestions that will fulfil the specific patient and departmental requirements which can then be accepted, or changed, as required. The data available about patient care and hospital activity will open the way for modelling of the hospital system and rearranging activities to minimise the length of stay of patients. The relative timing of outpatient sessions, theatre sessions, ward rounds, and days for specialised examination can all lead to changes in the pattern of delay as patients pass through their period of care. These activities too can be planned to minimise the delay once the basics of health care have been studied and documented. Ultimately mathematicians with a sufficiently clear understanding of clinical decision making will be able to provide assistance with medical decision making and investigation - this will lead to systems based on past, computer based, medical records which can help the clinician in his exploration of particular medical problems.

These EXPERT systems(1), have already been mentioned in Chapter 3.3.

One of the major problems of evaluating health care computer systems is the lack of evaluation of health care systems, the lack of specified objectives and the lack of knowledge of the patient benefits or outcomes arising from the health care system.   In the U.K. evaluation of systems has been imported into the Health Service along with the computers. It is to be hoped that the continued analysis of the health care situation will enable a better understanding to be achieved of the outcome of medical care, its objectives and the relative value of differing types of care for differing groups of patients. This evaluation of alternative health care delivery systems and the use of feasible alternative medical technology is crucial to the planning of health care services.

Systematisation in Nursing

The discussion of the Nursing Process appears to be endeavouring to systematise the practical activity of nursing, laying emphasis on the cyclic activities of:-

        (a) Data collection
        (b) Creation of Care Plans
        (c) Implementation of Care
        (d) Evaluation of Care

These systematic concepts lend themselves readily to computerisation in the same way that the structured problem-oriented medical records (P.O.M.R.) are more amenable to computerisation and analysis than a page of scribbled medical case notes.   The search for structure under-pinning nursing care and the use of computers does not diminish the traditional caring role of the nurse and make nursing mechanical.   It rather provides a framework within which nurses can function more effectively using modern tools and insights to achieve results in more complex and difficult situation.   The process of systematisation in an activity is a gradual and long drawn out affair. Similarly, the utilisation of operations analysis is a gradual development.   It is rarely possible in examining a new area of activity to locate and solve its major problems rapidly. Time is required for inter-disciplinary discussion and mutual confidence building.   One profession will rarely trust another with confidential and possibly damaging information until it is confident that the information will be constructively used and that the results are likely to be productive. It is usual for the analysts to work on minor problems while developing his or her understanding of the new area. However, it would appear that nurses are now willing to utilise the tools and insights of operations analysts and indeed, their own nursing research is leading them in the direction of a systematisation which already provides a good starting point and is compatible with the lines of enquiry of an operations analyst.

The Development of Operational Research at The London Hospital

Although a considerable amount of operational research took place at The London Hospital during the period 1961-1965, it wasn't until 1966 when the first Elliott 803 computer system had settled down that the hospital's Operational Research Unit was formed.   Barr of the Oxford Regional Hospital Board had written a nurse allocation program and it was obviously of some interest to see if the hospital had a use for it since allocation is a standard O.R. technique that might have other applications. Preliminary discussion led to the author spending a weekend in the allocation office discussing and observing the process of nurse allocation. A broad approach was taken, deliberately exploring the boundaries of the problem areas and then any possible specific solutions to the problems thus exposed.

In a complex system it is possible to split a problem into component parts and find that the best arrangements of each component system does not provide the best arrangement for the total system. For instance, staffing of a ward may be kept at a constant level but this may disrupt the educational programme of student nurses or an ideal educational programme may be followed precisely but this may result in unacceptable ward staffing patterns. The total problem requires an acceptable balance between these component systems. One of the key arts of the operations analyst is that of finding the right structure of problem and the right subdivisions to enable useful solutions to emerge. Sub-optimisation, in which part of the system is improved at the expense of overall performance, is a constant worry.

Following the discussions, a short report was produced that ranged over many nursing problems beyond nurse allocation including part time staff, nurse banks, creches and recruitment. Regarding the allocation program the report recommended the creation of a clerical file for student nurses recording their various movements into wards, departments, study, leave and sickness. At least half of the allocation week-end was occupied in finding students who were due to move and placements that needed to be filled. Such questions could readily be answered from a routine batch processing system. Subsequently, this file could be used in conjunction with a suitable allocation programme if required.

The problem structuring was seen as shown in fig 1. The nursing activity file was the key to a great deal of useful information about the educational and service aspects of allocations as well as sickness/absence and recruitment quite apart from providing the basic material for computer allocations subsequently. This fundamental problem structuring was accepted.

Following this original report, the Operational Research department has been consulted at intervals on a variety of matters ranging from mathematics to computer systems. During the work of the Briggs Committee(2) the Director of Nurse Education, a member of the committee, enlisted help to explore some of the effects of implementing the committees recomendations regarding the education and training of nurses.

A study on the records of former nurses led to the conversion of the contents of 18 4-drawer filing cabinets into a jacketted-microfiche system contained in one cabinet. The senior staff put a great deal of effort into weeding the files and putting the new system onto a sound archival base - thus substantially reducing the cost of the project.

Tests were carried out with personal two way radios to see whether this facility would enable changes to be made in the night staffing requirements.

The O.R. department and the nurses were closely involved in the implementation of the hospital information system with its ward terminals located at the nursing station and isolated nursing dependency studies were carried out either as independent research studies or in association with the evaluation of the hospital information systems.

In 1972 the problems of nurse allocation became acute and a detailed study was carried out in the hope that a suitable system might be implemented on the hospital's main, real time, computer system. However, it proved impossible to obtain access to the necessary resources at that time.

It was agreed to develop the desired system on a batch processing basis, recognising that this would be very much a second best approach. The outline of the system has been described already (J20 and Chapter 12.1). In essence the plan was to use the computer as a communications system so that the rather tangled flow of data could be brought under control thus completing the first stage of the programme outlined in 1966.

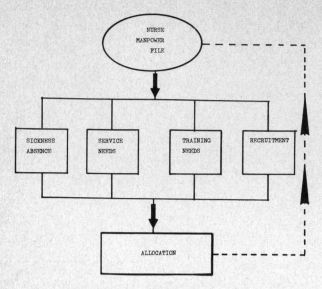

FIGURE 1   Nurse Training and Staff

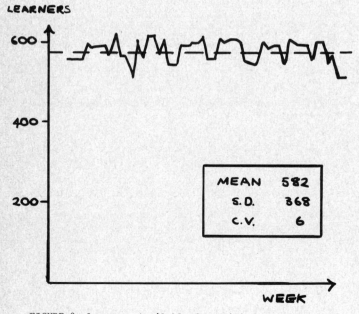

FIGURE 2   Learners Available for Clinical Experience

A substantial number of problems were encountered in getting and maintaining a satisfactory and accurate data base. It can be done, given sufficiently high computing and organisational priorities but it was always uncomfortable until the system was taken into the hospitals real time computing environment, in 1981 - at which time the opportunity was taken to extend the records to include all nursing staff not merely the trainees.

Having established a data base it is then possible to use it to make both short term and long term predictions of staff availability. As others have noted, the availability of staff was consequent upon the training programmes, the numbers of trainees in the various programmes, the pattern of sickness and the spacings between the start of various courses. Patterns such as that shown in fig 2 could be produced. In running her hospital, past Matrons will undoubtedly have been aware of these patterns but the availability of these estimates immediately enables the senior nurses to have constructive discussions with their medical and administrative colleagues. Furthermore, it puts the whole problem well in front of nurse managers and enables them to think constructively in day by day management and in both short term and long term planning. Such predictions are a routine part of the management of the District Health Authority and at intervals when there are clearly insufficient nurses to maintain the necessary standards of care, hard decisions have to be taken to reduce the workload at certain periods of shortage by closing beds or wards. The next obvious step was to explore the possibility of reducing the variability of the numbers of nurses available for ward work by modifying the components of the training programme, by changing the starting dates of various courses or by changing the number of courses run each year. A computer program was devised to enable nurses to explore these possibilities (J11). As a result of these studies and other discussion, the Director of Nurse Education decided to change the School from 4 intakes per year to 6 intakes per year and O.R. staff participated in preparing the plans for this changeover.

During 1981 an allocation programme for staff nurses was developed (J12) along lines that had previously been used for allocating House officers to jobs in medical school(3). This program only tackled a small part of the total problem and it has not yet been taken up routinely. At the present time work is being done on the problem of reducing the amount of night duty undertaken by trainee nurses, to conform with G.N.C. regulations.

Operational Research has become an integral part of the system by which the nursing staff examine and respond to at least some of their problems.

In Praise of Mathematics

Over the last decade National Health Service staff have become accustomed to the time required to produce computer systems and the voluminous systems reports associated with system development. Organisational problems do not become simple because computers are not used. The same study is required to elaborate and describe a particular situation but this description is then used to build a mathematical model of the situation. This model, which is often held in a computer for convenience of use, can then be manipulated to explore the various options for constructive action. Although an idea may emerge quickly, it may take days, weeks or months to implement according to the difficulty of the mathematics or the problem of obtaining data. By analysing the situation the discussion is lifted on to the practical plane of decision making. The various options and their implications can be set out and staff, in committee or individually, can select a course of action. Without an analyst available the discussion is confined to the hypothetical or the philosophical. It is necessary to nurse an analyst even if only to make sure that the treasurer has done his sums correctly!

Areas of O.R. Activity in Nursing

Nursing studies have been an important theme in the application of operations analysis to the health services. The main areas of activity are indicated below in terms of the problems being explored rather than the techniques used to solve them. This is not an exhaustive list as nurses are concerned with most health care activity and conversely most operations analysis in health care has some nursing implications. For more detailed study, a team at the Institute of Operational Research produced a very readable description of some aspects of their work(4) while a more recent and somewhat more mathematical approach to Nurse Staffing Management is given together with a bibliography of 60 papers in Boldy's book on "O.R. applied to the Health Services"(5). Flagle's group at the John Hopkins Hospital reviewed the total field in a valuable book O.R. in Health Care(6) in 1975 and Fries has produced a bibliography on "Applications of O.R. to Health Care Delivery Systems"(7). The question of implementation is frequently raised as it is much easier to design academic models than to get them into effective practice and this is discussed particularly by Stimson & Stimson(8).

The following gives a brief sketch of the main problem areas of interest so far.

1   Nursing Activity/Workload

An examination of nursing activity has revealed wide variations in workload for different patients. The early attempts to measure this led to the concepts of patient dependency, task analysis and activity sampling.

2   Staffing

Having obtained some measure of work it is then logical to attempt either to control it in some way or to adjust the staffing to the workload. The first objective can be achieved by control of admissions, routing of patients to different wards, or allocating priorities to either patients or activities. The adjustment of staffing can be achieved by having a pool of staff for immediate deployment according to work load or by adjustment over longer periods in response to workload predictions. The basic theory of allocating nurses to cope with workload has to be modified at off peak periods where staffing, sometimes above that required for the expected workload is needed to cope with emergency problems arising with patients in much the same way as the staffing of the emergency anaesthetic services is staffed(9).

3   Allocation

Having constructed a matrix of jobs to be done and, hopefully having staff to do them, a straight forward but relatively large allocation problem arises. This problem is exacerbated because the nurse training programmes involve repetitive and frequent job changes in order to provide the necessary training.

4   Rota Design

Taking the constraints imposed by the workload, staffing arrangements have to be made to provide nursing care at night and weekends. Regular patterns of activity are required for people, giving the best match to staffing and likely workload ensuring reporting overlap and staff where necessary but minimising excessive staff overlap.

5.   Timetable Design

Instead of trying to achieve the best arbitrary match between staff and jobs, one can attempt to design out the arbitrariness by designing school timetables that automatically provide a smooth flow of staff which can then be efficiently deployed.

6.   Records Systems Design

Part of the interest in Hospital Information Systems and in Nursing Records Systems arises from the hope that more reliable information systems will enable better system predictions and control to be achieved making the whole process more orderly and efficient. There will always be emergencies in health care but at least we might be able to avoid being caught out with predictable patterns of activity.

7.   Ward Design

The workload on a ward is clearly dependent on its design. Attention to design can improve the efficiency with which nurses carry out their tasks. Furthermore, some examination has been carried out of large ward designs to see whether the potential averaging effect of larger numbers allows the wards to be run at a higher average occupancy or a smoother pattern of workload.

8.   Manpower Planning

Having established the workload and staffing requirements the next step is concerned with recruitment and staff training in order to ensure that the right numbers of nurses are available to handle the workload.

In all these areas work has been done and interest moves between these areas according to the needs and interests of the various analysts and their nursing colleagues.   The main problem is that of structuring difficulties and the options available. If the logical structure is right then there is no escape from the organisations decision making. It is, however, vital that work should be preceeded by a thorough analysis of the situation at this level before embarking on the mathematical detail.   Decisions about what action may be feasible organisationally are of fundamental importance as they direct the course of the analysis but they may be reviewed in the light of the analysis.

Interesting O.R. Techniques

Most O.R. textbooks start by explaining that O.R. is not a set of techniques and then go on to describe the techniques.   However, there are some areas of analysis of particular interest even though a great deal of work can be done using school mathematics and statistics.   Mathematics is relatively cheap and knowledge of appropriate mmathematical approaches is far in advance of the corresponding knowledge of the operation of the health service.

1   Allocation and Programing

The fundamental problem of allocating available resources to handle activities in some optimal fashion is a mathematical programming problem and a variety of techniques exist for finding some best arrangement depending on the detailed structure of the problem. A key factor is concerned with some evaluation of the relative merits (or value) of using the various resources in different ways.

2   Simulation

Even when a particular situation has been studied in detail it may well be so complex as a result of the interaction of a variety of random factors that it is difficult to build a direct analytical model to enable one to find the best arrangement. In these circumstances, it can often be useful to build a computer model which deliberately incorporates all these random elements. In this way it is possible to test a variety of practical approaches to system management by running simulation trials on the computer model. This provides a very powerful way of exploring complex situations and modelling to assist with decision on course numbers at training schools, recruitment and pay structures. It can also be used as an educational tool for training managers in the effects of their decision making.

3   Manpower Modelling

A number of standardised manpower models are available as building blocks for developing work in manpower. Nurses were given some understanding of the basics of queueing theory so that they could manage their systems more effectively.

4   Decision Theory

There is a substantial theory available on decision making that is well worth exploring in nursing decision making as well as in medical decision making and this area of activity has been under-exploited so far. The construction of decision trees provides a good method of understanding the structure of the decision problem.

5   Queueing Theory

Much Health Care might be described theoretically by a sequence of inter-related queueing systems. It might be valuable if its results are readily intelligible to those concerned with handling the problem. Furthermore it may be structured into a user-friendly program and used as a training aid. Simulation has the merit that almost anything can be simulated and it always produces answers. The difficulties usually arise in selecting the most fruitful approach to the problem and in validating the model i.e. in proving that it does in fact represent the real situation.

6   Other Techniques

In the nature of things, it is impossible to provide a complete list of useful techniques. However, the limitations rest mainly on the formulation of problems rather than on the mathematics of their solution - only a small fraction of the available mathematical techniques are regularly utilised in this area.

8.   Conclusion

As an advocate of the term 'informatics' it is encouraging to see that operations analysts and systems analysts are discussing problems jointly more frequently than they did in the past and that quite a lot of operational research is now reported in the medical computing conferences and journals. It is hoped that the case has been made that there is a place for careful operations analysis as a means of solving some nursing problems rather than thinking that the computer alone will solve everything. It is necessary to nurse the analysts carefully so that they understand nursing requirements and can provide useful solutions.

REFERENCES

1.   Expert Systems - their nature and potential. Townsend H.R.A.,   Medical Informatics Europe 81, MIE-81,   Volume 11   Lecture Notes on Medical Informatics, Springer Verlag, Berlin, Heidelberg, New York, 1981. pp 898-907

2. Salmon Report, Report of the Committee on Nursing; Chaired by Briggs, A., H.M.S.O. CMD 5115, 1972

3. Pre- registration House Appointments; A Computer Allocation Scheme, Shah, A.R., Farrow, S.C., Medical Education, 1976, pp 10, 474-479

4. Patients Hospitals & Operational Research, Luck G.M., Luckman J., Smith B. W., & Stringer J., Tavistock Publications, London 1971. 172-193.

5. Operational Research applied to Health Services, ed. Boldy D., Croom Helm, London 1981. pp 189-220

6. Operations Research in Health Care, Shuman L.J., Dixon Spear R., & Young J.P., John Hopkins University Press. Baltimore & London 1975.

7. Applications of O.R. in Health Care Delivery Systems, Fries B.E., pp 107. Springer Verlag, Berlin, Heidelberg, New York, 1981. (Volume 10 in Series of Lecture Notes in Medical Informatics.)

8. Operations Research in Hospital: Diagnosis & Prognosis Stimson, D.H. & Stimson R.H., Health Research & Education Trust, Chicago, 1972

9. A Study of Emergency Anaesthetic Work, Taylor T. H., Jennings, A.M.C., Nightingale, D.A., Barber, B., Leivers, D., Styles, M. and Magner, J., Brit. J. Anaesth. 41 and 70-83, 167-175, 357-370, 1969.

The Impact of Computers on Nursing
M. Scholes, Y. Bryant and B. Barber (eds.)
Elsevier Science Publishers B.V. (North-Holland)
© IFIP-IMIA, 1983

15.2.

PERFORMANCE CRITERIA

William Abbott

In 1967 the Department of Health and Social Security initiated an experimental programme within the National Health Service which was intended to explore the use of real-time computing in hospital patient administration. The original objectives were:

    a)   Improve patient care
    b)   Improve clinical efficiency
    c)   Improve administrative efficiency
    d)   Provide facilities for research

Additionally, (as was the case with another major computer programme for Standardisation of systems e.g. Payroll), it was hoped to encourage an awareness of the benefits of computers through direct experience. A number of proposals were received by the Department and the first acceptance of a feasibility study was in 1969 and the first systems went live in 1971. Not all proposals received support as projects and not all projects actually implemented systems. Of the 15 projects actually accepted in the programme 13 implemented systems, 2 were terminated, 7 were heavily revised and only 4 kept to their original concepts.

At that time expertise in the application of real-time computing did not exist in either the D.H.S.S. or the N.H.S; indeed, it was only to be found in the very few installations worldwide that were using the then new technology of real time computing. In consequence the projects were given a high degree of operational freedom. The applications, the computer methodology and the user interactions were all selected locally according to local needs as perceived by local management. While virtually all the applications were within the general area of patient administration the major thrust of the programme was for integrated systems. Accordingly the more successful projects intended and in fact used the base of patient administration to extend their applications to other fields e.g. the nursing applications at the Queen Elizabeth Hospital, Birmingham and at The London Hospital.

It was appreciated almost from the beginning of the programme that there was a need to evaluate the benefits of the various projects(1).   Perhaps because of the Research and Development funding or of the obvious experimental nature of the programme the D.H.S.S. supported the concepts of evaluation(2), although other N.H.S. computing activities were not evaluated. The early projects formulated their own methodology(3) and after a progress review, guidance was issued supporting the concept of 'improved objectives'. This concept placed an emphasis on 'before and after' comparative data and the somewhat inconclusive results were published in 1977(4). Some methodological queries were raised(5) and finally a working group was set up to recommend a more appropriate methodology.

The working group observed that previous attempts at evaluation had tended to be unsuccessful for a variety of reasons but principally:-

1. The methodology employed was concerned with the local situation and thus did not reflect the potential of the computer systems for the national interest.
2. The 'before and after' concept was not fully enunciated until most projects that were to succeed were past the stage where the 'before' elements could be accurately measured.
3. Comparisons were difficult due to timescales and the dynamic nature of the institutions housing the projects.
4. Another local element was the efficiency of the system displaced by the computer system.
5. Probably most important, many of the projects had not been designed to meet the improvement objectives e.g. cost savings.

As a result of these considerations the working group considered a movement towards measuring performance rather than improvement, that is in assessing what a computer system will do and leaving a potential user to judge this performance against his own needs. It follows that the choice of performance measures should be made by consumers of computer services i.e. administrators, doctors, nurses, etc., and it was hoped that some half a dozen measures could establish performance for a particular application area. The working group envisaged that the judgement of the utility of a computer system for a particular application would be made by considering the various performance measures and the systems costs compared to the existing system to be replaced(6). This process was termed the shop window approach by the working group. Some pilot work in this area looked promising(7).

A national study was undertaken to identify the performance measures in a number of application or 'topic' areas. Nearly 1000 individuals stratified by discipline and type of hospital were interviewed in order to identify and then rank performance measures for the following topic areas:-

Inpatient Administration   Pathology Services
Outpatient Administration   Pharmacy Services
Waiting List Management   X-Ray Services
Medical Records   Health Care Records
Nursing Records

In the nursing records topic area, typical performance criteria are:-

(a) Completeness/accuracy of nursing records
(b) Effectiveness and a communication service

It is important to appreciate that these are criteria to apply to all systems. At this stage the various performance measures were ranked on the basis of the highest importance attached to them by any group. Originally it had been expected that some criteria would stand out and be adequate to provide a definitive performance. However, this was not so and the decision was made to measure criteria down to such a level as resources would permit. The method of measurement of each of the criteria was established by the working group and published in a handbook(8) to the evaluation teams.

During the measurement of performance criteria at the experimental project hospitals and other chosen sites (for comparison) it was found that there were some difficulties with particular criteria measurement methodology but these did not present insuperable problems. However, there was some adaptions to local situations with a consequent drift from standards and therefore comparability.

In general, the principal problem was the number of criteria and the complexity of the measurement. A comparability exercise was carried out in order to answer satisfactorily such questions as 'Are computer systems better than manual systems?' and 'Are some computer systems better than others?'.

The exercise resulted in full reports including detailed findings in five topic
areas (inpatients, outpatients, waiting lists, master index and pathology
laboratories) and three combined reports (nursing, primary care and medical
records).

The outcome of the exercise relating to nursing systems was that there were
distinct advantages accruing to the computer systems. Significant improvements
were recorded in a number of criteria and it was noted there were advantages to
the development of individual care plans rather than task orientated nursing
care. However, the exercise could only be carried out at two sites - Exeter and
Birmingham, although measurements were made on a 'before and after' basis thus
yielding manual and computer results in both cases.

In addition to the various reports mentioned previously a summary of all the
results has been published by the D.H.S.S.(9). Prior to this publication the
results of the exercise were presented to the N.H.S. at a Seminar. The
consensus of opinion was that performance criteria might be a useful tool but
that it was thought that such evaluation tools should not just be directed at
computer systems. Indeed the criticism was made that the subject matter was
somewhat dated.

This evaluation exercise represents the last major lesson from the experimental
programme. A scheme was outlined for an evaluation of the Programme as a
whole(10) and a review of the complete evaluation effort has been published(11).
The original objectives of the experimental programme were as stated previously
- four general aims and a specific. Without doubt the experimental programme
encouraged the build up of computer expertise in the N.H.S., both directly
within the projects and indirectly in fostering a spirit of competition with the
new Regional Board computer installations. While it could be argued that there
is still an overall shortage of skilled staff in the N.H.S. each Region has
within its own area an organisation of computer expertise.

The problem of communication between the builders of systems and the potential
users is well known, certainly a number of failures can be traced directly to
this fault. Performance criteria emphasise the user judgement of a system and
demonstrate the need to assess the value of an existing system in user terms -
whether that system be one in existence in the N.H.S. or a commercial package.
When a new system is being created then the involvement of the users becomes
essential from the beginning and the systems designers should take account of
performance measures by which the users will judge the systems.

Computing technology is, however, very dynamic and the situation viewed by the
performance criteria exercise has changed considerably. Systems are now being
designed that permit users themselves, easy access and manipulation of
information. Moreover such systems will be much easier to adapt as user
requirements vary. The very difficult financial climate now compared to the
time when the experimental programme was at its most intensive, results in a
much more stringent view being taken both of capital expenditure and the revenue
consequences. Most Regions now insist on a careful investment appraisal and
expect a cost benefit to be realised from changes of system. Side by side with
these harder attitudes are increasing demands for computer services and it may
be worth observing that all of the experimental sites that implemented a
computer system are still using computer systems. Perhaps at the end of the day
the best evaluation is to observe if an institution is prepared to continue with
a computer system when the life of the first equipment is at an end - especially
if it does so out of its own resources.

REFERENCES

(1) Uses for Computers in the N.H.S. Computers and Research Division, DHSS, May 1975

(2) Towards a methodology for evaluating new uses of computers, Sharpe. J. Proc. Medinfo 74, pp 137-143, 1975.

(3) An approach to an evaluation of The London Hospital Computer Project. Barber B. Proc. Medinfo 74, pp 155-165, 1975.

(4) The Evaluation of the N.H.S. Experimental Computer Programme: An Interim Report. Computers and Research Division, DHSS, March 1977.

(5) Evaluation of Computer Systems in Medicine, Cohen R.D., proc. Medical Informatics, Berlin 1979, pp. 931-937.

(6) A New Approach to the evaluation of the NHS Experimental Computer Programme, Molteno, B.W.H., proc. Medical Informatics, Europe 1978, pp 691-700.

(7) An Assessment of the use of performance criteria in the Evaluation of the NHS Experimental Computer Programme, Cundy A. D., & Nock, J.D., proc. Medical Informatics, Berlin 1979, pp 117-130.

(8) Handbook for the Measurement of Performance Criteria. Computers and Research Division, DHSS, 1979.

(9) The Evaluation of the N.H.S. Computer R & D Programme. Computers and Research Division, DHSS, 1982.

(10) An Approach to the Evaluation of the Experimental Computer Programme in England, Barber B., Abbott W., & Cundy A.D., proc. Medinfo 77, pp 913-916, 1977.

(11) Evaluating Evaluation - Some personal thoughts on a decade of evaluation in the NHS. Barber B., & Cundy A.. proc. Medinfo 80, pp 602-606, 1980 and in expanded form N.E. Thames R.H.A., M.S.D. Report 977.

The Impact of Computers on Nursing
M. Scholes, Y. Bryant and B. Barber (eds.)
Elsevier Science Publishers B.V. (North-Holland)
© IFIP-IMIA, 1983

15.3.

UNDERSTANDING DATA CAPTURE IN NURSING

Kathryn Erat

Introduction

The purpose of this paper is to bring into focus two different perspectives on nursing and computing. One is a personal observation on the involvement of nursing in computing and the other is the present and near-future state-of-the-art in computing. If in the past the state-of-the-art in computing has not been sufficiently developed that nursing could be conversant and comfortable with it, that is rapidly changing. Computing is rapidly extending itself to becoming a manageable and useful adjunct to the layman in every profession.

Nursing Profession Involvement with Computers

Computers can be useful to the typical clinical nurse, the administrator, the researcher, the planner (regional or agency), and the educator. However, if one scans the journals or conference proceedings concerned with the uses of computing in the health/medical area, it becomes strikingly clear that only a very small proportion of the accomplishments are related to nursing or have been pioneered or developed by nurses. For example, the United States National Center for Health Services Research Report, "Computer Applications in Health Care," published in June 1980, documents ten years of medical care computer applications research supported by the National Center for Health Services Research(B20). One-hundred thirty-eight projects were funded in response to applications from hospitals, clinics, community services, universities, corporations, and group practices. Of these 138 projects, approximately 7 projects heavily concerned nursing, and it seems likely that 3 to 5 were initiated by nurses. The titles of these projects are listed below:- (see pp 20-23 ref B20)

- Barnet, G., Massachusetts General Hospital, "Hospital Computer Project"
- Davis, E., Visiting Nurse Association of Vermont, "Demonstration of a Computerised Decision Support System in a Nurse Practitioner Staffed Rural Health Clinic."
- Gall, J., El Camino Hospital, "Demonstration of an Existing Hospital Information System."
- Huff, W., The Sisters of the Third Order of St. Francis, "Demonstration of a Shared Hospital Information System."
- Kittle, R., Lockheed Missiles Space Company, "Systems Analysis of Information Needs of Nursing Stations."
- O'Neill, J., The MITRE Corporation, "A Study of the Technology Required to Support Non-Physician Providing Health Care."
- Weed, L., University of Vermont, "Automation of a Problem-Oriented Medical Record."

This is both unfortunate and fortunate. What is unfortunate?

1. Nurses have not been able to take advantage on a large scale of the assistance that computers could give them.

2.   The practitioners in the medical/health computing field do not turn to nursing for leadership or even for insight on many routine computing projects.

3.   Nursing is, therefore, the passive recipient of systems designed for them by someone else with little or no consultation with them, the nurses, as users.

4.   As computerization becomes more and more relevant in the medical/health care field, a nursing profession lagging behind in its appreciation and expertise in the field may find itself effectively excluded from a domain of professionalism that they should be involved in.

Although there are several outstanding nurse computer specialists, the nursing profession, as a group, does not score high in computer literacy; is therefore not dynamic in the field; and accordingly is not perceived as an active initiator of the areas of computing that properly fall within the nursing domain.   And like any other sphere of life, if you are passive, someone else begins to make the decisions for you.   Nature abhors a vacuum.

Why has this happened?
What is the appropriate relationship of nursing to computing?
How can the appropriate relationship be brought about?
It is important to look at the reasons for the present situation:

1.   Most nurses are women and nurses are motivated by the interpersonal.

2.   Nurses have not had easy access to learning about computers.

3.   Nurses do not have access to large developmental budgets or discretionary funds.

4.   Nurses are timid about seeking funding to support the implementation of their creative ideas.

Let us look at the first contention: nurses are women.   Computing even though not necessarily highly mathematical, is nevertheless perceived as akin to mathematics and, indeed, computing does require precise logical abstract thinking.   It is a well-documented fact that large numbers of women express anxiety and avoidance when confronted with tasks, job requirements, or career paths that demand mathematical literacy and/or the practice of mathematical activities(1,2).   Indeed, the anxiety extends to those situations where women simply conjecture that maths is a requirement for successful performance.   For most women mathematical activities are not pleasurable activities.   Therefore, if computer activity is in some way related to mathematics or perceived as such, it is understandable that the same anxiety is invoked.   If there was a career path in nursing called nurse computer specialist, the vast majority of nurses would not seriously consider it as a career path.   Furthermore, this avoidance or lack of involvement in computing is also explained by the fact that nurses are primarily interested in the interpersonal.

The following is a list of random titles from the journals concerned with nursing education:

"Structure vs. People in Primary Nursing: An Inquiry" (3)
"Teaching Interpersonal Management for Effective Professional Nursing Practice"(4)
"Client Assessment: An Integrated Model"(5)
"Community Nursing - A Psychosocial Learning Experience"(6)
"Social Learning Theory as a Basis for Teaching Decisions"(7)
"Negotiating Group Process Experiences"(8)
"Patient Teaching as a Curriculum Thread"(9)

These titles are indicative of the emphasis and concerns of nurses and of those
that educate nurses. Indeed, there may be a temporal culture factor operating.
Sexual counselling, community health, patient education, team participation, and
preparation for death are presently relevant topics that were not prominent a
few years ago. They will, in the future, be replaced with other concerns that
are generically similar. The thread of emphasis running through all these
titles is concern and education for successful interaction on the interpersonal
level. That should surprise no one. Nurses literally take care of others.
Mothers take care of children, teachers take care of young students, and nurses
take care of people of all ages - a highly interpersonal activity. No wonder
that the curriculum and the journals are stressing the interpersonal and not the
abstract.

Let us look at the assertion that nurses have not had easy access to learning
about computers. In the United States, computers in nursing is barely
represented in the student curriculum. Therefore, most nurses have had no
structured exposure to learning about computing. Secondly, only now are
sections of medical computing conferences beginning to have sessions on
computers and nursing. And it is only in the last two years that nurses
themselves have begun to organize conferences on this topic. There have been
two conferences in the United States sponsored by the Clinical Center at the
National Institute of Health and the nursing personnel of the military
departments. These sessions have been extremely well attended, but they do not
provide in-depth training. The in-depth training tailored especially for
practicing nurses has not been readily available. That must be remedied
(L14,L13). Nursing education stresses the skills of observation and judgment -
two skills that if coupled with computer literacy could enable nurses to
contribute valuable insights on how computer systems should interface with users
from the human factors perspective.

There should also be some exposure for nursing students to computing. Even
though a student may not upon beginning a career become intimately involved with
computing, a good student-level introduction will make it that much easier later
on in her career to use computers. Student years are the easiest time to
confront and absorb different modes of thought and activity.

Let us examine the third point: nurses do not have access to large developmental
budgets. Computer developments in health and medicine have usually been funded
in the following ways:

1.   Government and/or foundation grants;
2   Centralized institutional investments;
3   Medical industry development.

Nurses traditionally have not usually been the petitioners or recipients of
funds via these channels. They are not usually the initiators of these large-
scale projects. Therefore, their participation on such projects has been
ancillary and/or consultative. Hence, computer system development related to
nursing needs has been initiated either mostly by non-nursing personnel or it
simply has not been done at all. When projects have been initiated by non-
nurses, sometimes close collaboration with nurses has been sought, and sometimes
it has not. Where there has not been close collaboration, the resultant systems
have not been as well designed or as usable as they should be. Invariably,
nursing consultation and effort must be sought after the fact to remedy the
situation. How much better if nursing personnel were involved from the very
beginning of the project. However, a nursing involvement demands an informed
involvement. Design and development have to eventually proceed from
generalities to specifics. For example, exactly how should a printed report
look? Should data presented in a report be arranged in rows or columns? How
often should a report be generated? These are examples of what seem to be

trivial questions, but are the type of questions that deserve serious design thought. They should not be left to the non-user to arbitrarily answer. Indeed, the wrong answers or even casual answers to these types of questions can make a system difficult to use if not totally unusable in some instances. It is clear then that the compulsive attention to petty detail is a must for system success. But alas is that all? Surely most of us do not want to devote our careers exclusively to answering questions like how many labels should be generated for a blood sample container or should the afternoon patient condition report display only changes in status or all known variables whether or not they have changed from the last report period. Indeed, even with the best forethought these answers may have to be changed. And that is just the point. Any system must have flexibility and modularity. Certainly, one role the nurse participant should aspire to when collaborating on system development teams is not only the role of the passive question answerer, but also one of overview conceptualizer. Her answer to the question of "How many labels?" may indeed be a specific number, but the very question should prompt her to respond that the generation of labels should be generic routine or module whose parameters such as number, content, size, etc., can be specified for each application that needs to generate labels. When asked about report contents and frequency, she should look at where reports fit into the total operation, what is needed, what is not needed, and what is the best way of receiving what is needed. Should it be routinely, on demand, by error/exception, hard copy, CRT display, or audio responses? Inadequate conceptializing usually leads to a plethora of paper that consumes manpower just to put it in neat piles in the right in-baskets or CRT displays that are confusing. Computer specialists will turn out all the reports you want. They are not the ones who have to file them. They also have a predilection for giving very little thought to how a CRT display should look for the user. The nurse should be assertive about conceptualizing the overall operation of her unit or office and specifying where and how computer support fits in.

And now for the assertion that nurses are timid about seeking funding to support the implementation of their creative ideas. Most women suffer from this timidity. Are we timid because we are afraid we will be refused support? Are we timid because we fear failure? Do we lack confidence in our ability to learn, to manage, and/or to implement? Do we lack confidence in our own ideas? Or do we wait for someone in a higher echelon to suggest that we start a project? There are creative, capable people in nursing who need to assert themselves, seek funding, and put their ideas to work.

Having discussed that it was unfortunate that nursing has not been heavily involved in medical computing, it is now the time to point out that it is also fortunate. Why?

1. Because nursing has not been involved, it has not been experimenting and developing with equipment that was initially extremely expensive and not always technologically well-suited for the job. Fortunately, nursing is not burdened with a heavy past investment in system concepts, design and equipment that is being rapidly made obsolete. They are coming into the field at a time when there is an abundance of technological power at very low cost and new concepts of systems organization.
2. The lack of training, previously lamented, can now be acquired in a much more effective environment.

Major Hardware and Software Developments that will increase the use of Computers in Health Care

Hardware:

1. The continuing decline in cost of computer hardware.

For example, in the U.K. Sinclair Research will market a personal computer for approximately £225 or $400 that will have 16K bytes of random access memory (RAM) and 16K bytes of read only memory (ROM). This will be a hand-held unit and have a 100K byte microfloppy disk drive, colour output high-resolution graphics, and a BASIC interpreter(10). Five years ago the microdisk did not exist; the computer itself would have occupied aproximately 1.5 cubic feet and would have cost $10,000.

2.   The increasing miniaturization of computer hardware.

Computer miniaturization has reached the point that hand-held units, briefcase units, and terminal centered units are all readily available. The only peripheral that is difficult to shrink to desktop size is the very high-speed printer.

3.   The progressive increase in the power and modularity of computer components: smaller systems that can do more work and possess great flexibility in system architecture. A system can be assembled from a vast array of vendor offering to meet almost any operation and cost criteria. There is a variety of devices from which to choose from an ever increasing number of vendors of both general-purpose and special-purpose components and systems. See Table 1.

Table 1

Proliferation of Personal Computers

	1975	1979
Manufacturers	5	55
Personal Computers Shipped	4,000	255,000
Sales	$6,000,000	$675,000,000
Number of Computer Retail Stores	1	1,000

Data presented at a forum at Massachusetts Institute of Technology, June 1982.
INFOWORLD July 5, 1982, Volume 4, 26, Pages 3, 6
MIT Forum Assesses Future of Personal Computers by David Needle(11)

4.   The progressing increase in the access speed and bit capacity of computer storage devices, such as memory, disks and tapes, with a parallel decrease in cost.

5.   Concurrent breakthroughs in ancillary technologies such as:

(a)   Digitization of visual images (video disks, optical disks)

Great progress has been made in the digitization of visual images. For example, it is envisioned that x-ray film will be replaced by digital storage of x-ray images. This means that the x-ray image can be transmitted and reproduced for whoever needs access to it. The video disk can be used to store text and visual information. As a read only device, it is fantastically inexpensive. For example, it is estimated that by 1992 a $10 disk could hold 1,000,000,000,000 bits of information(12). This is equivalent to the information in two-hundred 500-page books. With that kind or storage capacity, one can envisage entire special-purpose libraries being stored on optical disks. Coupled with the communications discussed below, the concepts of libraries, ready access to specialized information including pictorial information, and education can be rethought. However, even now there are available computer interfaces that allow computer control of display and visual material from prerecorded disks. Disks at present can hold 54,000 frames of visual information(13). For example, a student nurse could view visual presentation of surgical or birth procedures selectively as many times as necessary till she felt well informed about the procedure.

(b)   Communications

The merger of computers and communications has progressed rapidly in the last five years. There are external communications whereby computers are talking to other computers via phone lines, microwave transmission, and satellite transmission. Communications technology is rapidly developing the bandwidth capacity (speed of bit transmission) necessary to make data exchange on a large and popular scale financially feasible. For example, it is not unrealistic to assume that instead of having a journal delivered by mail we will have it delivered by telephone. In other words, it will be available electronically at a computer repository that we will use our personal terminal to dial into via a communication circuit. The individual journal pages will then be transmitted to our terminal for viewing and/or copying.

There are internal local area network communications whereby any computer and/or peripheral can communicate with any other computer and/or peripheral on the network. This gives us much greater flexibility to design any large health institution's computing/information system. It is not necessary to have one large central computer which requires a large capital investment. We can start with small units and link them as the plan grows.

(c)   Speech recognition and speech synthesis by computer.

Speech recognition by computer has sufficiently progressed that isolated word input from a speaker who has previously trained the computer to her voice for a specialized limited vocabulary is possible. This type of input is especially useful where one wants to enter information into the computer while her hands are busy performing another task. For example, one could dictate the results of a specialized patient examination while actually performing it. Speech synthesis is even further developed than speed recognition. Computers can now successfully be programmed to reply verbally. Both of these concepts have use in aids for the handicapped.

Software:

1.   Progress in the development of generalized database technology.
2.   Progress in the art of developing users' manuals (both in book form and computer form) that guide the unsophisticated user.
3.   Progress in the development of many generalized application programs such as:
     (a)   Word processing
     (b)   General ledger
     (c)   Patient billing for doctors' offices
     (d)   Budget tools such as VISICALC

4.   Progress in the development of software building tools such as frame
      generators, report generators, and complete database management systems
5.   Progress in the development of very high-level languages: program
      development tools, e.g. preprocessors to COBOL or FORTRAN that allow
      extremely high-level statements to be written that are then compiled into
      the several COBOL or FORTRAN statements
6.   Progress in the development of decision support system concepts such as
      rule-based systems and expert systems that incorporate artificial
      intelligence.

These developments can be summarized in general:

1.   More power, capacity and flexibility in smaller hardware packages for less
      cost.
2.   More user-ready packages for special software and/or hardware applications
      available at reasonable cost.
3   More flexibility for and less effort required of the user to develop her
      own applications.
4.   Users, applications, and information can be linked regardless of location.

How are these developments coalescing? What are they giving birth to? In
concrete terms, the individual workstation (the enhanced robust personal
computer) is becoming an office tool and a computational and communication
device. The typewriter is disappearing. I predict that within five years all
typewriters that are used for several hours per day will have been replaced by
personal computer workstations. In the United States, the word APPLE is
achieving the concept status and ubiquitousness that is comparable with such
household words as IBM and Kleenex. I suspect that in Europe the same thing is
happening to SINCLAIR and COMMODORE or similar microcomputer system names. See
Table 1. Indeed, many researchers believe we have just begun to develop the
personal workstation. At France's World Center Project an international group
of scientists is working on the ideal workstation. They have $20 million of
funding for this and related endeavours.

Along with the personal workstation are coming four things:

1.   Dedicated applications programs
2.   The capacity for tailoring special-purpose systems for various
      applications with a modest investment
3.   The capacity to link together many special-purpose units to build a large
      system
4.   The capacity to link workstations together and to both central and
      distributed databases across institutions or regions.

A workstation is a compact unit consisting of a CPU, approximately 64K bytes of
random access memory, display unit, input keyboard and ready access to hard
disk. This disk may or may not be shared with other workstations. A hard copy
of printer unit should be located within reasonable distance. The unit should
have sufficient I/O ports that it can communicate when necessary with other
workstations or a central computer. The workstation should not require special
environmental conditions such as air-conditioning, but be usable in the typical
office or nursing station environment. The workstation, if it has sufficient
memory, disk capacity, and I/O ports, may support more than one keyboard/display
unit via timesharing. The workstation operating system and locally stored
application programs should support all the computer activities relevant to that
geographic location. The workstation will collect and store data relevant to
its geographic location, transfer its data to other locations that require that
data, and solicit relevant data from other locations. Although many
workstations might perform many or all of their functions without communicating
with other workstations, others will need to communicate and can be considered

as part of a local area network. The advantages of using individual workstations in place of a large central computer are as follows:

1. The malfunction of one station affects only a small number of users.
2. Full equipment redundancy is expensive for a large centralized computer centre simply because a large central computer is so expensive. However, a large computing system composed of several small stations can be assured of minimal downtime by maintaining only a small number of spare workstations whose total cost is a fraction of a large computer. A spare workstation can quickly be substituted for a malfunctioning one. It can be statistically determined just how many extra workstations are required so that almost 100 percent up time is assured.
3. The communications burden that a centralized system must support is minimised when most of the work and data storage is shifted to workstations.
4. Response time should be excellent since only a small number of users are being serviced by a CPU and disk.
5. Since a workstation will primarily be used for specific functions, the overall systems organization for a particular workstation will probably be much less complex than it would be for a large central computer.
6. The application jurisdiction for user workstations could be parcelled out to many different responsible designers and users.

The communications among workstations and with a central computer, when necessary, can be greatly facilitated by the use of a local area network. Until recently, connectivity among computing devices had been point-to-point. That is, each device was hard-wired to each of the other devices it needed to communicate with. Generally, for each link there was one wire. For devices that had only one port (most terminals and printers) there was usually only one communication path and thus a profusion of wires was required to achieve multiconnectivity. The purpose of a local area network is to give any device access to any other device and at the same time minimize the wires. All devices are connected to one wire (cable) which traverses the locations of all devices. The devices then share the transmission capability of the wire by taking turns sending on the wire data addressed to the intended recipient device. Since all devices are connected to the one wire, any device can be addressed by another device. At present, most devices cannot interface directly to this single wire but require a network interface unit. At present, these interface units are fairly expensive, approximately $500, to give a device access to the wire. However, manufacturing competition and an expanding market for these devices should dramatically lower their cost over the next two to three years. At present, two approaches are being used to achieve the local area network:

1. Install a coaxial cable or other continuous wire.
2. Take advantage of the extended telephone network wires already in place within a building. In this approach a central switching device receives the addressed communication from the individual telephone wire the device is attached to and switches it to the wire of the addressed device.

It is this local network capability that makes it practical to let any workstation have access to data at any other workstation or central computer.

The common carriers, telephone companies, are moving rapidly and efficiently into the data transmission business. While we almost invariably think of voice conversations when we think of telephone, and indeed telephone companies are constantly expanding voice service, they are now also heavily involved in developing reliable high-speed, high-volume data communications services. See Table 2.

Table 2

Trends in Communication

                                                        Digital Techniques

                              Analog Techniques

                                                            EFTS

                                                            Electronic
                                                            Mail

                                                            Electronic
                                                            Newspapers

                                                            Information
                                                            Retrieval
                                          Radio
                                          Paging
                              Data   Video
                                          Conferencing
                                          View Phone
                    TV   Telemetry

          Telephone

Telegraph

1875   1900   1925 1950   1960   1975   2000

ELECTRICAL COMMUNICATION Volume 54, 4, 1979. Page 310
The Future for Standardization in Telecommunications by W. T. Jones(14)

Implications of Hardware/Software Developments for Nursing

Dedicated application programs, such as word processing, patient billing, and
accounting are becoming readily available. In the United States it is envisaged
that, in general, nurses working in health care settings involving only a small
number of physicians or other health care providers may more rapidly come face-
to-face with these administrative-related applications and their hardware for
two reasons:

a)   In a small health care setting it is easier to move into a new way of
     doing things - only a small number of people need to be informed, to
     agree, and to cooperate.
b)   In the past, computer innovation was expensive. Only large institutions
     with corresponding access to large financial resources could incorporate
     or innovate with computers. But with the dramatically lowered cost today,
     anyone with the most modest of budgets can both acquire a turnkey
     application or develop her own.

Which tools are brought into the health care setting, probably initially at the
behest of the office administrators or the physicians, may determine who has the
most immediate exposure to the potential of computers in the small health care
environment. The administrative personnel will, no doubt, be heavily involved
with the patient accounting. As a part of their daily routine, they will learn
about floppy disks, hard disks, letter quality printers, file storage, indexes,
tables, and screen formats. Where is the nurse in the midst of this? Aloof

from what is perceived as essentially a clerical task? A clerical task, yes, but one that can broaden the horizons of those who are willing to try to learn about it and use it. The nurse's responsibility may not be to keep track of patient appointments, but learning how the computer does it may spark her own creativity as to how the office computer might be more useful in patient care. For example, an infant health nurse, when demonstrated a file management capability on a workstation, caught on immediately and was intrigued with the idea of keeping track of the individual infants' feeding formulas and their weight patterns over time to build an experience base that provided statistical validity for recommendations of infant nursing formulas. Now that is the kind of spark that is not going to be struck much less ignite anything if the individual nurse ignores the equipment coming around her because basically it is someone else's responsibility or because she feels an insecurity about understanding it or learning to use it. It is the advantage of the small health care setting that there the nurse may indeed have a ready-made opportunity for a hands-on experience and where she may be more readily able to implement some of her own ideas of what would be useful on a health care computer.

But where does that leave our colleagues in the large health care settings, presumably where application decisions are made by a department or administrators remote from nursing? Three things are recommended:

1. Those in authority or at the level to be consulted about institutional computerization have the responsibility to either acquire the necessary background to contribute meaningfully and creatively to this decision or they should appoint others and see that they are properly educated to fulfill these functions. Nursing administrators demand that the staff education department assume responsibility for clinical and managerial updating of the nursing staff. There should be no less commitment to seeing that a core group of nurses within the institution are also computer literate. If need be, their education should be secured outside the institution. A further section of this paper will detail a computer literacy course for nurses. Once there is a core of computer literate nurses within the institution, they should:

    a. Insist that they be included in any institutional computer planning committees.
    b. Be active, committed participants in specifying and/or designing any clinical computer applications or administrative computer applications that affect the nursing department. Their participation must be general (overall goals, needed applications), specific (how many labels should be printed, how many can the institution afford to waste, the order of laboratory tests on a screen in a nursing unit, etc.), and dedicated (part-time commitment such as viewing a few demonstrations or visiting a few other institutions to see their systems, casting a vote and then leaving it to others simply will not work). Almost all systems, whether purchased from outside or developed in-house, should have flexibility for tailoring to the specific institution. It is in checking for that flexibility in candidate systems, and then in finally tailoring the system of choice that the computer nurse plays a unique and most inportant role. She must understand how her sister nurses go about their nursing tasks so that she can tailor whatever patient care systems they must use to their needs and the exigencies of the situations within which they work. This cannot be done from the ivory tower of the office. She must know the workings of each care and service area intimately in order to blend the requirements of all within the framework of the computer system at hand, and design input and output activities that assist her nurses and do not frustrate them or make them less efficient. For example,

an automated laboratory system may require the entry of a dozen items of information to order a laboratory test. If the nurse is going to do the ordering, how should that screen look? Should test codes be assigned according to frequency of order with easily remembered codes being assigned to CBCs and urinalysis or should all blood tests have a series of codes and all urine tests another series of codes, etc.? These are not the kinds of questions one should simply answer without some thought and research into how the nurses who will do the laboratory request entry think. Or consider instructing nurses how to use the computer terminal. What help messages are there on the systems? Are the messages such that the night shift nurse, who is relatively alone, can be guided by them alone successfully through whatever computer tasks she is required to perform. Again, those help messages should not be glibly designed but considered an important part of the system. No matter what wonderful thing the system can do, if the users cannot figure out how to make it work, the system is simply a failure.

2.   Any nurse within the large institution who is going to have computer hardware and software introduced into her area should at least be consulted for her ideas and opinions. The more familiar she is with CRTs, etc., from her past experience, the more relevant her comments will be.

3.   Any nurse anywhere who has an idea about a use for computers in health care should have the courage to discuss them with those working in the field. Indeed, she may find herself becoming the driving force behind getting the idea implemented. If she considers herself competent to implement the idea, she should not be hesitant to seek funding. Progress is made because we have the courage to try. We should not fear failure. Women have been traditionally afraid to initiate what they envisage as large massive projects. In the past because of the size, cost, and complexity of computer hardware and software, a computer project did indeed fulfil the criteria of a major undertaking. But that is no longer true. A modest budget can sustain hardware and software suitable for almost all nursing computer applications. There is no reason not to undertake these projects today.

Recommendations and Conclusion

Where can one acquire the education necessary? There are innumerable courses available via the usual institutions of learning of computer manufacturers. Three projects that undertaken together would create a quantum leap in nursing uses of computing at least as applied to the most routine and obvious clerical tasks, are:

1.   Software system developed so that it would be suitable for developing nursing station applications. This system should be resident on small personal-sized computers. Its software functions should include:
   a.   database management system
   b.   frame generator
   c.   report generator
   d.   high-level application language
   e.   VISICALC- or CLINFO-like calculation options.

These functions should be imbedded in a user-friendly operating system. The design should take advantage of cognitive learning theory and the rudiments of decision support theory(15).

2. Once this flexible software/hardware system is developed, intensive two-week seminars should be developed so that nurses could attend to become familiar with computing in a learning environment that has immediate relevance for their interests and recognizes their particular learning orientation of observing and doing.

3. In addition to an open attendance, selected regions and specialties within nursing should each be invited to send an attendee and her sponsoring organisation should be provided a single workstation for experimentation upon her successful completion of the course provided her sponsor agrees to allow her to devote 50 percent of work time for 18 months to integrating it into the nursing environment in whatever way she thinks best. Physicians have been able to work part time on their computer developments because they have been able to simultaneously work part time in patient care and administration. A similar means of support must be found to support nurses doing computer development.

Years ago, the United States government funded a similar activity to introduce physiologists to the power of computers in their laboratories. The U.S. National Institutes of Health have also taken a similar approach to encourage medical researchers to use computer data management and analysis to facilitate their clinical research. The CLINFO system was specifically developed with clinical researchers' needs as a specification, after careful study of these needs(16). The system consists of database management, worksheet or data manipulation section, a repertoire of statistical routines, interfaces to programs the user can construct in other languages, data entry via screen forms of the user's design, and reporting functions including graphing of data. The system is self-explanatory and forgiving. A key feature of the system is the worksheet section which strongly mimics the way researchers organize their research data for analysis.(17,18) This system has had excellent reception at the 16 medical centers in the United States that have been given a system by NIH. In other words, it was recognized that bringing a specifically tailored system to novice users is one of the best ways to rapidly integrate computing power into a particular environment. By seeding such systems at key installations, users are provided a facility long before their respective institutions might be prepared to provide them with such a facility. A similar approach for introducing nurses to the power of computing would be similarly successful and induce them to construct creative applications and such an endeavour should be undertaken for nursing in the near future.

REFERENCES
1. Schafer, Alice T., Brief Description of the Wellesley College Mathematics Project, A Component of Wellesley College - Wesleyan University Mathematics Project, Wellesley, Massachusetts (September 1978).
2. Tobias, Sheila
3. Shukla, R.K., Structure vs. people in primary nursing: an inquiry, in: Nursing Research 30, 4 (July-August 1981, pp. 236-41).
4. Wyatt, M.A., and Withersty, D.J., Teaching interpersonal management for effective professional nursing practice, in: Nursing Practice, Journal of Psychiatric Nursing 17, 6 (June 1979, pp. 23-7).
5. Hill, L. and Smith, N., Client assessment: an integrated model, in: Journal of Nursing Education 20, 9 (November 1981, pp. 16-23).
6. Rynerson, B.C., Community nursing - a psychosocial learning experience, in: Journal of Nursing Education 20, 1 (January 1981, pp. 12-17).
7. Brusich, J., Social learning theory as a basis for teaching decisions, in: Journal of Nursing Education 19, 5 (May 1980, pp. 27-31).
8. Wilson, M.F., Negotiating group process experiences, in: Nursing Outlook 28, 6 (June 1980, pp. 360-4).
9. Jenny J., Patient teaching as a curriculum thread, in: Canadian Nurse 74, 2 (February 1978, pp. 28-29).

10.   50 Handheld MC Will Feature 100K-Byte Microfloppy Drive, Editorial Note,
       in: EDN 27,   16 (June 9, 1982, p. 18).
11.   Needle, David, MIT forum assesses future of personal computers, in:
       INFOWORLD 4,   26 (July 5, 1982, pp. 3, 6), Data presented at a forum at
       Massachusetts Institute of Technology (June 1982).
12.   Optical Disks to Capture 67% of '92 Disk Market, Editorial Note, in: EDN
       27, (March 31, 1982, p. 229).
13.   Interface Links Low-Cost Video Disk Players with Computers, Editorial
       Note, in: Electronic Design 29, (July 9, 1981, p. 178).
14.   Jones, W. T., The Future for standardization in telecommunications, in:
       Electrical Communication 54,   4 (1979, p. 310).
15.   Henderson, J. D., and Martinko, M. J., Cognitive learning theory and the
       design of decision support systems, in: Young, Donovan and Keen, Peter G.
       W. (eds.), DSS-81 Transactions (First International Conference on Decision
       Support Systems sponsored by Execucom Systems Corporation, 1981, pp. 45-
       50).
16.   Palley, N. A., and Groner, G. F., Informational processing needs and
       practices of clinical investigators - survey results (AFIPS Conference
       Proceedings 44:717, 1975).
17.   Whitehead, Susan F. and Bilofsky, Howard S., CLINFO - a clinical research
       data management and analysis system, in: O'Neill, Joseph T. (ed.),
       Proceedings the Fourth Annual Symposium on Computer Applications in
       Medical Care, Vol. 2 (IEEE Computer Society, Los Alamitos, California,
       1980, pp. 1286-1291).
18.   An introduction to the CLINFO data management and analysis system (Bolt,
       Beranek and Newman, Inc., Cambridge, Massachusetts, 1979).

APPENDIX
Proposed Curriculum and Goals for an Intensive Two-week Seminar in Computing for Nurses

1.   Acquisition of the vocabulary of computer science

2.   Understanding of nature, function and interrelationships of
            CPU
            Storage
              Disk
              Tape
              Punched Card
            CRTs (VDU/Keyboard)
            Printers
            Communications
              Modems
              Multiplexers
              Network Interface Units

3.   Understanding of CPU operation
            Memory (bit, byte, word)
            Coding (binary, ASCII)
            Addressing
            Instruction set
            Stored program in machine language

4.   Understanding of programming techniques
            Arithmetic
            Comparisons and branches
            Loops
            Data arrays, indexing, pointers
            Tables
            Searches
            Sorts

Input/Output

5. Understanding of a higher level language
        BASIC
        LISP

6. Understanding of a file system (fields, records, indexes, pointers, directories)

7. Understanding of an operating system (resource management: memory, peripherals, I/O requests, users' applications, time-sharing, real-time)

8. Understanding of a database management system

9. Understanding of the system analysis task
        Data Load
        Data Flow
        Work Load
        Work Flow
        Input/Output
        Individual Functions

10. Understanding of the structure and heirarchy of the computer science profession and industry

All these concepts should be elucidated by student interaction with a workstation oriented to nursing applications. The laboratory part of the course, the second week, should be dedicated to class effort and individual effort in designing and implementing nursing applications.

The Impact of Computers on Nursing
M. Scholes, Y. Bryant and B. Barber (eds.)
Elsevier Science Publishers B.V. (North-Holland)
© IFIP-IMIA, 1983

15.4.

COMPUTER BASED QUALITY ASSURANCE FOR NURSING MANAGEMENT

Lillian Eriksen

Mackenzie (1979) described a conceptual framework (Figure 1) for thinking about the management process which is useful for examining one computerized approach to quality assurance in nursing. Mackenzie identified three basic components involved in the business of management: ideas, things, and people. The management of these three components is accomplished by five essentially sequential and cyclical processes. These processes include: planning, organizing, staffing, directing, and controlling. It is important to note that the control process provides the feedback to be used as the sequential cycle is begun again. In addition to the three components and five processes, Mackenzie (1979) noted there are three functions which continually occur when one is managing. These functions include: the analysis of problems, making decisions, and communicating.

FIGURE 1

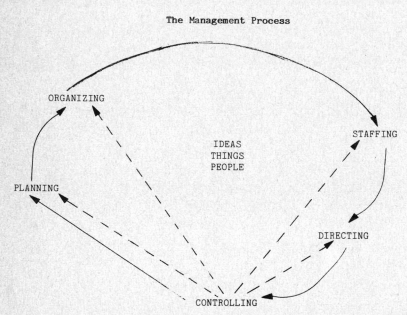

The Management Process

ORGANIZING

STAFFING

IDEAS
THINGS
PEOPLE

PLANNING

DIRECTING

CONTROLLING

PROBLEM ANALYSIS DECISION MAKING COMMUNICATION

For purposes of this paper, the control process and its inter-relationship to the other four processes will be emphasised. The purpose of the control process is to insure that organizational objectives are being achieved according to the managers plan. In order to accomplish this there are a number of tasks and activities which the manager must perform.

The first is to specify standards of performance. What are the indicators of a job well done? In quality assurance language this task relates to the identification of standards and specification of measureable criteria which will be used to assess whether or not the nursing care goals of the nurse manager have been achieved.

Following standard specification is the design of a suitable reporting system. The information needs of various levels of nurse managers will differ. The director of nursing will need broader comprehensive information while head nurses will require information specific to their particular units.

Devising a system for securing measurements of the expected performance is the third task in the control process of management. Who will measure what, when, and where needs to be decided and planned to insure smooth collection of the data.

Once the information is collected and the report generated, the nurse manager can evaluate the information, reward "good" performance and plan for corrective action in areas of performance requiring improvement. The analysis of the data regarding performance takes place in the context of previous planning, organizing, staffing and directing. Quality of nursing care cannot be addressed in isolation of these other processes. Thus the controlling process of the management function provides objective data on which decisions regarding planning, organizing, staffing and directing can be made.

An application of the use of a computer to assist in the analysis and reporting of data needed by nurse managers in the control process of management has been designed and used by Rush-Presbyterian-St. Luke's Medical Center in Chicago, Illinois. It is this application which will be used to exemplify a computerized quality assurance program as a control process for nurse managers.

As indicated in the model the first activity in the control process is specification of standards of performance. These standards are reflected in the methodology used to monitor the quality of nursing care being given to patients. The instrument used by this system is referred to as the Rush-Medicus Instrument as it was jointly developed by Rush-Presbyterian-St. Luke's Medical Center and Medicus Systems Corporation both of Chicago, Illinois.

The conceptual framework of the instrument is based on the nursing process. The nursing process was defined by the developers as "the comprehensive set of nursing activities performed in the delivery of a patient's care" (p.6). The conceptual structure of the instrument is presented in Table 1. There are six main objectives which organise the 32 subobjectives comprising the structure of the instrument. A total of 357 criteria, related to one of the subobjectives, are designed to provide measurement of the quality of nursing care in medical, surgical, pediatric, obstetric, psychiatric and emergency room areas of the hospital.

The first four main objectives are most specifically related to the nursing process. There are two additional objectives, the first of which assesses the unit's adherence to established policies and protocols. Included in this area are a number of situations which nurses might encounter, i.e., cardiac arrest, isolation of infectious disease and the handling of a fire on the unit. The second, that is number six, addresses support given to the patient care unit by

TABLE 1

OBJECTIVE AND SUBOBJECTIVE OF THE RUSH-MEDICUS INSTRUMENT

1.0. The Plan of Nursing Care is Formulated.

    1.1   The condition of the patient is assessed on admission.
    1.2   Data relevant to hospital care are ascertained on admission.
    1.3   The current condition of the patient is assessed.
    1.4   The written plan of nursing care is formulated.
    1.5   The plan of nursing care is coordinated with the medical plan of care.

2.0. The Physical Needs of the Patient are Attended

    2.1   The patient is protected from accident and injury.
    2.2   The need for physical comfort and rest is attended.
    2.3.   The need for physical hygiene is attended.
    2.4   The need for a supply of oxygen is attended.
    2.5   The need for activity is attended.
    2.6   The need for nutrition and fluid balance is attended.
    2.7   The need for elimination is attended.
    2.8   The need for skin care is attended.
    2.9   The patient is protected from infection.

3.0. The Non-Physical (Psychological, Emotional, Mental, Social) Needs of the Patient are Attended.

    3.1   The patient is oriented to hospital facilities on admission.
    3.2   The patient is extended social courtesy by the nursing staff.
    3.3   The patient's privacy and civil rights are honored.
    3.4   The need for psychological-emotional well-being is attended through interpersonal communication.
    3.5   The patient is taught measures of health maintenance and illness prevention.
    3.6   The patient's family is included in the nursing care process.
    3.7.   The need for psycho-emotional well-being is attended through therapeutic milieu.

4.0. Achievement of Nursing Care Objectives is Evaluated.

    4.1   Records document the care provided for the patient.
    4.2   The patient's response to therapy is evaluated.

5.0. Unit Procedures are Followed for the Protection of All Patients.

    5.1   Isolation and decontamination procedures are followed.
    5.2   The unit is prepared for emergency situations.
    5.3   Medical-legal procedures are followed.
    5.4   Safety and protective procedures are followed.

6.0. The Delivery of Nursing Care is Facilitated by Administrative and Managerial Services

    6.1   Nursing reporting follows prescribed standards.
    6.2   Nursing management is provided.
    6.3   Clerical services are provided.
    6.4   Environmental and housekeeping services are provided.
    6.5   Professional and administrative services are provided.

other services in the hospital such as the pharmacy, the dietary department and housekeeping. The developers of the instrument thought it necessary to assess these support departments as they directly impact the ability of nurses to carry out a number of functions related to meeting patient needs. Scores in this area provide information which assist in the interpretatiuon of the scores reflecting quality of nursing care.

Each patient care unit is randomly scheduled to be monitored for a four week period each quarter of the calendar year. Dependent on unit size and average length of stay, fourteen to eighteen patients are monitored on randomly assigned days and tours of duty during the four week data collection period.

The data are computer scored and printed as illustrated in Table 2. Each of the numerical figures in the report is an average of the criterion scores within each subobjective. Each criterion score represents the ratio of positive responses to all possible positive responses for each of the criteria. Percentage values for each objective are computed as averages of the subobjective score within each of the objectives. Thus 45 percent of the time Unit 1 assesses the condition of the patient on admission. The objective of formulating the nursing care plan is achieved 65 percent of the time.

TABLE 2

SAMPLE REPORT OF QUALITY SCORES FOR ONE OBJECTIVE

OBJECTIVE 1	UNIT 1
Condition is assessed on admission	45
Data relevant to care are ascertained	72
Current conditon is assessed	65
The written plan is formulated	60
Plan is coordinated with medical plan	84
	Nursing Care Plan is Formulated
	65

Another standard used in this sytem relates to staffing of the unit. Each unit has a staffing pattern based on its workload index. The workload index is formulated from the Rush-Medicus Patient Classification System. This classification system provides a checklist of indicators of nursing care required by each patient. These indicators reflect statements concerning the patient condition, basic care requirements and therapeutic needs.

Nurses check off those items which pertain to each patient for whom they are providing care. Each indicator has a point value. The total points accumulated for each patient determine the category or classification. There are four categories available, each representing an acuity level or the degree of the patient's dependence on nursing.

Using a Type 2 patient as the baseline, acuity values were ascribed to each patient type. The acuity values reflect the relative proportion of nursing time required for each patient type. The point range indicating patient type, the required number of nursing hours in 24 and the acuity value are presented in Table 3.

TABLE 3

CUMULATIVE POINT RANGE, REQUIRED HOURS AND ACUITY VALUE BY PATIENT TYPE

PATIENT TYPE	CUMMULATIVE POINT RANGE	REQUIRED HOURS PER 24	ACUITY VALUE
1	0 - 24	0 - 2	0.5
2	25 - 48	2 - 4	1.0
3	49 - 120	4 - 10	2.5
4	121+	10+	5.0

Based on prior experience with the data obtained from use of this classification system, each unit has a staffing plan to meet its expected workload. The classification system can be used on a daily basis to monitor staff utilization and on a long range basis to plan for staffing as patient care requirements change on a unit.

The workload on each unit is a function of the acuity of the patients and the census of the unit. The Workload Index (WI) is derived by multiplying the number of patients in each category by it's assigned acuity value as listed in Table 3. Thus the workload index is derived by the following formula: WI = Number of Type 1 Patients X 0.5 + Number of Type 2 Patients X 1.0 + Number of Type 3 Patients X 2.5 + Number of Type 4 Patients X 5.0. An average acuity for the patient care unit can also be determined by the following formula:

$$\text{AVERAGE ACUITY} = \frac{\text{Unit Workload Index}}{\text{Patient Unit Census}}$$

An example will be provided to illustrate the derivation of the Workload Index and Average Acuity for a patient care unit. Suppose the patient care unit has a census of 40 patients distributed across patient types as follows:

2	Patient Type	Number	Acuity Values		Workload Points	
	1		14	x	0.5	7.0
	2		15	x	1.0	16.0
	3		10	x	2.5	25.0
	4		1	x	5.0	5.0
			40			53.0

With a census of 40 patients the workload index on this unit is 53 or equivalent to having 53 Type 2 patients on the unit. The average acuity on the patients care unit would be 53/40 or 1.3 indicting that the average patient is demanding a little more nursing time than a Type 2 patient.

Each patient care unit has an assigned number of hours of nursing time for each unit of workload index. By multiplying the workload index by the assigned hours the number of nursing hours needed to staff the unit is determined. If the unit in the example above was assigned 3.8 hours of nursing time per workload index, then the nursing hours needed on that unit would be 53 x 3.8 or a total of 201.4 for a twenty-four hour period.

We now have two types of standards identified in this system: one for the quality of performance expected of the nursing system and one for the staffing projected to meet patient requirements for nursing care. With these two standards set, the next task of the nurse manager in the control process is to design a reporting system. Designing a useful reporting system is an arduous and ever changing project. As nurse managers become more familiar with and sophisticated in the use of management information, requests for format changes and special reports emerge. Presented here will be some examples of computer calculated and printed reports for nurse managers at the patient care unit level and the departmental (comprising multiple patient care units) level.

A unit summary report is illustrated in Figure 2. This report is issued every four weeks to each patient care unit and is cumulative with each report. Each item on the report represents data desired by nurse managers in this particular setting. In order to understand this report some discussion of each section is required.

The first section on the report, QUALITY SCORES (OBJ) represents the scores obtained by the unit on each of the six major objectives if the unit was monitored for its quality performance during the report period. A more detailed report of the quality scores is provided in a separate report which is illustrated in Figure 3.

The second section labeled UNIT STATISTICS, true to its title, relates a number of statistics about the unit including the average workload index and average acuity index for the four week period covered by the report.

The next section, STAFFING, identifies two groups of staff and reports the average number of actual hours worked in every twenty-four. Group 1 refers to fully oriented registered nurses while Group 2 would include everyone else such as licensed practical nurses, nurses awaiting licensure or completing orientation, and nursing assistants.

The TOTAL PERSONNEL section reports several statistics with regard to the staffing of the patient care unit. The first item indicates the average actual hours of nursing care provided for each 24 hours during the report period. The second item notes the average suggested number of hours, based on the workload index, per 24 hours. Subtracting the suggested staffing from the actual staffing indicates either the amount of oversupply or undersupply of nursing hours. In the three examples shown here the unit was understaffed during each period. The next two items relate to temporary staffing. The first represents a hospital "float pool" and the second outside agencies providing temporary staffing.

The % PERSONNEL DISTRIBUTION represents the ratio of the Group 1 nursing staff category to the Group 2 category. This may be useful in interpreting what is occuring on nursing units. If the Group 1 staffing declines while Group 2 increases, quality may be affected.

PRODUCTIVITY is defined here in a narrow sense, representing two commonly used statistics. The first is the average actual nursing hours provided per Workload Index. The second is the more common measure of the average actual nursing hours provided per patient day.

The MISCELLANEOUS section contains several statistics of importance to nurse managers. Included here are the average sick and absent time, vacation and holiday time, and overtime hours in every 24 hours.

FIGURE 2

NURSING SYSTEMS MANAGEMENT PROGRAM

Sample Unit Summary Report

Date: Today
Unit Name: My Unit

Reporting Period	2	4	7
Quality Scores (Objective)			
1. The Plan of Nursing Care is Formulated	62		65
2. The Physical Needs of the Patients are Attended	71		88
3. The Non-Physical Needs of the Patient are Attended	74		84
4. Achievement of Nursing Care Objective is Evaluated	47		65
5. Unit Procedures are Followed for the Protection of all Patients	83		87
6. The Delivery of Nursing Care is Facilitated	76		72
Unit Statistics			
Beds	30	30	30
Average % Occupancy (10 am)	90	93	96
Average Acuity	2.0	2.0	1.5
Average Workload Index	56.4	55.2	44.7
Average Total 10 am Census	28	28	29
Average Midnight Census	30	28	29
Staffing			
Group 1 Actual HRS/24 HRS	93.75	116.73	69.69
Group 2 Actual HRS/24 HRS	25.35	25.67	80.80
Total Personnel			
Actual HRS/24	119.10	142.40	150.49
Suggested HRS/24	214.32	209.76	169.86
Actual-Suggested/24	95.22-	67.36-	19.37-
Actual TPT/24	18.50	5.50	2.77
Actual Agency/24	10.50	0.00	3.38
% Personnel Distribution			
Group 1	78.72	81.97	46.31
Group 2	21.28	18.03	53.69

FIGURE 2 (Continued)

Reporting Period	2	4	7
Productivity			
Average Actual Total HRS/WI	2.4	2.7	3.4
Average Actual Total HRS/PD	4.91	5.28	5.28
Miscellaneous			
Sick/ABS HRS/24	12.50	16.35	5.64
VAC/HOL HRS/24	8.64	14.55	9.43
Overtime HRS/24	9.67	17.63	8.91
Personnel Cost			
Cost/Patient Day			
Payroll	47.64	69.25	64.17
Agency (Estimated)	4.49	0.00	1.57
TPT (Estimated)	6.33	1.68	0.76
Number Full Days			
Reported	16	24	26

The next to the last section PERSONNEL COST breaks down the average personnel costs for the three sources of nursing staff used at the hospital. The first is those nurses on the regular payroll of the hospital; the second is those nurses secured through an outside agency providing temporary staffing; and the third is the nursing staff used from the hospital's own temporary staffing system.

The final statistic reflects the number of days the unit completed the reports needed to complete the input data to generate this report. There are a total of 28 days in each reporting period.

Although quality of care scores are presented by the six major objective in the Sample Unit Summary Report illustrated in Figure 2, a more detailed report is provided as shown in Figure 3. In this report, scores are provided for each of the subobjectives comprising the total instrument. Thus, the nurse manager can examine performance standards more specifically.

With the information provided by the report a number of pictorial representations of the data can be done by the computer. Graphics provide assistance in seeing trends and relationships which are not as readily seen in the numbers of the report.

One of these pictorial displays is illustrated in figure 4. Here the suggested staffing based on the Workload Index of the Patient Care Unit is displayed in terms of full time equivalents (FTE's). The suggested staffing is represented by the letter S while the actual staffing is represented by an A.

Another pictorial representation of data is provided in Figure 5. This figure shows the changes which have occurred on one unit over the four periods in which the quality of nursing care was monitored in the past year. The scores are those reported for each of the six major objectives of the instrument used to measure quality.

At the departmental level, a departmental summary report of the same format as the unit summary report is provided to each nurse manager for each four week reporting period. This report differs in that data on all the units in the department are reported on the same page. This provides the Department Manager with an overview of the entire department at one time.

Graphic representations are also provided for the manager at the departmental level. A picture of staffing levels for each of the units in the department, the plot in Figure 6, is an example. Here the nurse manager can review the staffing situation on each unit for each reporting period in relation to the target level of staffing. In this particular department the staffing target level for units A, B, D, and J is 3.8 hours per Workload Index. This is indicated by the disconnected line across the graph.

In order to produce such reports a system for securing all the measurements needed for the reports, was devised by the nurse managers. Once the nurse managers decided on what information was desired, the best sources for the acquisition of the data were identified. The jobs of collection, co-ordination and production were then dealt with to make a workable system for all. As seemed most appropriate the work of data collection was divided into four basic sections. The first part takes place at the unit level where both nursing personnel and unit clerks are responsible for initiating the patient classification report which subsequently provides the data on which the Workload Index and staffing standards are figured by the computer.

FIGURE 3

NURSING SYSTEMS MANAGEMENT PROGRAM

Sample Unit Quality Report

Date: Today
Unit Names: My Unit

Reporting Period	2	7
Quality Scores		
The condition of the patient is assessed on admission	70	66
Data relevant to hospital care are ascertained on admission	80	79
The current conditon of the patient is assessed	44	20
The written plan of nursing care is formulated	42	55
The plan of nursing care is coordinated with the medical plan of care	75	70
1. Nursing Care Plan Formulated	62	65
The patient is protected from accident and injury	83	93
The need for physical comfort and rest is attended	80	88
The need for physical hygiene is attended	80	100
The need for a supply of oxygen is attended	78	96
The need for activity is attended	83	50
The need for nutrition and fluid is attended	17	83
The need for elimination is attended	33	100
The need for skin care is attended	33	75
The patient is protected from infection	100	80

Figure 3 (continued)

2. Patient Physical Needs Attended	71	88

The patient is oriented to hospital facilities
on admission ... 94 ... 77
The patient is extended social courtesy by the
nursing staff ... 88 ... 100
The patient's privacy and civil rights are honored ... 68 ... 92
The need for psychological-emotional well-being
is attended through interpersonal communication ... 88 ... 96
The patient is taught measures of health maintenance
and illness prevention ... 83 ... 69
The patient's family is included in the nursing
process ... 25 ... 56
The need for psycho-emotional well-being is
attended through therapeutic milieu

3. Non-Physical Needs Attended	74	84

Records document the care provided for the patient ... 29 ... 61
The patient's response to therapy is evaluated ... 75 ... 70

4. Achievement of Objectives Evaluated	47	65

Unit procedures followed for patient's protection ... 100 ... 100
The unit is prepared for emergency situations ... 83 ... 95
Medical-legal procedures are followed
Safety and protective procedures are followed ... 33 ... 0

Reporting Period ... 2 ... 7

5. Unit Procedures are Followed	83	87

Nursing reporting follows prescribed standards ... 68 ... 76
Nursing management is provided ... 76 ... 67
Clerical services are provided ... 85 ... 80
Environmental and housekeeping services are provided ... 76 ... 57
Professional and administrative services are
provided ... 77 ... 87

6. Delivery of Care Facilities	76	72

The departmental office secretary pulls together a daily report of patient
classification and staffing for each of the units in the department. The bulk
of co-ordination and preparation of the reports takes place in the office of
Nursing Systems Management. Here all the departmental data is reviewed for
completion and accuracy. In addition census reports are prepared along with
temporary personnel usage. Quality monitoring is also co-ordinated and done by
personnel associated with Nursing Systems Management.

Once all the data is secured and in order it is submitted to the data processing
department for the editing run. After the editing is completed by the Nursing
Systems Management office it is resubmitted to data processing for production of
the final management reports such as those illustrated earlier.

The nurse manager at each level, provided with the best objective data
available, can begin the process of analysis of the performance of staff within
each patient care unit or department. This data can be used to evaluate

FIGURE 4

NURSING SYSTEMS MANAGEMENT PROGRAM

SAMPLE ACTUAL VERSUS SUGGESTED STAFFING PLOT

Date: Today
Unit Name: My Unit

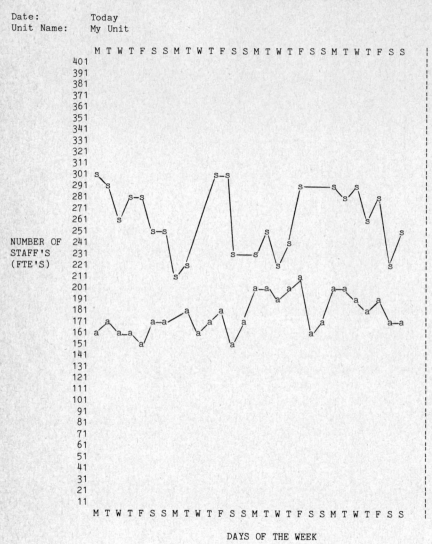

DAYS OF THE WEEK

FIGURE 5

NURSING SYSTEMS MANAGEMENT PROGRAM

SAMPLE QUALITY SCORE PLOT

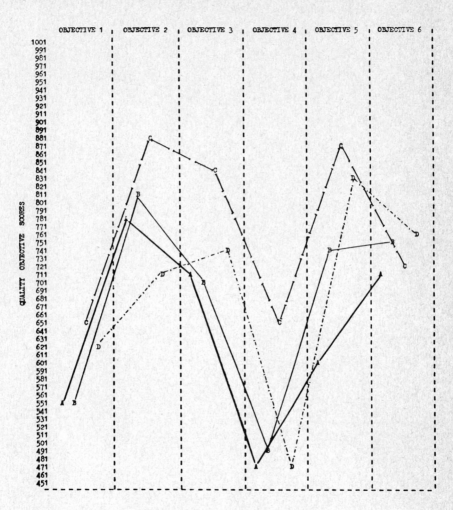

FIGURE 6

NURSING SYSTEMS MANAGEMENT PROGRAM

SAMPLE DEPARTMENT HOURS PER WORKLOAD INDEX PLOT

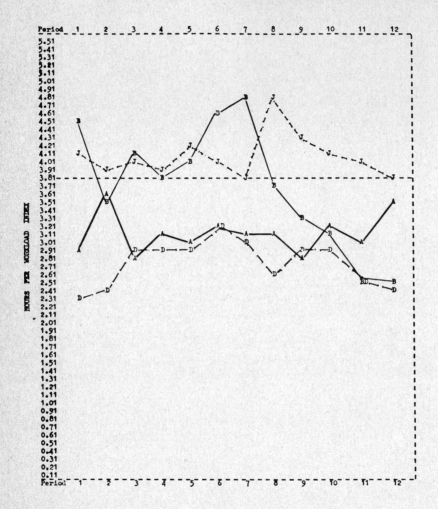

previous plans resulting in rewards and recognition for good performance or in changes for areas where performance has not met the expected standard. Thus feedback is provided for continuing the processes of planning, organizing, staffing, directing and controlling.

Thus a computer can assist the nurse manager in the control process of management. By providing a system whereby a set of standards, made measureable in the specification of a large number of criteria, nursing care quality can be measured. The collection of information regarding the context within which the nursing care is delivered provides additional important data for analysis of the system. The usefulness of the computer in generating a variety of reports and graphics has been illustrated.

As nurse managers have become more familiar with the use of the kind of information provided by the system, they have demanded more timeliness and flexibility in the system and the generation of reports to meet individual needs. Since the system is currently a batch approach it is difficult to conform to some of the nurse managers requirements. The area which is of particular interest on a day to day basis is the workload of the unit. In periods of acute staffing shortages this information becomes of paramount importance in making decisions regarding the allocation of scarce resources. For this purpose nurse managers may wish to use a micro or mini-computer. This would also afford them the opportunity of performing additional analyses or generation of specific reports not provided by the centralized services.

Based on these experiences it would seem that what would be helpful for nurse managers are some computer tools which are specifically designed to provide them with timely data, easy retrieval, useful analyses and a variety of reporting formats. Hardware and software which is user friendly could be developed for data collection, storage, retrieval and analysis. With the addition of word processing, findings could be communicated in the form of written reports to summarize or further discuss study results.

Today's nurse manager has a very useful and powerful tool in the computer. There is nothing like "seeing" on paper what is happening in patient care areas to assist in bringing about changes needed toward assuring quality of nursing care.

REFERENCES

1.   Mackenzie, R.A. The management process in 3D. **The Journal of Nursing Administration**, 1979, 9(11), 30-34.

2.   Haussmann, R.K., Hegyvary, S., & Newman, J.F. **Monitoring quality of nursing care, part 2, assessment and study of correlates** (DHEW Publication No. HRA 76-77). Washington, D.C.: U.S. Government Printing Office, 1976.

The Impact of Computers on Nursing
M. Scholes, Y. Bryant and B. Barber (eds.)
Elsevier Science Publishers B.V. (North-Holland)
© IFIP-IMIA, 1983

15.5.

COMBINED NURSING MANAGEMENT

Discussion

Before discussing the role of computers in nursing management it is appropriate to define nursing management. Each of the chapters deals with nursing management from a slightly different perspective yet the same themes often appear. Nursing management includes global management such as planning for an entire institution or district. It includes day-to-day unit operations and activities to analyse problems, establish priorities, goals and procedures and requires information gathering and dissemination to higher levels of heirarchy to insure that needed resources are forthcoming and to lower levels of heirarchy to insure that the institutions purposes are understood and achieved.

Nurse Managers require information:-

1. to reduce uncertainty, e.g. are her expenditures currently within budget?
2. to link together multiple variables that clarify a situation e.g. why is there a high staff turnover or what factors are affecting quality of patient care?
3. to assess patient needs and convert this assessment into a budget of resources to meet these needs
4. to support the rationale for organisational change and to reinforce the efforts of those implementing the change by providing them with feedback.

A continual nursing management responsibility is the balancing of manpower, finance and productivity where productivity includes quantity, quality and outcome. Productivity information is inevitably linked to patient assessment information which has been a subject of the patient care stream. It is these information needs in nursing management that computerisation should assist. Without well designed computer systems, nursing managers do not have:

1. data that is timely
2. data that is linked and presented in such a manner that it is readily interpreted
3. or in some instances do not have the data at all because it must be abstracted from some activity or data set that is not primarily within nursing jurisdiction and it would be exceedingly expensive in time and manpower to obtain it.

Nursing can turn to two sources to supply their information needs.

1. central computing departments (institutional or regional)
2. establish their own computer resources

Nursing management is quite willing to utilise central computer services provided the services are timely, relevant, responsive and adequate. Where they are not, the advent of the micro and the mini are making it possible for the individual nurse management department to undertake the computerisation of its own information needs. This has implications for the allocation of computing resources and the compatibility of diverse data bases.

In addition to the procurement of computer services nurse managers are increasingly sensitive to their staffs information needs in order to encourage superior nursing performance but at the same time they are concerned about the burden on their staff to generate, collect and record data that nurses and/or non-nurses require. As the data gathering burden grows, nurse managers are demanding that required information be produced as a by-product of nurses patient-care activities. Computerisation in many instances is the only possible way of achieving this.

Although nursing management can be defined as above for the countries represented at the conference, the administrative structure of the health service of each country is different. Therefore, each nurse manager must also carry out her tasks in relation to the particular administrative structure of her country. Her access to resources (financial, personnel and computers) will differ from country to country and here the protocol for obtaining computing resources will also differ. It must, therefore, be recognised that any international conference on nursing management and computers will inevitably have to discuss the management issues within the context of each countries health care system and the larger sociological orientation of the country (the role of unions, political cost consciousness, etc). Purely technological discussion and recommendations must be tempered with national insight. Therefore, although some conclusions and recommendations can be universal, others will pertain to particular countries.

The following questions were addressed in both papers and discussion.

Do the papers presented reflect current endeavours?

The range of papers was highly representative and it seemed they sufficed to elucidate nursing management computer activities and further discussion to enumerate other applications was considered to be not as productive as discussions on other questions.

Are there any specific areas that require research and the next step?

1. Nursing intention and nursing objectives should be well defined and their discrepancy from the reality of nursing understood. Computerised systems should be supporting the intention and objective of nursing yet be able to function in the real world. Nursing management cannot expect computer personnel to interpret nursing objectives and reality, they have an obligation to define it and communicate it.
2. Nursing must understand the role of finance departments and other supporting services so that their systems will relate appropriately. Nursing Management systems cannot proceed totally in isolation.
3. Standardised coding
4. How to evaluate systems
5. How to develop plans for computerisation, both short term and long term
6. Specific systems that should be worked on are:
    (a) patient dependency (also known as diagnostic coding), patient assessment. These concepts are different, but generally useful for nurse managers.
    (b) quality evaluation and assurance systems
    (c) manpower/financial linkage

Could the resources devoted to computing be more effectively deployed within health care?

It was impossible to answer this question directly since it can probably only be answered when one must compare a particular computerised system with other candidates needs, their respective budgets etc. The question is an important one and should be answered in particular situations. The group discussed related issues as follows :-

1. Opportunity costing should be part of the protocol to plan and evaluate computer systems.
2. Enthusiasm for new systems and technology should not impede unbiased evaluation
3. The present cost of doing things manually should be considered
4. The cost of not computerising should be considered
5. Can better use be made of existing computer resources?
6. Can better use be made of existing data?
7. Proposers of systems should not suffer from guilt about asking for resources. The assumption is they are convinced, at their level, of their appropriateness.
8. The allocation of resources is not only short term, but long term and both short term and long term computerisation plans should be prepared.
9. Computer resources will most likely be obtained if a nurse manager moves her proposal properly through the administrative hierarchy of planning and budgeting.
10. The buying powers of large health authorities such as the UK health service should be utilised to secure computer hardware and software well suited for their needs.

How do we facilitate the systems analyst/computer professional – nursing manager interaction to secure effective systems?

Both the nursing managers and the computer professionals emphasized the necessity for

1. communication
2. joint planning of systems
3. understanding of each others vocabulary, professional frame of reference, work setting, work problems.
4. feedback during implementation and use
5. the appropriate size of working groups
6. committee representatives and/or liaison personnel should:
    (a)   have the authority to definitively represent their group
    (b)   have the knowledge to explain their needs in detail
    (c)   the personality to relate to the other team members and to their own constituency in order to secure acceptance of decisions taken and systems designed.
7. The users should specify the functional aspects of systems, but in sufficient detail that there requirements are not ambiguous to the computer personnel.
8. The sharing of office space and mutual visits to each professions working environment is encouraged.
9. Manual systems, their protocol intent and content must be well understood before they are computerised.

The broad category of centralised systems versus decentralised ones was discussed from several viewpoints.

1. Computer services can be obtained through large centralised systems or by using mini and microcomputers sited locally or within units. There are technological arguments in favour of each approach. However, the impetus to the decentralised approach is either un-timeliness or non-existence of centralised support for local needs.
2. Centralised services are obviously needed for regional and national planning and, if local computer services are going to replace some centralised srvices, planning must assure data base compatibility and integrity in those situations where regional planning is dependent on the local data base.

3. The centralised/decentralised processing relationship leads to the concept of cascaded data. This is defined as follows: a cascaded system of information/data would proceed from ward --- department --- district --- region. Those data elements that are required at higher echelons will proceed upward from their regions in a standard form. Data elements not required at higher echelons will be controlled at their level of origin.
4. The centralised systems feedback is necessary to the local levels.
5. Centralised systems can achieve economy of scale. On the other hand, if centralised systems are separated from users by many bureaucratic or hierarchical layers it becomes difficult for users to obtain services suited to their needs.
6. It may be that the design of systems to service regions beyond a certain size effectively is extremely difficult because within increasing size of user population there is an attendant increase in numbers of diverse requirements.

System acceptance.

1. Installed systems must sometimes be modified to make them a success. This should not be a cause for discouragement, but seen as a learning experience.
2. The nursing staff must be educated about the benefits as well as the use of any systems installed in their area.
3. Non-nursing personnel will participate in nursing computer systems in proportion to the systems' usefulness to them.
4. The confidentiality of sensitive information must be guaranteed.

CHAPTER 16

RESEARCH

Many nurses have used computers as a tool for their research projects, but few have undertaken research into the impact of computers on nursing. Has the process of preparing data for computers made us think more systematically about Nursing? Has it focussed our attention on the individual patient's needs or the individual student's requirements - or has it returned us to lists of tasks to be completed?

The Impact of Computers on Nursing
M. Scholes, Y. Bryant and B. Barber (eds.)
Elsevier Science Publishers B.V. (North-Holland)
© IFIP-IMIA, 1983

16.1.

INFORMATION USE IN NURSING PRACTICE

Margaret R. Grier

The purpose of an information system is to provide data that are necessary for making decisions. In nursing the two major decisions are judgements about the patient's health state and choices of actions for the inferred health state.(1) Thus attention must be focused on the information needed to diagnose health problems and to choose nursing actions in developing a computerized system of information for nursing. A nursing information system can be modeled according to how humans process information or according to formal rules of logic, but given the lack of knowledge about information use in nursing, the former is prerequisite to the latter. The purpose of this paper is to present what research has revealed about how nurses identify, acquire, and use clinical data in making nursing decisions, and to discuss the implications of these findings for the computerization of nursing information.

Model

The model of information processing for making nursing decisions that will be addressed in the paper is depicted in Figure 1. As shown in the figure, the process begins with a patient situation (the vector X). Datum (d), from which information is derived, can be obtained on many patient variables, but data about the defining characteristics (d) of hypothesized health states (h:dx) are sought. The relationships of the hypotheses are determined and the hypothesis with the strongest association between the two becomes the inferred nursing diagnosis [dx=f(d ,d], and if confirmed, the selected diagnosis (dx*). Once a diagnosis is made, criteria (c) for measuring attainment of the desired outcomes of nursing care are established. Alternative nursing actions (a) expected to lead to the desired health state are specified and potential outcomes (o) of the set of actions identified. The optimal action is chosen by evaluating the potential outcomes or, in other words, by assessing the expected values (EVs) of the actions for achieving the desired outcome. The nursing action having the highest EV* is the one that will optimize benefits at the lowest risk or costs. After the chosen action is implemented, the resulting outcome data (o'd') are obtained and compared with the criteria for the desired state (o'd'<>c). The information derived from this calculation is returned to the information system for subsequent decision making.

Framework

Florence Nightingale, the eminent nurse scientist, provided a useful framework(2) for using clinical information as described in Figure 1. Nightingale said that observation and reflection were essential conditions of nursing practice, and implied that nursing judgements (or diagnoses), nursing actions, and evaluation resulted from these processes. To quote Nightingale:(3) 'Observation tells us the fact, reflection the meaning of the fact..... Observation tells how the patient is, reflection tells what is to be done.' (p.255) Other statements made by Nightingale that are relevant to this paper were:

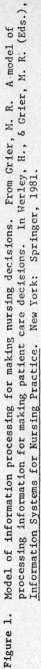

Figure 1. Model of information processing for making nursing decisions. From Grier, M. R. A model of processing information for making patient care decisions. In Werley, H., & Grier, M. R. (Eds.), Information Systems for Nursing Practice. New York: Springer, 1981.

'It is most important to observe the symptoms of illness; it is, if possible, more important still to observe the symptoms of nursing: of what is the fault, not of the illness, but of the nursing.' (p.255)(3) 'The most important office of the nurse is to take care to observe the effect of (a nursing action).' (p.75)(4) Training must show her (the nurse) how the effects on life of nursing may be calculated with nice precision - such care or carelessness, such a sick-rate; such a death rate.' (p.24-34)(5)   'Instead of asking 'has he had a good night' ask 'how many hours has he slept!' (p.105)(4) 'Observation may always be improved by training, will indeed seldom be found without training: for otherwise the nurse does not know what to look for.' 'Training and experience are, of course, necessary to teach us, too, how to observe, what to observe, how to think, what to think.' 'Reflection needs training as much as observation.' 'Telling the nurse what to do is not enough and cannot be enough to perfect her, whatever her surroundings.   The trained power of attending to one's own impressions made by one's own senses, so that these should tell the nurse how the patient is, is the **sine qua non** of being a nurse at all.' (p.254-255)(3)

Unfortunately, nursing has been so preoccupied with **what** nurses do that little attention has been given to the cognitive processes that Nightingale identified as fundamental to the practice of nursing: identifying what nurses should look for and observe, measuring the relevant dimensions of health, calculating the effects of nursing care and medical treatment, and most lacking, what and how to think about and analyze the data obtained. Beginning in the 1960s, however, attention has been given to the cognitive processes and information use that underlies nursing practice. These research findings will be presented within Nightingale's framework of:

Observation - Identifing and acquiring data on health states and the effects of nursing care and medical treatment.
Reflection - Weighing and combining information derived from the data to select nursing diagnoses, setting nursing goals, and choose nursing actions.

Observation

1.   Identifying Data

The lack of specifics about what nurses should observe is a major problem since such knowledge is the basis for nursing diagnoses which, in turn, are the focus of nursing actions!   Nurses are taught and expected to gather data about everything, a task that is inefficient and counterproductive in complex health care situations(6).   This expectation may have arisen from possible biological differences between males and females, from different job patterns for men and women, from the organization of clinical settings, and from the nursing goal of total patient care.

There are indications that the functioning of the right and left hemispheres of the brain differ between males and females, and that females are more skilled in divergent thinking (and thus information gathering and processing), while males are more skilled in convergent thinking (and thus decision making)(7,8). Female jobs were found to involve higher use of information sources and more information processing, while male jobs involve more decision making, presumably using the data gathered in the female positions(9).   Hammond(6) noted that nurses are expected to be observers for physicians, that they rely on perceptual rather than cognitive skills, because of the focus on acting rather than thinking and are nonselective in gathering data.   These characteristics of clinical practice probably lead to the information overload of nurses found by Bailey McDonald and Claus(10) and Gordon(11).

The use of nurses to gather data is not peculiar to nursing, but is characteristic of females and the jobs they hold. In addition, this function facilitates the nursing goal of providing and/or co-ordinating total patient care. It also is the source of much covert power in that nurses have more knowledge about the patient than other health care workers. Computerization will make it easier to expect others to handle clinical data, but such changes should be approached with a great deal of caution. Given our goal of caring for the total patient and the fact that power is associated with the amount of information, nursing should retain the responsibility for gathering clinical data. Rather than changing the pattern, efforts would be better placed toward improving nurses' skills and methods for acquiring, and processing clinical data, with a focus on identifying and using that information which is essential to nursing care.

First and foremost among these efforts is to describe precisely the dimensions of health and to identify specifically the human responses to disease and its treatment and care. The five National Conferences on Nursing Diagnoses, begun in 1973 within the United States, have begun this important work(12). With the 1982 Conference, 40 nursing diagnoses and their defining characteristics had been identified and a theoretical framework for the diagnoses had been set forth (Table 1). In addition, about 20 to 30 investigations of nursing diagnoses were underway.

Table 1: Nursing Diagnoses According to Characteristics of Unitary Man

1.	Anxiety	Feeling
2.	Body fluids, excess	Exchanging
3.	Fluid volume deficit, active loss	
4.	Fluid volume deficit, failure of regularity mechanism	
5.	Fluid volume deficit potential	
6.	Bowel elimination, alteration in: constipation	
7.	Bowel elimination, alteration in: diarrhea	
8.	Bowel elimination, alteration in: impaction	
9.	Bowel elimination, alteration in: incontinence	
10.	Cardiac output, alterations in	
11.	Circulation, interruption of	
12.	Comfort, alteration in: pain	Feeling
13.	Consciousness, altered levels of	Waking
14.	Coping patterns, family, ineffective	Choosing
15.	Coping patterns, individual, maladaptive	
16.	Functional performance, variations in	Moving
17.	Functional performance, variations in home maintenance	Moving Choosing
18.	Grieving	Valuing Feeling
19.	Impairment of significant others, adjustment to illness	Choosing Relating Feeling
20.	Injury, potential for	Exchanging
21.	Injury, susceptibility to hazard	Exchanging

22.	Knowledge, lack of	Knowing
23.	Mobility, impairment of	Moving
24.	Noncompliance	Choosing
25.	Nutrition, alterations in: less than body requirements	
26.	Nutrition, alterations in: more than body requirements	Exchanging
27.	Nutrition, changes related to body requirements	
28.	Nutrition, alterations in: actual or potential	
29.	Parenting, alterations in: actual or potential	Relating Communicating, Valuing
30.	Respiratory dysfunction	Exchanging
31.	Self-concept, alterations in body image, self-esteem, role performance, personal identity	Valuing
32.	Sensory/perceptual alterations	Perceiving
33.	Sexuality, alterations in patterns of	Relating, Communicating, Valuing
34.	Skin integrity, impairment of: actual	
35.	Skin integrity, impairment of; potential	Exchanging
36.	Sleep/rest activity	Waking
37.	Spirituality: spiritual concerns	
38.	Spirituality: spiritual distress	Valuing
39.	Spirituality: spiritual despair	
40.	Tissue perfusion, alteration, chronic	
41.	Urinary elimination, impairment of: alterations in patterns	
42.	Urinary elimination: incontinence	Exchanging
43.	Urinary elimination:..retention	

Note: From Kim, M. J., & Moritz, D. A. (Eds). Classification of nursing
diagnoses. New York: McGraw-Hill, 1982, p- 275-277.

The 37 nursing diagnoses listed in Table 1 were found to explain 52% of the
varients in nursing workload for 2,560 hospitalized patients (Table 2), as
compared to 26% of the varients explained by 31 diagnostic related grouping
(DRG's) of 383 medical diagnoses(13). A combination of the nursing diagnoses
and DRGs was the best predictor of nursing workload, with nursing diagnoses
explaining 45% of the variation, medical condition 15% and 40% unexplained.
Among the 37 diagnoses studied, five factors were the chief contributors to the
workload of the nurse: the patient's mental status, elimination patterns,
disabilities, post-surgical conditions, and cardiopulmonary conditions. The
psychosocial nursing diagnoses contributed little to the total variation in
nursing workload. A project is underway in New Jersey, United States, to
include nursing diagnoses with medical diagnoses for establishing hospital
charges.

TABLE 2:   PEARSON CORRELATIONS FOR NURSING DIAGNOSES AND DAILY NURSING WORKLOAD FOR 2560 PATIENTS

Nursing Diagnoses	r*
Altered Level of Consciousness	.520
Thought Process Impaired	.471
Altered Ability to Perform Self-Care	.467
Less Nutrition Than Required	.465
Altered Ability to Perform Hygiene	.447
Impairment of Mobility	.418
Sensory Perceptual Alterations	.388
Alteration of Urinary Pattern	.367
Dysrhythm of Sleep-Rest Activity	.361
Potential Impairment in Skin Integrity	.359
Depletion of Body Fluids	.353
Confusion	.351
Decreased Cardiac Output	.337
Bowel Incontinence	.317
Excess Body Fluids	.307
Respiratory Dysfunction	.275
Actual Impairment of Skin Integrity	.261
Urinary Retention	.255
Altered Self-Concents: Body Image	.252
Altered Composition of Body Fluids	.246
Moderate Anxiety	.214
Urinary Incontinence	.206
Severe Anxiety	.206
Non-compliance	.204
Bowel Impaction	.187
Bowel Constipation	.162
Diarrhea	.151
Pain	.142
Panic	.139
Potential Nutritional Alteration	.134
Acute Grieving	.116
Delayed Grieving	.113
Discomfort	.107
Manipulation	.092
Anticipatory Grieving	.078
Mild Anxiety	.074
More Nutrition Than Required	.061

Note: From Halloran, E.   Analysis of variation in nursing workload by patient medical and nursing condition.   Doctoral dissertation, University of Illinois Medical Center, 1981.

*$p < .01$

In addition to the work of the diagnoses conferences, The Visiting Nurse Association in Omaha, Nebraska, United States, is developing and computerizing a nursing classification system with funding from the Division of Nursing, United States Public Health Service, Department of Health and Human Services. Based on standard nursing practice in community health, 49 community health problems with descriptive signs and symptoms, and 580 outcomes with 2,125 criteria, have been identified and coded for computer processing. Work is continuing on identifying the nursing interventions and the actual outcomes of the nursing interventions for inclusion in the system.

While the reliability and validity of the identified nursing diagnoses of health problems have not been systematically tested, they have content validity as judged by nurses from across the United States, and pragmatic validity as shown by the above studies and by their wide acceptance in nursing practice within the United States.   Also, it is understood that the diagnoses are being used in Canada and Japan, although use in these countries is not yet described.   What is needed are formal studies of the reliability of the nursing diagnoses, as well as of their discriminant and predictive validity.

In describing nursing diagnoses the necessity of a standardized nomenclature for the diagnostic concepts and their various dimensions became obvious(14). Standardization of language is evolving haphazardly in the United States, but concerted and systematic effort to internationally standardize the labels and indicators for nursing diagnoses internationally is much needed.   The computerization of nursing data will make the standardization of nursing nomenclature more critical.

Nursing diagnoses should be the means for relating a nursing data base to data bases from other areas of health care, such as medical, pharmacy and social work.   Nursing diagnoses should be related to medical diagnoses in particular, because medical treatment and nursing care are inter-related with nursing sharing with physicians some responsibilities for medical diagnoses and treatments.   This stance does not negate the importance of defining independent nursing diagnoses, but in fact, makes clear delineation of those concepts more important if efficient and useful information systems are to be developed for all areas of health care.

Also, the development of theoretical frameworks for nursing diagnoses must continue.   Theory that describes nursing experiences, that explains facts about nursing, and that predicts circumstances occuring in practice, are necessary. These concepts then become specified and labelled as nursing diagnoses with associated nursing actions and outcomes.   Organizing a system of nursing information according to nursing theory gives meaning to the nursing process, and aids the thinking that accompanies that process.   The derived nursing diagnoses form the foundation and initiating frame of the system, to which nursing goals, nursing actions, and patient outcomes are related (See Figure 1).

While existing computerized information systems probably include nonstandard nursing diagnoses since they are based on plans of care for specific health problems, what is lacking in most systems is a conceptual framework for organising and integrating the information and directing its use.   Such a framework is essential to logical, efficient, and consistent use of information. Based on existing nursing theories, a framework of unitary man with constructs of interaction, action, and awareness was proposed by the National Conferences on Nursing Diagnoses; characteristics of these constructs are listed in Table 1. Faculty at the University of Maryland identified motion, sensation, cognition, and affiliation as concepts of nursing practice, and listed integration, associativity, ascendancy, and concurrence as expressions of health and illness associated with the concepts(15).   In addition, 10 nursing actions for these expressions were proposed as regulatory processes.   Descriptor terms for the concepts described by Neal(15) are being identified for a nursing information system retrieval system.

2.   Acquiring Data

Added to, or as a result of, the problem of undefined nursing data is the amount of data nurses collect.   The amount of data presented to nurses was described by Kelly(16) in a study of 118 cases of one nursing inference, pain.   Kelly found that nurses used 165 cues in diagnosing pain, that there were 58 doctors' orders for the pain, and that 17 nursing actions were implemented.   Gordon(11) found that nurses sought more data and were less accurate in their diagnoses when data were unrestricted than when data were restricted.

The nursing process directs nurses to collect data and then make judgements based on the vast amounts of data acquired. In keeping with this process, one of the first activities nursing students are taught is patient assessment before they learn what to assess! Thus nurses learn very early just to collect data without the tools for evaluating the data they collect. Grier, Johnson, and MacLean(17) found that if nursing students are taught strategies for making clinical decisions, the amount of data judged essential for making nursing judgements fell from an average of 55 to 41 items. While this reduction was significant, $F(1,89) = 16.43$, $P <.00$, information overload remains a problem since it is well established that the human brain can process only 7 ± 12 items of data at a given point in time.

While the large amount of data that nurses collect is a problem, a greater concern is the relevance of the data collected to the decision that must be made. None of the 165 cues to pain described by Kelly(16) conveyed more than trivial information, either singly or grouped; nurses selected data items sequentially, but the order of collection correlated only slightly ($r=.31$) with the information value of the cue. Elstein, Shulman, and Sprafka(18) found that the most common diagnostic error by physicians was using irrelevant data to confirm a diagnosis, a cognitive act they termed "overinterpretation". Cianfrani(19) found that increased amounts of irrelevant data decreased nurses' accuracy, both in hypothesizing possible diagnoses and in selecting the final diagnosis. Cianifrani concluded that identification of the data most relevant to nursing diagnoses would aid the diagnostic process in two ways: decrease the amounts of data as well as specify information that was essential for making a diagnosis.

Nondiagnostic, or irrelevant information, decreases the impact of relevant information, alters judgements, delays decision making, and can be hazardous to patients. The computerization of nursing data should help with this problem of an overload of irrelevant information since what data are to be included in a system must be identified and the system will do some of the processing. However, careful attention should be given to the diagnostic data included in a system, and this selection should be based on the relevance of the data to a given nursing diagnosis. The National Conferences on Nursing Diagnosis are specifying the patient characteristics that describe a nursing diagnosis, but once identified, the characteristics should be systematically addressed to determine their relationship to the diagnosis. Again, computerization can facilitate such work since the frequency with which a given characteristic occurs with a diagnosis can be determined from a computerized data base.

With computerization, data items that are the most highly correlated with nursing diagnoses can be differentiated from less relevant items, thus leading to a more precise and efficient information system. Data items which are irrelevent can be excluded, redefined, or included with other data bases. The goal 0 should be to include 5 to 9 items of diagnostic data, per diagnosis. This is because the human brain can process about $7<>2$ items of data at a given instance, although there are indications that about twelve items of related data can be processed by clustering or combining information(19,20). Certainly a computer can process larger amounts of data, but human capabilities is one approach to delimiting content of a nursing information system that will be exceptionally large, at best, given the current poorly defined data base.

Thus, a conceptual framework identifies those health problems about which information is needed in nursing practice. Standardized labels for those concepts, and a limited set of patient characteristics that define them, provide

the guide for acquiring data. As noted by Nightingale(3), knowing what to look
for is essention in skilled observation, but reflection also has a part.

Reflection

Deep and continued thought about clinical data is given little attention in
nursing, and even less opportunity in nursing practice. Computers can change
this because they require a logical sequencing of well-defined and precise data,
a necessary condition for diagnostic reasoning. From logically ordered data
about a patient, information is derived, from which a diagnosis is inferred,
then tested and concluded. While some computer systems support these decision
making processes (such as the system at Latter Day Saints Hospital in Salt Lake
City, Utah, United States) other systems only provide data they may or may not
be logically ordered, and many systems are primarily files for storing data.

1.   Weighing Information

To the extent that a computerized information system does not order data, derive
information, make and test decisions, these cognitive processes must be carried
out within the mind of the nurse. Cognitive strategies are needed that allow
the nurse to limit the information acquired and to use that information
efficiently in making choices. Hypothesizing possible diagnoses prior to
collecting data is one such strategy.

Arriving at possible diagnoses from data already gathered as currently expected
in nursing, requires personal or experimental observation and is inefficient in
complex situations. On the other hand, seeking data according to predetermined
hypotheses requires theoretical knowledge, but is a more efficient and accurate
strategy for the complexity of health care(6). Contrary to what is taught and
believed, physicians acquire facts about a patient with the aid of hypothesized
diagnoses.   Research has shown that experienced physicians generate 3 to 5
possible diagnoses during the first 1 to 5 minutes of patient encounter, and
then use these hypotheses as a guide for data collection(18). Because of the
lack of theoretical frameworks for nursing data, nurses first collect pages of
assessment data from which they are to generate hypotheses.   There is no
evidence that such hypothesizing occurs, and it is an ineffective and
inefficient strategy that probably leads to omission of the nursing diagnosis.

Once made, hypotheses can be tested singly or in groups. Testing each possible
diagnosis successively is slow but effective since each one is examined.
However, successive testing is cumbersome, cognitively taxing, and time
consuming, so only a few possible diagnosis can be individually examined, and
problems arise from limiting the number considered.   Hypotheses that are too
broad in scope may be retained, important diagnostic data that does not fit with
the hypotheses under consideration may be disregarded, while other data are
given undue importance to justify a possible diagnosis. On the other hand,
simultaneously testing of multiple hypotheses is more rapid than single
hypothesis testing (and thus may be necessary in complex situations), but is
difficult and risky.   Gordon(11) found that nurses use a mixed strategy of
testing multiple hypotheses in the first half of the diagnostic process and
single hypothesis testing in the latter half.   Initially nurses may examine
diagnoses simultaneousely to gain as much information as possible, to eliminate
hypotheses rapidly, and to reduce cognitive strain.   Elstein, Shulman, and
Sprafka(18) believed that the use of irrelevent data in confirming a medical
diagnosis, and the disregard of important data, resulted from the need to
simplify the diagnostic process and to restrict the number of hypotheses under
consideration.   Cianfrani(19) found that the number of incorrect hypotheses by
nurses increased as the amount of irrelevant data about a health problem
increased(See Fig 2).   Thus the optimal number of hypotheses to consider in
diagnosing health states remains unclear, and may vary with the skill of the
person making the judgement.

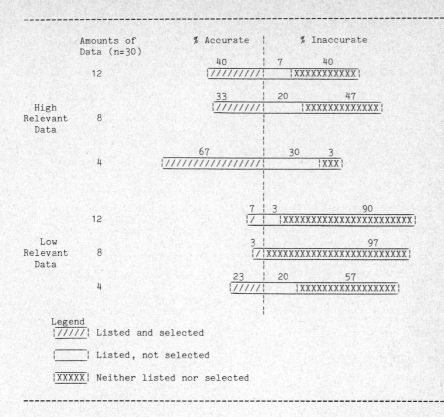

Figure 2
Nurses accurate in hypothesizing (listing) the health problem of alterations in comfort (chest pain) with varying amounts of relevance of data, and accurate in selecting the problem as their final diagnosis (N=180). From Cianfrani K, **The influence of amounts and relevance of data on identifying health problems.** Doctoral dissertation, University of Illinois Medical Center, 1982.

Another cognitive problem that occurs in the diagnostic process is the failure to revise existing hypotheses or to create new ones with new information. Hammond and his associates(6) found that nurses performed as well as a formal model in using new information for hypothesizing, but altered their final judgements only one third as much as the model. Johnson(21) found that nurses made decisions regarding pain relief measures prior to assessing the patient, and that these initial decisions were not modified with additional information. This is the problem of undue confidence on data that Elstein and his colleagues called overinterpretation.

A computer does not have the above limitations. It can sequentially search large or small amounts of data that are already in the system, or, by use of an algorythm request input of selected data. It can generate almost any number of hypotheses and systematically tests 1 or 20, with each item of data evaluated without bias. In carrying out these processes, the constraints of time and demands placed on busy clinicians are not factors, although even a computer can become overloaded and crash. If any group should make use of computers, nursing certainly should take advantage of such an aid.

2.   Selecting the Diagnosis

Whether hypotheses are generated early to guide data collection or generated from previously collected data, information must be derived from the data collected and weighed as to importance and relevance to the problem being considered. Based on the informational value, information is included or excluded into some clustering scheme(19). Within these clusters redundant and or related information are combined for selecting a diagnosis. These complex and unclear mental operations can be carried out logically, statistically, empirically, or intuitively(22,23), as well as by relating attributes or concepts(19). Whatever the strategy memory is an important element in this process. Research has shown that organized information is more easily retrieved from memory, which is another reason why a conceptual framework for an information system is so important. Physicians work with a hierarchy of hypotheses in diagnosing medical conditions(18), and Gordon(22) proposed a hierarchical structure for nursing diagnoses. The more limited, precise, and organised the information, the easier the selecting of a diagnosis.

3.   Setting Goals

Establishing goals that are related to the selected diagnosis is the first step in choosing a nursing action. From the standards of nursing practice and broad goals listed in most nursing texts, more specific outcomes that describe the state of health desired by and for the patient should be specified with criteria for their measurement. Criteria for measuring the desired outcomes should have three characteristics: related to the diagnosis, measurable, and realistic or achievable within a stated time. Research showed that goal setting is a major difficulty in nurse decision making. Althogh nurses minimize risk to patients, they do not optimize goals of nursing care(10,24). Johnson(21) found that risk to patients was the variable most frequently considered in choosing pain relief measures. Johnson(21) and Grier and Grier(25) found little relationship between nurses' varying goals and their selected measures for relieving pain. The Griers did find, however, that a systematic procedure for choosing analgesic medication led to choices more in keeping with the nurses' goals. In assessing recorded components of the nursing process, Sullivan(26) found that goals, evaluation, and reprocessing of evaluation data were omitted. In their recent 12-week study of teaching decision-making skills to undergraduate nursing students, Grier, Johnson and MacLean(17) were unable to show improvement in goal setting skills.

Measurement is the goal setting behaviour most in need of attention since this attribute directly effects the evaluation of nursing care. Measurement skills are needed, not only for gathering diagnostic data, but also for assessing outcomes. The lack of precise measurement presently limits the utility of computerized information systems, and will present increasing problems as attention turns to retrieval of data from these systems. Nightingale(4) remarked that nursing outcomes should be precisely calculated, implying that they should be quantified. Even with the model of Nightingale and her exceptional efforts to precisely measure health care, nursing has done little in this area, and indeed has not approached what Nightingale was doing in the last half of the 19th century.

4.   Choosing Actions

Once criteria are established, alternative actions for achieving the designated outcomes must be listed and potential outcomes of the set of actions must be specified. In choosing among the alternative actions it is the usefulness or utility of the potential outcomes in achieving the goal that is important.

Johnson(21) found that 11 of 29 nurses did not consider alternative pain relief measures even if the initial action was unsuccessful. Grier(27) found that there were different expectations about alternative living arrangements for an elderly person among visiting nurses, hospital nurses, and elderly people. Grier and Grier(25) found that one reason for undermedicating patients in pain was that nurses overestimated the occurrence of addiction. The average estimate for addiction occurring in cancer patients was 40% even though the literature reported less than 1% to 5%.   In their study of risk-taking, Grier and Schnitzler(24) found that nurses with associate degrees and diplomas made the same choices in a game where the outcomes depended on nursing skill as in a game where the choices depended on chance; this was not true for nurses with master's degrees, however. This difference in decision making skills resulted in nurses with master's degrees winning an average of $1.49 each while those with associate degrees and diplomas each lost $.47.

Nurses are capable of listing many alternative actions outside the clinical setting. In fact, the problem they have in listing possible actions is limiting the number sufficiently for analysis. In other words the problem of too much data occurs in choosing actions as well as in selecting a diagnosis. Once more, a theoretical framework by which optimal actions can be identified is lacking. The relationships among nursing diagnoses, goals, actions, and expected outcomes, have not been established. The computerized care plans used in the United States are propositions of such frameworks, but have not been systematically tested.

In addition, there are little data available on the potential outcomes of various nursing actions, although work on outcomes is proceeding(28). A major impediment to this work is the lack of skills and tools for measurement; attention is now being given to the development of tools for measuring outcomes. Improvements in choosing nursing actions will be limited to progress in this area, since the choice of actions should be based on this parameter. Just as computerized informations systems can aid in the identification of diagnostic data, they can also help to document the frequency with which an outcome follows a nursing science.

Evaluation of the potential outcomes of alternative actions requires knowledge of probabilities. Despite the fact that nursing situations are highly uncertain, nurses have little, if any, awareness of the probabalistic nature of nursing phenomena, and poor understanding of the concepts of probability. Although all humans have difficulty estimating probabilities, this should be of particular concern in nursing where health and illness are the focus. Certainly the basic concepts of probability should be taught at the secondary level, but professional nursing education programs must teach the relationship of probability to nursing science and must prepare students for its use.

Action

As described by Nightingale, the information processing depicted in Figure 1 is carried out by observing facts about the patient, by reflecting on what those facts mean about the patient's health, and by thinking about what should be done about the diagnosed state. Once the nursing diagnosis is selected, the action chosen and implemented, facts about the resulting health state must be observed; and reflected upon. Thus the use of information in nursing practice was described by Florence Nightingale 100 years ago as a process of observation, reflection, action, observation, and reflection.

Computerized systems of nursing information are needed to help with this process, and should be developed to provide the essential data for making nursing diagnoses, for choosing nursing actions, and for allocating resources to carry out the actions. Thus, data sets of nursing diagnoses, goals, actions,

and outcomes are needed, as well as data sets on nursing skills, supplies,
equipment, etc. These data sets should be well defined and limited, and items
should have standardized labels. These nursing data sets should be separated
from, but related to, data sets for medicine and other areas of health care.

Too frequently automated nursing information systems are developed by just
collecting data without considering how the data will be used or the value of
the data items included, the same problems found with manual systems. The
problems of too much irrelevant data, imprecision and omission in recording or
input, and no means of retrieval, are being reported in computerized systems.
If the information system is to be useful, the data sets must be clearly
identified, evaluated and refined; means for retrieving and using information
from the data base must be designed. Theoretical frameworks for the system must
be developed for logical, efficient and consistent use for the system.
Evaluation of the system should be based on the information provided for making
nursing diagnoses, choosing actions, and allocating resources. Systems of
nursing information that are logical and efficient will aid nursing practice and
contribute to the development of nursing.

REFERENCES

1.   Grier, M.R. The need for data in nursing. In H. H. Werley & M. R. Grier
     (Eds), **Information Systems for Nursing**, New York: Springer, 1981.
2.   Cianifrani, K.L. **Florence Nightingale's theory of nursing.** Unpublished
     manuscript, 1978.
3.   Nightingale, F. Training of nurses. In Quain (Ed.), **Dictionary of
     Medicine**, London: Longman's, Green & Co., 1894, p. 254-255. (Nutting, M.
     A. & Dock, L. A. **History of Nursing**, vol. II. New York: G. P. Putman's,
     1907.)
4.   Nightingale, F. **Notes on Nursing, what it is and what it is not.** New
     York Appleton-Century-Croft, 1946, p. 8, 75, 105.
5.   Nightingale, F. Sick nursing and health nursing. In Hampton et al.
     (Eds.) **Nursing of the Sick** (National League of Nursing Education). New
     York: McGraw-Hill, 1949, p 26, (Originally published, 1893)
6.   Hammond, K.R. Clinical inference in nursing: A psychologist's viewpoint.
     Nursing Research, 1966, 15, 27-38.
7.   Weintraub, P. The Brain: His and hers. **Discover,** April 1981, 14-20.
8.   Witting, M.A. & Petersen, A.C. **Sex-related differences in cognitive
     functioning.** New York: Academic Press, 1979.
9.   Barnhart, B. Job worth transcends pay issue. **Chicago Tribune,** April 12,
     1982, Section 6, p. 1.
10. Bailey, J.T., McDonald, F. J., & Claus, K.E. An experimental curriculum.
     In F.G. Abdellah et al. (Eds.), **New Directions in Patient Centered
     Nursing**, New York: Macmillan. 1973, 470-498.
11. Gordon, M. Information processing strategies in nursing diagnosis. Paper
     presented at the **ANA Ninth Nursing Research Conference**, San Antonio, March
     1973.
12. Kim, M.J., & Moritz, D.A., **Classification of nursing diagnoses.** New York:
     McGraw-Hill. 1980.
13. Halloran, E.J. Analysis of variation in nursing workload by patient
     medical and nursing condition (Doctoral dissertation, University of
     Illinois Medical Center, 1980).
14. Gordon, M. Nursing nomenclature. In H.H. Werley & M.R. Grier (Eds).
     Information Systems for Nursing, New York: Springer, 1981, p. 20-25.
15. Neal, M.K., A nursing retrieval system. In H.H. Werley & M.R. Grier
     (Eds.), **Information systems for Nursing**, New York: Springer, 1981, p. 300-
     350.
16. Kelly, K.J., Clinical inference in nursing: A nurse's viewpoint.
     Nursing Research, 1966, 15, 23-26.

17. Grier, M.R., Johnson, J.H., McLean, S. Helping nurses reduce information overload. Paper in preparation, 1982.

18. Elstein, A.C., Shulman, L.S., & Sprafka, S.A., **Medical problem solving.** Cambridge: Harvard University Press, 1978.

19. Cianifrani, K.L., The influence of amounts and relevance of data in identifying health problems (Doctoral dissertation, University of Illinois Medical Center, 1982).

20. Shanteau, J., & Phelps, R.H., Judgment and swine Approaches and issues in applied analysis. In M.F. Kaplan & S. Schwartz (Eds)., **Human Judgement and Decision Processes: Applications in Problem Settings.** New York: Academic Press, 1977, 255-272.

21. Johnson, J.H. Nurses' use of the decision making process in patients with short term and long term pain (Master's thesis, University of Illinois Medical Center, 1974).

22. Gordon, M. **Nursing diagnosis.** New York: McGraw-Hill, 1982.

23. Grier, M.R. Decision making about patient care. **Nursing Research**, 1976, 25, 105-110.

24. Grier, M.R., & Schnitzler, C.P. Nurses' propensity to risk. **Nursing Research**, 1979, 28, 186-190.

25. Grier, M.R., & Grier, J.B. The patients pain, the doctor's order, and the nurse's choice. In B.T. Williams (Ed.), **Fourth Illinois Conference on Medical Information Systems**, Urbana, Illinois: Regional Health Resource Center, 1978, 79-93.

26. Sullivan, M. Recordings of the nursing process. In H. Werley & M.R. Grier (Eds)., **Information Systems for Nursing**, New York: Springer, 1981, 250-260.

27. Grier, M.R. Choosing living arrangements of the elderly. **International Journal of Nursing Studies**, 1977, 14, 69-76.

28. Lang, N.M., & Werley, H.H. (Eds.) Evaluation research: Assessment of nursing care. **Nursing Research**, 1980, 29, 68-133.

The Impact of Computers on Nursing
M. Scholes, Y. Bryant and B. Barber (eds.)
Elsevier Science Publishers B.V. (North-Holland)
© IFIP-IMIA, 1983

16.2.

SOME THOUGHTS ON THE FUTURE DIRECTION OF NURSING

Maureen Lahiff

1.   Some Thoughts on the Future Directions of Nursing

The aim of this paper is that it should promote discussion about the impact of computers on nursing from a rather different perspective than the majority of papers presented at this workshop. The perspective chosen is that of a philosophical one, and it is anticipated that it will be provocative. Drawing only briefly on the literature relating to the uses of computers in nursing it will examine aspects of nursing which have precluded the development of a philosophical approach to nursing and it will outline some of the uses which such a perspective might have. Finally, it will outline briefly what other writers have contributed to the crystal ball scene before presenting the author's predictions about the future directions which the nursing profession might take.

A literature review based on the Rcn Nursing Bibliography 1979/1981 was conducted together with a MEDLINE search 1980-1982. It is not intended to review this material here; much of it has already been examined by other contributors. However, since this paper has a somewhat different aim, many papers were put aside precisely because of their omissions. On the whole, the published papers assume that their readers know, among other things, the meaning of such terms as nursing and health; that nurses are competent decision makers; that nurses can describe useful criteria for measuring the quality of care. In other words, that nurses have conceptual skills. One author was found, however, who opened her paper by drawing attention to the need for a philosophical approach to a computerised information system. McNeill begins her comprehensive paper by saying:

> 'Computers are simply tools that facilitate the accomplishment of tasks
> and the attainment of goals. An underlying philosophy is required to
> decide which goals and tasks are appropriate for computer
> application'(O 16).

The essence of the second sentence of this statement could be applied to many of the changes which surround the nursing profession today, and which have surrounded it in the past. The failure to recognise the need for, or the value of, an underlying philosophy on which decisions may be based could be said to have been a major factor in the comparative lack of achievement by the nursing profession as it has negotiated change in the past.

There is considerable rhetoric in the nursing press about the changes which are occurring in nursing. Some change is organisational, such as is being experienced in the National Health Service at the present time; other examples are the high turnover of patients in the acute sector of health care, or the adoption of the policy of community care rather than institutional care; the application of a scientific method to the delivery of nursing care - otherwise known as the nursing process - is yet another. On closer examination however, the nursing profession has contributed less to the initiation of change than it has as a respondent to it. Economics, politics and pressure groups all contribute to the major shifts in the delivery of health care.

The case to support the proposition that the nursing profession has failed to influence change effectively has been made by several writers. Davies,(1a,b,c); Menzies(2); Towell(3). For the purposes of this discussion it is appropriate to focus attention on what Davies(1c) calls 'A Constant Casulty' - nurse education. In a cross-cultural comparison between Britain and the USA, Davies argues that in both countries, albeit for different reasons, nurse education has failed to achieve the aspirations of its leaders. She chose to explore this aspect of the nursing profession firstly because she was aware that some British nurses are critical of nurse education yet feel powerless to change it. Secondly, these same nurses look enviously towards the USA where provision is somewhat different. Davies(1a) maintains that the choice of an apprenticeship training system in the nineteenth century was a compromise, probably the only one possible, given the power of the medical profession and the economics of hospital management. Although reviewed at intervals, this position is always maintained, ostensibly for other reasons, because to change it is to challenge the politics and economics of health care.

By comparing different cultures Davies has enlarged the agenda in the consideration of the forces which have been assembled to prevent many changes from occurring at all. She concludes her case by asking;

> 'Why didn't British nurses see the education problem in the way that American nurses did and vice versa?'

The answer, she maintains, will lie in a much deeper understanding of the economic, political and social structure than she has outlined. To which may be added - and to which most nurses in the U.K. are educated at present.

It can be concluded that nurse education today, in spite of some superficial changes with the curriculum, assessment procedures and the relationship between theory and practice, continues to suffer from the original compromise. Although experimental courses have been set up and evaluated, the case for nurses receiving a broad-based education has not been made with sufficient strength by the nursing profession to challenge the economic or professional forces which operate within the health care system. Nurse entrants are still an important component of the labour force; qualified nurses only receive limited opportunities for continuing education. How do we explain this position? Usually by arguing that nursing can only be learned on the job and by experience. Valuable though experience is, it is not true to say that everything can be learned through experience. Trial and error learning is slow, can be dangerous to the recipient of the service, and can result in the wrong things being learned. It is dependant on the learner being able to make appropriate judgements about the outcome of actions. Furthermore, when we say **nursing** can only be learned by experience what do we mean by **nursing**? Is nursing the only thing which needs to be learned? If we cannot define it, how do we teach it, or assess that it has been learned?

The ability to ask and attempt to answer such questions has not been an integral part of basic nursing courses in Britain. Thinking is not considered an essential attribute. Decision-making has not been seen as central to the nursing role. Both activities have been the prerogative of another, more powerful professional group. Drawing again on Davies(1a) and the sociological perspective of professional groups, autonomy and control is gained by the creation of dependency. Occupational strategies used by nurses include subordination to doctors, acceptance of a wide range to tasks and the routinisation of work. The reasons for this are both historical and contemporary. Historically, the occupational strategies made sense. A hundred years ago the medical profession was established, with Parliamentary support; the position of women in society was a subordinate one to men, reflected in their lack of educational and therefore work opportunities. Those who challenged this state of affairs risked the loss of public sympathy and did not gain State support.

Why has this state of affairs continued into the present time, when other professions have improved their educational preparation to the extent that nursing is alone among the professions in its continued use of the apprenticeship system? Three reasons can be considered. Firstly, the socialisation process inherent in an apprenticeship system is more resistant to change, since the ideologies held by the practitioners rub off on the initiates at an early stage. The ideologies may conflict with those expressed in the school of nursing, but commonsense and sociology tell us that teachers will be secondary to ward staff as role models. Secondly, nursing continues to be a predominately female profession, and the routine work is consistent with the image of feminine work in the family, for which education is not considered necessary. Thirdly, there is evidence to suggest that the nursing profession itself perpetuates this position for what are mostly unrecognised reasons.

Mention was made earlier of the dangers of trial and error learning. Knowledge of the consequences of mistakes can produce stress among nurses, as does the witnessing of pain, disfigurement and death. Menzies(2) in a case study of the nursing service in a teaching hospital, described a series of social defence mechanisms operated by the nurses, by depersonalising patient care, splitting the nurse-patient relationship, checking and counter-checking procedures to spread the responsibility of decision making, nurses could deal with the stress, to some extent. However, Menzies went on to argue that the nursing profession recruited able young women and then failed to use their abilities; recruited far more nurses than would ever be employed once they were qualified, hence the profession required a considerable drop-out rate during training; that the nurse administrators recognised the disadvantages of some of their actions but felt powerless to change anything. It is interesting to note that this study, although considered a classic among sociologists, and beginning to be known among educated nurses is hardly known among nurses generally. It was apparently rejected by the nurses who had commissioned it. While sympathising with those people who find the challenge it presents uncomfortable, the nursing profession must examine how and why it functions now before it can make appropriate choices about future changes.

Returning to education, it can be argued that the nursing profession in general, is against it. Although a minority group of nurse leaders have pioneered and led the way into further and higher education their impact on the profession, numerically speaking, is small. Graduate nurses describe difficulties of acceptance, both during and after training, somewhat similar to American nurse graduates. Early follow up evidence demonstrates that a relatively high proportion of nurse graduates opt to work away from health care institutions, finding more scope to use their skills and knowledge in the community. Again, the question must be asked - why? How does the nursing profession perceive education?

In the 1960's Reinkemeyer, an American nurse was struggling with similar questions(4). On the basis that American and British nursing has similar foundations she thought it worthwhile to explore the attitudes prevailing in this country at the time when the first steps were being taken to integrate university education and basic nurse training. Four integrated courses had been started by then and Reinkemeyer met nursing and non-nursing teaching staff, students, nurse leaders, exploring their views on the value of an association with the academic world. She concluded that the prime contributions of higher education to a profession - novel ideas, critical thought, independant judgement and innovative behaviour - were precisely what nurses did not want.

Most British nurses assume that any change in the traditional hospital training system would spell disaster because,

> 'perfect British nursing was what had always been practised within the framework of the system, and the skilled British bed-side nurse, the best in the world, was anyone recruited to and operating for, any period of time **in conformity to the prescriptions of the system.**'

Both these assumptions negated the need for university education and legitimised the denouncement of such programmes as potentially harmful to the 'high standards' of British nursing. University students and graduates faced depreciation by evaluation according to impossible standards and unrealistic expectations - to be 'better' than the ordinary nurse - but behave in exactly the same way as her! To move into leadership positions - yet not pose the threat of doing so! Faced with such dilemmas, students 'hideout' - or join the system. 'Hence their impact on nursing was fated to remain minimal' states Reinkemeyer.

From the forgoing discussion it can be concluded that the nursing profession in the past has played a subordinate role in health care, and has been relatively content with that position. Although attempts were made to influence policies when the National Health Service was founded in 1948, they were unsuccessful. (Davies, 1978)(1b). The nursing press regularly publishes correspondence suggesting that nursing is about doing things rather than about politics, although articles are increasingly written expounding the need for nurses to acquire a better understanding of politics in general, and of health care in particular.

Meanwhile, society has unmet health care needs. The National Health Service is dominated by a medical model of disease management, biased towards cure. The rise of patient pressure groups is clear evidence that after initial medical interventions, continuing support has been non-existent or sparse. The age distribution of the population demands that every nurse has the knowledge and skills relevant to the care of the elderly. Policies of community care mean that every nurse should understand about social groups - families and communities - why they are valuable assets in some instances and not in others, and should know how to assess the difference. Numerically, mental illness and handicap is more likely to affect a family than an acute illness. Yet none of these major needs in society are central to all nurse education. That they are present in the curriculum at all may be due more to external pressures, like the EEC Regulations, rather than through our own ability to recognise society's needs and to respond to them. Attempts are being made to change nurse education through the addition of sociology, and the use of the nursing process, for example. Hopes are pinned on the UKCC that it will improve matters in the future. Unless we take heed of some of the uncomfortable evidence of the past it is unlikely that the future will be fundamentally different.

Returning to the title of this paper - some future directions in nursing - what knowledge, skills and attitudes will nurses need to develop an underlying philosophy on which to base their decisions about goals and tasks which are appropriate for the use of computers, or for any other tool, for that matter? The first step in this process is to achieve a philosophy of nursing, whether it be based on a definition, a theory or a model. This abstract exercise requires that individuals develop the ability to analyse and define concepts and terms like nursing, health, illness, care, cure. One practical advantage of such a philosophy is the assistance it can give to decisions about the extended role of the nurse. We know that doctors, nurses and patients have differing perceptions of the nursing role. (Anderson, 1972)(5). Since all three participate in patient care it is necessary, for effective teamwork, for those perceptual differences to be explored and some congruence achieved.

Although Henderson has provided us with a definition of nursing which many nurses find acceptable, less well-known are the corollaries she has added. Firstly, that no one health worker should stake out a claim to their share of the burden of health care without reference to their co-workers and to the effect it will have on human welfare, less some essential task is shunned by all. (Henderson, 1979)(6). Secondly, that having established a unique, or prime, function, each health worker may perform overlap functions as human needs demand. However, should overlap functions exclude any workers prime function, reassessment must be made. (Henderson, 1966)(7). Put more simply, instead of automatic acceptance of the doctors's discarded tasks nurses should analyse the effect it will have ultimately on their unique function. Traditionally nurses have had a hierarchy of tasks - a suitable arrangement when nursing is mainly undertaken by unqualified staff such as learners and auxiliaries - where those discarded by the doctor are high status and those which are discarded down the line to others, are low status. By defining nursing, it should be possible to make better assessments with regard to what **should** be done, rather than what **could** be done.

A philosophy of nursing could contribute to nurse education in two ways. Firstly, by changing the focus of the curriculum from a disease orientated one to a holistic view of man's health needs and resultant nursing interventions. Secondly, by adding an abstract component to the curriculum, nurses will be enabled to develop the attributes of conceptual analysis and logical thinking which are necessary for their decision making function. A theoretical basis for nursing has the potential for improving the quality of nursing care by helping practitioners focus more sharply on their contribution to health care, within the total health care team.

Finally, a philosophy of nursing can contribute to research. Conceptual frameworks are essential for the guidance and interpretation of research data. British nursing research has been criticised for its lack of theoretical perspectives. (Macguire, 1969; Inman, 1975)(8,9). A further criticism by Macguire in her review of over sixty research reports impinging on attrition among student and pupil nurses was the extent to which so many individual projects had been carried out without much reference to any previous work.

> 'There is little or no sense of the accumulation of information or the growth of understanding,' She states. (p 121)

The twenty-five year span of the studies present a remarkably static picture. It could be argued that part of this problem has been the failure, or perhaps the reluctance, to pose a different question, to analyse the data against a broader theoretical background, or to compare with other occupational groups, for example.

To recap, the case for a better understanding of the external and internal social factors and processes which have, and still are, affecting the nursing profession, has been made, using research findings. The need for a philosophical basis for the assessment of any tool and its potential contribution to nursing has been outlined. It is not, as some practitioners might think, just an abstract pastime to occupy nurses in academic institutions. As Schrock has stated:

> 'A rational defence of nursing knowledge and beliefs .... is an urgent necessity in the face of its fundamental and often jealously guarded, irrationality, that sooner rather than later might lead it beyond the present crisis of confidence into social and political upheavals in which it would be unable to survive as a recognisable entity.' (Schrock, 1981)(10).

Turning to the future, the literature on nursing in the year ???? somewhere in the future has been explored.   Notable lectures have been given by Nuttall (1976)(11), Hockey (1978)(12)   and Collins (1981)(13).   Nuttall predicts the possible demise of the clinical nurse, because of undue emphasis being placed on the managerial role and undue reliance being placed on untrained staff.   She proposed that stress be laid on the clinical task, through the recognition and identification of the nursing process.   Hockey highlighted the dilemma which would be faced by the nursing profession if it prepared nurses for irrelevant roles which did not meet patient demands.   Her proposals included a common portal of entry for all health care workers, with subsequent diversion into the different professions.   Drawing on a descriptive historical perspective, Collins looked towards research and education as the tools which would enable the nursing profession to adapt its function to the changing needs of society, whilst preserving the essential role of caring.

The most revolutionary account of nursing in the future, however, would appear to be that by Bartholomew (1958)(14).   Looking ahead forty years she predicted the demise of the professional nurse.   Although an American, she described a health service dominated largely by a group known as health visitors.   Holding degrees, these workers would have undergone a 5-6 year educational programme, of which 4 years were concentrated on studying the Humanities and Social Sciences. Bartholomew described a revolution in the medical science field which had taken place in the 1970's, which had ultimately forced the public and the professions to examine the different disciplines as they were forced to cope with change. Many nurses, she said, were caught napping, their skills in the biological field were no longer required.   In a society which no longer needed medical technology to assist in its health needs, this new health worker evolved.   The health visitor is described as

> 'a composite of the "good-old-nurse", the disciplined-thinking social worker, and the "learning-process speciality" of the educator.' (p 303)

The health visitors of 1998 have found their way to the bedside and into the home of the patient.

Where are the computers? They did not get a mention in any of these glimpses of the future. However, it is not necessary to assume from this omission that they will not have a place. Clearly, the wide variety of tasks which can be undertaken by computers demonstrate that it has enormous potential as a nursing tool. Using both basic and continuing education nurse educators must prepare nurses to choose appropriate tools and strategies to meet the challenges of change in whatever form they may be.

For this writer the future offers the potential for the nursing profession to demonstrate that it is a discrete health discipline, responsible for the planning, organising, implementing and evaluating of nursing care.   As a discipline it will be based on a synthesis of the relevant knowledge and techniques from the behavioural and biological sciences which will be related to professional expertise.   Through the development of theories of nursing which have been explored, expanded and built upon by nursing research, the quality of nursing care of patients, clients, families and communities will be improved. Research, maintains Colton (1980)(15), will help the nursing profession to come of age.   Nurses in leadership positions will create a climate which fosters free enquiry, and encourages nurses to exercise the degree of assertiveness and forcefulness necessary to initiate and engage in research.   These same attributes will be required if the nursing profession is to manage change more successfully than it has in the past, which it must do, if it is to use any tools to the maximum advantage of the patient.

'Pure fantasy?   A sheer dream?   Who can tell?   As
unpredictable as tomorrow's children? Perhaps.

Yet the fabric of the day after is woven from
the fibers of the day before, and the fibers of the day
before were
grown from the seedlings of the day before that.

A tapestry of the day after can only be woven from the
skeins of the present - the colors of which may seldom
seem to match.

Yet elements of time assure us that events **will** and do
occur and take their shape from the now, the yesterday
and the day before that.

Events we once thought impossible are even now so well
accepted, that the resistance and the drama which
accompanied their arrival are already forgotten;   for
the social anxieties and fears of today are but the
heralders of the changes awaiting the new tomorrow, the
day after, and the day after that'(14).

REFERENCES

1a   Davies C. Experience of dependency and control in work;   the case of
      nurses, Jrnl of Advanced Nursing, (1976) I, 273-282
1b   Davies C.   Four events in nursing history: a new look, Nursing Times
      (1978) 74, 17, 65-68, 18 69-71
1c   Davies C. (ed) Rewriting Nursing History (Croom Helm, London 1980)
2   Menzies I.E.P.   A casestudy in the functioning of social systems against
      anxiety. Human Relations (1960) 13, 95-121
3   Towell D. A 'social Systems' approach to research and change in nursing
      care, Int. Jrnl. Nurs. Stud., (1979) 16, 111-121
4   Reinkemeyer M.H.   The limited impact of university programs in nursing,
      PhD Thesis, Univ. of California (June 1966)
5   Anderson E. The Role of the Nurse (Rcn. London, 1972)
6   Henderson V. The essence of nursing, Nursing Standard (1979)
7   Henderson V. The Nature of Nursing (Macmillan, London 1966)
8   Macquire J. Threshold to Nursing (Bell and Sons, London, 1969)
9   Inman U. Towards a Theory of Nursing Care (Rcn. London, 1975)
10   Schrock R.   Philosophical Issues, in Hockey, L (ed), Current Issues in
      Nursing (Churchill Livingstone, Edinburgh, 1981)
11   Nuttall P. Nursing in the year AD 2000, Jrnl of Advanced Nursing, (1976),
      I, 101-110
12   Hockey L. The future nurse: selection and training;   autonomy;   should
      her health-care role be modified for future patient demands?   Jrnl of
      Advanced Nursing, (1978) 3, 571-582
13   Collins S.M.   Nursing - the next 100 years, Jrnl of Advanced Nursing,
      (1981) 6, 165-171
14   Bartholomew C. And the day after that, in Reinhardt A. & Quinn, M (eds)
      Family Centered Community Nursing (Mosby, St Louis, 1973)
15   Colton M.R.   Research: Will it help us come to age as a profession?
      Supervisor Nurse, (1980) Dec

CHAPTER 17

CONCLUSIONS
Barry Barber

General

This book has attempted to tie together a platform on which it is possible to develop a new discipline of nursing informatics. By its nature the development can only be partial but it appears sufficient to justify the interest and aspirations of many specialists concerned with this area of activity whether as nurses or as informaticians.

There is little value in trying to recapture in brief the material presented at length earlier in the book. Undoubtedly, nursing systems will be developed and used increasingly. More powerful computers will become available, thus enabling more ambitious educational and service systems to be implemented and more convenient means will be devised to enable nurses to communicate with their computer systems. The designers of these systems can draw on existing hard-won expertise or learn it afresh for themselves. However, there are three issues which are perhaps the most important to bear in mind; they are the issues of multidisciplinary symbiosis, of the development of the institutions of collaboration, and of the perspective of human needs.

Collaboration between Nurses and Informaticians

In order to develop this new activity of nursing informatics it is important that there should be extensive collaboration between nurses and computer professionals, each contributing differing expertise to the joint development and each gaining insights from the other. This multidisciplinary symbiosis will eventually result in specialists with joint qualifications as has happened in so many other activities in health care. Although the participants at the workshop were mainly nurses concerned with computer systems, there were also other professionals with relevant backgrounds.

Informatics, like medicine and nursing, has a very broad range. It covers the full range of specialties from operations analysis and system modelling to systems design and implementation. It covers computer hardware design, engineering and selection as well as software structuring, writing and implementation in such diverse areas as operating systems, data base management systems, language compilers and application program suites. It covers the full range of equipment selection and maintenance as well as all facets of computer operations and systems and data management. Their vast range of activity must be understood as providing the technical back-up for nursing systems. Appropriate specialists can only be brought in as required if their specialist role and expertise is appreciated and understood; thus understanding is best achieved by collaboration on common projects.

There is a need for computer specialists in nursing, that is, members of a computer science team who understand and work with nurses developing and installing information systems and software for nursing, just as there are computer specialists for many facets of business. Another way to provide necessary input about nursing to computer systems designers is by bringing together "think tanks" of nurses with computer specialists during the planning, development, and implementation of projects.

Ways also need to be found for nurses to be released from some other duties when they are designated to work with computer specialists in developing and implementing systems. These responsibilities should not be "added on" to their existing duties.

Development of Institutions

As with medical informatics it is necessary to build up the basis of the discipline of nursing informatics with national and international meetings, seminars, workshops and conferences in order to exchange and develop ideas and explore the practical implementation of these ideas. Furthermore, these research and development ideas must be fed back into the training courses appropriately to prepare the next generation of nurses and informaticians for the challenges and opportunities ahead. This institutional development is necessary to underpin the multidisciplinary nature of the developing profession of nursing informatics and to give it coherent expression.

Nursing input into computer management courses would help computer specialists understand health care, hospitals, nursing needs and issues more thoroughly. Correspondingly, suitable courses have to be devised to provide nurses with an understanding of informatics at varying levels of detail. An understanding of systems and systems design implications is often much more important than immersion in the intricacies, and exhilaration, of programming.

Human Element

The implementation of computer systems must not be allowed to remove the human element from decisions that affect people and result in lowered staff morale. This issue needs to be considered when moving to such automation as, for example, a computerised staffing system. The systems must liberate people to do the things they can do best by providing increasingly effective educational, and managerial tools, together with systems to assist in the provision of patient care and ultimately assisting with decision making. The human needs of individuals must not be lost in the elegance of systems.

Nurses must control nursing and computing systems must not lure them into making decisions incompatible with good nursing practice. The role of the computer must be kept in proper perspective and not viewed as a magical entity. Its usefulness for nursing lies in its ability to improve the effectiveness or efficiency of nursing systems thus enabling nurses to concentrate on the development of nurse education, the management of resources, and the delivery of patient care. The computer has the potential of expanding the roles of individual nurses but it will certainly not replace them!

CHAPTER 18

GLOSSARY

This list of common computing terms is an extract from "A Glossary of Computing Terms for introductory courses." published by British Computer Society, 13 Mansfield Street, London W1M OPB. March 1982.

ACOUSTIC COUPLER: is a data communications device which enables a digital signal to be transmitted over the telephone network using an ordinary telephone handset.

ALGORITHM: is a finite set of rules giving a sequence of operations for solving a specific type of problem.

ANALOGUE COMPUTER: is a computer in which data is represented by a continuously variable physical quality such as voltage or angular position.

ARTIFICAL INTELLIGENCE: is the concept that computers can be programmed to assume some capabilities normally thought to be like human intelligence such as learning, adaption and self correction.

ASSEMBLY LANGUAGE: is a low-level programming language, generally using symbolic addresses, which is translated into machine code by an assembler.

BACKING STORE: is a means of storing large amounts of data outside the immediate access store; also known as secondary storage.

BATCH PROCESSING: is a technique in which computer processing does not begin until all the input (data and/or programs) has been collected together (i.e. batched).

BAUD: is the unit, one bit per second, used to measure the speed of transmission in a telegraph or telephone line.

BIT (BInary DigiT): is one of the digits used in binary notation, i.e. 0 or 1. It is also the smallest unit of storage.

BUFFERING: is the use of a store area (buffer) to temporarily hold data being transmitted between a peripheral device and the central processor, to compensate for differences in their working speeds. Buffering can also be used between two peripheral devices.

BUG: is an error in a program or a fault in equipment.

BUS: is a common pathway shared by signals from several components of the computer; e.g. all input/output devices would be connected to the I/O bus. Also called a Highway or a Data Bus.

BYTE: is a fixed number of bits, often corresponding to single character. In some computers, bytes may be individually addressed.

COMPUTER ASSISTED LEARNING (CAL):   is the use of the computer in education as an aid in routine presentation of material, testing.

CENTRAL PROCESSING UNIT(CPU):   is the main part of the computer consisting of the Immediate Access Store, Arithmetic Unit and Control Unit. Also called the Central Processor.

CODE: is a set of program instructions.

COMPILER: is a program which translates a high-level language program into a computer's machine code or some other low-level language. Each high-level instruction is changed into several machine-code instructions. It produces an independent program which is capable of being executed by itself. This process is known as compilation.

COMPUTER: is a machine which, under the control of a stored program, automatically accepts and processes data, and supplies the results of that processing. With continuing development, terms relating to size, speed and capability can only be relative, but at the time of writing the following terms have generally accepted meanings.

                                        MAINFRAME: is a computer with a variety of peripheral devices, a large amount of backing store and a fast CPU. The term is generally used in comparison to a smaller or subordinate computer.

MICROCOMPUTER: is a computer whose CPU is a microprocessor. Generally this is a cheap and relatively slow computer with a very limited access store, a simple instruction set and only elementary backing store (e.g. cassette tapes, floppy disks).

MINICOMPUTER: is a computer whose size, speed and capabilities lie between those of a mainframe and a microcomputer. The term referred originally to a range of computers cheaper and less well equipped than contemporary mainframe machines. With the advent of even cheaper microcomputers, the term is becoming more vague.

CONFIGURATION: is the particular choice of hardware and its connections making up a computer system.

CORE STORE: is a storage device consisting of a matrix of ferrite rings (called cores) with an interlacing system of sensing and energising wires. Each core can be energised in either of two directions, to represent a single bit of data.

CORE SIZE: is the amount of core store (or main store) measured as the number of storage locations; it is usually given as (e.g.) 32K words of store.

CP/M (CONTROL PROGRAM MONITOR): is an operating system for microcomputers which are based on the Z80 microprocessor chip.

CURSOR: is a character that indicates the current display position on a visual display unit. On many devices it flashes on and off.

DATA PREPARATION: is the translation of data into machine readable form.

DATA PROCESSING: is the complete operation of collecting data, processing it, and presenting results. The term is normally applied to business tasks where the use of the computer is involved. Also called Automatic Data Processing (ADP) or Electronic Data Processing (EDP).

DATA PROTECTION: is the establishment of safeguards to preserve the integrity, privacy and security of data.

DATA TRANSMISSION: is the process of using a data link.

DATEBASE MANAGEMENT SYSTEM
DBMS)

is a system which allows a systematic approach to the storage and retrieval of data in a computer often coordinating data from a number of files.

DECISION TABLE:

is a particular kind of table showing the relationship between certain named variables and specifying the actions to be taken when certain conditions arise.

DEDICATED SYSTEM:

is a computer system used for a single application.

DEFAULT OPTION:

is a specific alternative action to be taken automatically by the computer in the event of the omission of a definite instruction or action.

DIGITAL COMPUTER:

is a computer in which the data is represented by combinations of discrete pulses denoted by 0's and 1's.

DIRECT ACCESS:

is the process of storing or retrieving data items without the necessity of reading any other stored data first. Also called Random Access.

DIRECT DATA ENTRY:

is the input of data directly to the computer using, normally, a key-to-disk unit. The data may be validated while held in a temporary file, before being written to the disk for subsequent processing.

DOWN TIME:

is a period of time during which a computer is out of action ("down").

DUMP:

is to copy the contents of a file, or the contents of the immediate access store, to backing store or to an output device. The output is known as the dump, and may be used to ensure the security of the data in a file, or to assist in program error detection.

EMULATOR:

is the software, and sometimes associated hardware, in a computer system which permits it to imitate another computer system (usually a less sophisticated machine).

ERGONOMICS:

The analysis and consideration of the psychological and physiological factors related to the man-machine interface.

EXECUTIVE PROGRAM:

is a control program which schedules the use of the hardware required by the program being run. Also called Monitor, Supervisor Program.

FILE: is an organised collection of related records.

FLAG: is an indicator which can be set or unset. Its state indicates a condition (e.g. whether or not a list of numbers has been sorted or whether an interrupt has been sensed).

FLOWCHART: is a graphical representation of the operations involved in a data processing system. Symbols are used to represent particular operations or data, and flow lines indicate the sequence of operations or the flow of data.

FRONT END PROCESSOR: is a small computer which receives data from a number of input devices, organises it and transmits it to a more powerful computer for processing.

HARD COPY: is a computer output printed on paper.

HIGH-LEVEL PROGRAMMING: LANGUAGE: is a problem-orientated language, in which instructions may be equivalent to several machine-code instructions, and which may be used on different computers by using an appropriate compiler. Some of the commoner high-level languages are: ALGOL, BASIC, COBOL, FORTRAN, PASCAL, PL/1.

HYBRID COMPUTER: is a computer which uses both analogue and digital techniques.

INFORMATION: is the meaning given to data by the way in which it is interpreted.

INITIALISE: is to set counters or variables to zero, or some other starting value, usually at the beginning of a program or subprogram.

INPUT/OUTPUT DEVICE: is a peripheral unit which can accept data, presented in the appropriate machine-readable form, decode it and transmit it as electrical pulses to the central processing unit OR/ translates electrical pulses from the computer into a human-readable form or into a form suitable for re-processing by the computer at a later stage.

INTEGRATED CIRCUIT: is a solid state microcircuit consisting of interconnected semiconductor devices diffused into a single silicon chip.

INTELLIGENT TERMINAL: is one where software within the terminal allows a certain amount of computing to be done without contact with a central computer (e.g. data vetting on a VDU used for data entry).

INTERACTIVE COMPUTING: is the mode of operation of a system which allows the computer and the terminal user to communicate with each other.

INTERFACE: is the hardware and associated software needed, between a central processor and a peripheral device, in order to compensate for the difference in their operating characteristics (their speeds, codes, etc.).

KEY: is the record identifier used in many information retrieval systems.

LISTING: is the printing out, in sequence, of program statements or data.

MACHINE CODE INSTRUCTION: is one which directly defines a particular machine operation and can be recognised and executed without any intermediate translation.

MAINFRAME.   See Computer

MEDIA: is the collective name for materials (tape, disk, paper, cards etc.) used to hold data

MEMORY: is that part of a computer where data and instructions are held.

MICROCOMPUTER   See Computer

MINI COMPUTER   See Computer

MODEM (Modulator/Demodulator)   is a device to allow the conversion of bits into analogue electrical impulses for transmission over telephone-type circuits and vice versa.

MODULAR PROGRAMMING: is one aspect of structured programming in which individual tasks are programmed as distinct sections or modules (subprograms). One advantage is the ease with which individual sections can be modified without reference to other sections.

NETWORK: is a linked set of computer systems, usually geographically dispersed, each capable of drawing on the computing power or storage facilities of others within the network.

OBJECT PROGRAM: is the translated version of a program that has been assembled or compiled.

OFF-LINE PROCESSING: is processing carried out by devices not under the control of the central processor.

ON-LINE PROCESSING: is processing performed on equipment directly under the control of the central processor.

OPERATING SYSTEM:

is an advanced form of control program which allows a number of programs to be run on the computer without the need for operator intervention.

PASSWORD:

is a sequence of characters which must be presented to a computer system before it will allow a user access to the system or parts of that system (e.g. a particular file). The use of passwords is in connection with considerations of security and privacy of data.

PERIPHERAL DEVICE:

is the term used to describe any input, output, or backup storage device which can be connected to the central processing unit.

PIXEL:

is a contraction of 'picture element'. As used in graphics it is the smallest element of a display.

PROGRAM:

is a complete set of program statements structured in such a way as to specify an algorithm.

PROGRAMMER:

is the person responsible for writing computer programs.

PROGRAMMING LANGUAGE:

is an artificial language constructed in such a way that people and programmable machines can communicate with each other in a precise and intelligible way.

RAM (Random Access Memory):

is memory which may be read from and written to by the programmer. It is usually made on a chip.

ROM (Read-Only Memory):

is memory which may not be written to by the programmer. The software in the ROM is fixed during manufacture. PROM (Programmable Memory) is a type of ROM where the program may be written after manufacture by a customer but which is fixed from that time on. EPROM (Erasable PROM) is a type of PROM Memory which can be erased by a special process (for example, by exposure to ultra-violet radiation) and written as for a new PROM.

REAL-TIME SYSTEM:

is a system which is able to receive continuously changing data from outside sources and which is able to process that data sufficiently rapidly to be capable of influencing the sources of data (e.g. process control, air-traffic control, airline bookings).

RECORD:

is a collection of related items of data, treated as a unit.

SCRATCH FILE:

is a temporary storage area, usually held in backing store, for use by a program during execution. Also called a Work File.

SCREEN EDITING:

is the process of changing stored data or programs by the alteration of characters displayed on a VDU, using a cursor to indicate position.

SCROLLING:

is the action of a VDU when displaying text of 'rolling-up' the screen: as each new line of text appears at the bottom, a line of existing text disappears from the top.

SEMANTICS:

is the meaning attached to words or symbols in programming statements.

SEQUENTIAL (SERIAL) ACCESS:

is the process of storing or retrieving data items by first reading through all previous items to locate the one required.

SOFTWARE PACKAGE:

is a fully documented program, or set of programs, designed to perform a particular task.

SOURCE LANGUAGE:

is the language in which the source program is written.

SPOOLING:

is the temporary storage of input or output data on magnetic disc or tape, as a means of compensating for the slow operating speeds of peripheral devices or when queueing different output streams to one device.

SYNTAX:

is the set of rules for combining the element of a programming language (e.g. characters) into permitted constructions (e.g. program statements). The set of rules does not define meaning, nor does it depend on the use of the final construction.

SYSTEM ANALYSIS AND DESIGN:

is the analysis of the requirements of a job, a feasability study of potential computer involvement, and the design of an appropriate system to do the job.

TELETEXT:

is a computer based information retrieved system which uses screen messages either broadcast by television like the BBC system, Ceefax, or the ITV system, Oracle, or provided interactively like British Telecom's Prestel which allows information to be both accessed and stored. These messages are organised into "pages" allowing a modified domestic television to display the messages.

TERMINAL:	is the term used to describe any input/output device which is used to communicate with the computer from a remote site.
TIME-SHARING:	is a means of providing multi-access to a computer system. Each user is, in turn, allowed a time slice of the system's resources, although each appears to have continuous use of the system.
UTILITY PROGRAM:	is a systems program designed to perform a commonplace task such as the transfer of data from one storage device to another or sorting a set of data.
VALIDATION:	is an input control technique used to detect any data which is inaccurate, incomplete or unreasonable.
VERIFICATION:	The act of checking transferred data usually at the stage of input to a computer, by comparing copies of the data before and after transfer; e.g. repeating the keyboard operations to check that the data has been correctly transferred in a key-to-disk system, or when punching cards or paper tape. Where a separate device performs this task, it is called a verifier.
VIRTUAL STORAGE:	is a means of apparently extending main storage, by allowing the programmer to access backing store in the same way as immediate access store.
VISUAL DISPLAY UNIT (VDU):	is a terminal device, incorporating a cathode ray tube, on which text can be displayed. It is usually used in conjunction with a keyboard.
VOLATILE STORE:	is store holding data only while power is supplied.
WORD PROCESSOR:	is a computer system which is capable of assisting with the secretarial tasks of editing and production of typed letters and documents including the addition of stored text, for example for personalised circulars.

U: UNITS

SYMBOL		MEANING/VALUE		
		Fraction	Decimal	Power of 10
M	mega-	one million	1 000 000	$= 10^{6}$
K	kilo-	one thousand*	1 000	$= 10^{3}$
m	milli-	one thousandth	$^{1}/(1000)$	0.001	$= 10^{-3}$
μ	micro-	one millionth	$^{1}/(1\ 000\ 000)$	0.000 001	$= 10^{-6}$
n	nano-	one thousand millionth	$^{1}/(1\ 000\ 000\ 000)$	0.000 000 001	$= 10^{-9}$
p	pica-	one million millionth	$^{1}/(1\ 000\ 000\ 000\ 000)$	0.000 000 000 001	$= 10^{-12}$

* Note: K in computer storage the value of K is 1024 ($=2^{10}$), for example 8k of store is 8192 storage locations.

CHAPTER 19

BIBLIOGRAPHY

Compiled by Yvonne M. Bryant

INTRODUCTION

This bibliography was sponsored by the London Medical Specialist Group of the British Computer Society as a special project to meet the need for a comprehensive directory of literature available, in English, on the subject of using computers in nursing. It is intended that the material contained in this chapter will form the basis of an annotated bibliography to be published separately.

In the past, other disciplines have produced detailed bibliographies to enable them to readily access the published material about their subjects. It is intended that this work will bring together many of the papers, articles and books that have been written about our subject during the past fifteen years.

The references included in this bibliography have been selected on the basis that they described the use of computers in a nursing environment. It has sometimes been difficult, on this basis, to determine whether or not a particular publication should be included. The author therefore apologises in advance for any unintended omissions.

The bibliography has been organised so that it corresponds directly with the content of the preceding chapters. However, certain references naturally overlap the content of more than one chapter. The reader should be aware of this and cross-check in other possible subject areas when searching for particular information.

Where several papers have been published in the same book or proceedings of an international conference, abbreviated references have been used to avoid unnecessary duplication as follows:

NISYS - Werley H H, Grier M R, (eds) Nursing Information Systems. 1981, Springer.

Proc Medcomp 77 - Medcomp 77 Berlin, 1977, Online Conferences Ltd, Uxbridge, England.

Proc MEDINFO 74 - Anderson J, Forsythe J M, (eds), MEDINFO 74, 1974, North Holland.

Proc MEDINFO 77 - Shires D B, Wolf H, (eds), MEDINFO 77, 1977, North Holland.

Proc MEDINFO 80 - Lindberg D A B, Kaihara S, (eds), MEDINFO 80, 1980, North Holland.

Proc MIE 78 - Anderson J, (ed), Medical Informatics Europe 78, 1978, Springer-Verlag.

Proc MIE 79 - Barber B, Gremy F, Uberla K, Wagner G, (eds), Medical Informatics Berlin 79, Springer-Verlag.

Proc MIE 81 - Gremy F, Degoulet P, Barber B, Salamon R, (eds), Medical Informatics Europe 81, 1981, Springer-Verlag.

Proc MIE 82 - O'Moore R R, Barber B, Reichertz P L, Roger F, (eds), Medical Informatics Europe 82, 1982. Springer-Verlag.

The bibliography is arranged as follows:

A. General
B. Computer Technology in Health Care
C. Nursing Records
D. Measurement of Care
     Care Plans
     Dependency
E. Patient Monitoring
F. Drug Management
G. Community Based Care
H. Implications for Nurse Education
I. Computer Assisted Learning
J. Education Programmes and Records
     Education Programmes and Allocation
     Record Systems
K. Planning the Nursing Service
L. Resource Management
M. Management Sciences and the Nursing Service
N. Research
O. Health Care Systems
P. Unclassified References.

Within each category, the references are arranged alphabetically by first author's surname. It has been necessary to include a section of unclassified references. These are references that appear relevant by virtue of their titles, but which the author has been unable to trace to-date. An author index is included giving the category letter and reference numbers for each author.

The author points out that although considerable efforts have been made to ensure a fully comprehensive bibliography, it should in no way be considered complete for the time period covered.

In conclusion, the author wishes to express her thanks to John Bryant for his help in preparing the bibliography, and to her colleagues on the organising committee for their help in suggesting and obtaining many of the references.

A GENERAL

A1.   Ashton C C, Bryant Y M. A review of nursing systems in the United Kingdom. Proc MIE 79, 1979, :207-218.
A2.   Atack C C. Computers in nursing. WHO Fellowship Report. Queen Elizabeth Hospital, Birmingham, 1972.
A3.   Barber B, Cohen R D, Scholes M. A review of the London Hospital computer project. Med Inform, 1976, 1(1):61-72.
A4.   Barber B, Scholes M. Learning to live with computers. Nursing Mirror, 1979, Jul 5.
A5.   Barber B, Scholes M. Health services and the computer. Health Trends, 1970, July.

A6.   Bryant Y M. The role of the nurse in systems design. Royal Society of Health Journal, 1979, 99(1):9-11,27.

A7.   Butler E A. An automated hospital information system. Nursing Times, 1978, Feb 9, :245-247.

A8.   Butler E A. Computers in the ward situation. Nursing Times, 1973, Jan 25, :119-121.

A9.   Gatewood L C. Nursing interfaces to health care information systems. NISYS, 1981, :297-313.

A10.   Hammersley P. A review of hospital auxiliary systems. Proc MEDINFO 77, 1977, :171-178.

A11.   Hannah K J. The relationship between nursing and medical informatics. Proc MIE 78, 1978, :721-728.

A12.   Lindop N. Report of the Committee on Data Protection. HMSO (Cmnd 7341), 1978.

A13.   Pocklington D B, Guttman L. Computer technology in nursing: a comprehensive bibliography. 1980, US Dept of Health and Human Services (DHHS Publ No HRA 80-65).

A14.   Prendergast J A. Computerization of data for nursing practice. NISYS, 1981, :123-127.

A15.   Regester W D. A practicing physician's view of a community hospital's use of a computerized medical information system with emphasis on how it impacts the hospital's three most important areas. Proc MEDINFO 80, 1980,:67-69.

A16.   Scholes M. An overview of the use of computers in nursing. Royal Society of Health Journal, 1979, 99(1):8-9.

A17.   Scholes M. The role of computers in nursing. Nursing Mirror, Sep 23, 1976.

A18.   Scholes M, Barber B. Towards nursing informatics. Proc MEDINFO 80, 1980, :70-73.

A19.   Slack P. Changing to computers. Nursing Times, 1979, December 20/27, :2189

A20.   UK Government. The White Paper - Data Protection. HMSO (Cmnd 8359), 1982.

A21.   UK Government. The White Paper - Computers and Privacy. HMSO (Cmnd 6353), 1975.

A22.   Younger K. Report of the Committee on Privacy. HMSO (Cmnd 5012), 1972.

B COMPUTER TECHNOLOGY IN HEALTH CARE

B1.   Baker J D. The key to the vault. DIMENSIONS in Health Service, 1978, Apr, :24-25.

B2.   Barnett G O. Quality assurance through computer surveillance and feedback (Editorial). American Journal of Public Health, 1977, 67(3):230-231.

B3.   Bartoszek V. The potential of data processing in improved health care. J New York State Nurses' Association, 1975, 5:14-16.

B4.   Birckhead L M. The need for nurse support systems in affecting computer systems. J Nurs Admin, 1978, 8(3):51-53.

B5.   Birckhead L M. Nursing and the technetronic age. J Nurs Admin, 1978, 8(2):16-19.

B6.   Birckhead L M. Automation of the health care system: implications for nursing, part 1, dangers to nursing practice in the automation of the health care system. International Nursing Review, 1975, Jan/Feb, 22(1):28-31.

B7.   Brown P T S. Computers and the nurse. International Journal of Nursing Studies, 1978, 7(2):91-97.

B8.   Castledine G. Hardware on the ward. Nursing Mirror, 1981, Mar 5, 152(10):14.

B9.   Creighton H. The diminishing right of privacy: computerized medical records. Supervisor Nurse, 1978, 9(2):58-61.

B10.   Dingwall R. Are you ready for the microchip. Nursing Times, 1979, Jun 7, :975-976.

B11.   Donald L. All in a day's work. Nursing Mirror, 1981, Apr 9.

B12.   Eisler J, Goering P, Tierney J. Strangers in computerland. Am J Nurs, 1972, 72(6):1120-1123.

B13.   Franklin C B. Living with someone else's computer. In Payne J P and Hill D W (ed.), Real-time computing in patient management. Peregrinus, England, 1976, :119-131.

B14.   Goodwin J O, Edwards B S. Developing a computer program to assist the nursing process: phase 1 - from systems analysis to an expandable program. Nursing Research, 1975, 24(4):299-305.

B15.   Goshen C E. Your automated future. Am J Nurs, 1972, 72(1):62-67.

B16.   Hannah K J. The computer and nursing practice. Nursing Outlook, 1976, 24(9):555-558.

B17.   Hannah K J. Computers change role of nursing. CIPS Review, Toronto, 1979, Oct/Nov, 3(5):20-22.

B18.   Martindale A, Steele B. Keeping it confidential. Health and Social Service Journal, 1982, Aug 5, :937-940.

B19.   McLaughlin L. Nursing in telediagnosis. Am J Nurs, 1969, 69(5):1006-1008.

B20.   National Centre for Health Services Research. Computer Applications in Health Care. 1980, US Dept of Health and Human Services (DHHS Publ No PHS 80-3251).

B21.   Pritchard K. Computers: implications of computerisation. Nursing Times, 1982, Mar 24, 78(12):491-492.

B22.   Pritchard K. Computers: possible applications in nursing. Nursing Times, 1982, Mar 17, 78(11):465-466.

B23.   Pritchard K. Computers: systems analysis. Nursing Times, 1982, Mar 10, 78(10):414-415.

B24.   Pritchard K. Computers: an introduction. Nursing Times, 1982, Mar 3, 78(9):355-357.

B25.   Rappoport A E, Gennaro W B. You get the blood, computer does CBC. Modern Hosp, 1969, Nov, :103-107.

B26.   Sofaly K J. The nurse and electronic data processing. Medical Instrumentation, 1981, 15(3):169-170.

B27.   Tate S P. Automation of the health care system: implications for nursing, part 2, change strategies for nurses. International Nursing Review, 1975, Mar/Apr, 22(2):39-42.

B28.   Taylor D B, Johnson O H. Systematic nursing assessment: a step toward automation. (DHEW Publication No (HRA)74-17), Washington, U.S.Government Printing Office, 1974 viii, :164-240.

B29.   Tomasovic E R. Turning nurses on to automation. Hospitals, 1972, 46:80-86.

B30.   Unknown. Choosing your first computer - a practical introduction. Practical Computing, 1979, July, :53-60.

B31.   Watkin B R. A pocket computer in the ward. Nursing Times, 1982, Sep 1, :1468-1471.

B32.   Westwood B. Beam me up, nurse. Nursing mirror, 1981, 152(25):24-26.

B33.   Zielstorff R D. The planning and evaluation of automated systems: a nurse's point of view. J Nurs Admin, 1975, 5(6):22-25.

B34.   Zielstorff R D. Nurses can affect computer systems. J Nurs Admin, 1978, 8(3):49-51.

C NURSING RECORDS

C1.   Ashton C C. A developing nursing record system. Symposium on Computer Applications in the Field of Medicine, Sperry Univac, Rome, Oct 19-21, 1976.

C2.   Ashton C C. The computerised nursing information system at the Queen Elizabeth Hospital, Birmingham. Proc MIE 78, 1978, (unpublished).

C3.   Ashton C C. A nursing record system. Symposium on Computers in Health Care, Sperry Univac, Nice, May 15-17, 1979.

C4.   Froment A, Michard P, Milon H, Dechanoz G, Dupuy M, Magnon R, Melinon S, Bouveret C, Chorobik T, Falcoz H. Computer-assisted patient-care management. Med Inform 1979, 4(2):119-125.

C5.   Head A E. Maintaining the nursing record with the aid of a computer. Proc Medcomp 77, 1977, :469-483.

C6.   Henney C R, Bosworth R N. The nurse and the computer. Nursing Mirror, 1977, Nov 17.

C7.   Henney C R, Bosworth R N, Brown N, Crooks J. Can a computer improve communication in the ward area. Proc MEDINFO 77, 1977, :953-956.

C8.   Knight J E, Streeter J. The computer as an aid to nursing records. Nursing Times, 1970, 66:233-235.

C9.   McDonald C J, Murray R, Jeris D, Bhargava B, Seeger J, Blevins L. A computer-based record and clinical monitoring system for ambulatory care. Am J Public Health, 1977, 67(3):240-245.

C10. Olssen D E. Automating nurses' notes - first step in a computerized record system. Hospitals, 1967, 41(12):64-78

C11. O'Rourke M. A practical system of computerized medical records for documentation and decision making in the coronary care ward. Medical Journal of Australia, 1975, 1:301-304.

C12. Procter P M, Head A E, Jarvis J. A computerised nursing record - an effective means of communication. Proc MIE 82, 1982, :309-316.

C13. Rosenberg M, Carriker D. Automating nurses' notes. Am J Nurs, 1966, 66(5):1021-1023.

C14. Rosenberg M, Glueck B C. Automated nursing notes and psychiatric care. Canada's Mental Health, 1967, 15:25-26.

C15. Simborg D W. The development of a ward information-management system. Methods of Information in Medicine, 1973, 12(1):17-26.

C16. Smith B. Computer in the ward. Nursing Times, 1970, Nov 5, 64: 1426-1429.

C17. Smith E J. Computer and nursing practice. Supervisor Nurse, 1974, 5:55-62.

C18. Stein R F. An exploratory study in the development and use of automated nursing reports. Nursing Research, 1969, 18:14-21.

C19. Stroebel C F, Glueck B C. Computer derived global judgements in psychiatry. Am J Psychiatry, 1970, 126(8):1057-1066.

D MEASUREMENT OF CARE

Care Plans

D1.   Cornell S A, Brush F. Systems approach to nursing care plans. Am J Nurs, 1971, 71(7):1376-1378.

D2.   Cornell S A, Carrick A G. Computerized schedules and care plans. Nursing Outlook, 1973, 21(12):781-784

D3.   DeSanders N. Computer's basic plans help doctors initiate rehabilitation regimen. Modern Hospital, 1969, Nov, :98-100.

D4.   Henney C R. Chips with everything. Nursing Mirror, 1981, Feb 26, 152(9):35-36.

D5.   Hughes S J. Developing a patient care planning system for automation. NISYS, 1981, :143-148.

D6.   Kumpel Z, Davis A. Quantitive evaluation of the effects of computerisation on the nursing record. Proc MIE 82, 1982, :336-342.

D7.   Murray E, Curtis S, Anderson J. The role of a computerised information system in the nursing care of the elderly. Proc MIE 82, 1982, :343-347.

D8.   Parsons R. Computer technology and clinical nursing practice. The Lamp, 1976, 33(6):24-34.

D9.   Speed E L, Young N A. SCAN - data processed printouts of a patient's basic care needs. Am J Nurs, 1969, 69(1):108-110.

D10. Somers J B. A computerized nursing care system. Hospitals, JAHA, 1971, 45(8), :93,96-99.

D11. Wesseling E. Automating the nursing history and care plan. J Nurs Admin, 1972, 2(3):34-3

Dependency

D12. Bryant Y M, Hammersley P. Systems for nursing administration in a teaching hospital. Proc Toulouse Conference, IRIA, 1975, (2):299-324.
D13. Bryant Y M, Heron K. Monitoring patient-nurse dependency. Nursing Times (Occasional Paper), 1974, May 9/16.
D14. Harman R J. Nursing services information system. J Nurs Admin, 1977, 7(3):14-20.
D15. Henney C R, Bosworth R N. A computer-based system for the automatic production of nursing workload data. Nursing Times, 1980, 76(28):1212-1217.
D16. Moores B, Moult A. Patterns of nurse activity. J Advanced Nurs, 1979, 4:137-149.
D17. Rhys Hearn C, Young B. Experience with the Rhys-Hearn geriatric workload package - a regional survey. Nursing Times,1981, 77(3):9-12.
D18. Rhys Hearn C. Nursing needs and nursing resources. Proc Medical Data Processing Symposium, Toulouse, Taylor & Francis, 1977.

E PATIENT MONITORING

E1. Acton J C, Sheppard L C, Kouchoukos N J, Kirklin J W. Automated care systems for critically ill patients following cardiac surgery. National Institute of Health Conferences on Computers in Cardiology, 1974, Oct 2-4, Bethesda, Maryland.
E2. Allwood J M. A computerised system to monitor fluids in an intensive therapy unit. Loughborough Grammar School. Unpublished Report.
E3. Ashcroft J M. Computers in intensive care units. Nursing Mirror, Jun 28, 1974.
E4. Ashcroft J M, Berry J L. The introduction of a real-time patient data display system into the cardio-thoracic department at Wythenshawe Hospital. Proc MEDINFO 74, 1974, :101-107.
E5. Chow R. Postoperative cardiac nursing research: a method for identifying and categorizing nursing action. Nursing Research, 1969, 18(1):4-13.
E6. Christopherson K I. Microprocessor technology adds new dimension to patient monitoring systems. Hospital Administration in Canada, 1976, 18(5):50-51.
E7. Drazen E, et al. Guidelines for computer-based patient monitoring systems (Contract HSM 110). Arthur D Little Inc, 1975, :70-406.
E8. Drazen E, Wechsler A, Wiig K. Requirements for computerized patient monitoring systems. Computer, 1975, 8(1):22-27.
E9. Endo A S. Using computers in newborn intensive care settings. Am J Nurs, 1981, 81(7):1336-1337
E10. Gerbode F. Computerized monitoring of seriously ill patients. J Thorac and Cardiovasc Surg, 1973, 66:167-174.
E11. Gordon M, Wardener de H E, Venn J C, Webb J, Adams H. A graphic microcomputer system for clinical renal data. Proc MIE 81, 1981, :543-545.
E12. Greenburg A G. Computerization of the surgical intensive care unit: a new view for design. Proc MEDINFO 77, 1977, :901-905.
E13. Greenburg A G, McClure D K, Fink R, Stubbs J A, Peskin G W. Computerization of the surgical intensive care unit: improvement of patient care via education. Surg, 1975, 77(6):799-806.
E14. Greenburg A G, McClure D K, Janus C A, Stubbs J A. Nursing intervention scoring system: a concept for management, research and communication. Proc MIE 78, 1978, :729-738.
E15. Joshi M. The computer in coronary care. Nursing Times, 1982, Mar 3, :358-360
E16. Landucci L, Macerata C, Marchesi C, Chierchia S, Lazzari M, Maseri A. Real time computer based electrocardiographic and hemodynamic monitoring in CCU. Proc MIE 79, 1979, :325-339.

E17. Martz K Y, Beaumont J O. Computer-based monitoring in an intensive care unit (ICU): implications for nursing education. Heart Lung, 1972, 1(1):90-98.

E18. Miller J, Preston T D, Dann P E, Bailey J S, Tobin G. Charting v computers. Nursing Times, 1978, Aug 24, :1423-1425.

E19. Morrison S M J. Electronics in nursing. Biomedical applications of space related technology. New Zealand Nursing Journal, 1972, 65(6):12-16.

E20. Nielson B S, Anderson P. Implementation of a patient monitoring system at Herlev Hospital. Proc MIE 78, 1978, :739-744.

E21. Norlander O. Computerised information systems in intensive care units. Advances in Medical Computing, J Rose and J H Mitchell (eds), Churchill Livingstone, 1975, :150-157.

E22. Osborn J J, Beaumont J O. Computerized intensive care. Hospitals, JAHA, 1970, 44:49-53.

E23. Perlstein P H, et al. Computer-assisted newborn intensive care. Pediatrics, 1976, 57:494-501.

E24. Rawles J M. Automation in action. Nursing Mirror, 1970, 130:34-35.

E25. Robicsek F, Masters T N, Reichertz P L, Daugherty H K, Cook J W. Computer-based intensive care of patients following cardiovascular surgery. Proc Medcomp 77 1977, :71-81.

E26. Sabean R, Schillings H, Ehlers C T. Computer support of therapy in intensive care. Proc MIE 79, 1979, :345-358.

E27. Scot D. Whose hand rocks the cradle? Practical Computing, Jan 1980.

E28. Siesel J H, Strom B L. The computer as a "living textbook" applied to the care of the critically injured patient. The Journal of Trauma,Baltimore, 1972, 12(9):739-755.

E29. Taylor D E M. Human computer assisted measurement and diagnosis in an intensive care unit. Health Bulletin, 1976, 34(3):180-182.

E30. Tobin G. Nurse-patient-computer interaction. Scientific Aids in Hospital Diagnosis, :175-178.

E31. Tolbert S H, Pertuz A E. Study shows how computerization affects activities in ICU. Hospitals, Chicago, 1977, 51(17):79-82,84.

E32. Walleck C. The neurosurgical nurse and computer work together. Journal of Neurosurgical Nursing, 1975, 7(2):102-106.

E33. Woolff G A. Computer watches heart beat while nurse watches patient. Modern Hospital, 1971, 117:135-136.

F DRUG MANAGEMENT

F1. Beeley L, Bishop J M, Leach R H, Walker G F. A realtime system for drug prescribing. Proc IRIA Symposium on Medical Data Processing, Toulouse, 1974.

F2. Cohen S N, Armstrong M F, Crouse L, Hunn G S. A computer-based system for prospective detection and prevention of drug interactions. Drug Information Journal, 1972, Jan/Jun, :81-86.

F3. Derewicz H J, Zellers D D. The computer-based unit dose system in the John Hopkins Hospital. Am J Hospital Pharmacy, 1973, 30(3):206-212.

F4. Henney C R, Brodlie P, Crooks J. The administration of drugs in hospital - how a computer can be used to improve the quality of patient care. Proc MEDINFO 74, 1974, :271-276.

F5. Hulse R K, Clark S J, Jackson J C, Warner H R, Gardner R M. Computerized medication monitoring system. American Journal of Hospital Pharmacy, 1976, 33:1061-1064.

F6. Johnston S V, Henney C R, Bosworth R N, Brown N, Crooks J. The doctor, the pharmicist, the computer and the nurse: the prescription, supply, distribution and administration of drugs in hospital. Med Inform, 1976, 1(2):133-144.

F7. Parker E, Whelan K. A prescription chart survey. Nursing Times, Feb 5, 1981.

F8.   Simborg D W, Derewicz H J. A highly automated hospital medication system. Five years' experience and evaluation. Ann Intern Med, 1975, 83(3):342-346.

F9.   Souder D E, Zielstorff R D, Barnett G O. Experience with an automated medication system. Proceedings of Conference on Computer Aid to Drug Therapy and to Drug Monitoring, Ducrot et al (eds). New York: North Holland Publishing, 1978, :291-301.

F10.   Tatro D S, Briggs R L, Chavez-Pardo R, Feinberg L S, Hannigan J F, Moore T N, Cohen S N. Online drug interaction surveillance. Am J Hosp Pharm, 1975, 32(4):417-420.

G   COMMUNITY BASED CARE

G1.   Ashford J R, Pearson N G. A community based medical computing system. Community Health, 3(1).

G2.   Bates T, Dobra S A, Harding L. Regional study of community nursing policy. Proc MIE 82, 1982, :329-335.

G3.   Bradshaw-Smith J H. A computer record-keeping system for general practice. BMJ, 1976, Jun 5, :1395-1397.

G4.   Brown V, Mason W, Kaczmarski M. A computerized health information service. Nurs Outlook, 1971, 19(3):158-161.

G5.   Bussey A L. A Computer-based medical information system for child health. Proc Medcomp 77, 1977, :393-410.

G6.   Eccles T. Community nurses and the computer. Queens Nursing Journal, 1977, 19(14):391-392.

G7.   Gluck J. The computerized medical record system: meeting the challenge for nursing. J Nurs Admin, 1979, 9(12):17-24.

G8.   Griffith R. Nursing in the home - a suitable case for treatment. Computing, 1974, 10 October, :10.

G9.   Hannah K J. The relationship between nursing and medical informatics in community health care settings. Proc MEDINFO 77, 1977, :487-491.

G10.   Highriter M E. A computerized nursing management information system for identification and community follow-up of high-risk infants. NISYS, 1981, :162-178.

G11.   Hoskins D J. The computer assisted school health program (CASH): a field unit's viewpoint. Canadian Journal of Public Health, 1973, 64:521-536.

G12.   Hughes J, Stockton P, Roberts J A, Logan R F L. Nurses in the community: a manpower study. Journal of Epidemiology and Community Health, 1979, 33:262-269.

G13.   Livesay F H. Getting child health records "off the mark". Proc MEDINFO 77, 1977, :539-543.

G14.   McLoone M, Hunter A. A community care information system. Proc MIE 82, 1982, :706-712.

G15.   Meluish G W. A standard register and recall system for child health purposes. Proc MEDINFO 77, 1977, :501-505.

G16.   Meyer D R. What do we need today in a data processing system for nursing? (National League for Nursing Publication No 21-1506). New York, 1973.

G17.   National League for Nursing, Report of conference: state of the art in management information systems for public health/community health agencies (National League for Nurses Publication No 21-1637), 1976.

G18.   Parker M, Ausman R K, Ovedovitz I. Automation of public health nurse reports. Public Health Reports, 1965, 80:526-528.

G19.   Parkinson J S. A review of the national standard child health computer system and its potential benefits. Proc MIE 78, 1978, :745-755.

G20.   Richards I D G, Nicholson M F. The Glasgow linked system of child health records. Developmental Medicine and Child Neurology, 1970, 12(3):357:361.

G21.   Saba V K, Levine E. Patient care module in community health nursing. NISYS, 1981, :243-262.

G22.   Saba V K, Levine E. Management information systems for public health nursing services. Pulic Health Reports, 1978, 93(1):79-83.

G23.   Suffolk Area Health Authority. Suffolk community nursing (Research Project No 26). Suffolk AHA, Ipswich, 1977.

G24.   Walker M, Geller D. Ambulatory pediatric assessment: a computerized system for nurses. Pediatric Nurs, 1977, 3(5):37-41.

G25.   Whelan K M. Blake Fellowship 1980 report on developments in computing. Charing Cross Hospital, 1980.

G26.   Wiseman J. Activities and priorities of health visitors. Nursing Times (Occasional Papers), 1979, 75(24,25).

G27.   Wiseman J. Community nurse records - primary health care nurse. Proc MIE 81, 1981, :421-428.

H   IMPLICATIONS FOR NURSE EDUCATION

H1.   Huckabay L M, et al. Effect of specific teaching techniques on cognitive learning, transfer of learning and affective behaviour of nurses in an in-service education setting. Nurs Res, 1977, 26:380-385.

H2.   Jenkinson V M. The nurse and the computer. British Hospital Journal & Social Services Review, London, 1966, Apr 15, :688.

H3.   Meadows L S. Nursing education in crisis: a computer alternative. J Nurs Educ, 1977, 16(5):13-21.

H4.   Mirin S. The computer's place in nursing education. Nursing and Health Care, 1981, Nov, :500-506.

H5.   Norman S E, Townsend E. Computers in nurse education - a focussed bibliography. Sheffield City Polytechnic, 1982.

H6.   Price E M. A nurse looks at data processing. Pelican News, 1967, 23:6-9.

H7.   Price E M. Responsibility of nurses for data processing services. Chart, 1968, 65:257-260.

H8.   Ronald J S. Computers and undergraduate nursing education: a report on an experimental introductory course. J Nurs Educ, 1979, 18(9):4-9.

H9.   Runck H W. Information: systems need nurses. Datamation, 1968, 14:56-59.

H10.   Tornyay de R. Industrial technology and nursing education. J Nurs Educ, 1970, 9:8.

I   COMPUTER ASSISTED LEARNING

I1.   Bitzer M D. Clinical nursing instruction via the PLATO simulated laboratory. Nurs Res, 1966, 15(2):144-150.

I2.   Bitzer M D, Bitzer D L. Teaching nursing by computer: an evaluative study. Comput Biol Med, 1973, 3:187-204.

I3.   Bitzer M D, Boudreaux M C. Using a computer to teach nursing. Nurs Forum, 1969, 8(3):234-254.

I4.   Bitzer M D, Boudreaux M C, Avner R A. Computer-based instruction of basic nursing utilizing inquiry approach. Urbana, Illinois, Univ of Illinois, Computer-based Education Research Laboratory, 1973.

I5.   Buchholz L M. Computer assisted insruction for the self-directed professional learner. J Contin Educ Nurs, 1979, 10(1), :12-14.

I6.   Collart M E. Computer-assisted instruction and the teaching-learning process. Nurs Outlook, 1973, 21(8):527-532.

I7.   Conklin D. Computers in nursing education. Proc COACH Nursing Workshop, Mimeograph, 1978.

I8.   Finch A J. For students only: a system for learning. Nurs Outlook, 1971, 19(5):332-333.

I9.   Grobe S. CAI: a tie to nursing research. Proc Dr Mabel A Wandelt Conference, Univ of Texas at Austin School of Nursing, 1982.

I10.   Grobe S. The authoring system approach for developing CAI on nursing process. Proc ADCIS, Denver, Colorado, 1982.

I11. Hannah K J. Report of the computer assisted instruction project in the
      faculty of nursing at the University of Calgary. New Directions in
      Educational Computing, J Hirschbuhl (ed), ADCIS Publications, Bellingham,
      Washington, 1978, :289-294.

I12. Hannah K J. Overview of computer assisted learning in nursing education at
      the University of Calgary. Perspectives: Nursing Education, Practice and
      Research, M C Stainton et al (eds), University of Calgary, 1978, :43-56.

I13. Hannah K J, Conklin D N. The CAI microcomputer project in the faculty of
      nursing at the University of Calgary. Computer Literacy: Intelligent CAI,
      E Attala (ed), ADCIS Publications, Bellingham, Washington, 1982, :136-140.

I14. Hoffer E P, Mathewson H O, Loughrey A, et al. Use of computer-aided
      instruction in graduate nursing education: a controlled trial. J Emerg
      Nurs, 1975, 1(2):27-29.

I15. Huckabay L M D, Anderson N, Holm D M, Lee J. Cognitive, affective, and
      transfer of learning consequences of computer assisted insruction. Nurs
      Res, 1979, 28(4):228-233.

I16. Kamp M, Burnside I M. Computer-assisted learning in graduate psychiatric
      nursing. J Nurs Educ, 1974, 13(4):18-25.

I17. Kirchhoff K T, Holzemer W L. Student learning and a computer-assisted
      instructional program. J Nurs Educ, 1979, 18(3):22-30.

I18. Kuramoto A M. Computer-assisted instruction: will it be used? Nursing
      Leadership, 1978, 1(1):10-13.

I19. Landureth L J, Lamendola J A. Computers in nursing education. Hospitals,
      1978, 47(5):99-100,102.

I20. Levine D, Wiener E. Let the computer teach it. Am J Nurs, 1975,
      75(8):1300-1302.

I21. Lidz C G. Computer-managed instruction in nursing. New York: National
      League for Nursing, 1974.

I22. Naber S. Computerized nurse-midwifery management: its usefullness as a
      learning-teaching tool. J Nurse-Midwifery, 1975, 20(3):26-28.

I23. Norman S E. Computer-assisted learning - its potential in nurse education.
      Nursing Times, 1982, Sep 1, :1467-1468.

I24. Olivieri P, Sweeney M A. Evaluation of clinical learning by computer.
      Nurse Educator, 1980, 5(4):26-31.

I25. Porter S F. Application of computer-assisted instruction to continuing
      education in nursing: review of the literature. J Contin Educ Nurs, 1978,
      9(6):5-9.

I26. Reed F C, et al. Computer assisted instruction for continued learning. Am
      J Nurs, 1972, 72(11):2035-2039.

I27. Ross G R, Ross M C. Using the computer to prepare multiple choice
      examinations: a simplified system. J Nurs Educ, 1977, 16(5):32-39.

I28. Sumida S W. A computerised test for clinical decision making. Nurs
      Outlook, 1972, 20(7):458-461.

I29. Tymchyshyn P, Helper J. PLATO goes to the hospital. Nursing Careers, 1981,
      2(2):16-19.

I30. Unknown. A guide for authoring and programming computer-assisted
      instruction. Chemeketa Community College, Salem, Oregon, 1982.

I31. Valish A U, Boyd N J. The role of computer-assisted instruction in
      continuing education of registered nurses: an experimental study. J Cont
      Educ Nurs, 1975, 6(1):13-32.

I32. Ward J A, Griffin J M. Improving instruction through computer-graded
      examinations. Nurs Outlook, 1977, 25(8):524-529.

I33. Watkins C. Student evaluation by computer. Nurs Outlook, 1975, 23(7):449-
      452.

J   EDUCATION PROGRAMMES AND RECORDS

Education Programmes and Allocation

J1. Barlow A J. Nurse allocation by computer. Nursing Mirror, 1972, 134(4):43-45.

J2. Bosworth R N, Henney C R, Crooks J. A computer-based system for the automatic production of nursing workload data. Nursing Times, 1980, 76(28):1212-1217.

J3. Butler E A, Howarth M A. A computer system for student nurse allocation during training. Proc MIE 79, 1979, :219-229.

J4. Goldstone L, Collier M. Targets for quality. Health and Social Service Journal, 1982, Mar 25, :362-365.

J5. Henney C R, Bosworth R N, Chrissafis I, Crooks J. Nurse allocation by computer. Proc MIE 79, 1979, :244-252.

J6. Maguire G, Roberts J. Nursing allocation with computer assistance - extension to a manpower planner. Proc MIE 82, 1982, :317-321.

J7. Moriuchi J, et al. Juggling staff to reduce costs. Dimensions in Health Service, 1978, 55(4):13-14.

J8. Morrish A R, O'Connor A R. Cyclic scheduling. Hospitals, JAHA, 1970 (44):67-71.

J9. Moores B, Wood I. Nursing Allocation. Nursing Times, 1977, Aug 18, :109-112.

J10. Murray D J. Computer makes the schedules for nurses. Modern Hospital, 1971, 117:104-105.

J11. Shah A R. A computer-aided interative procedure to improve nurse-training programmes. Med Inform, 1979, 4(4):209-218.

J12. Shah A R, Hollowell J A. An optimal allocation of newly qualified nurses to wards. Proc MIE 81, 1981, :389-395.

J13. Smith L D, Bird D A. Designing computer support for daily hospital staffing decisions. Med Inform, 1979, 4(2):69-78.

J14. Smith L D, Bird D A, Wiggins A C. A computerized system to schedule nurses that recognizes staff preferences. Hospital and Health Services Administration, 1979, Fall, :19-35.

J15. Smith L D, Wiggins A. A computer-based nurse scheduling system. Computers and Operations Research, 1977, 4:195-212.

J16. Smith L D, Wiggins A, Bird D. Post-implementation experience with computer assisted nurse scheduling in a large hospital. INFOR, Canadian J Operational Research and Information Processing, 1979, 17(4):309-321.

J17. Soulsby A. Computer nurse allocation. Northern Regional Health Authority, Internal Report, 1975, Apr.

J18. Trent RHA. Schools of nursing computer system - user system specification (allocation). Internal Report No. C81 Trent Regional Health Authority, Aug 1981.

J19. Warner D M. Scheduling nursing personnel according to nursing preference: a mathematical programming approach. Operations Research, 1976, 24(5):842-856.

Records Systems

J20. Collins S M, Cundy A D, Shah A R. A computer based record system for nursing-learners. Proc MIE 79, 1979, :230-243.

J21. Dixon J M, Gouyd N, Varricchio D T. Computerized education and training record. J Cont. Educ Nurs, 1975, 6(4):20-23.

J22. Dwyer R N, Schmitt J A. Using the computer to evaluate clinical performance. Nursing Forum, 8(3), 1969, :266-275.

K PLANNING THE NURSING SERVICE

K1. Barnett G O, Zielstorff R D. Data systems can enhance or hinder medical, nursing activities. Hospitals, JAHA, 1977, 51:157-161.

K2.   Brady F K. A head nurse's viewpoint of automation. A.N.A Regional Clinical Conference, 1967, :46-50.
K3.   Brown R L. Computerised nursing. Nursing Mirror, 1976, 142(6):56.
K4.   Brunt van E E, Collen M F. Nursing station subsystems. Hospital Computer Systems, Collen M (ed.), Wiley, 1974, :114-147.
K5.   Campbell C M. Automatic data processing: information system for a short-term hospital. Hospitals, 1964, 38:71-75.
K6.   Cook M, McDowell W. Changing to an automated information system. Am J Nurs, 1975, 75(1):46-51.
K7.   Farlee C, Goldstein B. A role for nurses in implementing computerized hospital information systems. Nursing Forum, 1971, 10:339-357.
K8.   Flynn E D. The computer: an aid to nursing communication. Nursing Clinics of North America, 1969, 4:541-548.
K9.   Huff W S. Shared computer time: big benefits for small hospitals. Modern Hospital, 1979, Nov, :88-94.
K10.   Inman D W, Henry J, Melville P. Simulation and queing models to assist planning of accident and emergency services. Proc MIE 81, 1981, :266-274.
K11.   Jenkinson V M. Student nurses and the computer. Nursing Times, 1972, Mar 2, :254-255.
K12.   Mather B S. Nursing staff attitudes. The Australian Nurses Journal, 1973, 3(1):20-22.
K13.   Miller R A, DeLeon R F. Development of a computerized pharmacy control system. Am J Hospital Pharmacy, 1979, (29):963-966.
K14.   Reeves T J. Automation at the nurses' station. American Nurses' Association Regional Clinical Conference, American Nurses' Association, 1967, :41-45.
K15.   Sloane R. Computer-assisted manpower planning. Health and Social Services Journal, 1981, Jan 16, :49-51.
K16.   Zielstorff R D. Designing automated information systems. J Nurs Admin, 1977, Apr, :14-19.
K18.   Zielstorff R D. Orienting personnel to automated systems. J Nurs Admin, 1976, Mar/Apr, :14-16.

L RESOURCE MANAGEMENT

L1.   Ahuja H, Sheppard R. Computerized nurse scheduling. Industrial Engineering, 1975, 1(10):24-29.
L2.   Alderson M. Health information systems. Proc MEDINFO 77, 1977, :595-601.
L3.   Anderson J. Education of health staff in information processing techniques. Proc MEDINFO 77, 1977, :975-978.
L4.   Bahr J, Badour G, Hill H L. Innovative methodology enhances nurse deployment, cuts costs. Hospitals, JAHA, 1977, 51(8):104ff.
L5.   Ballantyne D J. Computerized scheduling system with centralized staffing. J Nurs Admin, 1979, :38-45.
L6.   Brooks A H. Training and organization of hospital personnel for a hospital communication system. Proc MEDINFO 77, 1977, :989-992.
L7.   Bryant Y M, Bryant J R. Towards an integrated system for nursing administration. Proc Medcomp 77, 1977, :439-451.
L8.   Butler E A, Hay B J. The passionate statistician: a computerised record of nursing sickness and absence. Nursing Times (Occasional Paper), 1977, Nov 24, Dec 1, :149-156 - Also published in Proc. Medcomp 77, 1977, 453-467).
L9.   Clark N. Automation as it affects the general nurse and her patients. Journal of West Australian Nurses' Association, 1968, 34:8-10.
L10.   Community Nursing Services of Philadelphia. Development of a computerized record system to store and summarize information relevant to administration, evaluation and planning of nursing services, (Contract NO1 NU-241271). Washington DC, Division of Nursing, Health Resources Administration, DHEW, 1976.

L11. Cook M. Introduction of a user-orientated THIS into a community hospital setting - nursing. Proc MEDINFO 74, 1974, :303-304.

L12. Duraiswamy N, Welton R, Reisman A. Using computer simulation to predict ICU staffing needs. J Nurs Admin, 1981, 11(2):39-44.

L13. Erat K E. The Use of Clinfo as a teaching tool to introduce health care personnel to computers and their applications. Proc MIE 82, 1982, :348-354.

L14. Erat K E, McGrath S. Developing a teaching/learning experience for nurses in fundamentals of computer programming preliminary to nursing research. Proc NECC 1979, D Harris (ed), University of Iowa, 1979, :316-325.

L15. Ernst E A, Hoppel C L, Lorig J L, Danielson R A. Operating room scheduling by computer. Anesth Analg, 1977, 56(6):831- 35.

L16. Finlayson H. The NUMBRS approach to nursing management. Dimensions in Health Service, 1976, May.

L17. Garrison G P. Computerization - implications for nursing service departments. New York, National League for Nursing, 1970.

L18. Gebhardt A N. Utilizing an on-line computer system for patient classification and staff determination.Proc MIE 82, 1982, :322-328.

L19. Gillam R. The use of computers in nursing. International Nursing Review, 1968, 4(15):308-352.

L20. Greenburg A G. The role of the computer in patient care. Surgery Annual, 1974, 6:61-71.

L21. Hale P, Hall J. Computers and their application to senior management - nursing division. The Lamp, 1977, 34(8):39-47.

L22. Hannah K J. Computers and nursing. Hospital Administration in Canada, 1978, 20(5):20-23.

L23. Hartmann B. The Impact of computers in nursing. Proc MEDINFO 74, 1974, :305-308.

L24. Hershey J C, Moore J R Jr. Use of an information system for community health services planning and management: Livingston, California. Medical Care, 1975, 13(2):114-125.

L25. Jackson R M, Kortge C. Automated proficiency reports. Hospitals, JAHA, 1971, 45(1):76-78.

L26. Jelinek R C, Zinn T K, Byra J R. Tell the computer how sick the patients are and it will tell how many nurses they need. Modern Hospital, 1973, Dec.

L27. Johansen S, Orthoefer J E. Development of a school health information system. American Journal of Public Health, 1975, 65(11):1203-1207.

L28. Johnson M E, Jackson R M. An integrated medical-financial hospital information system: utilization of the ancillary services as the basic modules. Hospital Information Systems, R H Shannon (ed), North Holland, 1979.

L29. Langill G, et al. A computer-assisted nursing audit program. Dimensions in Health Service, 1978, 55(3):36-37.

L30. Levy A H, Baker R L, Carrick J M. Electronic information programs: an inhospital system. Hospital and Community Psychiatry, 1970, 21:7-10.

L31. Mather B S. Use of an automated register in the administration of an operating theatre suite. Anaesthesia and Intensive Care, 1976, 4(3):211-216.

L32. Morooka K, Ogawa I. A quality control plan for nursing service. Proc International Conference on Systems Science in Health Care, Montreal, July 14-17, 1980.

L33. Paton M H, Ward K. The hospital nurse and electronic data processing. New Zealand Nurses' Journal, 1970, 63:11-13.

L34. Peel V J, Male R S, Gunawardena A. Computers in in-patient information systems - an alternative local approach. Hospital and Health Services Review, 1981, Jan, :5-11.

L35. Rhys Hearn C, Bishop J M. Computer model simulating medical care in hospital. BMJ, 1970,3:396-399.

L36. Saba V. Yesterday, today, and tomorrow in community health management information. In State of the Art in Management Information Systems for Public Health/Community Health Agencies: Report of the Conference. New York: National League for Nursing, 1976, :61-69.

L37. Scholes M. Education of health staff in computing. Proc MEDINFO 74, 1974, :213-215.

L38. Scholes M, Forster K V, Gregg T. Continuing education of health service staff in computing. Proc Medcomp 77, 1977, :639-648.

L39. Slack P. SNIPPET - a computerised nursing information bank. Nursing Times, 1981, Apr 9, :656-659.

L40. Smith J L. The computer: its impact on the physician, the nurse, and the administrator. Hospitals, 1969, 43:61-65.

L41. Somers J B. Purpose and performance: a system analysis of nurse staffing. J Nurs Admin, 1977, Feb, :4-9.

L42. Squire P. Monitoring a sick pattern. Nursing Mirror, 1982, Feb 10, :20-22.

L43. Squire P. Name, rank and number. Nursing Mirror, 1982, Feb 3, :30-33.

L44. Thomson M E. An automated ward census and reporting system. How computers help nurses. The Australian Nurses Journal, 1973, 3(1):16-19.

L45. Toussaint J R. Why not schedule labor with the computer? 1970 , Feb, :14-17,32.

L46. Ulett G A, Sletten I W. A statewide electronic data processing system. Hospital and Community Psychiatry, 1969, 20:74-77.

L47. Unknown. Computer systems spread to patient care (Special Report). Modern Hospital, 1979, Nov, :84-85.

L48. Verzi M A. Task audit program (TAP) pinpoints staffing needs. Hospitals, JAHA, 1966, 40(1):56-59,121.

M MANAGEMENT SCIENCES IN THE NURSING SERVICE

M1. Barber B. Patients' perspectives in hospital information systems. Hospital Information Systems, R H Shannon(ed), North Holland, 1979, :31-39.

M2. Liebman J S, Young J P, Bellmore M. Allocation of nursing personnel in an extended care facility. Health Services Research, 1972, 7(3):209-220.

M3. Luck G M, Luckman J, Smith B W, Stringer J. Planning surgery: a computer simulation. Patients, Hospital, and Operational Research, Chap 10, Tavistock Publication 1971.

M4. Monaco R J, Smith T T. How supervisors can put systems to work in day to day management. Hospital Topics, 1977, Sep/Oct, :34-41.

M5. Wolfe H. A multiple assignment model for staffing nursing units. Operations Research Division, The John Hopkins Hospital, Baltimore.

N RESEARCH

N1. Beggs S, Vallbona C, Spencer W A, Jacobs F M, Baker R L. Evaluation of a system for on-line computer scheduling of patient care activities. Computers and Biomedical Research, 1971, 4:634-654.

N2. Murphy J R. Preparing research data for computerization. Am J Nurs, 1979, 79(5):954-956.

N3. Stein R F. Use of automated nursing reports. Indiana Nurse, 1970, 34:6-11.

N4. Sweeney M A, Olivieri P, An Introduction to Nursing Research, Part V - Using the Computer, :297-386.

O HEALTH CARE SYSTEMS

O1. Barker M. The era of the computer and its impact on nursing. Supervisor Nurse, 1971, 2:26-36.

02. Bartel G J, Fahey J J. Nursing station is home base for phone printer system. Modern Hospital, 1969, 113:85-88.

03. Chodoff P, Gianaris C. A nurse-computer assisted preoperative anesthesia management. Computers and Biomedical Research, 1973, (6):371-392.

04. Clarkson D McG, Gray R H, Jones D H A, Smith P H S, Jones I W. Microcomputer system in an accident unit. BMJ, 1982, 284:722-724.

05. Collen M F. (ed). Hospital computer systems. Wiley, 1974.

06. Cook M, Mayers M. Computer-assisted data base for nursing research. NISYS, 1981, :149-156.

07. DeMarco J P. Automating nursing's paper work. Am J Nurs, 1965, 65(9):74-77

08. Haessler H A, Cooper C G. Staff reaction to a hospital information system. Proc Medcomp 77, 1977, :625-638.

09. Johnson D S, Ranzenberger J. A computer-based system for hospital-based patient monitoring. NISYS, 1981, :196-213.

010. Jotwani P. A nursing-centred patient information system. NISYS, 1981, :179-195.

011. Keliher P. The standardized form. Supervisor Nurse, 1975, (11):40-41,44-45.

012. Kelly J, Roberts J, Harvey P W. A simple data-processing system for the monitoring of cross-infection in a district general hospital. Med Inform, 1979, 4(1):29-34.

013. King Faisal Hospital. Computers aid patient care. Middle East Health Service & Supply. 1977, Feb, 1(2):26-28,31.

014. Lilford R J, Chard T. Microcomputers in antenatal care: a feasibility study on the booking interview. BMJ, 1981, (283):533-536.

015. McIntyre N. Instant information. Health and Social Service Journal, 1981, Aug 14, :980-984.

016. McNeil D G. Developing the complete computer-based information system. J Nurs Admin, 1979, 9(11):34-46.

017. Maresh M, Steer P J, Dawson A M, Beard R W. The logical development of a perinatal data base for clinicians. Proc MIE 78, 1978:156-161.

018. Monagle W J, Lasalle T D. Computerized multiphasic screening: more tests, more speed - but not more cost. Modern Hospital, 1979, Nov, :100-103.

019. Norwood D D. A patient care quality assurance system overlayed on a hospital-wide medical information system (El-Camino Hospital-Phas 2), Proc MEDINFO 77, 1977, :23-27.

020. O'Dwyer T V. The establishment of a perinatal notification system in Ireland. Proc MIE 78, 1978, :180-187.

021. Ohsato A, Sekiguchi T, Nakai T, Yamazaki K. Information processing for nursing by fuzzy relation. Proc MEDINFO 80, 1980, :62-66.

022. Prendergast J A, Inns J E. Spectra: a computerized medical information system. NISYS, 1981, :214-220.

023. Price E M. Data processing: present and potential. Am J Nurs, 1967, 67:2558-2564.

024. Rankin J W. Four Carolina hospitals go on-line with computer. Modern Hospital, 1968, 111:86-89.

025. Saunders M, Campbell S, White H, Coats P. A unique real-time method of obstetric data collection. Proc MIE 78, 1978, :143-155.

026. Schmitz H H, et al. Study evaluates effects of new communication system. Hospitals, 1976, 50(21):129-130,132,134.

027. Simborg D W, Macdonald L K. Liebman J S, Musco P. Ward information management system - an evaluation. Computers and Biomedical Research, 1972, 5:484-497.

028. Sofaly K J. The nurse and the computerized history. NISYS, 1981, :157-195.

029. Taylor D B. A clinical information system: a tool for improving nurses' decisions in planning patient care. In ANA Clinical Sessions American Nurses' Association, 1970.

030. Walker C H M. Neonatal records and the computer. Archives of Disease in Childhood, 1977, 52:452-461.

O31.   Warford H S, Jennett R J, Gall D A. A computerized perinatal data system.
        Med Inform, 1979, 4(3):133-138.

P   UNCLASSIFIED REFERENCES

P1.   Chodoff P, Helrich M. Construction of an automated system for the
        collection and processing of preoperative data. Anesth Analg, 1969,
        48:870-876.
P2.   Given C W, Given B. Automation and technology: a key to professional care.
        Nursing Forum, 1969, 8(1).
P3.   Jacobs S E. Growth in hospital computer usage. Computer Medicine, 1975,
        5(8):1,3.
P4.   Opit L J, Woodroffe F J. Computer-held clinical record system. BMJ, 1970,
        4, 76.
P5.   Randall A M. The nursing system - a computer challenge of the 80's.
        Computers in Hospitals, 1982, 3:50-53.
P6.   Singer J P. Hospital computer systems: myths and realities. Hospital
        Topics, 1971, 49.

AUTHOR INDEX FOR BIBLIOGRAPHY

Acton J C...E1
Adams H...E11
Ahuja H...L1
Alderson M...L2
Allwood J M...E2
Anderson J...D7,L3
Anderson N...I15
Anderson P...E20
Armstrong M F...F2
Ashcroft J M...E3,E4
Ashford J R...G1
Ashton C C...A1,C1,C2,C3
Atack C C...A2
Ausman R K...G18
Avner R A...I4

Badour G...L4
Bahr J...L4
Bailey J S...E18
Baker J D...B1
Baker R L...L30,N1
Ballantyne D J...L5
Barber B...A3,A4,A5,A18,M1
Barker M...O1
Barlow A J...J1
Barnett G O...B2,F9,K1
Bartel G J...O2
Bartoszek V...B3
Bates T...G2
Beard R W...O17
Beaumont J O...E17,E22
Beeley L...F1
Beggs S...N1
Bellmore M...M2
Berry J L...E4
Bhargava B...C9
Birckhead L M...B4,B5,B6
Bird D A...J13,J14,J16
Bishop J M...F1,L35
Bitzer D L...I2
Bitzer M D...I1,I2,I3,I4
Blevins L...C9
Bosworth R N...C6,C7,D15,F6,J2,J5
Boudreaux M C...I3,I4
Bouveret C...C4
Boyd N J...I31
Bradshaw-Smith J H...G3
Brady F K...K2
Briggs R L...F10

Brodlie P...F4
Brooks A H...L6
Brown N...C7,F6
Brown P T S...B7
Brown R L...K3
Brown V...G4
Brunt van E E...K4
Brush F...D1
Bryant J R...L7
Bryant Y M...A1,A6,D12,D13,L7
Buchholz L M...I5
Burnside I M...I16
Bussey A L...G5
Butler E A...A7,A8,J3,L8
Byra J R...L26

Campbell C M...K5
Campbell S...O25
Carrick A G...D2
Carrick J M...L30
Carriker D...C13
Castledine G...B8
Chard T...O14
Chavez-Pardo R...F10
Chierchia S...E16
Chodoff P...O3,P1
Chorobik T...C4
Chow R...E5
Chrissafis I...J5
Christopherson K I...E6
Clark N...L9
Clark S J...F5
Clarkson D McG...O4
Coats P...O25
Cohen R D...A3
Cohen S N...F2,F10
Collart M E...I6
Collen M F...K4,O5
Collier M...J4
Collins S M...J20
Community Nursing Services of
  Philadelphia...L10
Conklin D...I7
Conklin D N...I13
Cook J W...E25
Cook M...K6,L11,O6
Cooper C G...O8
Cornell S A...D1,D2
Creighton H...B9

Crooks J...C7,F4,F6,J2,J5
Crouse L...F2
Cundy A D...J20
Curtis S...D7

Danielson R A...L15
Dann P E...E18
Daugherty H K...E25
Davis A...D6
Dawson A M...O17
DeLeon R F...K13
DeMarco J P...O7
DeSanders N...D3
Dechanoz G...C4
Derewicz H J...F3,F8
Dingwall R...B10
Dixon J M...J21
Dobra S A...G2
Donald L...B11
Drazen E...E7,E8
Dupuy M...C4
Duraiswamy N...L12
Dwyer R N...J22
Eccles T...G6
Edwards B S...B14
Ehlers C T...E26
Eisler J...B12
Endo A S...E9
Erat K E...L13,L14
Ernst E A...L15
Fahey J J...O2
Falcoz H...C4
Farlee C...K7
Feinberg L S...F10
Finch A J...I8
Fink R...E13
Finlayson H...L16
Flynn E D...K8
Forster K V...L38
Franklin C B...B13
Froment A...C4

Gall D A...O31
Gardner R M...F5
Garrison G P...L17
Gatewood L C...A9
Gebhardt A N...L18
Geller D...G24
Gennaro W B...B25
Gerbode F...E10
Gianaris C...O3
Gillam R...L19
Given B...P2
Given C W...P2
Gluck J...G7
Glueck B C...C14,C19
Goering P...B12
Goldstein B...K7
Goldstone L...J4
Goodwin J O...B14
Gordon M...E11

Goshen C E...B15
Gouyd N...J21
Gray R H...O4
Greenburg A G...E12,E13,E14,L20
Gregg T...L38
Griffin J M...I32
Griffith R...G8
Grobe S...I9,I10
Gunawardena A...L34
Guttman L...A13

Haessler H A...O8
Hale P...L21
Hall J...L21
Hammersley P...A10,D12
Hannah K J...A11,B16,B17,G9,I11,
   I12,I13,L22
Hannigan J F...F10
Harding L...G2
Harman R J...D14
Hartmann B...L23
Harvey P W...O12
Hay B J...L8
Head A E...C5,C12
Helper J...I29
Helrich M...P1
Henney C R...C6,C7,D4,D15,F4,F6,J2,J5
Henry J...K10
Heron K...D13
Hershey J C...L24
Highriter M E...G10
Hill H L...L4
Hoffer E P...I14
Hollowell J A...J12
Holm D M...I15
Holzemer W L...I17
Hoppel C L...L15
Hoskins D J...G11
Howarth M A...J3
Huckabay L M D...H1,I15
Huff W S...K9
Hughes J...G12
Hughes S J...D5
Hulse R K...F5
Hunn G S...F2
Hunter A...G14
Inman D W...K10
Inns J E...O22
Jackson J C...F5
Jackson R M...L25,L28
Jacobs F M...N1
Jacobs S E...P3
Janus C A...E14
Jarvis J...C12
Jelinek R C...L26
Jenkinson V M...H2,K11
Jennett R J...O31
Jeris C...C9
Johansen S...L27
Johnson D S...O9
Johnson M E...L28

Johnson O H...B28
Johnston S V...F6
Jones D H A...O4
Jones I W...O4
Joshi M...E15
Jotwani P...O10

Kaczmarski M...G4
Kamp M...I16
Keliher P...O11
Kelly J...O12
King Faisal Hospital...O13
Kirchhoff K T...I17
Kirklin J W...E1
Knight J E...C8
Kortge C...L25
Kouchoukos N J...E1
Kumpel Z...D6
Kuramoto A M...I18

Lamendola J A...I19
Landucci L...E16
Landureth L J...I19
Langill G...L29
Lasalle T D...O18
Lazzari M...E16
Leach R H...F1
Lee J...I15
Levine D...I20
Levine E...G21,G22
Levy A H...L30
Lidz C G...I21
Liebman J S...M2
Lilford R J...O14
Lindop N...A12
Livesay F H...G13
Logan R F L...G12
Lorig J L...L15
Loughrey A...I14
Luck G M...M3
Luckman J...M3

Macdonald L K...O27
Macerata C...E16
Magnon R...C4
Maguire G...J6
Male R S...L34
Marchesi C...E16
Maresh M...O17
Martindale A...B18
Martz K Y...E17
Maseri A...E16
Mason W...G4
Masters T N...E25
Mather B S...K12,L31
Mathewson H O...I14
Mayers M...O6
McClure D K...E13,E14
McDonald C J...C9
McDowell W...K6
McGrath S...L14

McIntyre N...O15
McLaughlin L...B19
McLoone M...G14
McNeil D G...O16
Meadows L S...H3
Melinon S...C4
Meluish G W...G15
Melville P...K10
Meyer D R...G16
Michard P...C4
Miller J...E18
Miller R A...K13
Milon H...C4
Mirin S...H4
Monaco R J...M4
Monagle W J...O18
Moore J R Jr...L24
Moore T N...F10
Moores B...D16,J9
Moriuchi J...J7
Morooka K...L32
Morrish A R...J8
Morrison S M J...E19
Moult A...D16
Murphy J R...N2
Murray D J...J10
Murray E...D7
Murray R...C9

Naber S...I22
Nakai T...O21
National Centre for Health Services
    Research...B20
National League for Nursing...G17
Nicholson M F...G20
Nielson B S...E20
Norlander O...E21
Norman S E...H5,I23
Norwood D D...O19

O'Connor A R...J8
O'Dwyer T V...O O
O'Rourke M...C11
Ogawa I...L32
Ohsato A...O21
Olivieri P...I24,N4
Olssen D E...C10
Opit L J...P4
Orthoefer J E...L27
Osborn J J...E22
Ovedovitz I...G18

Parker E...F7
Parker M...G18
Parkinson J S...G19
Parsons R...D8
Paton M H...L33
Pearson N G...G1
Peel V J...L34
Perlstein P H...E23
Pertuz A E...E31

Peskin G W...E13
Pocklington D B...A13
Porter S F...I25
Prendergast J A...A14,022
Preston T D...E18
Price E M...H6,H7,023
Pritchard K...B21,B22,B23,B24
Procter P M...C12

Randall A M...P5
Rankin J W...024
Ranzenberger J...09
Rappoport A E...B25
Rawles J M...E24
Reed F C...I26
Reeves T J...K14
Regester W D...A15
Reichertz P L...E25
Reisman A...L12
Rhys Hearn C...D17,D18,L35
Richards I D G...G20
Roberts J...J6,012
Roberts J A...G12
Robicsek F...E25
Ronald J S...H8
Rosenberg M...C13,C14
Ross G R...I27
Ross M C...I27
Runck H W...H9

Saba V K...G21,G22,L36
Sabean R...E26
Saunders M...025
Schillings H...E26
Schmitt J A...J22
Schmitz H H...026
Scholes M...A3,A4,A5,A16,A17,A18,L37,L38
Scot D...E27
Seeger J...C9
Sekiguchi T...021
Shah A R...J11,J12,J20
Sheppard L C...E1
Sheppard R...L1
Siesel J H...E28
Simborg D W...C15,F8,027
Singer J P...P6
Slack P...A19,L39
Sletten I W...L46
Sloane R...K15
Smith   ...C16
Smith B W...M3
Smith E J...C17
Smith J L...L40
Smith L D...J13,J14,J15,J16
Smith P H S...04
Smith T T...M4
Sofaly K J...B26,028
Somers J B...D10,L41
Souder D E...F9
Soulsby A...J17
Speed E L...D9

Spencer W A...N1
Squire P...L42,L43
Steele B...B18
Steer P J...017
Stein R F...C18,N3
Stockton P...G12
Streeter J...C8
Stringer J...M3
Stroebel C F...C19
Strom B L...E28
Stubbs J A...E13,E14
Suffolk Area Health Authority...G23
Sumida S W...I28
Sweeney M A...I24,N4

Tate S P...B27
Tatro D S...F10
Taylor D B...B28,029
Taylor D E M...E29
Thomson M E...L44
Tierney J...B12
Tobin G...E18,E30
Tolbert S H...E31
Tomasovic E R...B29
Tornyay de R...H10
Toussaint J R...L45
Townsend E...H5
Trent RHA...J18
Tymchyshyn P...I29

UK Government...A20,A21
Ulett G A...L46
Unknown...B30,I30,L47

Valish A U...I31
Vallbona C...N1
Varricchio D T...J21
Venn J C...E11
Verzi M A...L48

Walker C H M...030
Walker G F...F1
Walker M...G24
Walleck C...E32
Ward J A...I32
Ward K...L33
Wardener de H E...E11
Warford H S...031
Warner D M...J19
Warner H R...F5
Watkin B R...B31
Watkins C...I33
Webb J...E11
Wechsler A...E8
Welton R...L12
Wesseling E...D11
Westwood B...B32
Whelan K M...F7,G25
White H...025
Wiener E...I20
Wiggins A C...J14,J15,J16

Wiig K...E8
Wiseman J...G26,G27
Wolfe H...M5
Wood I...J9
Woodroffe F J...P4
Woolff G A...E33

Yamazaki K...O21
Young B...D17
Young J P...M2
Young N A...D9
Younger K...A22
Zellers D D...F3
Zielstorff R D...B33,B34,F9,K1,K16,K18
Zinn T K...L26

ORGANIZING COMMITTEE AND CONTRIBUTORS

William Abbott, MBCS AHA is Management Services Officer for the North East Thames Regional Health Authority, UK. He has been involved in the National Health Service for 36 years and with computing for 25. Currently UK representative and secretary of the International Medical Informatics Association. **Organising Committee Treasurer.**

John Anderson, MD MA BSc FRCP FBCS is Professor of Medicine at Kings College Hospital Medical School, Denmark Hill, London, UK. He is chairman of the London Medical Specialist Group of the British Computer Society, has a keen interest in Medical Informatics in Education and is chairman of the Editorial Board of Medical Informatics.

Clare Ashton, SRN is a systems designer in the computer services department at the Queen Elizabeth Hospital, Birmingham, UK where she has worked for over 10 years in designing and implementing wardbased computer systems. She is currently Chairman of the Computer Projects Nurses Group (DHSS). **Organising Committee, Joint Co-ordinator Care Stream.**

Barry Barber, PhD MA FInstP FBCS FSS worked at The London Hospital UK for 21 years as a medical physicist, an operations analyst and a computer scientist before moving to the North East Thames Regional Health Authority. His specialties are health care informatics and health care planning. **Organising Committee Secretary, Joint Editor.**

Constance Berg, RN BA MBA has been in the 'computers in health care' industry since 1972. Her experience with Technicon Data Systems Corporation, California, USA includes design, training, implementation and marketing of medical information systems.

Joy Brown, SRN SCM RN is a nursing analyst at the York Central Hospital, Ontario, Canada. She has been involved with computers in nursing for the past 4 years and has extensive background knowledge in design and coding, nursing workload measurement and nursing administration in IBM patient care systems.

Yvonne M Bryant, SRN MBCS spent eight years as the nursing adviser to the Computer Unit at Addenbrookes Hospital, Cambridge, UK. Part of her work included liaison with nursing staff to ensure communication at all levels. She is a member of the Computer Projects Nurses Group (DHSS). **Organising Committee, Joint Editor.**

Elizabeth Butler, SRN ONC MChs CMBPart 1 is senior nursing officer, computing, at St. Thomas' Hospital, London, UK. This post has an advisory/co-ordinating function between the division of nursing and the computing services department. She is a member of the Computer Projects Nurses Group (DHSS). **Organising Committee, Joint Co-ordinator Management Stream.**

Jim Cartwright OBE, Executive, NHS Training Centre, Harrogate.

Joan Cobin, PhD RN FAAN is a professor occupying the chair of the nursing department, California State University, USA. She has received awards as an outstanding educator and she supports several projects enhancing the learning environment for all students and faculty.

Sheila M. Collins OBE, BA SRN RSCN RNT FRCN, is a nurse educator who has been involved in the advancement of professional education for nurses in the UK since 1960. As a member of a multidisciplinary team she has developed computer based systems at The Princess Alexandra School of Nursing, The London Hospital, which have improved the design of courses, for the benefit of nursing students and for nursing management.

Margo Cook, RN MA is Director, Medical Information System, El Camino Hospital, California, USA. She has experience in patient care records, care planning, medication systems, and a large integrated information system.

Catherine V Cunningham, RGN SCM MTD was a mature entrant to nurse training at The Royal Infirmary, Stirling in 1964. Since then she has been a nurse, a midwife, a teacher and a researcher. She is now in a staff post as adviser to the Chief Area Nursing Officer, Glasgow, UK.

Kathryn Erat, BA is systems manager for the CLINFO system at Brigham Women's Hospital, USA and has spent 25 years in computers, the last 18 years in medical computing. Her specialties include modular design of computer health systems, computer bases in health care and research and computer communication interfaces.

Lilian Eriksen, BSN MN is currently in the faculty of the college of nursing of the University of Wyoming, USA and has 6 years of experience in quality assurance in nursing. She has worked extensively with nurse managers in developing and using information for management processes.

Colin Fildes, BSc is a senior systems analyst with the Trent Regional Health Authority, UK. He has been responsible for the design and implementation of a computer system for learner nurse allocation and lectures on systems design and implementation during computer appreciation courses held in his region.

Anne N. Gebhardt, RN is presently director of special projects in nursing USA, with the main focus on developing and implementing computer applications in nursing. Her past experience has primarily been in nursing service administration in medical and surgical nursing.

Ulla Gerdin-Jelger, RN was a user of the computer system in the thoracic intensive care unit at the Karolinska Hospital, Stockholm, Sweden for 6 years. She then spent 2 years as a consultant to a computer company and is currently employed by the Stockholm County Council and responsible for the co-ordination and development of computer systems within the area. She is a member of the SHSTF's computer group.

Deirdre M Gossington, MSc SRN HV QIDN is senior nursing officer (administration) in North Staffordshire Health Authority, UK. Her job responsibilities include manpower, operational and service planning. She acts as a link between the computer department and nurses, ensuring that the users are represented in all aspects of computer developments in the authority. She is a member of the Computer Projects Nurses Group (DHSS).

Margaret R Grier, PhD MS BSN is associate professor at the College of Nursing, University of Illinois, Chicago, USA. She was editor of the award winning book 'Information Systems for Nursing Practice' and has published several articles on decision making in nursing.

Margaret Griffiths, SRN is a ward sister at the Queen Elizabeth Hospital, Birmingham, UK. She has been a ward sister for the past 7 years and participated in the pilot study as well as the development of the wardbased computer systems.

Susan Grobe, PhD RN MSN is currently a project director of HHS, Division of Nursing Special Projects Grant entitled "Developing Authoring Models for CAI on Nursing Process" in the USA. She has been involved in professional nursing organisations and nursing education. Her special interest and preparation in nursing and communications (i.e. T.V., film and electronic media) has been an important foundation for her teaching activities in associate degree, baccalaureate and higher degree programs for nurses.

Bernard Groves, AIDPM is the chief systems analyst at the North East Thames Regional Health Authority, UK. He has spent 16 years in the computer field and 6 years in the Health Service.

Dame Catherine Hall DBE Hon D Litt SRN SCM FRCN is chairman of the UK Central Council for Nursing, Midwifery and Health Visiting. She was general secretary of the Royal College of Nursing of the United Kingdom from 1957-1982. Her work has had a significant impact on the development of the nursing profession in the UK and she has served on numerous national and international committees on nursing.

Brian Hambleton, SRN RMN NAHCert DipAdminMgt is secretary of the National Staff Committee for Nurses and Midwives, Hannibal House, Elephant and Castle, London, UK. **Organising Committee, Joint Co-ordinator Education Stream.**

Kathryn J Hannah, PhD RN Dip NursEd BSN MSN is associate professor and assistant dean, research and development in the Faculty of Nursing, University of Calgary, Canada. She has conducted numerous workshops and seminars on computers and nursing.

Patricia Hardcastle, RN RM Dip N Admin Dip Ed is senior nursing service manager at the Groote Schuur Hospital, Cape Town, South Africa. She is responsible for the clinical nursing services in all departments with a particular interest in workload measurement linked to staff deployment and staffing in general.

Alison Head, BSc is senior systems analyst at the Royal Devon and Exeter Hospital, UK. She has a background of mathematics, computing and operational research. She joined the Health Service in 1970 and has worked closely with nurses developing systems for their use.

Christine R Henney, RGN SCM was a ward sister and a research nurse prior to introducing and designing the computerised nursing system at Ninewells Hospital, Dundee, UK. She has recently written a book on Drug Notes for Nurses, and is a member of the Computer Projects Nurses Group (DHSS).

Ronald Hoy, SRN Dip MS AMBIM LHA RNT is director of nurse education at The MacDonald Buchanan School of Nursing, Middlesex Hospital, London, UK. He is currently investigating the possibility of setting up a system for computer assisted learning. **Organising Committee, Joint Co-ordinator Education Stream.**

Shirley J Hughes, RN was a manager of Medical Information Systems Development at Nebraska Methodist Hospital, USA, and was responsible for implementation, co-ordination of departmental systems and on-going development of computerised hospital information systems from 1973-1981.

Pirjo Hynninen, RN MN is director of nursing services in The Health Centre of the District of Varkaus, Finland. She has been involved in the computer project running in the health centre for the 3 years 1979-1981 and is currently working for a masters degree in nursing.

Jean Jarvis, SRN HV is chief nursing officer, Swindon Health Authority, UK. Previously divisional nursing officer at The Royal Devon and Exeter Hospital where she was instrumental in the implementation of the nursing systems on all wards and also in the development of the personnel record system.

Dickey Johnson, RN BSN is a computer co-ordinator in the Department of Medical Biophysics at the LDS Hospital, Salt Lake City, USA. She has previous experience as an intensive care unit staff nurse and also as a computer research assistant.

John Kwok, MBCS AMIDPM is project leader of microcomputing development at the West Midlands Regional Health Authority, UK. He has been involved in various aspects of computing, programming, systems analysis, project management, research and development since 1965, and has worked in the National Health Service since 1969.

Maureen E Lahiff, SRN SCM BTA(Cert) HV CHNT has extensive experience in continuing education for nurses having been a health visitor tutor prior to the development of the BSc(Hons) Nursing Studies course for qualified nurses at the North East Surrey College of Technology, UK, of which she is now course director. She also teaches undergraduate nurse students at the University of Surrey.

Brian Layzell, Senior Executive Officer, Management Support and Computers Division, Department of Health and Social Security, London, UK. **Organising Committee, Joint Co-ordinator Management Stream.**

Jill Martin, SRN SCM RSCN was the nursing officer responsible for the implementation and development of the computer system whilst working as a nurse member of a team with the intensive therapy unit at Wythenshawe Hospital, UK. Her current post is nurse tutor at the Queen Elizabeth Hospital, King's Lynn, Norfolk, UK.

Susan Mirin, RN MS teaches science writing at Boston University's school of Public Communication and is director of Public Information at Action for Boston Community Development (ABCD), Boston's official anti-poverty agency. She is also adjunct assistant professor in the Department of Continuing Education at the Boston University School of Nursing, USA.

Sally J Mizrahi, RN Dip Ward Mgt Dip Nurse Admin, has a background of paediatric nursing. Her current post at the Royal Children's Hospital, Melbourne, Australia is that of a supervisory nurse in the Nursing Department, liaising closely with the computer services department. The specific functions of the job are to maintain and develop general interest in nursing programmes within the hospital.

Susan E Norman, SRN NDN RNT is a nurse educator at the Nightingale School, St Thomas' Hospital, London, UK. She visited the USA in 1981 on a Florence Nightingale Scholarship, working on computer assisted instruction.

Fotine O'Connor, BA MN is director of nursing services and education at the Los Angeles County University of Southern California Medical Center, USA. Her previous positions have included director of nursing, director of inservice education, and instructor positions in schools of nursing.

Fumiko Ohata, RN, is a chief instructor at the Perfect Liberty Nursing School, Osaka, Japan.

Josephine A Plant, JP SRN SCM BSc is the chief nursing officer of Lewisham and North Southwark Health Authority, UK. She is a member of the Körner working group on confidentiality.

Elly Pluyter-Wenting, SRN is assistant director of nursing at the University Hospital, Leiden, Holland having become involved with computer systems in 1973. Together with a computer scientist, she developed a computer system for allocation of student nurses. She is a member of the hospital board for computerised information systems.

Gerd de Pooter, RN works in the department of nephrology/hypertension at the Akademisch Ziekenhuis, Antwerpen Wilrykstraat, Belgium.

Doreen T Redmond, SRN RMN TD is nursing adviser to the Department of Health and Social Security, London, UK on the policy and management of computing for the National Health Service. **Organising Committee, Joint Co-ordinator, Care Stream.**

Barbara Rivett, SRN SCM RNT is currently principal nursing officer, nursing division, Department of Health and Social Security, London, UK. Formerly a nursing officer associated with the development of the Department of Health's experimental computer programme (regional liaison and planning).

Jean Roberts, BSc MBCS is computer services officer with the Lancaster Health Authority, UK. She is involved in making computer facilities available to a multidisciplinary health care team on a local basis. **Organising Committee, Exhibition Organiser.**

Judith S Ronald, PhD BN EdD BA BSN MN, is an associate professor of nursing at the State University of New York at Buffalo, USA. Prior to entering nursing, Dr Ronald was a systems engineer for the IBM corporation.

John E M Rowson, BSc MBCS joined the NHS in 1969 as a systems analyst working on the development of real time patient administration services at The London Hospital, UK. He is currently director of computing, Tower Hamlets District Authority.

Maureen Scholes, SRN CMBPart 1 NAHCert MBCS is senior nursing officer at The London Hospital, UK. She has been a member of the computer executive within the hospital since 1967. She was chairman of the Computer Projects Nurses Group (DHSS) 1975-80 and a member of the Evaluation Working party (DHSS) 1981. **Organising Committee Chairman, Joint Editor.**

Michael G Sheldon, MB BS FRCGP MBCS is senior lecturer in general practice in the Department of Community Health at Nottingham University. His research interests include information systems and use of computers in primary care.

Peter Squire, SRN is district nursing officer with the South Warwickshire Health Authority, UK. He studied for the Diploma in Health Service Administration and has held a number of posts in nursing management.

Jackie Streeter, SRN NAHCert is a member of the Computer Projects Nurses Group (DHSS). **Organising Committee, Co-ordinator Management Stream*.**

Mary Anne Sweeney, PhD BS RN MS is an associate professor at the Boston College School of Nursing, USA. She has written a number of articles on computers and a book entitled 'Introduction to Nursing Research'. Dr Sweeney conducts workshops for faculty members on the application of research and computers in nursing.

Charles Tilquin, PhD is associate professor of systems analysis/operations research at the University of Montreal, Canada. He is interested in systems science in health and social services, particularly nursing care and care of the elderly and disabled, assessment of need, design of programs, co-ordination of resources, appropriate orientation of clients and planning of a network of resources.

Ian Townsend, MA NDET CertEd joined the National Health Service Learning Resources Unit, Sheffield, UK in 1974, since when he has been widely involved in supporting and developing innovation in nurse education. He has written on many subjects concerned with teaching and learning from experimental education to computer assisted instruction.

Richard D Turner, MB ChBEd is regional specialist in community medicine (information and research), with the Yorkshire Regional Health Authority, UK.

Patricia Tymchyshyn, PhD BSc MS is a nursing instructor at Parkland College, Champaign, Illinois, USA and a computer design consultant for the Statewide Nursing Program at the Consortium of California State University, USA. Her particular interest is computer assisted learning in nursing.

Beryl Warne OBE, SRN SCM RNT is a nursing adviser for the Wessex Regional Health Authority, UK. She has been a clinical nurse, nurse teacher, officer and member of the General Nursing Council for England and Wales, and lately a nurse administrator. She is convinced of the need for accurate, timely information systems for all nurses from ward to administrative level. She is a member of the Computer Projects Nurses Group (DHSS).

Joyce Wiseman, MSc SRN SCM HV DN Dip Mgt Stud is director of the North West Region, Nurse Staffing Levels Project UK. She has a strong health visiting background and since 1975 her interest and knowledge has developed in research, with a responsibility for developing a managerial tool to assist managers with their allocation of nurse staffing and planning of resources.

* (Withdrew due to family illness.)

AUTHOR INDEX OF CONTRIBUTORS

Abbott, W., 492
Anderson, J., 126
Ashton, C.C., 105, 175

Barber, B., xvii, 24, 482, 551
Berg, C.M., 42
Broe, M.E. de, 163
Brown, J.L., 412
Bryant, Y.M., xvii, 563
Butler, E., 421

Carle, J., 136
Cobin, J., 269
Collins, S., 350
Cook, M., 84, 172
Cunningham, C.V., 457

Elseviers, M.M., 163
Erat, K., 496
Eriksen, L., 510

Fildes, C.J., 356

Gebhardt, A.N., 95
Gerdin-Jelger, U., 389
Gossington, D.M., 406
Grier, M.R., 530
Griffiths, M., 120
Grobe, S.J., 307
Groves, B., 476

Hall, C., 5
Hambleton, B., 265
Hannah, K.J., 280
Hardcastle, P., 374
Head, A.E., 115
Henney, C.R., 147
Hoy, R., 257
Hughes, S., 91
Hynninen, P., 207

IMIA, xix

Jarvis, J.G., 445
Johnson, D., 394

Kwok, J., 16

Lahiff, M.E., 544
Lambert, P., 136
Lewis, J., 269
Lins, R.L., 163

Martin, J.M., 156
Mirin, S., 291
Mizrahi, S., 438

Norman, S.E., 327

O'Connor, F.D., 470
Ohata, F., 222

Plant, J.A., 74
Pellicom, J. van, 163
Pluyter-Wenting, E., 430
Pooter, G.M. de, 163

Redmond, D.T., 59
Rivett, B., 370
Roberts, J., 364
Ronald, J.S., 248
Rowson, J.E.M., 34

Saulnier, D., 136
Scholes, M., xvii, 1
Sheldon, M.G., 230
Squire, P., 382
Stewart, L.H., 147
Sweeney, M.A., 240, 288

Tilquin, C., 136
Townsend, I., 334
Turner, R.D., 12
Tymchyshyn, P., 300

Verpooten, G.A., 163

Waeleghem, J.P., 163
Warne, B.E.M., 200
Wiseman, J., 215